Revision Notes for FRCEM Intermediate SAQ Paper

B

WITHDRAWN FROM LIBRARY

D1339270

1001302

Revision Notes for FRCEM Intermediate SAQ Paper

SECOND EDITION

Ashis Banerjee
Consultant and Honorary Senior Lecturer in Emergency Medicine
Barnet Hospital, Royal Free London NHS Foundation Trust, London, UK

Clara Oliver
Specialist Registrar in Emergency Medicine,
North East London Higher Training Programme

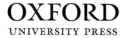

OXFORD
UNIVERSITY PRESS

OXFORD

UNIVERSITY PRESS

Great Clarendon Street, Oxford, OX2 6DP,
United Kingdom

Oxford University Press is a department of the University of Oxford.
It furthers the University's objective of excellence in research, scholarship,
and education by publishing worldwide. Oxford is a registered trade mark of
Oxford University Press in the UK and in certain other countries

© Oxford University Press 2017

The moral rights of the authors have been asserted

First Edition published in 2012
Second Edition published in 2017

Impression: 1

All rights reserved. No part of this publication may be reproduced, stored in
a retrieval system, or transmitted, in any form or by any means, without the
prior permission in writing of Oxford University Press, or as expressly permitted
by law, by licence or under terms agreed with the appropriate reprographics
rights organization. Enquiries concerning reproduction outside the scope of the
above should be sent to the Rights Department, Oxford University Press, at the
address above

You must not circulate this work in any other form
and you must impose this same condition on any acquirer

Published in the United States of America by Oxford University Press
198 Madison Avenue, New York, NY 10016, United States of America

British Library Cataloguing in Publication Data

Data available

Library of Congress Control Number: 2017935054

ISBN 978–0–19–878687–0

Printed and bound by
CPI Group (UK) Ltd, Croydon, CR0 4YY

Oxford University Press makes no representation, express or implied, that the
drug dosages in this book are correct. Readers must therefore always check
the product information and clinical procedures with the most up-to-date
published product information and data sheets provided by the manufacturers
and the most recent codes of conduct and safety regulations. The authors and
the publishers do not accept responsibility or legal liability for any errors in the
text or for the misuse or misapplication of material in this work. Except where
otherwise stated, drug dosages and recommendations are for the non-pregnant
adult who is not breast-feeding

Links to third party websites are provided by Oxford in good faith and
for information only. Oxford disclaims any responsibility for the materials
contained in any third party website referenced in this work.

Preface

Successful completion of the Fellowship of the Royal College of Emergency Medicine (FRCEM) examination is a requisite for obtaining a Certificate of Completion of Specialist Training in Emergency Medicine in the United Kingdom. A new examination structure has been introduced as of August 2016.

The FRCEM Primary replaces the MRCEM Part A, and comprises a paper of 180 single-best answer questions lasting three hours. The FRCEM Intermediate replaces the MRCEM Part B with a 60 three-mark short-answer question (SAQ) paper lasting three hours. The FRCEM Intermediate also will include a Situational Judgement Paper, replacing MRCEM Part C and being phased in from autumn 2017.

This book provides candidates with a comprehensive revision tool for the FRCEM Intermediate SAQ paper, the curriculum being the same as the erstwhile MRCEM Part B, which is being continued overseas.

The chapters are divided into systems and the content is based on the Royal College of Emergency Medicine Curriculum for 2015. The format for each topic follows a similar layout incorporating pathophysiology (when relevant), clinical features, investigations, scoring systems (where they exist), ED management, and definitive management (when applicable). National clinical guidelines are often used as the basis for questions and, where relevant, these are summarized. Within each chapter there are 'exam tips' boxes and 'key points' boxes. The exam tips provide advice for the exam and the key points summarize the main learning points from a section. Where, to my knowledge, previous subjects have appeared in a SAQ paper, they will be highlighted. We would like to thank Geraldine Jeffers and Rachel Goldsworthy of the Oxford University Press for guiding this project through to its conclusion and for their meticulous attention to detail. At the end of each chapter are sample SAQs and suggested answers, to enable the candidate to practice questions and reinforce key facts from the chapter.

Ashis Banerjee
Clara Oliver

Acknowledgments for the First Edition

Author of the First Edition:

Victoria Stacey, Consultant in Emergency Medicine, Cheltenham General Hospital, UK

Contributors to the First Edition:

Dr Robert Stacey, Consultant in Emergency Medicine, Gloucestershire Royal Hospital, UK
Dr Sarah Wilson, Consultant in Emergency Medicine, Wexham Park Hospital, UK

Contents

Abbreviations

AAA	abdominal aortic aneurysm	**COPD**	chronic obstructive pulmonary disease
AAGBI	Association of Anaesthetists of Great Britain and Ireland	**CPAP**	continuous positive airways pressure
		CPP	cerebral perfusion pressure
ABG	arterial blood gases	**CPR**	cardiopulmonary resuscitation
ACCS	acute care common stem	**CRAO**	central retinal artery occlusion
ACEI	angiotensin converting enzyme inhibitors	**CRF**	corticotrophin-releasing factor
		CRP	C-reactive protein
ACS	acute coronary syndrome	**CRRT**	continuous renal replacement therapy
ADH	antidiuretic hormone	**CRVO**	central retinal vein occlusion
AF	atrial fibrillation	**CSF**	cerebrospinal fluid
AKI	acute kidney injury	**CVP**	central venous pressure
ALS	advanced life support	**CXR**	chest X-ray
ALTE	apparent life-threatening event	**DI**	diabetes insipidus
APLS	advanced paediatric life support	**DIC**	disseminated intravascular coagulation
ARB	angiotensin receptor blockers	**DIPJ**	distal interphalangeal joint
ARDS	adult respiratory distress syndrome	**DKA**	diabetic ketoacidosis
		DNAR	Do Not Attempt Resuscitation
ASA	American Society of Anaesthesiologists	**DVLA**	Driver and Vehicle Licensing Agency
		DVT	deep vein thrombosis
ASW	approved social worker	**ECG**	electrocardiogram
ATLS	advanced trauma life support	**ED**	emergency department
ATN	acute tubular necrosis	**EGDT**	early goal-directed therapy
BASH	British Association for the Study of Headache	**EM**	erythema multiforme
		ENT	ear, nose, and throat
BiPAP	bi-level positive airways pressure	**EPAP**	expiratory positive airway pressure
BLS	basic life support	**EPLS**	European Paediatric Life Support
BPPV	benign paroxysmal positional vertigo	**ESR**	erythrocyte sedimentation rate
		ETT	endotracheal tube
BSA	body surface area	**FAST**	face arm speech test
BSPED	British Society of Paediatric Endocrinology and Diabetes	**FAST**	focused assessment with sonography in trauma
BTS	British Thoracic Society	**FBC**	full bood count
CAFCASS	Children and Family Court Advisory and Support Service	**FDP**	Flexor digitorum profundus
		FDS	Flexor digitorum superficialis
CAP	community-acquired pneumonia	**FRC**	functional residual capacity
CCDC	Consultant in Communicable Disease Control	**FRCEM**	Fellowship of the Royal College of Emergency Medicine
CES	cauda equina syndrome	**FVC**	forced vital capacity
CK	creatine kinase	**GABA**	gamma-aminobutyric acid
CNS	central nervous system	**GCS**	Glasgow coma scale
CO	cardiac output	**GFR**	glomerular filtration rate

GMC	General Medical Council	**PCI**	percutaneous coronary intervention
GRACE	Global Registry of Acute Cardiac Events	**PCR**	polymerase chain reaction
		PD	peritoneal dialysis
HELLP	haemolysis, elevated liver enzymes, and low platelets	**PE**	pulmonary embolism
		PEA	pulseless electrical activity
HHS	hyperosmolar hyperglycaemic state	**PEF**	peak expiratory flow
		PEFR	peak expiratory flow rate
HSV	herpes simplex virus	**PEP**	post-exposure prophylaxis
IBD	Inflammatory bowel disease	**PID**	pelvic inflammatory disease
ICHD	International Classification of Headache Disorders	**POCS**	posterior circulation stroke
		PVC	premature ventricular contractions
ICP	intracranial pressure	**RCEM**	Royal College of Emergency Medicine
ICU	intensive care unit	**RCOG**	Royal College of Obstetricians and Gynaecologists
IMCA	independent medical capacity advocates	**RIPL**	Rare and Imported Pathogens Laboratory
IO	intraosseous		
IPAP	inspiratory positive airway pressure	**RMO**	responsible medical officer
		ROSC	return of spontaneous circulation
IPJ	interphalangeal joint	**ROSIER**	recognition of stroke in the emergency room
ITP	idiopathic thrombocytopenic purpura		
		RRT	renal replacement therapy
IVC	intravenous	**RSI**	rapid sequence induction
IVC	inferior vena cava	**RTC**	road traffic collisions
LACS	lacunar stroke	**SAQ**	short-answer question
LAT	lidocaine, adrenaline, tetracaine	**SBP**	spontaneous bacterial peritonitis
LMA	laryngeal mask airway	**SCD**	sudden cardiac death
LMN	lower motor neuron	**SCT**	supervised community treatment
LMWH	low molecular weight heparin	**SIGN**	Scottish Intercollegiate Guidelines Network
LPA	Lasting Power of Attorney		
MAP	mean arterial pressure	**SIRS**	systemic inflammatory response syndrome
MRCEM	Membership of the Royal College of Emergency Medicine		
		SJS	Steven-Johnson Syndrome
MHRT	Mental Health Review Tribunal	**SSC**	Surviving Sepsis Campaign
MI	myocardial infarction	**SSRI**	selective serotonin reuptake inhibitors
MSCC	metastatic spinal cord compression		
		SSSS	Staphylococcal scalded skin syndrome
NAI	non-accidental injury	**STEMI**	ST-elevation myocardial infarction
NCEPOD	National Confidential Enquiry into Patient Outcomes and Death	**TACS**	total anterior circulation stroke
		TCA	tricyclic antidepressant
NEXUS	National Emergency X-Radiography Utilization Study	**TEN**	toxic epidermal necrolysis
		TIA	transient ischaemic attack
NG	nasogastric	**TIMI**	thrombolysis in myocardial infarction
NICE	National Institute for Health and Care Excellence	**TIPS**	transjugular intrahepatic portosystemic shunting
		TLoC	transient loss of consciousness
NIHSS	National Institute for Health Stroke Score	**TLS**	tumour lysis syndrome
		TNF	tumour necrosis factor
NIV	non-invasive ventilation	**TRH**	thyrotropin-releasing hormone
Nok	next of kin	**TSH**	thyroid stimulating hormone
NR	nearest relative	**UMN**	upper motor neuron
NSAID	non-steroidal anti-inflammatory drug	**UTI**	urinary tract infection
		VF	ventricular fibrillation
NSTEMI	non-ST-segment elevation myocardial infarction	**VHF**	viral haemorrhagic fevers
		VT	ventricular tachycardia
NYHA	New York Heart Association	**WCC**	white cell count
OSCE	objective structured clinical examination	**WFNS**	World Federation of Neurological Surgeons
PACS	partial anterior circulation stroke		

Exam tips

CONTENTS

1.1 Structure of the exam

The Fellowship of the Royal College of Emergency Medicine (FRCEM) exam is a pre-requisite for obtaining the Certificate of Completion of Specialist Training in the United Kingdom. It consists of three sections, Primary, Intermediate, and Final FRCEM, as from August 2016.

The FRCEM Primary consists of a single best-answer question paper of 180 questions in three hours, and replaces the MRCEM Part A. A maximum of six attempts is allowed to pass the examination. Previous attempts at the MRCEM Part A examination will not be included in the number of available attempts for the FRCEM Primary examination.

The FRCEM Intermediate replaces MRCEM Parts B and C for Emergency Medicine trainees in the United Kingdom. It comprises a short-answer question (SAQ) paper consisting of 60 three-mark questions in three hours, and a situational judgement paper consisting of 120 single best-answer questions in two hours.

The regulations relating to the FRCEM examinations can be found on the Royal College of Emergency Medicine website (https://www.rcem.ac.uk).

This book is aimed at candidates sitting the FRCEM Intermediate SAQ paper.

1.2 Marking system

The FRCEM Intermediate consists of 60 SAQs in three hours. The questions are typically divided into three or four parts and are carefully constructed so that failure to answer the first part of the question does not preclude answering other parts. The available marks for each part of the question are displayed so that candidates can judge how much detail to write.

The exam is scored cumulatively and there is a pass mark, not a rate. The pass mark is determined before the exam, depending on the difficulty index of the exam. Examiners meet before the exam to determine the pass mark and ensure the questions are clear, unambiguous, and fair. The pass mark is roughly in the range 60–68%. There are no critical response or 'sudden death' questions.

It is often easier to gain the first 5 marks of a question than the last 5. Therefore, if you are struggling with a question, it is worth moving on. Questions will frequently indicate the number of responses expected. Examiners will mark the answers in the order written, therefore ensure your first answer is your 'best answer' and do not give more answers than requested. If the question asks for four answers and you write five, only the first four will be marked, even if the fifth is correct. Marks will not be gained for repeating an answer in the same question or reiterating information given in the stem of the question.

It is very important to read the stem of the question carefully. Had this scenario been that the patient had recently fractured his or her femur and asked for four other risk factors, then 'recent lower limb trauma' would not gain a mark.

Answers must be legible and any corrections made clearly so the examiner knows which answer is to be considered. The exam is written in pencil, which sometimes surprises candidates, so it is worth practising writing in pencil beforehand.

EXAM TIP

Example question:

Give four risk factors for a pulmonary embolism (4 marks)

Recent immobilization	Correct (1 mark)
Recent lower limb trauma	Correct (1 mark)
Diabetes	Incorrect
Clinical deep vein thrombosis	Correct (1 mark)
Malignancy	(not marked because fifth answer)

This answer would score 3 out of a 4 possible marks because, despite having four correct answers, only three of the first four are correct.

1.3 Content

Emergency Medicine encompasses many specialties, and national guidance and evidence-based medicine protocols often appear in the examination. This is done to ensure that the exam is up-to-date, but also to encourage candidates to keep up-to-date with recently published scientific evidence. If there are multiple guidelines, then allowance is made for this in the marking scheme.

The basic sciences are primarily examined in the FRCEM Primary but may also be assessed in FRCEM Intermediate. There is not a separate basic sciences chapter in this book but, where relevant, information on basic sciences is included.

Some topics appear more commonly in exams than 'real-life' practice (e.g. dermatology and ophthalmology). This is particularly true in the FRCEM Intermediate examination, because questions based around visual images are relatively easy to design for a SAQ, but more difficult to include in an objective structured clinical examination (OSCE).

1.4 Curriculum

The College of Emergency Medicine published a new curriculum in August 2015, replacing the June 2010 curriculum.

The curriculum is divided into major and acute presentations. Due to this design, certain conditions are applicable to several different presentations; for example, pulmonary embolism is relevant to the major presentations of cardiorespiratory arrest and shock, and the acute presentations of breathlessness, chest pain, blood gas interpretation, and cyanosis. Therefore, to avoid unnecessary repetition, this book's chapters are written by system and not by presenting complaint. To enable the candidate to use this book in conjunction with the new curriculum, the following tables list the presentations and corresponding chapters that trainees are expected to cover in their first three years of UK Emergency Medicine training (i.e. the curriculum that is used for the FRCEM examination).

The paediatric curriculum is largely covered in Chapter 20 with cross-referencing to other chapters, where necessary.

1.4.1 Major adult presentations

Table 1.1 lists the chapters covering the major adult presentations.

Table 1.1 Chapters covering the major adult presentations

CMP1—Anaphylaxis	Chapter 2
CMP2—Cardiorespiratory arrest	Chapter 2
CMP3—Major trauma	Chapter 4
CMP4—Septic patient	Chapter 15
CMP4—Shocked patient	Chapter 2
CMP5—Unconscious patient	Chapters 4 and 11

1.4.2 Acute adult presentations

Table 1.2 lists the chapters covering the acute adult presentations.

Table 1.2 Chapters covering the acute adult presentations

CAP1—Abdominal pain, including loin pain	Chapter 6
CAP2—Abdominal swelling, mass, constipation	Chapter 6
CAP3—Acute back pain	Chapter 5
CAP4—Aggressive/disturbed behaviour	Chapters 18 and 21
CAP5—Blackout/collapse	Chapters 9 and 11
CAP6—Breathlessness	Chapter 10
CAP7—Chest pain	Chapter 9
CAP8—Confusion/acute delirium	Chapters 11 and 18
CAP9—Cough	Chapter 10
CAP10—Cyanosis	Chapter 10
CAP11—Diarrhoea	Chapter 13
CAP12—Dizziness and vertigo	Chapters 7 and 11
CAP13—Falls	Chapter 11
CAP14—Fever	Chapter 15
CAP15—Fits and seizures	Chapter 11
CAP16—Haematemesis and melaena	Chapter 13
CAP17—Headache	Chapter 11

(continued)

Table 1.2 Continued

CAP18—Head injury	Chapter 4
CAP19—Jaundice	Chapter 13
CAP20—Limb pain and swelling (atraumatic)	Chapter 5
CAP21—Neck pain	Chapter 4
CAP22—Oliguric	Chapter 6
CAP23—Pain management	Chapter 3
CAP24—Painful ears	Chapter 7
CAP25—Palpitations	Chapter 9
CAP26—Pelvic pain	Chapter 8
CAP27—Poisoning	Chapters 17 and 18
CAP28—Rash	Chapter 16
CAP29—Red eye	Chapter 7
CAP30—Mental health	Chapter 18
CAP31—Sore throat	Chapter 7
CAP32—Syncope and pre-syncope	Chapter 9
CAP33—Traumatic limb and joint injuries	Chapters 4 and 5
CAP34—Vaginal bleeding	Chapter 8
CAP35—Ventilatory support	Chapters 3 and 10
CAP36—Vomiting and nausea	Chapter 13
CAP37—Weakness and paralysis	Chapters 4 and 11
CAP38—Wound assessment and management	Chapter 5

1.4.3 Major paediatric presentations

Table 1.3 lists the chapters covering the major paediatric presentations.

Table 1.3 Chapters covering the major paediatric presentations

PMP1—Anaphylaxis	Chapter 19
PMP2—Apnoea, stridor, and airway obstruction	Chapter 19
PMP3—Cardiorespiratory arrest	Chapter 19
PMP4—Major trauma	Chapter 19
PMP5—The shocked child	Chapter 19
PMP6—The unconscious child	Chapter 19

1.4.4 Acute paediatric presentations

Table 1.4 lists the chapters covering the acute paediatric presentations.

Table 1.4 Chapters covering the acute paediatric presentations

PAP1—Abdominal pain	Chapters 6 and 19
PAP2—Accidental poisoning, poisoning, and self-harm	Chapters 17 and 18
PAP3—Apparent life-threatening events (ATLE)	Chapter 19
PAP4—Blood disorders	Chapters 19 and 20
PAP5—Breathing difficulties	Chapter 19
PAP6—Concerning presentations	Chapter 19
PAP7—Dehydration secondary to diarrhoea and vomiting	Chapter 19
PAP8—Ears, nose, and throat (ENT)	Chapter 7
PAP9—Fever in all age groups	Chapters 15 and 19
PAP10—Floppy child	Chapter 19
PAP11—Gastrointestinal bleeding	Chapter 19
PAP12—Headache	Chapters 11 and 19
PAP13—Neonatal presentations	Chapter 19
PAP14—Ophthalmology	Chapter 7
PAP15—Pain in children	Chapter 3
PAP16—Painful limbs in children—atraumatic	Chapter 19
PAP17—Painful limbs in children—traumatic	Chapters 5 and 19
PAP18—Rashes in children	Chapter 16
PAP19—Sore throat	Chapter 7

1.5 Glossary

The questions for the FRCEM examinations are put through a rigorous refinement process. Every word of the SAQ clinical scenario is carefully considered. Candidates are provided with a glossary of terms used in the exam, which can be downloaded from the College website (https://www.rcem.ac.uk) and is worth looking through before the exam.

The terms commonly used in exam questions are summarized.

- **Abnormality:** any feature in an examination or investigation that is outside the standard deviation of the population being studied. A clinical abnormality relates to a pathologically relevant abnormality (e.g. the presence of facial burns and not the presence of an endotracheal tube).
- **Assessment:** history-taking, physical examination, and use of investigations.
- **Clinical findings:** these may include symptoms, signs, and vital signs. It is information gleaned from the clinical evaluation, but not the results of investigations, even bedside ones (e.g. blood glucose or urine dipstick).
- **Criteria:** refer to the fact that there is a formal international/national guideline or scoring system that allows you to define the seriousness of a condition (e.g. CURB-65 score for pneumonia).

- **Definitive management:** this may include things you would do in the emergency department but usually requires you to list the operation or procedure that will cure or contain the condition.
- **Emergency department (ED) management:** this requires you to list actions that are life or limb-saving or that might improve the course of the condition if done within the ED. It is not definitive management. This may, however, include analgesia, referral to specialty team, and so on.
- **Essential:** this indicates life-saving treatments/management steps that are the priority, and would not normally include things like analgesia, communication, and so on.
- **Features:** in the context of a medical history, may be either a symptom or a sign. If asked for key features, you should give the symptoms or signs that are definitive for that condition, rather than general abnormalities that might be present. When asked for in the context of an electrocardiogram (ECG) or chest X-ray (CXR), it might be a pathological abnormality or might simply be the presence of an endotracheal tube (ETT) or central line.
- **Investigations:** specific tests undertaken to make a diagnosis or monitor the patient's condition. They may include bedside tests such as urine dipstick or blood glucose, unless otherwise specified.
- **Management:** aspects of care, including treatment, supportive care, and disposition. This does not include investigations.
- **Pathophysiological sequence of events:** this requires you to list in chronological order, the events that happen on a cellular or hormonal level, leading to the current condition. For example, if a lactate is high in the presence of sepsis, you could suggest:
  - hypotension;
  - poor organ perfusion;
  - tissue hypoxia;
  - anaerobic metabolism;
  - glycolysis and lactate build-up.
- **Treatment:** measures undertaken to cure or stabilize the patient's condition. This includes oxygen, fluids, drugs, and may also mean surgery. It does not include investigations.

Throughout this book, terminology has been used in keeping with the College glossary to help you become familiar with how the terms are used.

1.6 Making the most of your knowledge

Having reached this stage in your medical career, you are already well-versed in sitting exams. However, it may have been several years since your last written exam. A consistent theme of feedback from examiners is that candidates let themselves down through their exam technique. Practising questions before the exam is crucial to achieve the best result possible.

Each chapter of this book has practice SAQs, which will help refine your technique. It is also useful to sit mock exams to get used to performing under exam conditions. Such mocks are available via revision courses or frequently from regional Emergency Medicine training schemes.

When answering questions, think carefully about what is being asked. Long lists of investigations or differential diagnoses are unlikely to be acceptable. If asked to give investigations, try to use ones that will help differentiate between causes or be useful in the risk assessment of the disease. Often questions will ask you to justify why you want a certain investigation; for example, measuring urea in pneumonia so that a CURB 65 score can be calculated. Similarly, when answering questions on treatments, the mechanism of action may be asked for (e.g. salbutamol is a beta-agonist and used in asthma as a bronchodilator).

Knowledge of drug doses often worries candidates because they are uncertain which ones they need to remember. As a general rule, drugs doses that are used in the emergency resuscitation setting should be known because in practice there is often not enough time to look these up. Similarly, commonly used drugs (e.g. analgesics, antibiotics) should be known. Other questions may ask for the drug plus the dose and route. Candidates often lose marks on these questions because they write the drug name, but don't write the dose or route because they are uncertain of the dose. Remember there is no negative marking, so it is worth a guess and even if you are uncertain of the dose, the route is usually known, so don't forget to include it in your answer.

No matter how much preparation is done before the exam, there will always be unexpected questions. It is important to remember that these will be unexpected for the majority of candidates and not to panic. There is usually something that can be remembered about the topic and it is worth having a guess because there is no negative marking.

1.7 How to use this book

The chapters are divided into systems and the content is based on the Royal College of Emergency Medicine Curriculum 2015. Each chapter has a contents page listing the main topic headings, which are numbered numerically to enable easy reference. Section 1.4 in this chapter, 'Curriculum', provides a cross-reference between each book chapter and presenting complaint, as laid out in the new curriculum.

The format for each condition within a chapter follows a similar layout incorporating pathophysiology (when relevant), clinical features, investigations, scoring systems (where they exist), ED management, and definitive management (when applicable). The exception to this are conditions that require a more practical knowledge (e.g. resuscitation, airway management, and so on).

Increasingly, the College is using national guidelines as the basis for questions. Where relevant, this book summarizes established UK guidelines (e.g. National Institute for Health and Care Excellence (NICE), Scottish Intercollegiate Guidelines Network (SIGN), British Thoracic Society (BTS), and so on). If UK guidance does not exist, then European guidelines may be used. The guidelines used are clearly identified and website addresses provided so that the candidate can check for any updates prior to the exam.

Within each chapter there are 'exam tips' boxes and 'key points' boxes. The exam tips provide advice for the exam and the key points summarize the main learning points from a section.

EXAM TIP

Always ensure you read the question carefully, remain calm, and write clear, concise answers.

Previous subjects known to have appeared in previous examinations will be highlighted.

Previous MRCEM question

At the end of each chapter are sample SAQs and suggested answers. The SAQs can be used for exam practice and will reinforce key facts from the chapter.

Further reading

Royal College of Emergency Medicine. Available at: www.rcem.ac.uk [Online].

KEY POINTS

The FRCEM exam has three sections, Primary, Intermediate, and Final, which have to be passed in succession to be awarded Fellowship of the Royal College of Emergency Medicine.

The FRCEM Intermediate focuses on data interpretation skills and is a short-answer question (SAQ) paper. The paper consists of 60, 3 -mark questions. The exam lasts three hours.

There is no negative marking.

There are no critical response or 'sudden death' questions.

Examiners will mark the answers in the order written, therefore ensure your first answer is your 'best answer' and do not give more answers than requested.

The Royal College of Emergency Medicine published a new curriculum in August 2015.

Section 1.4 in this chapter, 'Curriculum', provides a cross-reference between book chapter and presenting complaint as laid out in the new curriculum.

The questions for the FRCEM examinations use specific terms which are defined in a glossary that the candidate is provided with in the exam and is available on the College website. Look through the glossary before the exam so that you are familiar with the terms.

Resuscitation

CONTENTS

2.1 Advanced life support

2.1.1 Introduction

Completion of an advanced life support (ALS) course is a mandatory requirement of Acute Care Common Stem (ACCS) training and all candidates would be expected to be ALS providers prior to sitting the FRCEM Intermediate examination.

This section is based on the 2015 Resuscitation Council Guidelines. It includes the ALS algorithms and focuses on cardiac arrest in special circumstances. The aim is to highlight the main features of, and changes in, the 2015 guidance and focus on areas that could be questioned in an short-answer question (SAQ) paper.

EXAM TIP

The Resuscitation Council manuals are a good resource for revision. The latest guidance is freely available on their website https://www.resus.org.uk/.

ALS is most likely to be examined in the OSCEs of the Final FRCEM but knowledge of the guidance could appear in a SAQ.

2.1.2 ALS algorithm

Figure 2.1 shows the adult ALS algorithm and the main features of the 2015 guidelines are presented in Table 2.1.

2.1.3 Shockable rhythms (VF/VT)

The first monitored rhythm in approximately 28–35% of cardiac arrests out of hospital is ventricular fibrillation (VF) or pulseless ventricular tachycardia (VT) with approximately 21% surviving to hospital discharge. In hospital, VF/VT accounts for approximately 18% of cardiac arrests, with approximately 44% surviving to discharge.

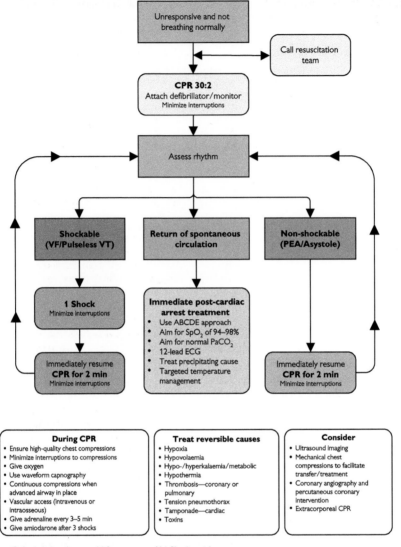

Figure 2.1 Adult advanced life support (ALS) algorithm.
Reproduced with the kind permission of the Resuscitation Council (UK).

Defibrillation strategy

- The 2005 guideline first introduced the single-shock strategy instead of the previously used three-stacked shocks protocol. The 2015 guidelines continue to recommend a single-shock strategy in order to minimize interruptions to chest compressions.
- In a few very specific circumstances, three initial stacked shocks have been reintroduced: patients who have just had cardiac surgery; patients in the cardiac catheter laboratory; and patients who have a witnessed monitored arrest and are already connected to a manual defibrillator. If given, the three initial stacked shocks should be considered as the first shock in the ALS algorithm, and both adrenaline and amiodarone should be given after a further two defibrillation attempts (i.e. delayed until after the fifth shock).

Table 2.1 Main features of the 2015 Resuscitation Council Adult Guidelines

BLS	• Minimally interrupted high-quality chest compressions remain essential to improving outcomes and should be to a depth of 5–6 cm and at a rate of 100–120 per minute ('push hard and fast'). After each compression, the chest should be allowed to recoil completely. When providing rescue breaths/ventilations, about 1 s should be spent inflating the chest with sufficient volume to ensure visible chest wall rise. The ratio of chest compressions to ventilations remains 30:2. Chest compressions should not be interrupted for more than 10 s to provide ventilations.
	• The routine use of mechanical chest compression devices is not recommended, however they may be useful in certain situations, where sustained high-quality manual chest compressions are impractical or compromise patient safety.
Defibrillation	• Interruptions to chest compressions should be kept to a minimum and pauses should only occur briefly to enable specific planned interventions (e.g. defibrillation, intubation).
	• Chest compressions should continue during charging of the defibrillator to reduce the pre-shock pause to less than 5 s.
	• Chest compressions should be continued immediately after delivering a shock, as it is very rare for a pulse to be palpable immediately after defibrillation, and as the duration of asystole can be longer than 2 minutes in as many as 25% of successful shocks.
	• The focus on using self-adhesive pads for defibrillation continues, although it is recognized that defibrillator paddles are used in some settings.
Drugs	• Peripheral venous access is quicker, easier to perform, and safer. If intravenous (IV) access is not achievable, intraosseous (IO) access should be used.
	• In the shockable ventricular fibrillation/ventricular tachycardia (VF/VT) algorithm, adrenaline 1 mg is given after the third shock, once chest compressions have resumed. Adrenaline is then given every 3–5 min (alternate cycles).
	• Amiodarone 300 mg is given after the third shock in VF/VT cardiac arrests. Consider a further dose of amiodarone 150 mg after a total of five shocks. Lidocaine 1 mg/kg may be used as an alternative if amiodarone is not available but should not be given if amiodarone has been given already.
	• There is greater equipoise (uncertainty regarding the therapeutic benefits) concerning the role of drugs in improving outcomes from cardiac arrest. Drugs are of secondary importance to high-quality uninterrupted chest compressions and early defibrillation.
Airway	• A stepwise approach to airway management based on patient factors, the phase of the resuscitation attempt and the skills of the rescuer is recommended. This includes compression-only CPR, compression-only CPR with the airway held open, mouth-to-mouth breaths, mouth-to-mask, bag-mask ventilations with simple airway adjuncts, supraglottic airways, and tracheal intubation.
	• The use of waveform capnography to monitor end-tidal CO_2 is recommended to confirm and continually monitor tracheal tube placement, quality of chest compressions during CPR, and to provide an early indication of return of spontaneous circulation (ROSC). ROSC can be detected without pausing chest compressions and bolus adrenaline injection can be avoided as a result.
Ultrasound	• The potential role of ultrasound in identifying reversible causes of cardiac arrest continues to be emphasized (e.g. cardiac tamponade; pulmonary embolism (PE); myocardial infarction (regional wall motion abnormality); aortic dissection; hypovolaemia; and pneumothorax).

(continued)

Table 2.1 Continued

Post-resuscitation care	• Hyperoxia may be harmful after ROSC, therefore oxygen should be titrated to maintain saturations of 94–98%. • There is a greater emphasis on urgent coronary catheterization and primary percutaneous coronary intervention (PCI) in patients with ROSC following out-of-hospital cardiac arrest of likely cardiac cause. • Blood glucose levels >10 mmol/L should be treated, but hypoglycaemia should be avoided. • Targeted temperature management or temperature control should be considered in comatose survivors of cardiac arrest associated with non-shockable, as well as shockable, rhythms. There is an option to target a temperature of 36 C instead of the previously recommended 32–34 C. • Extracorporeal life support techniques may be used as a rescue therapy in selected patients where standard ALS measures are not successful, or to facilitate specific interventions (e.g. coronary angiography, PCI, or pulmonary thrombectomy).

• The recommended initial biphasic shock should be at least 150 J. Recommendations for subsequent shocks depend on the manufacturer of the machine and may be fixed at 150 J or escalate. When using a monophasic machine, all shocks should be at 360 J.

Fine ventricular fibrillation

Fine VF that is difficult to distinguish from asystole should be treated as asystole with good-quality closed chest compression. This may improve the amplitude and frequency of the VF and improve the chances of successful defibrillation. Repeated defibrillation of fine VF is very unlikely to restore a perfusing rhythm and will increase myocardial injury, both directly by the electrical current and indirectly by interruptions in chest compressions.

2.1.4 Non-shockable rhythms (pulseless electrical activity and asystole)

Pulseless electrical activity (PEA) and asystole are the commonest initial cardiac arrest rhythms and have a less favourable outcome than shockable rhythms (8% of out-of-hospital patients and 7% of in-hospital patients surviving to discharge). Unless a reversible cause can be found and treated, survival is unlikely.

2.1.5 Reversible causes

Potential reversible causes should be considered and treated in both shockable and non-shockable cardiac arrests.

• **Hypoxia**—should be corrected by delivering high-concentration oxygen to the patient via a bag-valve-mask, supraglottic airway device, or endotracheal tube. Effective ventilation should be confirmed by chest wall movement and auscultation.
• **Hypovolaemia**—is usually due to severe haemorrhage (e.g. trauma, GI bleeding, aortic aneurysm rupture). Intravenous fluids should be infused rapidly if hypovolaemia is suspected. Crystalloid (0.9% sodium chloride or Hartmann's) is appropriate because there is no clear advantage for colloid.
• **Hyper/hypokalaemia, hypocalcaemia, and other metabolic disorders**—are usually detected on arterial blood gas analysis, recent blood results, or suggested by the patient's history. The management of electrolyte disturbances is discussed in the special circumstances section (section 2.2).

- **Hypothermia**—should be checked for with a low-reading thermometer. If the patient is hypothermic, they should be rewarmed to 36°C.
- **Tension pneumothorax**—can be detected clinically or via ultrasound. Needle thoracocentesis should be performed to decompress the pneumothorax and followed up with a chest drain.
- **Cardiac tamponade**—can be difficult to detect clinically in an arrested patient. There should be a high index of suspicion for patients suffering penetrating thoracic trauma. Echocardiography may be used to confirm the diagnosis. If present, resuscitative thoracotomy should be performed.
- **Toxins**—the history is important in determining whether therapeutic or toxic substances could have precipitated the arrest. If an appropriate antidote (e.g. naloxone for opiates) exists, it should be administered.
- **Thromboembolic**—a massive pulmonary embolism (PE) can cause circulatory obstruction and cardiac arrest. The diagnosis is difficult and may be based purely on the patient's history prior to the arrest. If rapid echocardiography is available, this may support the diagnosis (dilated right heart). The use of thrombolysis in cardiac arrest is decided on a case-by-case basis. If thrombolysis is given, it may take up to 90 minutes to be effective and should only be administered if it is appropriate to continue cardiopulmonary resuscitation (CPR) for this length of time.

2.1.6 Drugs used in cardiac arrest

Table 2.2 shows the drugs used in cardiac arrest.

Table 2.2 Drugs used in cardiac arrest

Drug	Actions	Dose/Indications
Adrenaline	• Direct-acting sympathomimetic amine. • Stimulates α and β adrenergic receptors. • Stimulation of α receptors produces vasoconstriction, increasing systemic vascular resistance, and improving cerebral and coronary perfusion during CPR. • Stimulation of β_1 receptors increases heart rate and the force of contraction (in a beating heart).	• Adrenaline dose 1 mg. • Give as soon as possible in PEA/asystole. • Give after the third shock in VF/VT. • Repeat every 3–5 min (alternate cycles).
Amiodarone	• Membrane-stabilizing anti-arrhythmic drug. • Increases the duration of the action potential and refractory period in atrial and ventricular myocardium, and slows AV conduction. • Slight negative inotropic action and can cause peripheral vasodilatation.	• Amiodarone dose 300 mg bolus after the third shock in VF/VT. • A further 150 mg may be given for refractory VF/VT followed by a 900 mg infusion over 24 h.
Magnesium	• Constituent of many enzyme systems, especially those involved with generating adenosine triphosphate (ATP) in muscle. • Decreases acetylcholine release and reduces the sensitivity of the motor end plate. • Improved contractility of the stunned myocardium and limits infarct size (mechanism unknown). • Bronchodilator.	• Magnesium dose 2 g. Indications: • Shock refractory VF/VT if hypomagnesaemia suspected. • Ventricular tachyarrhythmias if hypomagnesaemia suspected. • Torsades de pointes. • Digoxin toxicity.

(continued)

Table 2.2 Continued

Drug	Actions	Dose/Indications
Sodium bicarbonate	<ul><li>Alkalinization to correct pH.</li><li>Bicarbonate administration generates carbon dioxide, which diffuses rapidly into cells.</li></ul> Effects include: <ul><li>Exacerbation of intracellular acidosis.</li><li>Negative inotropic effect on ischaemic myocardium.</li><li>Large, osmotically active, sodium load to an already compromised circulation and brain.</li><li>Shifts the oxygen dissociation curve to the left inhibiting the release of oxygen to the tissues.</li></ul>	<ul><li>Bicarbonate dose 50 ml of 8.4% (50 mmol).</li></ul> Indications: <ul><li>Hyperkalaemia.</li><li>Tricyclic acid overdose.</li></ul>
Calcium	<ul><li>Involved in the cellular mechanisms underlying myocardial contraction.</li></ul>	<ul><li>Calcium chloride dose 10 ml of 10%.</li><li>Can be repeated PRN.</li><li>Indications:</li><li>Hyperkalaemia.</li><li>Hypocalcaemia.</li><li>Overdose of calcium channel blocking drugs.</li></ul>

KEY POINTS

Pauses in chest compressions should be kept to a minimum.

When defibrillating, the pre-shock pause should be kept to a minimum (<5 s) by planning ahead, continuing chest compressions during charging, and using a very brief safety check.

Adrenaline 1 mg should be given as soon as IV/IO access is gained in asystole/PEA and after the third shock in VF/VT.

Amiodarone 300 mg IV is given after the third shock in VF/VT.

Waveform capnography should be used, if available, in an intubated patient to confirm and continually monitor tube placement, quality of CPR, and to provide an early recognition of return of spontaneous circulation (ROSC).

If thrombolysis is given for a massive PE in cardiac arrest, CPR should be continued for 60–90 min.

Targeted temperature management remains important with a target of 33–36 C depending on local policy.

2.2 Cardiac arrest in special circumstances

2.2.1 Introduction

Good-quality CPR is paramount, regardless of the cause of cardiac arrest; however, certain circumstances require additions and modifications to the resuscitation algorithm. These 'special circumstances' could well appear in an SAQ.

2.2.2 Electrolyte disorders

Hyperkalaemia

Hyperkalaemia is defined as a K$^+$ >5.5 mmol/L. The management of hyperkalaemia in the non-arrested patient is discussed in Chapter 12, section 12.4. The modifications for ALS in the arrested hyperkalaemic patient are:

- Calcium chloride: 10 ml of 10% given as a rapid bolus
- Sodium bicarbonate: 50 ml of 8.4% given as a rapid injection
- Insulin/glucose: 10 units of short-acting insulin and 50 ml of 50% glucose given as a rapid infusion
- Haemodialysis: considered in resistant hyperkalaemia

Hypokalaemia

Hypokalaemia is defined as a K$^+$ <3.5 mmol/L and severe hypokalaemia as a K$^+$ <2.5 mmol/L. Causes of hypokalaemia include:

- Gastrointestinal losses (e.g. diarrhoea)
- Drugs (e.g. diuretics, laxatives, steroids, adrenaline, and so on)
- Renal losses (e.g. renal tubular acidosis, diabetes insipidus, dialysis)
- Endocrine disorders (e.g. Cushing's syndrome, hyperaldosteronism)
- Metabolic alkalosis
- Hypomagnesaemia

Clinical features of hypokalaemia include:

- Fatigue
- Weakness
- Cramps
- Constipation
- Rhabdomyolysis
- Ascending paralysis

Electrocardiogram (ECG) features of hypokalaemia are:

- U waves
- T-wave flattening
- ST segment elevation
- Arrhythmias
- VF/VT, asystole, PEA

Management of hypokalaemia includes:

- Stopping any causative agent(s).
- K$^+$ supplementation—the speed of replacement depends on the K$^+$ level, the patient's symptoms, and presence of ECG changes. The maximum recommended IV infusion rate is 20 mmol/h. More rapid infusions can be given via a central line in a critical care setting. Continuous ECG monitoring is essential during the infusion.
- In a cardiac arrest, K$^+$ can be given more rapidly (2 mmol/min for 10 minutes, followed by 10 mmol over 5–10 minutes).
- Patients may also be deficient in magnesium. Repletion of magnesium stores will facilitate more rapid correction of hypokalaemia and is recommended in severe cases (magnesium sulfate 2 g IV).

Hyper/hypocalcaemia

The management of calcium disorders is discussed in Chapter 14, section 14.10.

In the event of cardiac arrest secondary to hypocalcaemia or a calcium channel blocker overdose, a bolus of calcium chloride 10 ml of 10% should be given. Hypocalcaemia is difficult to correct if hypomagnesaemia is not corrected, therefore patients should also receive magnesium sulfate 2 g IV.

2.2.3 Poisoning

Poisoning is a leading cause of cardiac arrest in patients younger than 40 years old. Toxicology is discussed in more detail in Chapter 17.

Opiates

Opiate poisoning causes progressive depression of the central nervous system leading to coma, respiratory depression, and eventually respiratory arrest. Cardiac arrest is the consequence of hypoxia. The pupils are usually equal and pin-point. The antagonist to opiates is naloxone, which can be given IV, intraosseous (IO), intramuscularly (IM), intranasally (IN), or via an endotracheal tube.

Management of opiate poisoning:

- The priority is airway management, oxygenation, and ventilation.
- The initial dose of naloxone is 400 mcg IV (800 mcg IM and 2 mg IN). It should be repeated if there is no response within two minutes. Naloxone is a competitive antagonist and large doses (4 mg) may be required in the seriously poisoned patient. The empirical administration of naloxone to all unresponsive victims of possible opiate-associated life-threatening emergency may be reasonable.
- The plasma high-life of naloxone is shorter than all opiate analgesics and an intravenous infusion of naloxone may be required. This involves adding 2 mg of naloxone to 500 ml of normal saline or 5% glucose, giving a final concentration of 4 mcg/ml. The usual infusion rate is 25–100 ml/hour (100–400 mcg/hour).
- In the event of cardiac arrest, standard resuscitation guidelines should be followed.

Tricyclic antidepressants

The management of tricyclic antidepressant (TCA) overdose is discussed in Chapter 17, section 17.6. In the event of cardiac arrest secondary to a TCA overdose sodium bicarbonate (50 ml of 8.4%) should be given and prolonged resuscitation attempts of up to one hour may be required.

Cocaine toxicity

Cocaine is a sympathomimetic, which may cause agitation, tachycardia, hypertension, hyperthermia, and myocardial ischaemia.

Management of cocaine toxicity:

- Intravenous benzodiazepines (diazepam or lorazepam) are the first-line agents to manage agitation, convulsions, hypertension, and chest pain.
- Persisting hypertension can be treated with IV nitrates. Calcium channel blockers (e.g. nifedipine, diltiazem, and verapamil) are second-line agents. Beta-blockers should be avoided due to the risk of paradoxical hypertension and vasoconstriction from unopposed alpha-adrenergic effects. Phentolamine is an alternative in patients with hypertension but it can cause a precipitous fall in blood pressure and should be avoided in those with a history of cardiac ischaemia.
- Cocaine causes coronary artery vasospasm and chest pain should be treated with aspirin, diazepam, and nitrates. If chest pain continues despite these treatments and the ECG shows

changes suggestive of myocardial infarction, conventional reperfusion management should be followed (e.g. thrombolysis or primary angioplasty).
- In the event of cardiac arrest, standard resuscitation guidelines apply.

2.2.4 Hypothermia

Hypothermia exists when the core body temperature is less than 35°C. It can be classified as:

- Mild 32–35°C
- Moderate 30–32°C
- Severe <30°C

A low-reading thermometer is needed to measure the core temperature. Hypothermia may develop rapidly (e.g. sudden immersion in cold water) or gradually due to immobility or impaired conscious level secondary to illness, alcohol, or drugs. The elderly and very young are more suitable to hypothermia due to impaired thermoregulation. Hypothermia in cardiac arrest may be the primary cause, or it may be secondary to a normothermic cardiac arrest followed by cooling due to the environment. Hypothermia can exert a protective effect on the brain after cardiac arrest. Confirmation of death should not be made until the patient has been rewarmed, or attempts to rewarm the patient have failed.

Modifications to the ALS algorithm in a hypothermic cardiac arrest:

- Palpate a major artery for a pulse and look for signs of life for up to one minute before concluding that there is no cardiac output. If possible, use echocardiography or Doppler ultrasound to confirm the presence or absence of cardiac output. If there is doubt about the presence of a pulse, begin CPR.
- The drug regime should be modified in a hypothermic cardiac arrest because the heart may be unresponsive to cardioactive drugs and drug metabolism is slower, leading to potentially toxic plasma concentrations of drugs. Withhold cardioactive drugs until the core temperature is >30°C. Once 30°C has been reached, double the interval between doses until the temperature returns to normal (>35°C).
- If VF/VT is detected, the patient should be defibrillated. If VF/VT persists beyond three shocks, further attempts at defibrillation should be postponed until the temperature is >30°C.
- Interventions such as central line placement and intubation should be performed by an expert to avoid excessive movement of patient and the risk of precipitating VF.
- Rewarm the patient to 32–34°C, a target temperature of 36°C is an alternative. A period of therapeutic hypothermia may be beneficial post-arrest.
- Patients may require large volumes of IV fluids as they rewarm and vasodilate.

Hypothermia in patients with a pulse

As the core temperature falls, cerebral and cardiovascular function deteriorates. Patients become ataxic, dysarthric, and their conscious level falls, progressing to coma. The blood pressure falls and arrhythmias develop; typically sinus bradycardia becomes atrial fibrillation, followed by VF and asystole.

Investigations in hypothermia:

- Renal function—risk of rhabdomyolysis
- FBC and clotting studies—hypothermia may precipitate a coagulopathy
- Toxicology screen
- Blood glucose—risk of hypoglycaemia
- Amylase—hypothermia may precipitate pancreatitis
- ABG—to determine the level of oxygenation, effectiveness of ventilation, and presence of metabolic acidosis

- ECG—prolonged PQRST complex, J waves (delayed repolarization), and arrhythmias may develop
- CXR—to look for evidence of aspiration, pneumonia, or pulmonary oedema
- CT head—if a head injury or cerebrovascular accident (CVA) is suspected

Management of hypothermia:

- Patients should be rewarmed. This may be a combination of active and passive rewarming techniques, depending on the severity and duration of hypothermia, and available facilities. Aim for a rate of 0.5–2°C per hour. Rapid rewarming may precipitate pulmonary and cerebral oedema, especially in the elderly (Table 2.3).

Table 2.3 Rewarming techniques

Passive	• Remove cold or wet clothing. • Dry the patient. • Cover with blankets/hot air blanket. • Warm room (overhead heaters, if available). • Forced-air warming system (e.g. Bair Hugger).
Active	• Warmed, humidified oxygen. • Warmed IV fluids. • Gastric, peritoneal, pleural, or bladder lavage with warmed fluids. • Cardiopulmonary bypass.

- ECG monitoring is necessary to detect the development of arrhythmias. Most arrhythmias other than VF tend to revert spontaneously as the core temperature increases and do not usually require immediate treatment.
- Regular blood glucose levels should be checked to monitor for hypoglycaemia. If present, it should be corrected with 50% glucose.
- IV fluids may be required as the patient rewarms. If the blood pressure falls, 300–500 ml of warmed 0.9% sodium chloride should be given. There is a risk of pulmonary oedema and unstable patients should be monitored with a central venous pressure (CVP) line and urinary catheter.

2.2.5 Hyperthermia

Hyperthermia develops when the body's ability to thermoregulate fails and the core temperature exceeds that normally maintained by homeostatic mechanisms (controlled by the hypothalamus).

The pathophysiology of fever and hyperthermia are discussed in Chapter 15, section 15.2.

Causes of hyperthermia

Exogenous:

- Environmental conditions—high temperatures/humidity.

Endogenous:

- Prolonged muscular activity—seizures, marathon running, excessive dancing secondary to recreational drugs (e.g. ecstasy).
- Drugs—ecstasy, cocaine, amphetamines, and so on.
- Neuroleptic malignant syndrome—idiosyncratic drug reaction to antipsychotics. (Discussed further in Chapter 18, section 18.5.)

- Malignant hyperthermia—rare autosomal dominant condition related to the use of suxamethonium or inhaled anaesthetic agents. (Discussed further in Chapter 3, section 3.3.5).

Severity of hyperthermia

Heat cramps
The core temperature is 37–39°C. Heat cramps are typically seen during exercise where insensible fluid losses (sweating) are replaced with hypotonic fluids. Sodium levels fall and the patient develops muscle cramps. Management is with oral rehydration fluids.

Heat exhaustion
The core temperature is <40°C. Patients have both sodium and water depletion. Symptoms include weakness, fatigue, headache, dizziness, nausea, vomiting, and syncope. The patient's homeostatic mechanisms still function but are overwhelmed.

Patients should be removed from the heat. Treatment ranges from oral rehydration fluids in mild cases to IV rehydration in more severe cases.

Heat stroke
The core temperature is >40.6°C. Early symptoms are similar to heat exhaustion but progress to confusion, seizures, coma, hypotension, and arrhythmias. All thermoregulatory control is lost and ultimately multiorgan damage occurs.

Complications of heat stroke include:

- CNS—cerebral oedema and petechial haemorrhages
- Renal—acute kidney injury due to hypovolaemia and rhabdomyolysis
- Liver—raised liver enzymes and jaundice after 24 hours
- Haematological—thrombocytopenia and disseminated intravascular coagulation (DIC)
- Metabolic—hyper/hypokalaemia, metabolic acidosis, hypoglycaemia
- Muscle—rhabdomyolysis

Management of hyperthermia

- Cooling: remove the patient from the hot environment and take off any clothing. Evaporative cooling should be employed; spray the patient with tepid water and blow air over them with fans. Ice packs can be used in the neck, axillae, and groins. Aim to rapidly reduce the core temperature to 39°C. Advanced cooling techniques can be used as for therapeutic hypothermia after cardiac arrest: cold IV fluids, intravascular cooling catheters, surface cooling devices, and extracorporeal circuits, if available.
- Monitor for hypoglycaemia and treat accordingly.
- IV fluids should be given cautiously due to the risks of pulmonary/cerebral oedema. If the blood pressure remains low despite a reduction in temperature, titrate 0.9% sodium chloride cautiously (consider the use of a CVP line and urinary catheterization). IV fluids will need to be given more rapidly if there is evidence of rhabdomyolysis.
- There is no evidence for the use of antipyretics (paracetamol, NSAIDSs) in heat stroke.
- If the hyperthermia is due to neuroleptic malignant syndrome or malignant hyperthermia, dantrolene can be given.

2.2.6 Trauma

The ERC 2015 guidelines highlight the fact that traumatic cardiac arrest carries a high mortality but survival with a good neurological outcome is more likely with ROSC.

Causes of cardiac arrest in trauma

- Severe traumatic brain injury
- Hypovolaemia from massive haemorrhage
- Hypoxia from respiratory arrest
- Direct injury to major organs or vessels
- Tension pneumothorax
- Cardiac tamponade
- Commotio cordis (blunt chest wall trauma leading to VF)

Modifications to the ALS algorithm in trauma

- In the presence of a history of trauma, it is important to determine whether this is a primary traumatic arrest or whether there a medical event that has led to secondary trauma.
- In primary traumatic cardiac arrest, the emphasis is on correction of reversible causes, which takes priority over chest compressions, which are not likely to work in the presence of hypovolaemia, cardiac tamponade, or tension pneumothorax.
- Hypoxia—early tracheal intubation should be undertaken, if possible.
- Hypovolaemia—external haemorrhage should be controlled (e.g. direct pressure, elevation, splinting, tourniquets, and haemostatic agents). In cardiac arrest, aggressive IV fluid resuscitation should be given. If the patient has a pulse, fluids should be given more cautiously (NICE guidance on pre-hospital fluid replacement in trauma recommends 250 ml boluses of crystalloid until a radial pulse is achieved). The emphasis is on rapid surgical control of bleeding. Tranexamic acid loading 1 G IV followed by a 1 G infusion over eight hours should be considered.
- Tension pneumothorax—can be difficult to diagnose in a cardiac arrest. Decompression should be performed by lateral or anterior finger thoracostomy (incision in the chest wall through to the pleural cavity) in the fourth intercostal space. A thoracostomy is likely to be more effective than needle decompression and quicker than inserting a chest drain.
- Cardiac tamponade—consider resuscitative thoracotomy.

Resuscitation Council guidance on when to consider an emergency department thoracotomy:

- Penetrating cardiac injuries who arrive, after a short pre-hospital time, with witnessed signs of life or ECG activity.
- Penetrating non-cardiac thoracic injuries.
- Exsanguinating abdominal vascular injury to enable cross-clamping of the descending aorta.
- Only in blunt trauma when there are vital signs on arrival and a witnessed cardiac arrest.

2.2.7 Asthma

Asthma still causes many deaths in young adults. Asthma management is discussed further in Chapter 10, section 10.1.

Causes of cardiac arrest in asthma

- Hypoxia—severe bronchospasm and mucous plugging leading to asphyxia.
- Cardiac arrhythmias—due to hypoxia, stimulant drugs (e.g. salbutamol, aminophylline), or electrolyte abnormalities.
- Dynamic hyperinflation (gas trapping)—can occur in ventilated asthmatic patients. The increased intrathoracic pressure decreases cardiac output.
- Tension pneumothorax (may be bilateral).

Modifications to the advanced life support algorithm in asthma

- Standard basic life support (BLS) should be performed although ventilation may be hindered by increased airway resistance.
- Patients should be intubated early to reduce the risk of gastric inflation and hypoventilation.
- If dynamic hyperinflation is suspected, compression of the chest wall and/or a period of apnoea (disconnection of tracheal tube) may relive gas trapping.
- Dynamic hyperinflation increases transthoracic impedance. In VF/VT, higher shock energies for defibrillation may be necessary.
- Pleural ultrasound may allow rapid bedside detection of tension pneumothorax. Tension pneumothorax should be treated with needle thoracocentesis (performed in the second intercostal space, mid-clavicular line). A chest drain will then be required. In a ventilated patient a thoracostomy may be quicker and more effective.

2.2.8 Pregnancy

Cardiac arrest is fortunately rare in pregnant patients.

Causes of cardiac arrest in pregnancy

- Pre-existing cardiac disease
- Thromboembolism
- Suicide
- Eclampsia
- Sepsis
- Ectopic pregnancy
- Uteroplacental haemorrhage
- Amniotic fluid embolism

Modifications to the advanced life support algorithm in pregnancy

- Supine positioning will result in aortocaval compression. Aortocaval decompression is achieved by manual displacement of the uterus to the left or by using a 'Cardiff wedge' to support the pelvis and thorax, to achieve the left lateral position, if the fundal height is at or above the level of the umbilicus.
- The hand positioning for chest compression may have to be slightly higher than normal to adjust for elevation of the diaphragm and abdominal contents caused by the gravid uterus.
- Patients should be intubated early due to the risk of pulmonary aspiration of gastric contents.
- Defibrillator pad position may have to be adjusted due to the left lateral tilt and large breasts.
- Consider hypovolaemia as a cause and give a large fluid challenge.
- Consider giving magnesium (4 g IV) in the event of cardiac arrest in eclampsia.
- Emergency delivery of the foetus (>20 weeks gestation) via caesarean section should occur within five minutes of cardiac arrest, when initial resuscitation attempts fail. The rationale is to decompress the inferior vena cava (IVC) for the mother and remove the foetus from the hypoxic environment, providing it with the best chance for survival. The team should not wait for surgical equipment if not immediately available, as only a scalpel is required to start the procedure. Emergency caesarean for gestational age <20 weeks is not necessary because a gravid uterus of this size is unlikely to compromise maternal cardiac output.

KEY POINTS

Good-quality CPR is paramount, regardless of the cause of cardiac arrest, and the ALS algorithm should be followed.

Consideration and treatment of the reversible causes is the mainstay of treatment.

Here is a summary of the main additions and modifications to the resuscitation algorithm for cardiac arrest in special circumstances:

- Hyperkalaemia—calcium chloride 10 ml of 10%, sodium bicarbonate 50 ml of 8.4%, and insulin/glucose infusion (10 units of insulin and 50 ml of 50% glucose).
- Hypokalaemia—K^+ 2 mmol/min for 10 minutes, followed by 10 mmol over 5–10 minutes. Plus magnesium sulfate 2 g IV, if concurrent hypomagnesaemia suspected.
- Hypocalcaemia—calcium chloride 10 ml of 10%, plus magnesium sulfate 2 g IV, if concurrent hypomagnesaemia suspected.
- Opiates—naloxone 400 mcg IV. Repeated doses up to a total of 4 mg may be required.
- Tricyclic antidepressants—sodium bicarbonate 50 ml of 8.4%.
- Local anaesthetic toxicity—20% lipid emulsion IV bolus (1.5 ml/kg). Further details can be found in Chapter 3, section 3.7.5.
- Hypothermia—palpate a pulse/look for signs of life for up to 1 minute (if possible use Doppler). Withhold drugs until temperature >30°C and then double the dosing interval until >35°C. If VF/VT persists beyond three shocks, postpone further attempts at defibrillation until the temperature >30°C. Rewarm to 32–34°C.
- Hyperthermia—active cooling (cold IV fluids, intravascular cooling catheters, surface cooling devices, and extracorporeal circuits). Dantrolene if hyperthermia is due to neuroleptic malignant syndrome or malignant hyperthermia.
- Trauma—intubate early. Manage hypovolaemia with haemorrhage control and fluids. Emergency department (ED) thoracotomy is only indicated in very specific circumstances.
- Asthma—intubate early. Consider the possibility of tension pneumothorax (possibly bilateral) and treat accordingly.
- Pregnancy—place the patient in the left lateral position. Emergency delivery of the foetus (>20 weeks gestation) via caesarean section should occur within five minutes of cardiac arrest.

2.3 Anaphylaxis

2.3.1 Introduction

Anaphylaxis is a severe, life-threatening, systemic, type 1 hypersensitivity reaction. Anaphylaxis is triggered when an antigen binds to immunoglobulin E (IgE) antibodies on mast cells, causing degranulation and the release of inflammatory mediators.

An anaphylactic reaction is likely when all of the following three criteria are met:

- Sudden onset and rapid progression of symptoms.
- Life-threatening airway and/or breathing and/or circulation problems.
- Skin and/or mucosal changes (flushing, urticaria, angioedema).

The diagnosis is supported by exposure to a known allergen for the patient. Anaphylaxis can be triggered by a broad range of substances, but those most commonly identified are food, drugs, and venom.

- Food—most commonly nuts
- Drugs—antibiotics, radiological contrast media, muscle relaxants, NSAIDs
- Venom—wasp or bee stings

The speed of onset will depend upon the trigger. Intravenous medications will cause a more rapid onset than stings, which, in turn, tend to cause a more rapid onset than orally ingested triggers.

2.3.2 Clinical features of anaphylaxis

- Airway—swelling resulting in pharyngeal and laryngeal oedema. This can cause difficulty in breathing and swallowing, a hoarse voice, and stridor.
- Breathing—dyspnoea, wheeze, cyanosis, and ultimately respiratory arrest.
- Circulation—tachycardia, hypotension, dizziness, collapse, reduced level of consciousness, and ultimately cardiac arrest.
- Disability—A, B, and C problems can lead to decreased cerebral perfusion resulting in confusion, agitation, and loss of consciousness.
- Exposure—skin and mucosal changes (urticaria and angioedema) occur in 80% of anaphylactic reactions but may be subtle or absent. Skin changes without life-threatening A, B, or C problems do not signify an anaphylactic reaction.
- Other features—patients may have gastrointestinal symptoms of vomiting, abdominal pain, and diarrhoea.

2.3.3 Management of anaphylaxis

An ABCDE approach should be followed and life-threatening problems treated as they are identified. Initial treatments should not be delayed by the lack of a complete history or definite diagnosis. If possible, the trigger should be removed by stopping any drug or fluid infusions, or removing the sting.

The anaphylaxis algorithm (Figure 2.2 and Table 2.4) details the Resuscitation Council guidance.

Fluids—large volumes of fluid may be required due to vasodilatation and capillary leak. Fluid should be given as 500 ml boluses and repeated as necessary. There is no evidence for colloid over crystalloid in this setting. If the patient is receiving colloid at the time of developing anaphylaxis, consider it as a possible cause and stop the infusion.

Glucagon—adrenaline may fail to reverse the clinical manifestations of an anaphylactic reaction in patients taking β-blockers. Glucagon (1–2 mg IV) can be useful in this situation.

Cardiac arrest—if cardiac arrest occurs, the usual ALS algorithm should be followed and adrenaline should no longer be given IM but IV at a dose of 1mg.

2.3.4 Investigations in anaphylaxis

Anaphylaxis is a clinical diagnosis. The specific investigation which may help confirm the diagnosis retrospectively is measurement of the mast cell tryptase.

Mast cell tryptase

Tryptase is the major protein component of mast cell secretory granules. In anaphylaxis, mast cell degranulation leads to increased blood levels of tryptase. The investigation is useful for follow-up in suspected cases of anaphylaxis but will not alter ED management. However, the timing of the levels is very important.

Tryptase levels may not increase significantly until more than 30 minutes after the onset of symptoms and peak one to two hours later. The half-life of tryptase is short (approximately two hours) and levels will return to normal within six to eight hours. A sample for serum tryptase testing should be obtained as soon as possible after emergency treatment, with a second sample ideally within one to two hours (no later than four hours) from the onset of symptoms. Ideally, a third sample can be taken at 24 hours or in convalescence (e.g. in a follow-up allergy clinic) to establish baseline tryptase levels. Not all patients will have a documented tryptase rise and the absence of a rise does not reliably exclude anaphylaxis.

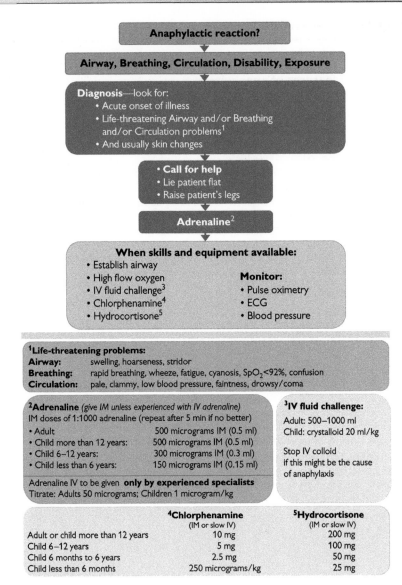

Figure 2.2 Anaphylaxis algorithm.
Reproduced with the kind permission of the Resuscitation Council (UK).

2.3.5 Discharge and follow-up after anaphylaxis

Patients recovering from anaphylactic reactions may be cared for by the ED on a clinical decision unit or equivalent. It is therefore possible that a SAQ will include elements of the discharge advice and follow-up care.

- Patients who have had a suspected anaphylactic reaction should be observed for at least 6–12 hours.

Table 2.4 Drugs used in the treatment of anaphylaxis

Drug	Actions	Indications	Dose
Adrenaline	α-agonist—reverses peripheral vasodilatation and reduces oedema. β-agonist—bronchodilation, positive inotrope, suppresses histamine and leukotriene release. $β_2$ actions also inhibit the activation of mast cells, attenuating the severity of IgE-mediated allergic reactions.	Give as soon as the diagnosis of anaphylaxis is made.	0.5 mg IM (the best site is the anterolateral aspect of the middle-third of the thigh). Repeat after 5 minutes if no improvement. IV adrenaline (50 mcg boluses) should only be used by those experienced in the use and titration of vasopressors.
Antihistamines	H_1-antihistamine may help counter histamine-mediated vasodilatation and bronchoconstriction. H_2-antihistamine (e.g. ranitidine) there is little evidence to support the use in the initial treatment of anaphylaxis.	Second-line treatment.	10 mg chlorpheniramine IV or IM.
Corticosteroids	May prevent or shorten protracted reactions.	For use after the initial resuscitation.	200 mg hydrocortisone IV or IM.
Bronchodilators	β-agonist (salbutamol) and/or antimuscarinic (ipratropium bromide).	If evidence of wheeze on auscultation.	Salbutamol 5 mg and ipratropium bromide 500 mcg nebulizer.

- Patients should be warned of the risk of recurrence, being informed about anaphylaxis, including the signs and symptoms of a biphasic reaction in the next 24 hours. The risk of a biphasic reaction is greater in the following groups:
  - Severe reactions with slow onset caused by an unknown trigger.
  - Reactions in patients with asthma.
  - Reactions with possible continuing absorption of the allergen.
  - Reactions in a patient with a history of biphasic reactions.
- Patients should be reviewed by a senior clinician prior to discharge and if at risk of a biphasic reaction observed for longer (e.g. 24 hours).
- Patients may be discharged with a three day prescription of oral steroid and antihistamines.
- All patients who have had an anaphylactic reaction should be prescribed two adrenaline autoinjector devices as an interim measure before their specialist allergy appointment.
- Patients should be educated on the likely trigger, how to avoid it, and what to do in the event of a future attack.
- All patients should be referred on to an age-appropriate specialist allergy service for follow-up.

KEY POINTS

Patients who have an anaphylactic reaction have life-threatening airway and/or breathing and/or circulation problems usually associated with skin and mucosal changes.

Early recognition of anaphylaxis and treatment with adrenaline 0.5 mg IM is paramount.

The most important investigation in suspected anaphylaxis is the collection of timed serum samples for mast cell tryptase.

Patients should be observed for a minimum of 6–12 h after an anaphylactic reaction.

Patients suspected of having an anaphylactic should be referred on to an allergy specialist.

Urticaria and angioedema can be caused by more than just anaphylaxis. Angioedema can be classified as allergic, hereditary, acquired, drug-induced, or idiopathic. Further details on the different types of angioedema can be found in Chapter 16, section 16.2.5.

2.4 Post-resuscitation care

ROSC is only the first step in recovery from a cardiac arrest. Patients may develop post-cardiac-arrest syndrome, the severity of which varies according to the duration and cause of cardiac arrest.

The post-cardiac-arrest syndrome comprises brain injury, myocardial dysfunction, systemic ischaemia/reperfusion response, and persistence of the precipitating pathology.

- Post-cardiac-arrest brain injury—manifests as coma, seizures, myoclonus, varying degrees of neurocognitive dysfunction, and brain death. It can be exacerbated by microcirculatory failure, impaired autoregulation, hyperoxia, hypoxia, hypercarbia, pyrexia, hyperglycaemia, and seizures.
- Post-cardiac-arrest myocardial dysfunction—manifests as hypotension, arrhythmias, cardiogenic shock, and potentially further cardiac arrest. It usually recovers after two to three days.
- Systemic ischaemia/reperfusion—results in activation of the immunological and coagulation pathways contributing to multiorgan failure and increasing the risk of secondary infection.

The 2015 Resuscitation Council Guidelines continue to emphasize the treatment of the post-cardiac-arrest syndrome. The ABCDE approach to management is recommended (Table 2.5).

Table 2.5 Post-resuscitation care

	Recommendation	Rationale
Airway and breathing	Advanced airway. Waveform capnography. Aim for normocarbia. Aim for normoxia (SpO2 94–98%). Consider sedation, intubation, and ventilation in any obtunded patient.	Hypoxia and hypercarbia increase the likelihood of further cardiac arrest and may contribute to secondary brain injury. Hyperoxia may cause oxidative stress and harm post-ischaemic neurons. Controlled oxygenation and ventilation enable normocarbia and normoxia to be achieved.

Table 2.5 Continued

	Recommendation	Rationale
Circulation	12 lead ECG. Aim for SBP > 100 mm Hg. Crystalloid to restore normovolaemia. Intra-arterial blood pressure monitoring. Consider vasopressor/inotrope to maintain SBP. Patients with ST-elevation should undergo early reperfusion therapy, ideally PCI. Patients without ST-elevation, who are suspected of having coronary artery disease as the cause of their arrest, should be considered for early PCI. Myocardial dysfunction should be managed with IV fluids and inotropes. If this is insufficient, an intra-aortic balloon pump should be considered.	Primary PCI is the preferred treatment in ST-elevation myocardial infarction (STEMI) if it can be performed in a timely manner (within 90 min of first medical contact). If primary PCI is not feasible, thrombolysis should be given (CPR is not a contraindication). Chest pain and ST-elevation are relatively poor indicators of acute coronary occlusion post-cardiac-arrest. Therefore, a low threshold for early PCI is warranted.
Disability	Seizures should be controlled with benzodiazepines, phenytoin, sodium valproate, propofol, or a barbiturate.	Seizures increase cerebral metabolism up to 3-fold and may cause cerebral injury.
Glucose control	Blood glucose should be maintained ≤10 mmol/L. Hypoglycaemia should be avoided.	Hyperglycaemia post-cardiac arrest is associated with a poorer neurological outcome. Intensive glucose control (4.5–6.0 mmol/L) has not been shown to be superior to conventional glucose control and increases the risk of hypoglycaemia, which is associated with increased mortality in the critically ill.
Temperature control	Hyperthermia should be avoided with antipyretics and active cooling. Control shivering. Targeted temperature management or control (32–36°C) is recommended for comatose survivors of both non-shockable and shockable cardiac arrests. Targeted temperature management should be initiated in the ED. Techniques include ice packs and/or wet towels, cooling blankets or pads, water- or air-circulating gel-coated pads, transnasal evaporative cooling, intravascular heat exchanger (via femoral or subclavian vein), and extracorporeal circulation (cardiopulmonary bypass, ECMO).	There is an association between post-cardiac-arrest pyrexia and poor outcome. Mild hypothermia is neuroprotective and improves outcome after a period of global cerebral hypoxia. Cooling suppresses apoptosis and reduces the cerebral metabolic rate (~6% for each 1°C reduction). Hypothermia may reduce the release of excitatory amino acids and free radicals. Animal data indicate that earlier cooling after ROSC produces better outcome.

2.5 Peri-arrest arrhythmia management

2.5.1 Introduction

Arrhythmia management is a subject that many candidates find difficult. The 2015 Resuscitation Council Guidelines have tried to simplify the management as much as possible. Knowledge of this guidance should be sufficient for the MRCEM examination.

2.5.2 Generic management of peri-arrest arrhythmias

- All patients should be assessed using the ABCDE approach. Patients should be given oxygen, have an IV line inserted, and assessed for adverse features.
- If time allows, patients should have a 12-lead ECG.
- Any electrolyte abnormalities (e.g. K^+, Ca^{2+}, Mg^{2+}) should be corrected.
- If there is an underlying condition (e.g. MI, sepsis), this must also be treated.
- The two main questions to answer when managing an arrhythmia are:
  - Is the patient stable?
  - What is nature of the arrhythmia?

Adverse features in peri-arrest arrhythmias

There is now a single set of adverse features for tachy- and bradyarrhythmias. If adverse features are present, it suggests that the patient is potentially unstable from their arrhythmia.
   The adverse features are:

- Shock—hypotension (systolic BP <90 mmHg), pallor, sweating, cold extremities, clammy, confusion, or impaired level of consciousness.
- Syncope—transient loss of consciousness due to a reduction in cerebral perfusion.
- Myocardial ischaemia—ischaemic chest pain and/or evidence of ischaemia on the ECG.
- Heart failure—pulmonary oedema and/or raised jugular venous pressure (with or without peripheral oedema and liver enlargement).

If the patient is unstable, the treatment of choice is electricity: cardioversion for tachyarrhythmias and pacing for bradyarrhythmias (see Figure 2.3). Table 2.6 details the drugs used in peri-arrest arrhythmias.

2.6 Peri-arrest tachycardias

2.6.1 Stable versus unstable tachyarrhythmias

If the patient is unstable, due to their tachyarrhythmia, synchronized cardioversion is the treatment of choice. Cardioversion should be carried out under general anaesthesia or conscious sedation. The defibrillator should be set to synchronized mode. The recommended energies vary slightly depending on the type of tachyarrhythmia, but 120 J biphasic would be an appropriate initial energy for any tachyarrhythmia. If this fails, a further two shocks at increasing increments should be tried.

   If electrical cardioversion fails to restore sinus rhythm, and the patient remains unstable, amiodarone 300 mg IV should be given over 10–20 minutes. Electrical cardioversion can then be repeated. The loading dose of amiodarone can be followed by an infusion of 900 mg over 24 hours.

   If the patient is stable and has no adverse features, then there are several possible treatment options depending on the nature of the arrhythmia. The ECG assessment should include whether the QRS is broad or narrow, and whether it is regular or irregular.

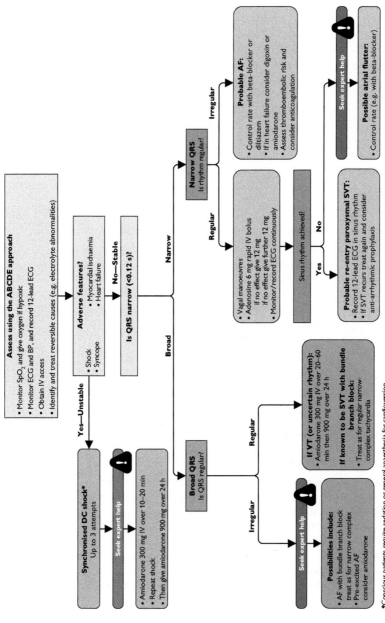

Figure 2.3 Adult tachycardia (with pulse) algorithm.

Reproduced with the kind permission of the Resuscitation Council (UK).

Table 2.6 Drugs used in peri-arrest arrhythmias

Drug	Actions	Indications/Dose
Adrenaline	• As detailed in Table 2.2.	• Treatment of cardiogenic shock. Dose 0.05–0.1 mcg/kg/min • Bradycardia if there is a delay for pacing. Dose 2–10 mcg/min IV.
Amiodarone	• As detailed in Table 2.2	• Stable VT and wide-complex tachycardias of unknown origin. • To control a rapid ventricular rate in pre-excited AF. • Following unsuccessful electrical cardioversion in unstable arrhythmias. Dose: 300 mg IV over 10–60 min. Followed by 900 mg over 24 h.
Adenosine	• Blocks transmission across the AV node. • Very short half-life (10–15 s). Must be given as a rapid bolus into a large cannula, in a large vein with a 20 ml saline flush.	• Paroxysmal SVT. Dose 6 mg IV bolus. If unsuccessful a further two doses at 12 mg IV may be tried.
Atropine	• Antagonizes the action of the parasympathetic neurotransmitter acetylcholine at muscarinic receptors. • Blocks the action of the vagus nerve at the SA and AV nodes, increasing sinus automaticity, and facilitating AV node conduction.	• Unstable bradycardia. Dose 500 mcg IV bolus. Repeated up to a maximum of 3 mg.
Magnesium	• As detailed in Table 2.2	• Polymorphic VT (Torsades de pointes). • Digoxin toxicity. • Ventricular tachyarrhythmias if hypomagnesaemia suspected. Dose 2 g IV over 10 min.

2.6.2 Broad-complex tachycardia (QRS >0.12 seconds)

Broad-complex tachycardias are usually ventricular in origin but may also be caused by supraventricular rhythms (SVT) with aberrant conduction (bundle branch block). There are several features on the ECG that can help distinguish VT from SVT with aberrant conduction (Figure 2.4 and Table 2.7). If there is doubt about the source of the arrhythmia and the patient is unstable, assume the rhythm is ventricular in origin and perform electrical cardioversion.

Treatment options for regular broad-complex tachycardias in stable patients

• If a regular broad-complex is diagnosed as SVT with aberrant conduction, it can be treated with adenosine.
• If VT is diagnosed, the treatment is amiodarone 300 mg IV over 20–60 minutes, followed by an infusion of 900 mg for 24 hours.
• In a stable patient with a regular broad-complex tachycardia of uncertain origin, adenosine can be tried.

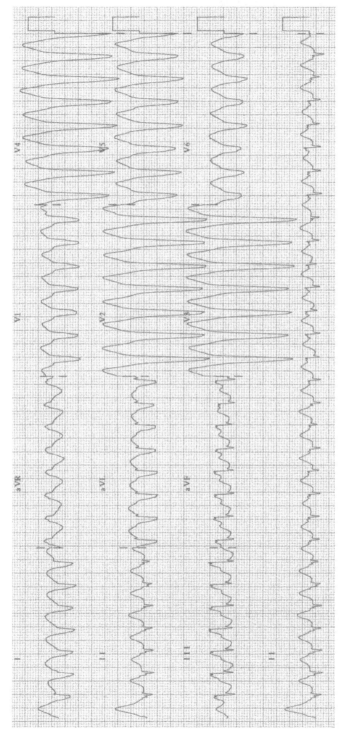

Figure 2.4 A broad-complex tachycardia with a ventricular rate of 180 bpm. AV dissociation is seen with buried P waves in V6. There is concordance across the chest leads.

Reproduced from Saul G. Myerson, Robin P. Choudhury, and Andrew R. J. Mitchell, *Emergencies in Cardiology*, 2010, Figure 21.35, p. 421, with permission from Oxford University Press.

Table 2.7 Distinguishing VT from SVT with aberrant conduction

Regularity	• Monomorphic VT originates from one area in the ventricle and therefore is regular. • SVT may be irregular if the underlying rhythm is atrial fibrillation, atrial flutter with variable block, or multifocal atrial tachycardia.
QRS width	• A broader QRS (>0.14 s) favours VT.
QRS concordance	• In monomorphic VT, all the precordial leads (V1–V6) point in the same direction. • SVT may have mixture of positive and negative QRS deflections in the precordial leads.
Beat-to-beat variability	• In VT there is often beat-to-beat variability of the QRS morphology.
Electrical axis	• VT normally has an axis in the extreme right quadrant. • SVT will have right axis deviation in right bundle branch block and left axis deviation in left bundle branch block.
AV dissociation	• In VT, the atria and ventricles are depolarizing independently and therefore the P waves (if seen) have no relationship to the QRS. • In SVT, if P waves are seen they correlate with the QRS.
Capture beats	• In VT, the AV dissociation is often intermittent and therefore occasionally the atria are able to conduct a beat through the AV node resulting in a normal QRS ('capture beat'). • In SVT, the AV node is already conducting maximally, so there is no opportunity for a capture beat.
Fusion beats	• In a similar mechanism to capture beats, the AV node conducts an atrial impulse that combines with the ventricular depolarization wave giving a fused complex on the ECG ('fusion beat').

Treatment options for irregular broad-complex tachycardias in stable patients

- Irregular broad-complex tachycardias are most likely to be atrial fibrillation (AF) with bundle branch block and should be treated as AF (if uncertain, amiodarone 300 mg IV over 20–60 minutes is usually a reasonable choice).
- Torsades de pointe (polymorphic VT) should be treated by stopping all drugs known to prolong the QT interval, correction of electrolyte abnormalities, and magnesium sulphate 2 g IV over 10 minutes. Overdrive pacing may be indicated to prevent a relapse once the arrhythmia has been corrected.

2.6.3 Regular narrow-complex tachycardias

The ECG should be examined to determine if the rhythm is regular or irregular. Causes of a regular narrow-complex tachycardia include:

- Sinus tachycardia—a physiological response to a stimulus. Treatment is of the underlying cause (e.g. sepsis, hypovolaemia, anaemia, and so on).
- Atrioventricular (AV) nodal re-entry tachycardia—the commonest type of regular narrow-complex tachycardia. Occurs due to a re-entry circuit within or just next to the AV node. The circuit usually involves two pathways: a slow pathway and a fast pathway. The slow pathway is usually the anterograde limb of the circuit and the fast pathway, the retrograde limb. The circuit is triggered by an atrial premature complex, which is able to conduct down the slow pathway due to a short refractory period, but not the fast pathway due to a longer refractory period. Once the impulse reaches the ventricle, the fast pathway has recovered from the

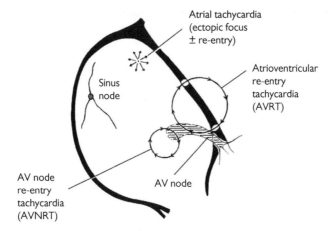

Figure 2.5 Types of supraventricular tachycardia.

Reproduced from Punit Ramrakha, Kevin Moore, and Amir Sam, *Oxford Handbook of Acute Medicine*, 2010, Figure 1.9, p. 69, with permission from Oxford University Press.

refractory period and is able to conduct the impulse retrogradely to the atrium and the atrial end of the slow pathway, perpetuating the circuit (Figure 2.5).

- AV re-entry tachycardia—usually due to Wolff–Parkinson–White (WPW) syndrome. An accessory pathway exists between the atria and ventricles. It is separate from the AV node and in conjunction with the AV node can set up a re-entry circuit.
- Atrial flutter with regular AV conduction (usually 2:1)—typically atrial flutter has a rate of 300, so atrial flutter with 2:1 conduction produces a tachycardia of 150 bpm. It may be indistinguishable from AVRT and AVNRT initially.

Treatment options for regular narrow-complex tachycardias depend on whether the patient is stable or not (Table 2.8).

Adenosine

Adenosine slows transmission across the AV node and therefore is highly effective at terminating AVNRT and AVRT. It has a very short half-life (10–15 seconds) and needs to be given as a rapid bolus into a large cannula, in a large vein (e.g. antecubital fossa) with a 20 ml saline flush.

Table 2.8 Treatment options in regular narrow-complex tachycardias

Unstable patient	If the patient is unstable, with adverse features, treat with synchronized electrical cardioversion. While preparations are being made to perform synchronized cardioversion, it is reasonable to try adenosine, provided it does not delay electrical cardioversion should it fail to restore sinus rhythm.
Stable patient	Step wise progression until sinus rhythm restored: • Vagal manoeuvres—Valsalva and/or carotid sinus massage. • Adenosine 6 mg as a rapid IV bolus. • Repeat adenosine at 12 mg and again at 12 mg if no response. • Consider verapamil 2.5–5 mg IV over 2 min (if adenosine is contraindicated).

Patients should be warned of transient unpleasant side effects including nausea, flushing, and chest tightness.

Cautions when using adenosine:

- Asthma due to the risk of bronchospasm.
- Patients with an accessory pathway (e.g. WPW) and AF due to the risk of promoting conduction down the accessory pathway and inducing VF.
- Patients with denervated hearts (e.g. heart transplant) who have a markedly exaggerated response to adenosine.
- Patients taking theophyllines because it blocks the effects of adenosine.
- Patients taking dipyridamole or carbamazepine due to a dangerously exaggerated response to adenosine.

If adenosine is contraindicated and the arrhythmia is known to be of supraventricular origin, verapamil (2.5–5 mg IV) can be used. Flecanide (2 mg/kg IV) is another alternative, but should not be used in patients with structural heart disease due to the risk of fatal arrhythmias.

Wolff–Parkinson–White (WPW) syndrome

WPW syndrome is due to an accessory pathway (bundle of Kent) between the atria and ventricles (Figure 2.6). It can often be diagnosed incidentally on the ECG of an asymptomatic patient, due to a short PR interval and a widened QRS complex due to the slurred upstroke (delta wave).

Patients may remain asymptomatic their entire life but they are at risk of tachyarrhythmias. Medications that block the AV node (e.g. adenosine, diltiazem, verapamil, and digoxin) should be avoided in patients with an accessory pathway who develop AF or atrial flutter because they can lead to a relative increase in pre-excitation. Treatment options for such situations include amiodarone, electrical cardioversion, or flecanide (if the heart is known to be structurally normal).

2.6.4 Irregular narrow-complex tachycardias

An irregular narrow-complex tachycardia is likely to be AF or, less commonly, atrial flutter with a variable AV block. If the patient is unstable, with adverse features caused by the arrhythmia, they should be treated with synchronized electrical cardioversion.

In stable patients there are several treatment options:

- Rate control by drug therapy (e.g. beta-blocker or rate-limiting calcium antagonist)
- Rhythm control by drug therapy (e.g. amiodarone or flecanide)
- Rhythm control by electrical cardioversion
- Anticoagulation to prevent thromboembolism (should be considered in all patients)

The management of AF is discussed in more depth in Chapter 9, section 9.5.

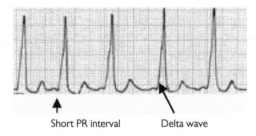

Short PR interval   Delta wave

Figure 2.6 Wolff–Parkinson–White syndrome.

Reproduced from Nick Dunn, Hazel Everitt, and Chantal Simon, *Cardiovascular Problems*, 2007, Figure 3.9, p. 91, with permission from Oxford University Press.

2.7 Peri-arrest bradycardias

2.7.1 Introduction

Patients with bradycardia (heart rate <60 beats per minute) should be assessed using the ABCDE approach. Bradycardia may be:

- Physiological
- Cardiac in origin (e.g. AV block, sinus node disease, post-MI)
- Non-cardiac in origin (e.g. vasovagal, hypothermia, hypothyroidism, raised intracranial pressure)
- Drug-induced (e.g. β-blockade, calcium channel blockers (diltiazem), digoxin, amiodarone)

See Table 2.9 and Figures 2.7 and 2.8.

2.7.2 Unstable bradycardias

The same adverse features are used for bradyarrhythmias as for tachyarrhythmias:

- Shock
- Syncope
- Myocardial ischaemia
- Heart failure

If adverse features are present, treatment should be started immediately.

Table 2.9 Types of bradyarrhythmias

First-degree heart block	Delayed conduction between the atria and ventricles resulting in a prolonged PR interval (>0.2 s).
Second-degree heart block	Only a proportion of the P waves are conducted to the ventricles.
	There are two main types: • Mobitz type I (Wenckebach)—the PR interval gets progressively longer until a P wave fails to conduct. • Mobitz type II—constant PR but occasionally a P wave fails to conduct. This may be in a regular pattern (e.g. 2:1 or 3:1 block) or irregular.
Third-degree heart block (complete heart block)	Atrial activity is not conducted to the ventricles. The atria and ventricles work independently of each other (P waves and QRS complexes are not related to each other).
	The rate and breadth of the QRS complexes depends upon level of the block. With a proximal block (e.g. at the AV node) the escape rhythm will arise from the AV node or bundle of His resulting in a narrower QRS complex and a rate of approximately 50 bpm. With a more distal block, the escape rhythm will produce broader QRS complexes at a slower rate (approximately 30 bpm).
Sick sinus syndrome	Due to ischaemia or fibrosis/degeneration of the SA node.
	Resulting in sinus pauses (>2 s) or sinus arrest. Junctional or other escape rhythms (e.g. AF) may emerge, often known as 'tachy-brady' syndrome. Patients ultimately need a pacemaker to manage the bradyarrhythmias and medical therapy (e.g. β-blockers) to manage the tachyarrhythmias.

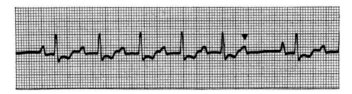

Figure 2.7 Second-degree heart block, type I (Wenckebach). The PR interval progressively prolongs until there is a failure of conduction following a P wave (arrow).

Reproduced from David A. Warrell, Timothy M. Cox, and John D. Firth, *Oxford Textbook of Medicine*, 2010, Figure 16.4.8, p. 2693, with permission from Oxford University Press.

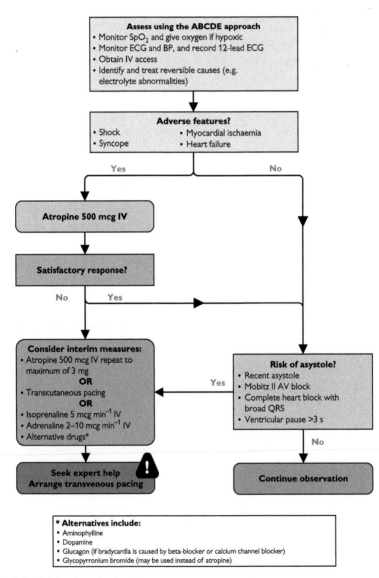

Figure 2.8 Adult bradycardia algorithm.

Reproduced with the kind permission of the Resuscitation Council (UK).

Treatment of unstable bradycardia

- **Atropine**—is the first-line agent in bradycardia (500 mcg IV boluses up to a total dose of 3 mg). Atropine antagonizes the action of the parasympathetic neurotransmitter acetylcholine at muscarinic receptors. It blocks the action of the vagus nerve at the SA and AV nodes, increasing sinus automaticity and facilitating AV node conduction. Atropine should be used cautiously in those with acute myocardial ischaemia or infarction because the increased heart rate may worsen ischaemia or increase infarction size. Atropine should not be given to patients with heart transplants because their hearts are denervated and will not respond to the vagal blockade by atropine; paradoxically they may develop sinus arrest or high-grade AV block.
- **Pacing**—should be started if bradycardia with adverse signs persists despite atropine. Transcutaneous pacing can be painful and the patient should be sedated. For pacing to be successful, there must be electrical capture (i.e. a QRS complex after each pacing stimulus) and mechanical capture (i.e. a palpable pulse corresponding to the QRS complexes). Transcutaneous pacing is a temporary intervention and arrangements should be made for placement of a transvenous pacing wire.
- **Other drugs**—may be appropriate if there is a delay for transcutaneous pacing or in certain clinical situations. If there is a delay for pacing, adrenaline 2–10 mcg per minute IV can be given. If the likely cause is β-blockers or calcium channel blockers, then IV glucagon (1–2 mg) can be tried. If the bradycardia is due to digoxin toxicity, then digoxin-specific antibody can be considered. Theophylline (100–200 mg slow IV) can be given for bradycardia complicating acute inferior wall MI, spinal cord injury, or cardiac transplantation.

2.7.3 Stable bradycardias

Patients without adverse features should be assessed for the risk of asystole. The risk of asystole is greater in patients with the following ECG findings:

- Ventricular pause >3 seconds
- Mobitz type II AV block
- Complete heart block
- Recent asystole

These patients should be considered for temporary transvenous pacing.

KEY POINTS

There is a single set of adverse features for all peri-arrest arrhythmias: shock, syncope, myocardial ischaemia, and heart failure.

If a patient is unstable from their arrhythmia, the treatment of choice is electricity: synchronized cardioversion in tachyarrhythmias and pacing in bradyarrhythmias.

Broad-complex tachycardias are usually ventricular in origin but may be SVT with aberrant conduction. Know the ECG features that help distinguish them.

Stable VT is treated with amiodarone 300 mg IV over 20–60 min.

Torsades de pointe is treated with magnesium 2 g IV over 10 min.

SVT is treated with vagal manoeuvres, followed by adenosine.

AF can be rate-controlled with β-blockers or calcium channel blockers.

Bradycardia is treated with atropine 500 mcg IV to a maximum dose of 3 mg.

2.8 Shock

Shock is an abnormality of the circulatory system resulting in inadequate tissue perfusion and oxygenation.

2.8.1 Physiology of cardiac output

Provided the haemoglobin level and oxygen saturation are adequate, the main determinant of oxygen delivery to the tissues is cardiac output. In order to understand shock, it is necessary to understand the physiology of the cardiac output.

Cardiac output

The cardiac output (CO) is the volume of blood pumped out by the heart each minute:

$$CO = Heart Rate(HR) \times Stroke\ Volume\ (SV).$$

Stroke volume

The stroke volume is the amount of blood pumped out per cardiac contraction. Stroke volume is determined by the following:

- Preload
- Myocardial contractility
- Afterload

Preload

Preload is the volume of venous return to the heart and is defined as the ventricular wall tension at the end of diastole. It is determined by venous capacitance, volume status, and the difference between venous systemic pressure and right atrial pressure.

The volume of venous blood returned to the heart determines the degree of ventricular filling and the length of myocardial muscle fibres. Muscle fibre length is related to the contractile properties of the myocardium (Frank–Starling law). Increased muscle fibre length results in a greater SV. However, above a certain point, the ventricle becomes overstretched and further filling results in a fall in SV.

Previous MRCEM question

Knowledge of the Frank–Starling curve (Figure 2.9) has appeared in previous SAQs.

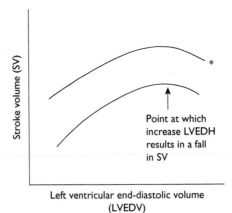

Point at which
increase LVEDH
results in a fall
in SV

Left ventricular end-diastolic volume
(LVEDV)

* Effects of increased contractility
independent of preload (e.g. effects
of a positive inotrope).

Figure 2.9 Frank–Starling curve.
Data from Frank 1918, and Starling 1919

Myocardial contractility

Myocardial contractility is the ability of the heart to work independent of the preload and after-load. Contractility can be increased by inotropes resulting in an increased SV for the same preload (Figure 2.9). Decreased myocardial contractility may result from intrinsic heart disease or from myocardial depression (e.g. caused by acidosis, hypoxia, sepsis, drugs, and so on).

Afterload

Afterload is defined as the ventricular wall tension at the end of systole. It is the resistance to forward blood flow.

2.8.2 Pathophysiology of shock

Shock can be the result of numerous pathophysiological processes and can be broadly divided into two groups: those that impair cardiac output and those that impair systemic vascular resistance (Table 2.10).

Irrespective of the cause of shock, inadequate delivery of oxygen to the tissues results in a failure of aerobic metabolism. Anaerobic respiration ensues, which is less efficient than aerobic, and results in the production of lactic acid. Eventually cell metabolism ceases, leading to cell death, and end organ dysfunction.

2.8.3 Clinical features of shock

Patients should be assessed and managed using the ABCDE approach. Any physiological derangements should be noted and corrected during the assessment. The underlying cause should be sought and treated.

The body has a range of compensatory mechanisms to cope with a reduction in oxygen delivery. These mechanisms account for some of the initial clinical features seen in a patient developing shock. Later features are those of organ dysfunction, as compensatory mechanisms fail (Table 2.11).

Shock due to acute blood loss

Shock secondary to acute blood loss can be classified into four groups depending on the estimated percentage blood loss (Table 2.12). The classification system is useful for demonstrating the clinical features of shock as the body compensates, and how late a fall in blood pressure can occur.

2.8.4 Investigations and monitoring in shock

Investigations should be guided by the suspected underlying cause (e.g. ECG in MI, FAST/CT scan in trauma, echocardiography in massive PE, septic screen in sepsis).

Certain investigations are generic and applicable to all causes of shock. This enables the severity of shock to be determined and monitoring of the response to treatment.

Table 2.10 Causes of shock

Cardiac output falls	Systemic vascular resistance falls
• Hypovolaemic (reduced preload), for example haemorrhage, diarrhoea and vomiting, burns. • Cardiogenic (reduced contractility), for example MI, myocardial contusion, myocarditis, late sepsis, overdose (e.g. β-blockers), complete heart block. Obstructive (increased afterload), for example PE, cardiac tamponade, tension pneumothorax.	• Sepsis. • Anaphylaxis. • Neurogenic—loss of sympathetic tone due to a spinal cord injury.

Table 2.11 Clinical features of shock

Clinical features	Compensatory response	Caveats
↑ Heart rate	Reduced CO results in sympathetic activation via arterial baroreceptors. This results in an increased heart rate to try and restore the CO.	Not all patients with a reduced CO develop a tachycardia. Patients taking certain medications (e.g. β-blockers) will not develop a tachycardia. Patients with a cardiogenic cause for their shock (e.g. complete heart block, β-blocker overdose) may not develop a tachycardia.
↑ Respiratory rate	Hypoxia may increase the respiratory rate (e.g. in pneumonia). Respiratory compensation for metabolic acidosis will raise the respiratory rate.	The respiratory rate may be normal or low in patients who are tiring and compensatory mechanisms are failing.
↓ Blood pressure	Blood pressure may not fall until 30–40% of the blood volume is lost in hypovolaemia (see Table 2.12). Blood pressure is often maintained by the release of catecholamines, which increases the systemic vascular resistance.	Before the BP falls, the pulse pressure may narrow due to a diastolic increase in response to vasoconstriction.
Cool peripheries, sweating	Vasoconstriction of cutaneous, muscle, and visceral circulation preserves blood flow to the heart, kidneys, and brain. Consequently the skin is pale and cool. Catecholamine release can result in sweating/clamminess.	In distributive shock (early sepsis, anaphylaxis, neurogenic) there is usually peripheral vasodilatation.
↓ Conscious level	Conscious level may be reduced due to decreased cerebral perfusion.	Do not assume a reduced conscious level is related purely due to shock. Ensure other causes are excluded (e.g. hypoglycaemia, intracranial bleed).
↓ Urine output	Urine output is typically reduced and patients should be catheterized early.	Urine output is of limited use in the initial assessment of patients in the ED.

Table 2.12 Classification of shock due to acute blood loss

Class of shock	Class I	Class II	Class III	Class IV
Volume of blood loss (ml)	Up to 750	750–1500	1500–2000	>2000
Volume of blood loss (%)	0–15%	15–30%	30–40%	>40%
Heart rate	<100	>100	>120	>140
Blood pressure	Normal	Normal	Decreased	Decreased
Pulse pressure	Normal or increased	Decreased	Decreased	Decreased
Respiratory rate	14–20	20–30	30–40	>35
Mental state	Slightly anxious	Mildly anxious	Anxious, confused	Confused, lethargic

Reproduced with permission from the American College of Surgeons, Committee on Trauma Advance Trauma Life Support program. 2008. *Advanced Trauma Life Support Course: Student Manual*, 8th edn. Copyright American College of Surgeons.

- **Lactate**—is produced by anaerobic respiration. It is a useful marker of the severity of shock. Elevated lactate levels (>4 mmol/L) are associated with increased intensive care unit admissions and mortality in sepsis. The normalization of lactate in trauma and post-cardiac arrest patients correlates with improved survival.
- **Central venous pressure monitoring**—enables measurement of right heart filling pressures and guides fluid resuscitation. A CVP line also allows delivery of inotropic drugs and the measurement of central venous oxygen saturations.
- **Central venous oxygen saturations ($ScvO_2$)**—allows a measure of the oxygen content of blood returning to the heart. As oxygen is extracted from the blood, the oxygen saturation falls and the level can give an indication of total body oxygen extraction. The oxygen concentration in the mixed venous blood of the pulmonary artery (SvO_2) is usually 70–75%. If the SvO_2 is lower than this, it indicates that oxygen extraction has increased and in shocked states this is usually because oxygen delivery has become inadequate (demand > supply).

In the ED it is impractical to sample blood form the pulmonary artery (SvO_2) and consequently the central venous oxygen saturation ($ScvO_2$) is used. The $ScvO_2$ is about 5–7% higher than the SvO_2. Early goal-directed therapy in sepsis has incorporated the $ScvO_2$ as a guide for blood transfusion and inotropic support. Sepsis management is discussed in more detail in Chapter 15, section 15.1.

- **Invasive arterial pressure monitoring**—allows beat-to-beat measurement of the arterial blood pressure and easy serial blood gas analysis. Significant variation in the amplitude of the arterial pressure wave ('respiratory swing') is characteristic of hypovolaemia.

2.8.5 Management of shock

The management of shock should be directed at treating the underlying cause and correction of the physiological derangement. Specific treatments for the various causes of shock are dealt with in other chapters (e.g. Chapter 4, Chapter 9, Chapter 10, and Chapter 15).

Resuscitation to correct the physiological deficit is a dynamic process guided by the patient's clinical features, investigations, and monitoring. Resuscitation should occur in conjunction with the ABCDE assessment.

Airway and breathing

- Patients should receive high-flow oxygen to ensure oxygen delivery to the tissues is maximal.
- Intubation and ventilation should be considered early in the management of shocked patients. Positive pressure ventilation can dramatically reduce the work of breathing and therefore oxygen consumption. Patients requiring large volumes of fluid resuscitation are at risk of pulmonary oedema due to increased capillary permeability, especially in sepsis, and may require intubation.

Circulation

- Adequate fluid resuscitation is critical in shock. Patients should be given fluid boluses of 250 ml IV and reassessed after each. There is no evidence that colloid is superior to crystalloid (0.9% sodium chloride or Hartmann's is appropriate).
- In certain circumstances (e.g. penetrating chest trauma), cautious fluid resuscitation is appropriate until haemostasis is achieved.
- Haemoglobin is critical in determining adequate oxygen delivery to tissues. As a general rule, transfusing to haemoglobin of 7–9 g/dl is a reasonable target in otherwise healthy patients.
- Inotropes and vasopressors may be required if hypotension persists despite adequate intravenous fluid resuscitation.

Table 2.13 Effects of agonists on vasoactive receptors

Receptor	Effect
α_1	Vasoconstriction
β_1	Inotropic (increased force of contraction) and chronotropic (increased heart rate)
β_2	Vasodilatation (and bronchodilation)
Dopamine	Splanchnic and renal vasodilatation

2.8.6 Inotropes and vasopressors

Vasoactive drugs can be classified as:

* inotropes—which increase cardiac contractility, or
* vasopressors—which increase systemic vascular resistance.

Combinations of vasoactive drugs are often used to optimize cardiac output and perfusion pressure (Table 2.13).

The ACCS curriculum includes knowledge of vasoactive drugs used in shocked patients (Tables 2.14 and 2.15). The most commonly used inotrope in the ED is adrenaline, because it is the most useful in hypotensive states when the overall haemodynamic status is unclear.

Table 2.14 Actions of inotropic agents

Inotrope	Actions
Adrenaline (epinephrine)	Stimulates α and β receptors.
	At low doses, the β effects predominate—increasing CO and vasodilatation.
	At higher doses, α_1 effects predominate—increasing systemic vascular resistance.
	It also causes splanchnic vasoconstriction, hyperglycaemia ($\uparrow$ glycogenolysis and gluconeogenesis), increases myocardial oxygen consumption, and increases lactate.
Dobutamine	Stimulates β_1 and β_2 receptors.
	β_1 actions increase the heart rate and force of contraction.
	β_2 actions cause peripheral vasodilatation.
	It is useful in low CO states (e.g. post-MI) when vasomotor tone is reasonably maintained. It is frequently used in combination with noradrenaline, which provides the peripheral vasoconstriction to maintain systemic vascular resistance.
Dopamine	Stimulates dopamine, α_1 and β_1 receptors. It also releases noradrenaline from adrenergic nerves.
	At low doses, it acts predominantly on dopamine receptors resulting in increased splanchnic and renal perfusion.
	At higher doses, it acts on α_1 and β_1 receptors leading to vasoconstriction and increased CO.

Table 2.15 Actions of vasopressor agents

Vasopressor	Actions
Noradrenaline (norepinephrine)	Stimulates α_1 receptors.
	Causes peripheral vasoconstriction.
	Excessive use can increase afterload and reduce CO, reduce renal blood flow, reduce splanchnic blood flow, and impair peripheral perfusion.
Phenylephrine	Stimulates α_1 receptors.
	Causes peripheral vasoconstriction.
Metaraminol	Stimulates α_1 receptors.
	Causes peripheral vasoconstriction.
	Can be given peripherally. Often used in cardiovascularly unstable patients during induction of anaesthesia.

KEY POINTS

Shock is an abnormality of the circulatory system, resulting in inadequate tissue perfusion and oxygenation.

Blood pressure = Cardiac output (CO) × Systemic vascular resistance (SVR).

CO = Heart rate × Stroke volume.

Stroke volume is determined by the preload, myocardial contractility, and afterload.

Global oxygen delivery is determined by CO and arterial oxygen content, but perfusion of individual organs depends on many other factors.

Shock can be classified by causes that reduce the CO and causes that reduce the SVR:

- CO reduced—hypovolaemia, cardiogenic, obstructive
- SVR reduced—sepsis, anaphylaxis, neurogenic

Initial compensatory responses can conceal the development of shock. Do not be falsely reassured by a normal heart rate and blood pressure.

Lactate, $ScvO_2$, and urine output are useful adjuncts to the initial clinical assessment and to guide ongoing resuscitation.

Inotropes and vasopressors should not be used as a substitution for adequate fluid resuscitation. In a shocked patient of unknown aetiology, adrenaline is the inotrope of choice.

2.9 SAQs

2.9.1 Tachycardia

A 34-year-old lady attends, having developed palpitations three hours ago while walking the dog. She has never experienced these symptoms before. Figure 2.10 shows her ECG.

a) What is the rhythm on the ECG (Figure 2.10)? (1 mark)
b) What four adverse features should you assess her for according to the Resuscitation Council Guidelines? (2 marks)
c) (i) She has no adverse features and vagal manoeuvres are unsuccessful. What is the recommended first-line drug to try and cardiovert the patient? What is the initial dose of this drug and the two subsequent doses, if this is unsuccessful? (1 mark for drug, 2 marks for doses)
   (ii) List four relative contraindications for the drug in answer c(i). (2 marks)
d) Name two other drugs, and the doses, you might use to try and achieve cardioversion in this patient. (2 marks)

Suggested answer

a) What is the rhythm on the ECG? (1 mark)
   Supraventricular tachycardia or narrow-complex tachycardia
b) What four adverse features should you assess her for according to the Resuscitation Council guidelines? (2 marks)
   Shock
   Syncope
   Myocardial ischaemia
   Heart failure

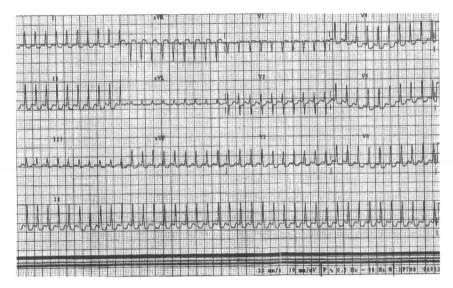

Figure 2.10 Tachycardia in a 34-year-old woman.

c) (i) She has no adverse features and vagal manoeuvres are unsuccessful. What is the
        recommended first-line drug to try and cardiovert the patient? What is the initial dose
        of this drug and the two subsequent doses if this is unsuccessful?
        Adenosine
        Doses: 6 mg, 12 mg, 12 mg
        (1 mark for drug; 1 mark for 6 mg; 1 mark for both 12 mg doses)
   (ii) List four relative contraindications for the drug in answer c (i). (2 marks)
        Asthma
        Heart transplant (denervated heart)
        Sick sinus syndrome
        AF/flutter with accessory pathway or WPW
        Dipyridamole use
        Carbamazepine use
        Theophylline use
        Second- or third-degree heart block

d) Name two other drugs, and the doses, you might try to achieve cardioversion in this
    patient. (2 marks)
    Amiodarone 300 mg IV over 20–60 minutes
    Flecainide 2 mg/kg IV over 10 min or 100–200 mg PO
    Verapamil 5 mg IV over two minutes, repeat after five minutes
    Beta-blockers, for example sotalol 20–60 mg IV or 80–160 mg PO; or metoprolol 5 mg IV
       repeat after five minutes or 50 mg PO.

2.9.2 Cardiac arrest in special circumstances

A 55-year-old man is brought to the ED in cardiac arrest. He was seen to fall through the ice on
a lake and took 10 minutes to be rescued. Figure 2.11 shows his ECG following a ROSC.
(a) List four modifications to the ALS algorithm for patients in a hypothermic cardiac arrest.
     (2 marks)
(b) Name two methods of passive rewarming and two methods of active rewarming. (2 marks)

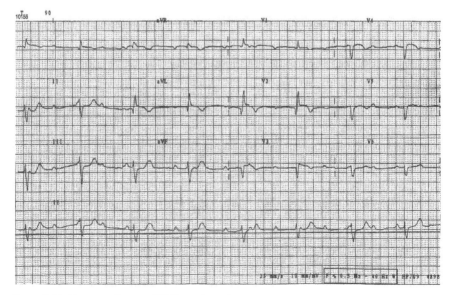

Figure 2.11 Electrocardiogram (ECG) in a hypothermic patient.

(c) He has a ROSC and his temperature is 31°C. What temperature should he be rewarmed too and why? (1 mark for temperature, 1 mark for reason)

(d) (i)   What is the rhythm on his ECG? (1 mark)

    (ii) What are your three main treatment options for managing this arrhythmia in this patient? (3 marks)

Suggested answer

a) List four modifications to the ALS algorithm for patients in a hypothermic cardiac arrest. (2 marks)

Pulse check/look for signs of life for up to one minute.

Consider Doppler/echocardiography to confirm the presence or absence of cardiac output.

Withhold cardioactive drugs until the core temperature is >30°C.

>30°C double the interval between doses of cardioactive drugs (until >35°C).

If VF/VT persists beyond three shocks, postpone further shocks until the temperature is >30°C.

Patients may require large volumes of IV fluids as they rewarm and vasodilate.

Give drugs via a central or large proximal vein if possible.

Monitor glucose regularly due to the risk of hypoglycaemia.

Confirm the temperature with a low-reading thermometer.

Warm the patient actively and passively.

Perform interventions (e.g. CVP insertion or intubation) carefully to avoid excessive movement and precipitating VF.

b) Name two methods of passive rewarming and two methods of active rewarming. (2 marks)

Passive: Remove cold or wet clothing; dry the patient; cover with blankets/hot air blanket; warm room (e.g. overhead heater); forced-air warming system (Bair Hugger).

Active: Warmed humidified oxygen; warmed IV fluids; gastric, peritoneal, pleural, or bladder lavage with warmed fluids; cardiopulmonary bypass.

c) He has a ROSC and his temperature is 31°C. What temperature should he be rewarmed too and why? (1 mark for temperature, 1 mark for reason)

Between 32–34°C. In comatose survivors, a period of therapeutic hypothermia may be beneficial.

d) (i)   What is the rhythm on his ECG? (1 mark)

    Complete (third-degree) heart block.

    (ii) What are your three main treatment options for managing this arrhythmia in this patient? (3 marks)

    Rewarm the patient—most arrhythmias revert spontaneously with rewarming.

    Drugs—atropine 500 mcg IV boluses, to a total of 3 mg (only if rewarming fails) (adrenaline IV if atropine fails and pacing is delayed).

    Pacing—only indicated if the bradyarrhythmia persists after rewarming.

Further reading

National Institute for Health and Care Excellence, December 2011. NICE clinical guideline 134. Anaphylaxis: assessment and referral after emergency treatment. Available at: https://www.nice.org.uk/guidance/CG134 [Online].

Resuscitation Council (UK), 2015. Resuscitation Guidelines. Available at: https://www.resus.org.uk [Online].

CHAPTER 3

Anaesthetics and pain management

CONTENTS

3.1 Emergency airway care

3.1.1 Introduction

Effective airway management is a key skill of an emergency physician. Good airway care is paramount in the care of critically ill and injured patients. The theoretical aspects of acute airway assessment and management are likely to feature in the Intermediate FRCEM examination.

3.1.2 Indications for intubation

The decision to intubate or not is often the first key decision in the management of a critically ill patient. This does not detract from the need to provide supplemental oxygen and good basic airway management.

The advantages of intubation include:

- A secured airway protected from obstruction by swelling, blood, or vomit.
- Lungs protected from aspiration.
- Optimized oxygenation.
- Improved ventilation, which can assist in the correction of respiratory or metabolic acidosis.
- Removal of the work of breathing, reducing metabolic demands.
- Safe sedation of the patient without the risk of respiratory compromise.
- Minimization of the risk of gastric insufflation.
- Ventilation without interrupting chest compressions in cardiac arrest.

The risks of intubation include:

- Failed intubation.
- Inability to intubate or ventilate the patient following induction of anaesthesia.
- Misplaced endotracheal tube. This may be during the intubation itself or subsequently dislodged. This is catastrophic if not identified.
- Cardiovascular instability following the use of induction agents.
- Raised intracranial pressure.
- Precipitating laryngospasm.

- Trauma to the lips, teeth, oropharynx, larynx, and trachea.
- Interruptions to chest compressions while intubating in cardiac arrest.

There are four main situations when intubation may be indicated:

- Apnoeic patient in respiratory arrest.
- Patient with a partially or completely obstructed airway, where basic airway management is ineffective (e.g. burns, facial trauma, actively vomiting, or bleeding).
- Patient requiring invasive respiratory support for oxygenation or ventilatory failure (e.g. severe pneumonia, chest trauma, overdose).
- Patient whose predicted clinical course includes a high probability of airway obstruction, aspiration, or ventilatory failure (e.g. epiglottis, early burns); or, a patient requiring transport where airway management will be difficult (e.g. CT scanner, ambulance transfer).

The urgency of the intubation may vary depend on the clinical situation:

- Immediate intubation—patient is deteriorating rapidly and definitive airway care is required with a minimum of delay (e.g. a hypoxic patient with partial airway obstruction secondary to burns).
- Urgent intubation—basic techniques are maintaining adequate oxygenation and ventilation at present but will only do so for a short time (e.g. a head-injured patient with a Glasgow coma scale (GCS) <8 whose airway obstruction can be relieved with a jaw thrust).

Intubation is indicated when the risks of continuing basic airway support are greater than the risks of intubation. The difficulty of intubation must be factored into the decision, and a patient with an anticipated 'difficult airway' may need to be postponed (if possible) until more senior help arrives and a difficult airway cart is available.

Reversible causes

In some patients there may be reversible causes for airway obstruction, respiratory compromise, or reduced conscious level. If a reversible cause is identified, it should be treated, which may negate the need for intubation (Table 3.1).

Table 3.1 Potential reversible causes of airway obstruction, respiratory failure, and reduced conscious level

Reversible cause	Treatment
Opiate overdose	Naloxone
Hypoglycaemia	10% or 50% glucose
Seizures	Benzodiazepines, phenytoin
Hypercapnia (e.g. in COPD)	Reduce inspired oxygen concentration ± non-invasive ventilation
Hypovolaemia	IV fluids, inotropes
Arrhythmia	Electrical cardioversion
Anaphylaxis	IM adrenaline
Asthma	Nebulizers (salbutamol, ipratropium bromide), magnesium, aminophylline, steroids
Heart failure	Diuretics, nitrates, non-invasive ventilation
Agitation (with impaired conscious level)	Analgesia, if in pain
	IV fluids if hypotensive
	Glucose if hypoglycaemic
	Ensure bladder empty

KEY POINTS

Intubation is always preceded by basic airway management and oxygenation.

Intubation is indicated when the risks of continuing basic airway support are greater than the risks of intubation.

The four main indications for intubation are:

- Apnoeic patient in respiratory arrest
- Patient with a partially or completely obstructed airway, where basic airway management is ineffective
- Patient requiring invasive respiratory support for oxygenation or ventilatory failure
- Patient whose predicted clinical course includes a high probability of airway obstruction, aspiration, or ventilatory failure

Reversible causes for airway obstruction, respiratory compromise, and reduced conscious level should be considered and treated, which may negate the need for intubation.

3.2 Identifying the difficult airway

Difficulties with the airway should be expected in all emergency patients. Patients requiring intubation in the ED are a different cohort to those patients undergoing elective intubation and the risks are greater. ED patients may have deranged physiology, poor cardiorespiratory reserve, and an unstable cervical spine.

Airway difficulties are more than just difficulties intubating and can be categorized according to the different components of airway management:

- Difficult basic airway manoeuvres; for example, neck immobility limiting the ability to perform a head tilt; facial fractures limiting a jaw thrust; trismus preventing insertion of an oropharyngeal airway; and nasal deformity preventing insertion of a nasopharyngeal airway.
- Difficult mask ventilation—gaining an adequate seal with a facemask may be prevented by facial hair, lack of teeth, cachexia, obesity, or trauma. Ventilation may be difficult in those with diaphragmatic splinting, abdominal distension, or increased airway resistance (e.g. asthma).
- Difficult laryngoscopy—classified by Cormack and Lehane (Figure 3.1). In grade 3 and 4 views, the vocal cords are not visible and intubation may be impossible without specialist equipment.

  - Grade 1—the vocal cords are visible
  - Grade 2—the vocal cords are only partially visible
  - Grade 3—only the epiglottis is seen
  - Grade 4—the epiglottis is not visible*

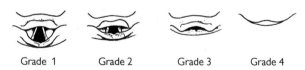

Grade 1   Grade 2   Grade 3   Grade 4

Figure 3.1 Cormack and Lehane classification of glottic visualization.

Reproduced with permission from R. S. Cormack, J. Lehane, Difficult tracheal intubation in obstetrics, *Anaesthesia*, Volume 39, Issue 11, pp.1105–11, Copyright © 2007 John Wiley and Sons. Reproduced from Keith Allman and Iain Wilson, *Oxford Handbook of Anaesthesia*, 2011, Figure 37.1, p. 867, with permission from Oxford University Press (2016).

---

* Reproduced with permission from R. S. Cormack, J. Lehane, Difficult tracheal intubation in obstetrics, *Anaesthesia*, Volume 39, Issue 11, pp.1105–11, Copyright © 2007 John Wiley and Sons.

- Difficult intubation—defined as occurring when an experienced laryngoscopist, using direct laryngoscopy, requires more than two attempts with the same blade; or a change of blade; or an adjunct (bougie); or an alternative device.
- Difficult cricothyroidotomy—an assessment of the patient's neck should be made prior to induction of anaesthesia to determine how difficult a surgical airway would be to perform if required.

3.2.1 Airway assessment

There are several tests described to predict difficult intubation. Unfortunately the sensitivity and specificity of them is fairly poor. A patient may have a positive test and not have a difficult airway, and, conversely, a patient with a negative test may have difficulties. However, they do provide a guide to identifying those with a potentially difficult airway and knowledge of such tests is included in the curriculum.

To help remember predictors of a difficult airway there are several different mnemonics. It is not essential to use a mnemonic but some candidates find it useful. A commonly used mnemonic is LEMON (Table 3.2).

Table 3.2 LEMON assessment of airway

Look— for characteristics that are known to cause difficult intubation or ventilation	• Obesity • Facial trauma • Excessive facial hair • Facial deformity • Sunken cheeks • Edentulous • Prominent upper incisors • High arched palate • Receding mandible • Short neck • Thick neck circumference (> 45 cm) • Narrow mouth • Macroglossia • Prognathia (inability to move lower teeth in front of upper teeth) • History of snoring (obstructive sleep apnoea)
Evaluate—mouth opening and thyromental distance (the 3–3–2 rule)	• 3 fingers breadth between incisors • 3 fingers between hyoid bone and the chin • 2 fingers between thyroid notch and floor of the mouth
Mallampati score (Figure 3.2)—used to assess how much of the hypopharynx is visible with the patient sitting, mouth fully open, and tongue protruding	• Class 1—faucial pillars, soft palate, and uvula visible • Class 2—faucial pillars and soft palate visible; tip of uvula masked by base of tongue • Class 3—only soft palate visible • Class 4—soft palate not visible
Obstruction—pathology within or surrounding the upper airway	• Peri-tonsillar abscess • Epiglottis • Retro-pharyngeal abscess • Trauma • Burns • Tumour

Table 3.2 Continued

Neck mobility—assessed by asking the patient to place their chin on their chest and extend their neck to look to the ceiling	• In-line stabilization • Rheumatoid arthritis • Osteoarthritis • Ankylosing spondylitis • Previous neck injuries or surgery • Neck extension undesirable: unstable cervical spine fracture; severe cervical stenosis; vertebral artery insufficiency; Chiari malformation

Reproduced from *Canadian Anaesthetists' Society Journal*, Clinical sign to predict difficult tracheal intubation (hypothesis), volume 30, issue 3, May 1983, pp. 316–17, S. Rao Mallampati, With permission of Springer.

3.2.2 Pre-anaesthetic assessment

In most emergency situations there is time to perform a pre-anaesthetic assessment. This is a more focused assessment than that used in elective anaesthesia and forms an important part of the preparation for rapid sequence induction.

The pre-anaesthetic assessment should include a relevant history and examination (Table 3.3).

KEY POINTS

Airway difficulties may be encountered during basic airway manoeuvres, bag-valve-mask ventilation, laryngoscopy, intubation, and/or cricothyroidotomy.

The LEMON mnemonic can be used to assess the airway and identify those with potential difficulties:

• **L**ook—for characteristics that are known to cause difficult intubation or ventilation.

• **E**valuate—mouth opening and thyromental distance (the 3–3–2 rule).

• **M**allampati—grades 1–4.

• **O**bstruction—is there evidence of pathology within or surrounding the upper airway.

• **N**eck mobility.

A pre-anaesthetic assessment should be performed, focusing on the relevant history and examination.

Adapted from *Canadian Anaesthetists' Society Journal*, Clinical sign to predict difficult tracheal intubation (hypothesis), volume 30, issue 3, May 1983, pp. 316–17, S. Rao Mallampati, With permission of Springer.

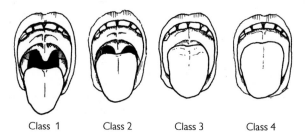

Class 1   Class 2   Class 3   Class 4

Figure 3.2 Mallampati test (Samsoon and Young modification).

Reproduced with permission from G.L.T Samsoon and J.R.B. Young, 'Difficult tracheal intubation: a retrospective study', Anaesthesia, 42, 5, pp. 487–490, Copyright Wiley, 1987.

Reproduced from *Canadian Anaesthetists' Society Journal*, Clinical sign to predict difficult tracheal intubation (hypothesis), volume 30, issue 3, May 1983, pp. 316–17, S. Rao Mallampati, With permission of Springer.

Table 3.3 Emergency pre-anaesthetic assessment

History	Examination
• History of events and current condition • Past medical and surgical history • Current medications • Allergies • Previous anaesthetics and any complications • Last oral intake	• Cardiorespiratory status • Assessment of face and neck • Assessment for pneumothorax • GCS • Focal neurological signs • Evidence of pathology in the chest, abdomen, and pelvis

3.3 Emergency airway drugs

Anaesthesia requires three components—'the triad of anaesthesia':

• Hypnosis
• Analgesia
• Muscle relaxation

3.3.1 Induction agents (hypnosis)

There are four main induction agents used in emergency rapid sequence induction (RSI) in the United Kingdom (Table 3.4). All of the agents have limitations and the drug used depends on the condition of the patient and the familiarity of the practitioner with the drug.

3.3.2 Muscle relaxation

Muscle relaxation is usually achieved with suxamethonium. However, occasionally a non-depolarizing agent, such as rocuronium, may be used.

Suxamethonium

Suxamethonium is a depolarizing muscle relaxant and the only one in clinical use today. Its rapid onset and short duration of action make it the drug of choice for muscle relaxation in emergency RSI (Table 3.5).

Non-depolarizing muscle relaxants

Occasionally a non-depolarizing muscle relaxant may be used instead of suxamethonium (e.g. if suxamethonium is contraindicated) (Table 3.6). Of the non-depolarizing muscle relaxants, rocuronium is the agent most likely to be used for a modified RSI. Other non-depolarizing muscle relaxants may be used for maintenance of paralysis following recovery from suxamethonium.

One of the main concerns about using a non-depolarizing muscle relaxant is the prolonged duration of action compared to suxamethonium. The short duration of suxamethonium is advantageous if a difficult airway is encountered and intubation and/or ventilation are not possible. However, in 2008, a reversal agent for rocuronium was licensed, sugammadex—the first selective relaxant binding agent. This has resulted in rocuronium being a much more feasible first-line agent for RSI. Reversal of non-depolarizing muscle relaxants prior to the introduction of sugammadex was with neostigmine, an anticholinesterase. Neostigmine is still in use but causes autonomic instability and bradycardia, so has to be given concurrently with an anti-muscarinic (e.g. atropine or glycopyrronium bromide). Sugammadex is associated with much greater cardiovascular and autonomic stability, and therefore is better suited to cardiovascularly compromised patients in the ED.

Table 3.4 Induction agents used in emergency RSI

	Indications	Dose	Onset/Recovery	Physiological effects
Thiopental	Most useful in cardiovascularly stable patients with an isolated head injury or seizures.	4–5 mg/kg IV (1.5–2 mg/kg if cardiovascularly unstable)	Onset: 5–15 s Recovery: 5–15 min	Cerebroprotective: • Decreases cerebral metabolic oxygen consumption. • Decreases cerebral blood flow. • Decreases intracranial pressure (ICP). • Maintains cerebral perfusion pressure. • Anticonvulsant properties. • Cardiovascular depression: • Venodilatation. • Myocardial depression.
Propofol	Most commonly used induction agent in elective anaesthesia. Can be used for maintenance of anaesthesia. Used for procedural sedation.	1.5–2.5 mg/kg IV	Onset: 20–40 s Recovery: 5–10 min	Marked hypotension in patients with cardiovascular compromise (due to vasodilatation and myocardial depression). Apnoea. Pain on injection. Anticonvulsant properties (although patient may have some involuntary movements on induction).
Etomidate	Useful in haemodynamically compromised patients.	0.3 mg/kg IV	Onset: 5–15 s Recovery: 5–15 min	Relative haemodynamic stability. Adrenocortical suppression. Attenuates increase in ICP on laryngoscopy. Reduces cerebral blood flow. Reduces cerebral oxygen demand.
Ketamine	Severe bronchospasm. Cardiovascularly unstable patients. Burns.	1–2 mg/kg IV 5–10 mg/kg IM	Onset: 15–30 s (IV) Recovery: 15–30 min	Analgesia. Sedation. Dissociative state. Amnesia. Sympathetic stimulation: ↑HR, ↑BP. Bronchodilation. Enhanced laryngeal reflexes (potential for laryngospasm). Increased respiratory secretions. Emergence phenomena.

Table 3.5 Summary of the properties of suxamethonium

Indication	Muscle paralysis for RSI
Dose	1–2 mg/kg IV
Induction characteristics and recovery	5–15 s: fasciculations
	45–60 s: paralysis
	3–5 min: first return of respiratory activity
	5–10 minutes: return of effective spontaneous ventilation
Physiological effects	Depolarizing muscle paralysis
	Metabolized by pseudocholinesterase
Adverse effects	• Hyperkalaemia (plasma concentration increased by up to 0.5 mmol/L)
	• Bradycardia (children are at the greatest risk)
	• Fasiculations resulting in muscle pain
	• Histamine release causing potential anaphylaxis
	• Malignant hyperthermia
	• Suxamethonium apnoea (patient has low or abnormal pseudocholinesterase activity and paralysis may last for several hours)
Contraindications	Hyperkalaemia—known blood result or ECG suggestive Risk of hyperkalaemia:
	• Severe trauma or infection
	• Desquamating skin conditions
	• Burns (risk greatest after 2 days)
	• Peripheral neuropathy (risk greatest after 5 days)
	• Spinal cord injury (risk greatest after 5 days)
	• Upper motor neurone lesions or structural brain disease
	• Muscular dystrophy

EXAM TIP

It is easy to become overwhelmed by the pharmacology of anaesthetic drugs. It is important to know the general pros and cons of the induction agents and muscles relaxants used in the resuscitation room. However, the exam is not an anaesthetic exam. In-depth pharmacological questions or knowledge of doses are unlikely to be asked and, if they were, they would only be worth 1 or 2 marks.

Table 3.6 Non-depolarizing muscle relaxants

	Dose	Onset/Duration	Metabolism
Rocuronium	Loading dose 0.6–1 mg/kg	Onset 60 s	Hepatic/renal
	Maintenance 0.1–0.5 mg/kg/h	Duration 30–60 min	
Atracurium	Loading dose 0.3–0.5 mg/kg	Onset 3–5 min	Hoffman elimination
	Maintenance 5–10 mcg/kg/min	Duration 20–35 min	
Vecuronium	Loading dose 0.05–0.1 mg/kg	Onset 3–5 min	Hepatic/biliary
	Maintenance 1–2 mcg/kg/min	Duration 20–35 min	

3.3.3 Analgesia in rapid sequence induction

Analgesia is part of the 'triad of anaesthesia' but is not part of the classic RSI technique. However, some practitioners will use opiates to attenuate the cardiovascular response to laryngoscopy and intubation. This is particularly advantageous in patients with raised intracranial pressure (ICP), severe hypertension, or ischaemic heart disease.

The commonly used opiates with RSI are fentanyl or alfentanil. They have a faster onset of action than morphine (alfentanil 1 minute; fentanyl 3 minutes; morphine 5 minutes). However, opiates cause respiratory depression, which may persist beyond the recovery from neuromuscular blockade, requiring reversal with naloxone, if intubation fails.

Analgesics are discussed in more detail in section 3.6.

3.3.4 Maintenance of anaesthesia

Following successful intubation, anaesthesia must be maintained. The commonly used infusions for this are propofol or midazolam and morphine. In the ED, paralysis is usually maintained with a non-depolarizing muscle relaxant.

3.3.5 Complications of anaesthetic drugs

There are a few well-recognized complications of anaesthetic drugs, which could appear in a short-answer question (SAQ).

- Malignant hyperthermia—is a rare autosomal dominant condition related to general anaesthesia (e.g. suxamethonium or gaseous agents). It results in uncontrolled skeletal muscle oxidative metabolism. Masseter muscle spasm may be an early sign of malignant hyperthermia, later effects include rhabdomyolysis, tachyarrhythmias, and pyrexia. Treatment involves stopping the precipitant, supportive management, and dantrolene.
- Suxamethonium apnoea—occurs when the patient has low or abnormal pseudocholinesterase activity. Muscle paralysis may last for several hours after a dose of suxamethonium. Treatment is continued ventilation and sedation until normal neuromuscular activity returns.
- Anaphylaxis—may occur with any anaesthetic agent. Management should be as per advanced life support (ALS) guidance detailed in Chapter 2, section 2.3.

KEY POINTS

Anaesthesia requires three components—'the triad of anaesthesia': hypnosis, analgesia, and muscle relaxation.

RSI involves giving an anaesthetic induction agent to achieve hypnosis, rapidly followed by a muscle relaxant to produce complete paralysis.

The four main induction agents used in emergency RSI in the United Kingdom are thiopental, propofol, etomidate, and ketamine.

Muscle relaxation is usually achieved with suxamethonium. However, occasionally a non-depolarizing agent, such as rocuronium, may be used.

3.4 Rapid sequence induction

RSI involves giving an anaesthetic induction agent to achieve hypnosis, rapidly followed by a muscle relaxant to produce complete paralysis. The drugs are given in quick succession to minimize time from loss of consciousness to intubation because the stomach is assumed to be full. Cricoid pressure is applied as the induction agent is given, to protect the airway from gastric regurgitation. To prevent inflation of the stomach, the lungs are not usually ventilated between induction and intubation.

3.4.1 Preparation for a rapid sequence induction

Prior to performing an RSI, preparations must be made to maximize the chance of success. Intubation rarely has to be achieved so urgently that basic preparatory steps cannot be taken (Table 3.7 and Figure 3.3).

Table 3.7 Preparation for RSI

Monitoring The minimum recommended standards are defined by The Association of Anaesthetists of Great Britain and Ireland.	• Inspired oxygen concentration (FiO_2). • Capnography. • Pulse oximetry. • Non-invasive blood pressure. • 3-lead ECG.
Equipment The airway equipment in the resuscitation room should be checked daily. The practitioner performing the RSI should prepare and check the equipment prior to induction.	Basic airway equipment: • Oxygen. • Oxygen masks and tubing. • Tilting trolley. • Suction. • Airway adjuncts (nasopharyngeal and oropharyngeal). • IV access. • Monitoring. Advance airway equipment: • System to pre-oxygenate the patient and provide ventilation (e.g. bag-valve-mask or Mapleson C anaesthetic circuit/ Waters circuit). • Laryngoscope handles and blades (usually a size 3 and 4 Macintosh). • Magill's forceps. • Intubating stylet and bougie. • Tracheal tubes in a range of sizes (women, 7–7.5 mm; men, 8 mm); tubes should be uncut if there is a risk of facial swelling (e.g. burns). • 20-ml syringe to inflate the cuff and lubricating gel for the tracheal tube. • Tie and/or adhesive tape. • Ventilator. • Drugs (labelled). Failed intubation equipment: • Supraglottic airway device (e.g. laryngeal mask airway sizes 3, 4, and 5). • Surgical cricothyroidotomy set. • Needle cricothyroidotomy set.
Positioning Alignment of the oral, pharyngeal, and laryngeal axes during laryngoscopy provides the best view of the laryngeal inlet.	'Sniffing the morning air' (neck flexed on the torso and head extended on the neck) is the best position in an adult. This position can be achieved by placing a pillow under the patient's head (flexes the neck) and then extending the patient's head. In obese patients, standard neck positioning may flex the head forwards forcing the chin onto the chest. The key to correct positioning in such a patient is to make sure the chin is higher than the highest point on the chest or abdomen (i.e. place a pillow under the shoulders and further pillows under the head to raise it further). If a cervical spine injury is suspected the neck must be maintained in a neutral position. In this situation manipulation of the larynx may improve the view, for example the 'BURP' manoeuvre (backwards, upwards, rightwards laryngeal pressure).

Table 3.7 Continued

Checks Prior to RSI a few final checks should be made to ensure the patient is optimized.	Briefly review the history to obtain relevant clinical information. The AMPLE mnemonic is a useful reminder for this: ● Allergies. ● Medications. ● Past medical history (including previous anaesthetics). ● Last ate/drank. ● Events. *Resuscitation*—ensure the patient is optimized as best as possible. *Final examination*—if time allows record the patients GCS, note any focal neurological signs, assess the abdomen, pelvis, and long bones for any evidence of pathology. *IV access*—ensure there are two functioning IV lines.
Staffing A RSI requires at least 3–4 practitioners to perform safely.	The roles required in a RSI include: ● An airway practitioner. ● An assistant to the airway practitioner who has knowledge of the equipment, techniques, and failed intubation drill. ● Cricoid pressure (this may be the airway assistant). ● Drug delivery (induction agent, muscle relaxant, and fluids/inotropes if required). ● Manual in-line stabilization, if a cervical spine injury is suspected. ● A practitioner to maintain responsibility for overall care of the patient. An appropriately experienced airway practitioner should also be available in case expert help is required.

3.4.2 Performing the rapid sequence induction

The skill of performing a RSI is most likely to be tested in the part C examination. The following section summaries the main stages of a rapid sequence induction.

Pre-oxygenation

The purpose of pre-oxygenation is to maximize the time before desaturation occurs, following the onset of apnoea. Effective pre-oxygenation replaces nitrogen in the alveoli with oxygen, which increase the oxygen reserve in the lungs. Ideally 100% oxygen should be given for three minutes before induction of anaesthesia.

In a breathing patient, this is best delivered via a Mapleson C or Waters circuit. A bag-valve-mask with a good seal can also be used, but the resistance to inspiratory and expiratory flow is high, making it less than ideal.

If the patient is agitated and will not tolerate oxygenation via a bag-valve-mask or Mapleson C circuit, an oxygen mask with a non-rebreathing bag can be used, at flow rates of 15 L, with a well-fitting mask—this provides approximately 90% inspired oxygen concentration.

If the patient is not spontaneously breathing, or breathing inadequately, then assisted ventilation will be required to achieve pre-oxygenation. The time to desaturation is related to the effectiveness of the pre-oxygenation and also the age, weight, and physiological status of the patient. In a healthy adult, the time taken to desaturate to 90% may be up to eight minutes. In a critically ill patient, this time is significantly reduced. Due to the shape of the oxyhaemoglobin dissociation curve (Figure 3.4), once the saturations reach 92%, the rate of desaturation accelerates. Therefore, when saturations of 92% are reached, corrective action is required, and the patient should be reoxygenated immediately.

Planning for intubation   Assessing
                                                                               urgency

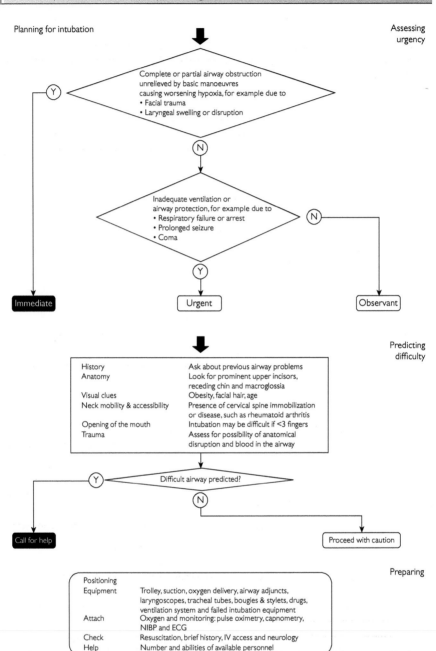

Figure 3.3 Patient assessment and preparation for intubation.
Reproduced with permission from Jonathan Benger, Jerry Nolan, Mike Clancy (eds), *Emergency Airway Management*
2009. © College of Emergency Medicine, London, published by Cambridge University Press.

Drugs

The induction agent and muscle relaxant are given in quick succession in pre-calculated doses. The choice of agents depends on the clinical status of the patient. The emergency airway drugs that are commonly used are discussed in section 3.3.

Cricoid pressure

Cricoid pressure is applied as the induction agent is given. The aim is to compress the upper oesophagus between the cricoid and the cervical vertebrae posteriorly. Cricoid pressure aims to stop passive regurgitation of gastric contents but should not be applied during active vomiting because of the risk of oesophageal rupture.

Technique of cricoid pressure:

- The cricoid is located below the thyroid cartilage and cricothyroid membrane.
- The cricoid ring is stabilized between the thumb and index finger.
- Firm pressure is applied directly backwards as the induction agent is given and consciousness lost.
- The correct pressure is 30–40 Newtons.
- Cricoid pressure is removed only on the instruction of the intubating clinician, once correct tube placement has been confirmed.

Laryngoscopy and intubation

The technique of laryngoscopy is best learnt as a practical skill and details of the technique are unlikely to be asked in an SAQ.

In order to gain the best view at laryngoscopy, the following techniques may be required:

- Suction.
- Adjustment of the cricoid pressure and/or the BURP manoeuvre (backwards, upwards, rightwards laryngeal pressure) may be required.
- Good laryngoscopy technique—clear identification of the epiglottis and insertion of the tip of the laryngoscope into the vallecula, followed by elevation of the laryngoscope in the line of the handle to bring the laryngeal inlet into view.
- Different laryngoscope—if the blade is too short the view can be poor, so generally a size 4 Macintosh is used from the start. If the practitioner is practised with alternative blades (e.g. McCoy blade or straight blade), these may be tried.

In order to increase the likelihood of successful intubation the following techniques can be used:

- Intubating stylet—used to stiffen and pre-shape the tracheal tube. The stylet should never protrude beyond the distal end of tracheal tube and should be withdrawn after the tip of the tube has passed through the vocal cords. This technique minimizes the risk of damaging the trachea.
- Intubating bougie—may be used routinely or in those with poor views (grade 3 or a difficult grade 2). The bougie is bent at one end (shaped like a hockey stick) to enable it to be passed behind the epiglottis and into the trachea. Confirmation of passage of the bougie into the trachea is provided by the detection of clicks as the bougie slides over the tracheal rings and hold-up of the bougie in the distal airways. Once the bougie is within the trachea, the tracheal tube is railroaded over the bougie with the help of an assistant, who stabilizes the bougie at the top end. The tracheal tube is then advanced into the trachea under direct vision and the bougie removed.

Confirmation of tube placement

Carbon dioxide detection is the gold standard for confirming tracheal tube placement. Ideally this should be by continual waveform monitoring of end tidal CO_2. If this is not immediately available, a disposable colourimetric CO_2 detector can be used.

Additional checks of tube placement include inspection and auscultation of the chest to confirm bilateral air entry.

Once tube position is confirmed, cricoid pressure can be removed and the tube secured. In a patient with raised ICP, adhesive tape is better than a tie to avoid impairing venous drainage and increasing intracranial pressure further. The position of the tube at the teeth should be noted for future reference (usually 22–24 cm for a woman and 24–26 cm for a man). An oropharyngeal airway can be used as a 'bite block'.

3.4.3 Failed airway management

Failure to place a tracheal tube correctly after an RSI is not a disaster, but failure to recognize an incorrectly placed tube, or persistent attempts to secure an airway resulting in patient harm, is. The old adage 'if in doubt, take it out' should be followed. The most important factor is to continue oxygenation of the patient (see Figure 3.5).

If the first attempt at intubation fails, there are a series of fundamental questions that should be asked to determine the most appropriate course of action (Table 3.8):

- Is the patient's arterial blood oxygenated enough to enable further attempts at intubation safely? If not, can it be improved?
- Were the intubating conditions ideal?

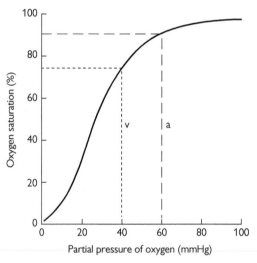

Figure 3.4 The haemoglobin–oxygen dissociation curve. (a) Partial pressure of oxygen of 8 kPa (60 mmHg), which is the definition of arterial hypoxia. (v) partial pressure of oxygen of 5.3 kPa (40 mmHg), which is typical of mixed venous blood. Note that once the PaO_2 falls below 8 kPa, small further falls dramatically decrease the arterial oxygen saturation.

Reproduced with permission from Chr. Bohr, K. Hasselbalch, August Krogh, Ueber einen in biologischer Beziehung wichtigen Einfluss, den die Kohlensäurespannung des Blutes auf dessen Sauerstoffbindung übt1, *Acta Physiologica*, Volume 16, pp.104–412, Copyright © 1904 John Wiley and Sons.

Reproduced from David A. Warrell, Timothy M. Cox, and John D. Firth, *Oxford Textbook of Medicine*, 2010, Figure 18.5.1, p. 3568, with permission from Oxford University Press.

Table 3.8 Treatment options in failed intubation

Reoxygenation	Bag-valve-mask ventilation with 100% oxygen.
	Use two-person technique and airway adjuncts to achieve the best seal possible.
	If this fails, the first rescue technique is a supraglottic airway device.
Improve intubating conditions	Ensure full muscle relaxation has occurred, otherwise jaw tone, gagging, and laryngeal spasm may prevent intubation.
Improve laryngeal view	Improve positioning ('sniffing the morning air'), with maximal head extension and maximal jaw thrust.
	Suction.
	External manipulation of larynx (BURP).
	Use an alternative laryngoscope blade (if appropriately skilled).
	Change practitioner.
Improve intubating technique	Intubating stylet.
	Intubating bougie.
Alternative techniques	Supraglottic airway device: classic or intubating laryngeal mask airway; i-gel
	Specialist techniques (e.g. fibreoptic laryngoscope, light-wand techniques, intubating supraglottic airway device, and so on).
Surgical airway	Surgical cricothyroidotomy.
	Needle cricothyroidotomy.

- Can the laryngeal view be improved?
- Can the intubation technique be improved?
- Should further attempts fail, are there suitable alternatives?
- Should further attempts fail, is a surgical airway necessary and possible?

There are no absolute rules for the length of time intubation can be attempted. The oxygen reserves are individual to each patient and depend upon the patient's age, weight, and physiological state. When the oxygen saturations reach 92%, intubation attempts should be stopped and the patient reoxygenated. Below 92% the oxyhaemoglobin curve falls steeply.

Supraglottic airway device

Supraglottic airway devices are used widely in emergency airway management. They are the recommend first-line airway device in cardiac arrest patients and are the recommended rescue device in the anaesthetic 'can't intubate, can't ventilate' situation. Examples include the laryngeal mask airway (LMA), the pro-seal LMA, and the i-gel.

The advantages of supraglottic airway devices include:

- Easy to insert with a high success rate after a short period of training.
- More effective ventilation and less gastric inflation than with a bag-valve-mask.
- A degree of protection from aspiration of gastric contents. A correctly placed device sits in the oesophagus and protects the glottic opening.
- Ability to insert into a spontaneously ventilating patient (provided they have an appropriately reduced level of consciousness).

The disadvantages of supraglottic airway devices include:

- Risk of hypoventilation due to leak around the cuff when airway pressures are high.
- Greater gastric inflation than a correctly placed cuffed tracheal tube.
- Theoretical risk of aspiration of gastric contents.
- Airway obstruction by folding the epiglottis down to cover the laryngeal inlet.
- Risk of inducing laryngospasm (in a non-paralysed patient).

Surgical airway

The commonest error when performing a surgical airway is performing the procedure too late. If a surgical airway is indicated, it must be performed rapidly and effectively to minimize hypoxic damage.

The choice between a needle cricothyroidotomy and a surgical cricothyroidotomy depends on the available equipment and the skills of the practitioner (Table 3.9). In the case of 'can't intubate can't ventilate', the Difficult Airway Society now recommend the use of surgical cricothroidotomy over needle cricothyroidotomy.

Needle cricothyroidotomy

A wide-bore, non-kinking cannula is inserted through the cricothyroid membrane. The technique enables oxygenation but not ventilation. A high-pressure oxygen source is required to deliver the oxygen, which may cause barotrauma. The technique is a temporizing measure (i.e. 30–45 minutes) until a more formal airway intervention is performed.

Technique:

- A stiff cannula (minimum 14 gauge) is attached to a syringe and inserted through the cricothyroid membrane into the airway at an angle of 45°, aiming caudally in the midline.
- Aspiration of air from the cannula confirms its position in the trachea. The cannula is then advanced over the needle into the trachea. The needle is removed and air aspirated again to reconfirm position.

Table 3.9 Advantages and disadvantages of different surgical airway techniques

Needle Cricothyroidotomy	
Advantages	Disadvantages
<ul><li>Quick</li><li>Easy</li><li>Enables oxygenation</li></ul>	<ul><li>Does not provide ventilation</li><li>Temporary measure (30–45 min)</li><li>Definitive airway still required</li><li>Risk of barotrauma</li><li>Risk of kinking of the cannula</li></ul>
Surgical cricothyroidotomy	
Advantages	Disadvantages
<ul><li>Definitive airway</li><li>Enables oxygenation and ventilation</li><li>Enables suctioning of the trachea</li></ul>	<ul><li>Trauma to the surrounding structures (e.g. thyroid, blood vessels, posterior wall of trachea)</li><li>Risk of creating a false passage in the soft tissues or oesophagus</li><li>Technically more difficult than a needle cricothyroidotomy</li></ul>

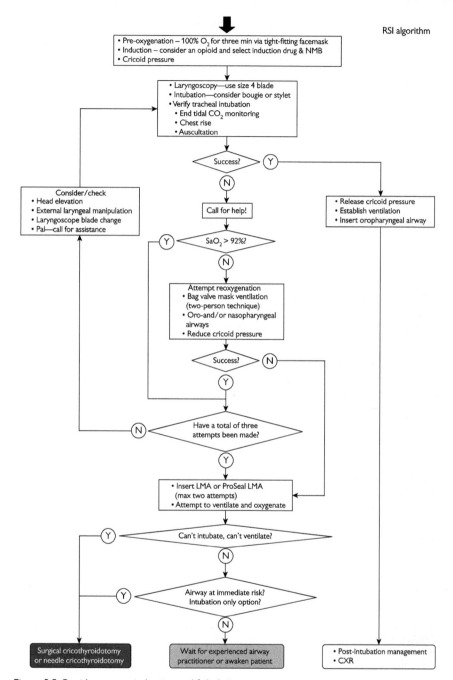

RSI algorithm

Figure 3.5 Rapid sequence induction and failed airway management.

Reproduced with permission from Jonathan Benger, Jerry Nolan, Mike Clancy (eds), *Emergency Airway Management 2009*. © College of Emergency Medicine, London, published by Cambridge University Press.

- An oxygen supply at a pressure of 400 kPa is required (wall oxygen is appropriate), at a flow rate of 15 L/minute. The oxygen is connected to the cannula via oxygen tubing with a Y-connector or side hole cut in the tubing. Intermittent insufflation is provided in the cycle, one second on and four seconds off.
- To minimize barotrauma, evidence of exhalation via the upper airway should be looked for during the four-second 'off period'.

Surgical cricothyroidotomy

This provides a definitive airway that can be used to oxygenate and ventilate the patient. The technique is more difficult than a needle cricothyroidotomy and the risk of damaging adjacent structures is greater (e.g. thyroid, posterior wall of the trachea, overlying blood vessels).

The technique:

- A horizontal stab incision is made through the cricothyroid membrane into the trachea.
- The incision is opened with tracheal dilators. Once a passage is made into the trachea, it should be occupied by an instrument until a tube is inserted to minimize the chance of losing the passage.
- A small endotracheal tube (e.g. 6 mm) or tracheostomy tube is inserted and the cuff inflated.
- Tube position is confirmed by capnography, plus observation, and auscultation of the chest.

KEY POINTS

Prior to performing an RSI, preparations must be made to maximize the chance of success. Intubation rarely has to be achieved so urgently that basic preparatory steps cannot be taken. Preparation for an RSI includes:

- Monitoring
- Equipment
- Checking the patient (resuscitation, brief history and examination, IV access)
- Positioning of the patient
- Having the correct personnel

The stages of RSI are:

- Preparation
- Pre-oxygenation
- Drugs (induction agent and muscle relaxant)
- Cricoid pressure (applied as the induction agent is given and consciousness lost)
- Laryngoscopy and tracheal intubation
- Confirmation of tube placement (capnography)
- Removal of cricoid pressure
- Tube secured and ventilation established
- Patient reassessed

The first attempt at intubation should be the best attempt.

If the first attempt at intubation is unsuccessful, the most important thing is to ensure adequate oxygenation of the patient.

If the oxygen saturations are greater than 92%, a further attempt at intubation may be attempted. If the saturations are below 92%, then reoxygenation is required.

A supraglottic airway device is the first-line rescue technique.

If oxygenation cannot be maintained a surgical airway is indicated.

3.5 Procedural sedation

3.5.1 Introduction

Procedural sedation has become widespread practice in UK EDs. It allows potentially painful and distressing procedures to be undertaken in a timely fashion with minimal distress to the patient. Sedation is not a substitute for adequate analgesia and should be combined with appropriate pain management and/or local anaesthetic techniques.

Procedures for which sedation may be required include:

- Joint reduction
- Fracture manipulation
- Electrical cardioversion
- Suturing
- Incision and drainage
- Wound care

Sedation is not without risks and potentially life-threatening complications include apnoea, hypoxia, hypotension, and pulmonary aspiration.

3.5.2 Levels of sedation

Sedation is the depression of a patient's awareness to the environment and reduction of their responsiveness to external stimulation. Sedation can produce a continuum of states, ranging from minimal sedation (anxiolysis) through to general anaesthesia (Table 3.10 and Figure 3.6).

Certain sedatives (e.g. ketamine) produce a dissociative state, which can be considered a type of moderate sedation. A disconnection is caused between the thalamoneocortical and the limbic systems preventing higher centres from receiving sensory stimuli. During dissociative states, airway reflexes, spontaneous ventilation, and cardiovascular function are maintained.

The depth of sedation required should be determined before the procedure is initiated. Generally, a level of moderate or deep sedation is required for procedures in the ED.

3.5.3 Drugs used in procedural sedation

The ideal sedative would exhibit all of the following qualities:

- Sedation
- Anxiolysis
- Amnesia
- Analgesia

Most sedatives do not possess all of these properties and one action may predominate. Therefore, sedation alone is not sufficient for painful procedures and should be supplemented with analgesia and/or local anaesthetic techniques.

Sedatives can be given orally, intramuscularly, intravenously, or by inhalation. In general, sedation is given intravenously in the ED due to its quicker onset of action, more predictable absorption, and better titration.

Sedative agents

Intravenous sedative drugs should be given in small, incremental doses that are titrated to the desired end-point of sedation. The most commonly used sedative agents in the ED are midazolam, propofol, and ketamine (Table 3.11). No one agent or regime is conclusively more effective than another and familiarity with a drug's effects and potential side effects is more important.

Table 3.10 Levels of sedation

	Minimal sedation	Moderate sedation ('conscious sedation')	Deep sedation	General anaesthesia
Verbal response	Normal response to verbal stimuli	Purposeful response to external stimuli (verbal or tactile)	Purposeful response to repeated or painful stimuli	State of unconsciousness
Airway reflexes	Maintained	Maintained	May require intervention	Intervention required
Respiratory effects	Unaffected	Unaffected	May be inadequate	Usually inadequate
Cardiovascular effects	Unaffected	Unaffected	Usually maintained	May be impaired

Excerpt from ASA Physical Status Classification System. Approved October 27, 2004, amended October 21, 2009 of the American Society of Anesthesiologists. A copy of the full text can be obtained from ASA, 1061 American Lane Schumburg, IL 60173-4973 or online at www.asahq.org.

| Minimal sedation → Moderate sedation → Deep sedation → General anaesthesia |

Figure 3.6 The continuum of sedation levels.

Inhaled sedative agents

The inhaled anaesthetic agent nitrous oxide, as a 30–70% mixture in oxygen, acts as a sedative and analgesic. The usual formulation in UK EDs is 50:50 nitrous oxide and oxygen, known as Entonox®. It is useful for short-term relief of severe pain and for performing short duration uncomfortable procedures.

The sedative properties of nitrous oxide are more noticeable clinically than its analgesic properties and therefore it should be coadministered with an analgesic. It has a rapid onset of action (30 seconds) and a short duration of action (one minute). It is thought to act by binding to opiate receptors in the central nervous system.

Adverse effects include vomiting and hypoxia, if not mixed with an adequate oxygen percentage. Nitrous oxide is more soluble than oxygen and nitrogen, so will tend to diffuse into any air-filled spaces in the body; therefore, it is contraindicated in patients with pneumothoraces, bowel obstruction, middle ear or sinus disease, and head injuries. Prolonged exposure may result in megaloblastic anaemia due to interference with the action of vitamin B12.

Analgesic agents

Sedation should be augmented by pre-procedure analgesia or local anaesthesia. The two most commonly used analgesics in procedural sedation are morphine and fentanyl.

Due to the time to onset of action, morphine should be given at least 10 minutes before sedation and fentanyl three minutes before. Both can cause respiratory depression and hypotension, especially when combined with a sedative agent. The properties of opiates are discussed further in the pain management section 3.6.

Antagonists

An antagonist should not be required if sedation and analgesia are given at appropriate doses and titrated slowly. However, some patients may have an unexpected exaggerated response. If a patient is oversedated, supportive management is the mainstay of treatment. Antagonists are available for benzodiazepines and opiates. There are no antagonists for propofol and ketamine. The need for flumazenil reversal for midazolan overdosage is now regarded as a 'Never Event'.

Flumazenil

- Competitive antagonist of benzodiazepines.
- Onset of action is 1–2 minutes after IV administration.
- Peak effect is within 10 minutes.
- Duration of action is shorter than longer-acting benzodiazepines (e.g. lorazepam or diazepam). Therefore, repeated dosing may be required.
- Dose of 0.2 mg IV, repeated up to 1–2 mg.
- Caution is required in patients receiving long-term benzodiazepines because it may precipitate acute withdrawal and seizures.
- Flumazenil should only be used to reverse sedation in medically administered benzodiazepines and not blindly in overdose patients who may have taken a mixture of medications, due to the risk of seizures.

Table 3.11 Sedatives used in procedural sedation

	Desired effects	Dose	Onset/Recovery	Adverse effects	Cautions
Midazolam (fast-acting water soluble benzodiazepine metabolized in the liver).	Anxiolysis. Sedation. Amnesia.	Total dose 0.05–0.1 mg/kg. Titrate slowly (1 mg increments) until desired affect achieved.	Onset 30–60 s. Peak effect 12 min. Duration 30 min.	Respiratory depression. Hypotension (although cardiovascular depression is not common at sedative doses). Risk of paradoxical disinhibition and increased agitation at low doses in children.	No analgesic properties. Elderly—enhanced and prolonged effect. Concurrent opioid use—enhanced respiratory and cardiovascular depression. Cirrhosis—metabolized by the liver.
Propofol (Alkylphenol derivative. Very lipid soluble. Clearance is not affected by renal or hepatic dysfunction because it has no active metabolites).	Sedation amnesia.	Total dose 0.5–1 mg/kg. Titrate carefully to sedation level and blood pressure.	Onset <1 min. Duration 10 min (dose-dependent).	Loss of airway reflexes. Respiratory depression (dose-dependent). Apnoea. venodilator.	No analgesic properties. No available antagonist. Elderly—enhanced and prolonged effect. Concurrent opioid use—enhanced risk of hypotension and apnoea. Patients with underlying cardiovascular disease or hypovolaemia are at greater risk of hypotension.
Ketamine (an antagonist for NMDA receptors. Most commonly used agent in paediatric ED sedation).	Dissociative anaesthetic. Anxiolysis. Amnesia. Analgesia. Airway reflexes maintained. Rarely produces haemodynamic compromise.	0.5–1 mg/kg slowly IV (2.5 mg/kg IM).	Onset 1–2 min. Duration 15–30 min.	Emergency phenomena (hallucinations may develop during recovery from the dissociative state). Laryngospasm. Increased salivary and respiratory secretions. Increased heart rate and blood pressure. Increased ICP.	Active respiratory tract infection—increased risk of laryngospasm. Risk of vomiting during recovery. Glaucoma or penetrating eye injury—increases intraocular pressure. Hyperthyroidism or thyroid medication—contraindicated.

Naloxone

- Competitive opiate antagonist. Reverses sedative and analgesic effects of opioids.
- Onset of action is two to three minutes.
- The duration of action is dose-related and may be shorter than longer-acting opiates.
- Initial dose of 400 mcg IV, which may need repeating up to a dose of 10 mg.
- It can also be given IM and IN.
- Administration by infusion may be required for longer-acting opiates.
- Metabolized in the liver and excreted by the kidney.
- Naloxone can be given as a diagnostic and therapeutic trial in an obtunded overdose patient.

3.5.4 Pre-sedation assessment

Prior to procedural sedation informed consent must be obtained and a full assessment of the patient's clinical condition must be made, appropriate to general anaesthesia, to include:

- Medical history
- Fasting status
- Airway assessment

Medical history

The medical history should include:

- History of events and current condition
- Past medical and surgical history
- Previous anaesthetics/sedation and any complications
- Current medications
- Allergies

A patient's pre-procedural health status is important in determining whether sedation is safe to perform in the ED or whether an alternative technique such as general anaesthesia in theatre or a regional anaesthetic technique is more appropriate. If sedation is appropriate, it also helps guide the most appropriate pharmacological agent to use.

Sedation is contraindicated in the following situations:

- Procedures that are more appropriately performed under general anaesthesia or under sterile conditions in theatre
- Patients requiring procedures in the mouth or oropharynx
- Patients with an American Society of Anaesthesiologists (ASA) grade >2 (see Table 3.12)
- Patients with a history suggestive of airway difficulties (e.g. tracheal surgery, tracheal stenosis, abnormal facial anatomy, and so on)
- Patients with active pulmonary infection or disease (increased risk of laryngospasm)
- Patients with significant cardiac disease
- Patients with a head injury associated with loss of consciousness, decreased level of consciousness, or vomiting
- Patients with central nervous system (CNS) masses, abnormalities, or hydrocephalus
- Patients with poorly controlled seizure disorders
- Patients with glaucoma or acute globe injury
- Patients with psychosis
- Patients with porphyria
- Patients with hyperthyroidism or on thyroid medications

Table 3.12 The American Society of Anaesthesiology (ASA) classification for assessing the fitness of patients before surgery (data from the ASA)

Class 1	A normal healthy patient
Class 2	A patient with mild disease
Class 3	A patient with severe disease
Class 4	A patient with severe disease that is a constant threat to life
Class 5	A moribund patient who is not expected to survive without the operation

Excerpt from *Continuum of Depth of Sedation: Definition of general anesthesia and levels of sedation/analgesia*. Approved October 27, 2004, amended October 21, 2009 of the American Society of Anesthesiologists. A copy of the full text can be obtained from ASA, 1061 American Lane Schumburg, IL 60173-4973 or online at www.asahq.org.

Fasting status

Emergency physicians frequently administer procedural sedation and analgesia to non-fasted patients and currently there are no specific guidelines to aid the pre-procedure risk stratification. Historically, general anaesthetic protocols for fasting have been followed: a minimum of six hours for solid food and milk; and two hours for clear fluids. The Royal College of Emergency Medicine ketamine guidelines for sedation in children state 'the fasting state of the child should be considered in relation to the urgency of the procedure, but recent food intake should not be considered as an absolute contraindication to ketamine use'. Therefore, a pragmatic approach is appropriate weighing the risks of sedation and fasting status against the urgency of the procedure.

Airway assessment

An airway assessment should be conducted, as for a RSI. The LEMON mnemonic (section 3.2) can be used to assess the airway and identify those with potential difficulties:

- **L**ook—for characteristics that are known to cause difficult intubation or ventilation.
- **E**valuate—mouth opening and thyromental distance (the 3–3–2 rule).
- **M**allampati—grades 1–4.
- **O**bstruction—is there evidence of pathology within or surrounding the upper airway.
- **N**eck mobility.

3.5.5 Performing procedural sedation

Staffing

The minimum staffing requirements for sedation are:

- One doctor to perform the procedure
- One doctor to perform the sedation (who has advanced airway skills and is trained in sedation)
- Another trained staff member to assist (e.g. ED nurse)

Clinical area

Procedural sedation and recovery should take place in the resuscitation room with immediate access to full resuscitation equipment.

Equipment

The equipment required for sedation includes:

- Oxygen
- Suction
- Tilting trolley
- Basic airway equipment (airway adjuncts and bag-valve-mask)
- Advanced airway equipment and difficult airway trolley
- Reversal agents (flumazenil and naloxone should be accessible)
- Secure IV access

Monitoring

Close observation and monitoring is required throughout procedural sedation and during recovery. Monitoring should include:

- Continuous oxygen saturations.
- Continuous 3-lead electrocardiogram (ECG).
- Continual monitoring of the respiratory rate and depth.
- Continual monitoring of level of consciousness.
- Regular monitoring of the blood pressure (e.g. every 3–5 minutes).
- Continuous quantitative capnography, with end tidal CO_2 monitoring, is mandatory wherever deep sedation or dissociative sedation occur.

The procedure for sedation

- A pre-sedation assessment should be made.
- The fasting status should be noted and a risk assessment made. Fasting is not needed for minimal sedation or moderate sedation where verbal contact with the patient is maintained. For deeper levels of sedation, the fasting rules for general anaesthesia apply.
- Written consent should be obtained and the patient should have the benefits, risks, and alternatives explained.
- The patient should be transferred to the resuscitation room with full access to resuscitation equipment.
- Monitoring should be attached and a baseline set of observations should be recorded.
- Three members of staff should be present: a doctor to manage the sedation and airway; a clinician to perform the procedure; and an experienced nurse.
- The patient should have appropriate analgesia.
- The sedative agent should be chosen based on the procedure being undertaken, the familiarity of the user with the agent, and the patient's health status. The appropriate dose should be calculated.
- The sedative agent should be given slowly IV with continual monitoring of observations (heart rate, respiratory rate, blood pressure, conscious level, and end tidal CO_2).
- Once the pre-determined level of sedation is achieved the procedure should be performed, while continually monitoring the patient.
- The patient should be monitored closely once the procedural stimulation is withdrawn because the level of sedation may deepen.
- After the procedure, the patient should be recovered in the resuscitation room until the pre-sedation level of consciousness and observations are achieved.
- If antagonists have been administered, the patient should be monitored for longer.
- Any post-procedure investigations should be performed (e.g. X-ray).

- The patient may be discharged from the ED once pre-sedation levels of verbalization, awareness, and mobility are achieved.
- The patient and carer should be given appropriate discharge advice.
- The sedation and procedure should be carefully documented and any audit documentation completed.

Discharge criteria

Prior to discharge the patient must:

- Have returned to baseline level of consciousness
- Have stable vital signs (within normal limits for the patient)
- Have no evidence of compromise of respiratory status
- Be able to walk without support/walk as well as prior to sedation
- Be able to tolerate oral fluids
- Be accompanied by a responsible adult
- Be advised not to drive, operate machinery, or sign legally binding documents for 24 hours
- Have follow-up arranged, including analgesia if required
- Have written information about aftercare given to the accompanying adult

---

KEY POINTS

Sedation is the depression of a patient's awareness to the environment and reduction of their responsiveness to external stimulation. It allows potentially painful and distressing procedures to be undertaken in a timely fashion with minimal distress to the patient.

Sedation can produce a continuum of states, ranging from minimal sedation (anxiolysis) through to general anaesthesia.

Sedation alone is not sufficient for painful procedures and should be supplemented with analgesia and/or local anaesthetic techniques.

The most commonly used sedative agents in the ED are midazolam, propofol, and ketamine.

No one agent or regime is conclusively more effective than another and familiarity with a drug's effects and potential side effects is more important.

Prior to procedural sedation, informed consent must be obtained and a full assessment of the patient's clinical condition and past medical history performed.

The fasting status should be considered in relation to the urgency of the procedure, but recent food intake should not be considered as an absolute contraindication to sedation.

Sedation should be performed in the resuscitation area with immediate access to full resuscitation facilities. Monitoring should include 3-lead ECG, blood pressure, respiratory rate, conscious level, and pulse oximetry. If available, monitoring of end tidal CO_2 is recommended.

At least three members of staff are required to perform procedural sedation (a doctor to perform the sedation, a clinician to perform the procedure, and an experienced nurse).

Patients may be discharged from the ED once pre-sedation levels of verbalization, awareness, observations, and mobility are achieved.

3.6 Pain management

3.6.1 Introduction

Pain is a disabling accompaniment of many medical conditions and can be defined as an unpleasant experience in response to a noxious stimulus. Pain is perhaps the most common complaint of

Table 3.13 Royal College of Emergency Medicine Clinical Standards for pain management

Moderate and severe pain

Time to analgesia

75% within 30 min

100% within 60 min

Re-evaluation of pain

90% of patients with moderate to severe pain should have documented evidence of re-evaluation and action within 120 minutes of the first dose of analgesic

If analgesia is not prescribed the reason should be documented in the notes

Data from the College of Emergency Medicine Pain Management Guideline (www.rcem.ac.uk).

patients presenting to the ED and pain control one of the most important therapeutic priorities. There is some evidence that pain relief is related to patient satisfaction.

The management of pain is a key ED priority and is given high importance by the Royal College of Emergency Medicine. Pain management is one of the clinical standards for EDs produced by the College's Clinical Effectiveness Committee. These standards detail the importance of pain scoring, early analgesia, and re-evaluation of pain (Table 3.13). The process of pain management should start at triage, be monitored during a patient's time in the ED, and finish ensuring adequate analgesia at, and if appropriate, beyond discharge.

3.6.2 Pain assessment

In order to make the appropriate choice of analgesic and monitor response, the level of pain needs to be assessed. Pain assessment forms an integral part of the National Triage Scale. Multiple assessment tools are in use for grading the level of pain; the ones detailed in this chapter are those recommended by the Royal College of Emergency Medicine in their guidelines on the management of pain in adults and children.

The benefits of using a pain-scoring system include:

- grading the severity of pain;
- guiding the choice of analgesic;
- monitoring the patient's response to analgesia; and,
- aiding audit and research.

Assessment of acute pain in adults

- The College guidance for management of pain in adults uses a scale that contains subjective and objective descriptions. Using this method of pain scoring it is possible to assess the patient into one of four categories and treat pain appropriately (Table 3.14).

Assessment of acute pain in children

The Royal College of Emergency Medicine guideline for pain management in children includes a composite assessment tool for pain scoring (Table 3.15). The assessment tool uses established pain-scoring scales including the faces score, ladder score, and behavioural scoring. Using this method of pain scoring, it is possible to assess the patient into one of four categories.

3.6.3 Managing pain

Pain management is multifactorial and involves pharmacological agents, the use of psychological strategies, and non-pharmacological adjuncts.

Table 3.14 Royal College of Emergency Medicine recommendations for assessing and treating pain in the emergency department

	No pain	Mild pain	Moderate pain	Severe pain
	0	1–3	4–6	7–10
Type/route of analgesia	Nil	Oral paracetamol +/– NSAID	As for mild pain plus oral NSAID (if not already given) or codeine phosphate	IV opiate or PR NSAID
Initial assessment	Within 20 minutes of arrival	Within 20 minutes of arrival	Within 20 minutes of arrival	Within 20 minutes of arrival
Re-evaluation	Within 60 minutes of initial assessment	Within 60 minutes of analgesia	Within 60 minutes of analgesia	Within 30 minutes of analgesia

Reproduced with kind permission of the Royal College of Emergency Medicine (2014).

Psychological strategies are important for all groups of patients but particularly children and those with learning disabilities. Such techniques include:

- Explanation with reassurance
- Involving parents or carers
- Quiet, calm environment
- Distraction techniques (toys, reading, story-telling, and so on).

Non-pharmacological adjuncts are detailed in Table 3.16

3.6.4 Pharmacological management of pain

Once a patient has had their level of pain assessed, it is possible to choose the appropriate analgesic(s). The pain relief or analgesic ladder is a commonly used method of controlling pain (Figure 3.7). It was first described by the World Health Organization for the management of cancer pain, but is now widely used by medical professionals for the management of all types of pain.

The general principle of the pain ladder is to start at the bottom rung of the ladder, and then to climb the ladder if the pain is still present. This pain relief programme groups drugs into three main categories:

- Non-opioid drugs (e.g. paracetamol) and other non-steroidal anti-inflammatories (NSAIDs) (see Table 3.17)
- Weak opioids (e.g. codeine phosphate)
- Strong opioids (e.g. morphine)

ED patients are a different cohort to those with cancer pain. ED patients often need rapid control of severe pain and therefore immediate treatment with a strong opiate may be required, rather than a gradual progression up the analgesic ladder.

Table 3.15 Royal College of Emergency Medicine composite method of assessing acute pain in children

	No pain	Mild pain	Moderate pain	Severe pain
Faces scale score	(a)	(b)	(c)	(d)
Ladder score	0	1–3	4–6	7–10
Behaviour	Normal activity No ↓ movement Happy	Rubbing affected area ↓ movement Neutral expression Able to play/talk normally	Protective of affected area ↓ movement/quiet Complaining of pain Consolable crying Grimaces when affected part moved/touched	No movement or defensive of affected part Looking frightened Very quiet Restless/unsettled Complaining of lots of pain Inconsolable crying
Injury example	Bump on head	Abrasion Small laceration Sprain ankle/knee Fracture fingers/clavicle Sore throat	Small burn/scald Finger tip injury Fracture forearm/elbow/ ankle Appendicitis	Large burn Fracture long bone/dislocation Appendicitis Sickle crisis

Reproduced with kind permission of the Royal College of Emergency Medicine (2015).

Table 3.16 Non-pharmacological techniques for pain relief

Method	Effect
Splinting	• Results in decreased pain and decreased analgesic requirements. • Splints include plaster, vacuum splints, box splints, and devices such as the Thomas splint for femoral fractures.
Elevation	• Swelling frequently causes increased pain and stiffness. • Essential for dependent injuries. • Can aid earlier mobilization.
Temperature	• Cooling burns can stop further tissue destruction as well as relieve pain. • Ice-packs can help with recent sprains and muscle injuries. • Muscle spasm may be eased with warm compresses (e.g. strains of back and neck).
Dressings	• The pain of minor burns can be dramatically reduced by the application of a dressing (air currents over exposed superficial dermis cause pain due to stimulation of exposed nerve endings).
Definitive treatment	• Early reduction of a dislocation will reduce total analgesic requirements. • Conditions such as pulled elbow may require no analgesia as treatment may give immediate relief of pain.

Paracetamol is a safe first-line treatment for the elderly, while NSAIDs should be used with caution and at the lowest possible dose, in order to avoid gastrointestinal, renal, and cardiovascular side effects, and drug–drug interactions. Paracematol is considered safe in all three trimesters of pregnancy, while ibuprofen is best avoided and can only be used in the second trimester (if essential). Morphine and codeine can be used in all three trimesters.

Figure 3.8 is an algorithm more suited to ED practice, which has been developed from the Royal College of Emergency Medicine recommendations on the treatment of acute pain.

Non-opioid analgesics

Opioid analgesics

Opioids bind to specific opioid receptors in the central and peripheral nervous system. They are commonly used in the ED to relieve moderate and severe pain (Table 3.18).

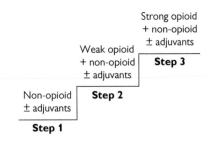

Figure 3.7 The analgesic ladder.

Reprinted from *Cancer pain relief: with a guide to opioid availability*, 2nd edition, World Health Organization, 1996.

Table 3.17 Commonly used non-opioid analgesics

Drug	Indications	Dose and route	Contraindications and cautions	Side effects
Paracetamol (inhibits cyclooxygenase 3)	Mild and moderate pain. Anti-pyretic.	Adult: 1 g every 4–6 h (maximum dose 4 g in 24 h). Children: 20 mg/kg as a loading dose (maximum 90 mg/kg daily in divided doses). Can be given PO/PR/IV.	Allergy. Severe hepatic impairment. Toxic in overdose. Look for any previous paracetamol use (including co-codamol and over-the-counter (OTC) preparations, as well as paramedic use prior to arrival in the ED).	Rare. May cause hypotension on infusion.
NSAIDs (Cyclooxygenase inhibitors. The non-selective agents are most commonly used in the ED).				
Ibuprofen	Mild and moderate pain.	Adults: 1.2–1.8 g daily in 3–4 divided doses. Children (>5 kg): 20–30 mg/kg daily in divided doses. Given PO.	Allergy. Hypersensitivity to aspirin. Severe renal impairment. Peptic ulceration. Asthmatics known to get worsening bronchospasm with NSAIDs. Elderly (>65 years)—risk of subclinical renal impairment. Used with caution in pregnancy and avoided in the last trimester.	Best side effect profile of NSAIDs. GI bleeding/irritation. Bronchospasm. Platelet inhibition. Fluid retention.
Naproxen	Moderate to severe pain—particularly musculoskeletal.	Adult 500 mg initial dose followed by 250 mg 6-8 hrly.	As for ibuprofen.	As for ibuprofen—relatively fewer side effect compared to other NSAIDs.
Diclofenac	Moderate and severe pain. Particularly useful PR for renal colic.	Adults: 150 mg daily in 2–3 divided doses. Children: 1mg/kg 8 hourly. Given PO or PR.	As for ibuprofen. Contraindicated in IHD/PVD/CVD/heart failure die to increased thrombotic risk.	As for ibuprofen.

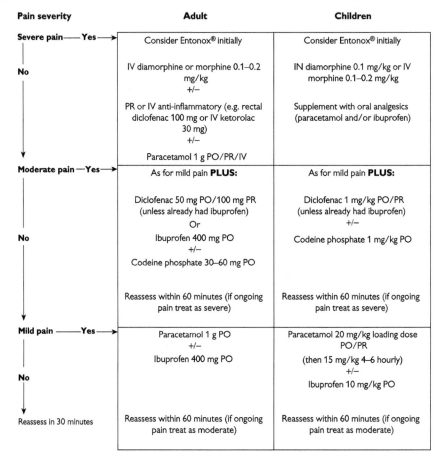

Pain severity	Adult	Children
Severe pain —— Yes →	Consider Entonox® initially	Consider Entonox® initially
No	IV diamorphine or morphine 0.1–0.2 mg/kg +/–	IN diamorphine 0.1 mg/kg or IV morphine 0.1–0.2 mg/kg
	PR or IV anti-inflammatory (e.g. rectal diclofenac 100 mg or IV ketorolac 30 mg) +/–	Supplement with oral analgesics (paracetamol and/or ibuprofen)
	Paracetamol 1 g PO/PR/IV	
Moderate pain —Yes →	As for mild pain **PLUS:**	As for mild pain **PLUS:**
No	Diclofenac 50 mg PO/100 mg PR (unless already had ibuprofen) Or Ibuprofen 400 mg PO +/– Codeine phosphate 30–60 mg PO	Diclofenac 1 mg/kg PO/PR (unless already had ibuprofen) +/– Codeine phosphate 1 mg/kg PO
	Reassess within 60 minutes (if ongoing pain treat as severe)	Reassess within 60 minutes (if ongoing pain treat as severe)
Mild pain —— Yes →	Paracetamol 1 g PO +/– Ibuprofen 400 mg PO	Paracetamol 20 mg/kg loading dose PO/PR (then 15 mg/kg 4–6 hourly) +/– Ibuprofen 10 mg/kg PO
No ↓ Reassess in 30 minutes	Reassess within 60 minutes (if ongoing pain treat as moderate)	Reassess within 60 minutes (if ongoing pain treat as moderate)

Figure 3.8 Algorithm for the treatment of acute pain in the emergency department.

KEY POINTS

Recognition and alleviation of pain should be a priority when treating ill and injured patients. The Royal College of Emergency Medicine consider pain management an important priority and therefore questions on pain management often appear in SAQs. The College's Clinical Effectiveness Committee has produced standards for pain management.

All patients should have a pain score recorded and receive appropriate analgesia based on their score. There are a variety of scoring systems, including visual analogue scales and verbal rating scales.

All patients with mild to moderate should have their pain re-evaluated within 60 minutes of their first dose of analgesia, while those in severe pain should be re-evaluated within 30 minutes

Pain management is multifactorial and involves pharmacological agents, the use of psychological strategies, and non-pharmacological adjuncts.

It is important to know about the analgesic ladder but ED patients often require a modified approach to pain management. ED patients may present with severe pain that requires rapid control and therefore immediate treatment with a strong opiate may be required, rather than a gradual progression up the analgesic ladder.

Table 3.18 Commonly used opioid analgesics

Drug	Indications	Dose and route	Contraindications and cautions	Side effects
Codeine (weak opioid)	Moderate pain.	Adults: 30–60 mg every 4–6 h up to 240 mg daily. Children: restricted >12 years only dose as per adults.	Allergy.	Nausea. Vomiting. Drowsiness. Constipation. Hypotension.
Morphine (strong opioid)	Severe pain. Anxiolysis. Cough suppression.	Adults and children: 0.1–0.2 mg/kg titrated to effect. Should be used IV for ED patients in severe pain. Onset of action within 10 min.—peak effect at 20 min. Duration approximately 4–5 h.	Allergy Acute respiratory depression. Head injury (may impair neurological assessment).	Respiratory depression. Bronchospasm. Hypotension. Drowsiness. Miosis. Histamine release. Constipation. Nausea and vomiting.
Diamorphine (twice as potent as morphine)	Severe pain.	Adults: 0.1 mg/kg IV titrated to effect. Children: typically used IN 0.1 mg/kg.	As for morphine.	As for morphine. (NB Nausea and hypotension may be less marked.)
Fentanyl (100 times more potent than morphine)	Severe pain. Particularly useful in procedural sedation due to a rapid onset of action.	1–2 mcg/kg IV. Onset of action within 1–2 min—peak effect at 4–5 min. Duration approximately 30 min.	As for morphine.	As for morphine. (NB Hypotension may be less marked than morphine and respiratory depression is uncommon.)

3.7 Local anaesthesia

3.7.1 Introduction

Local anaesthetic agents enable the emergency physician to achieve analgesia and anaesthesia, facilitating procedures and minor operations that would otherwise be difficult, impossible, or require general anaesthesia.

Local anaesthesia can be used for local infiltration, nerve blocks, intravenous regional blocks, or topically.

Indications for local anaesthesia:

- Topical use—venepuncture or venous cannula, arterial puncture or cannulation, wound cleaning and/or closure
- Local infiltration—cleaning, exploration, and closure of wounds
- Nerve block—such as femoral nerve block for a femoral shaft fracture (discussed in section 3.8)
- Intravenous regional block—such as Bier's block (discussed in section 3.9)

Contraindications to local anaesthesia:

- Allergy.
- Infection at the proposed injection site—may cause spread of the infection, can be painful, and may be ineffective due to the high tissue acidity reducing the effectiveness of the local anaesthetic. Hyperaemia at the site may also increase the rate of removal of the local anaesthetic reducing the duration of action and increasing the risk of toxicity.
- Bleeding disorder—anticoagulant therapy and thrombocytopenia are contraindications for nerve blocks in which there is a risk of inadvertent arterial puncture.
- Poor patient co-operation or patient refusal.
- Procedures that are more appropriately performed under general anaesthesia or under sterile conditions in theatre.

3.7.2 Local anaesthetic agents

The most commonly used local anaesthetic agents in the ED are lidocaine, bupivacaine, and prilocaine. Their mode of action is via reversible blockade of sodium channels in excitable/conducting neural tissue.

The onset of action is related to the lipid solubility, which is dependent upon the pKa. The pKa is the pH at which a drug is 50% ionized and 50% unionized. The closer the pKa is to pH 7.4 the more lipid soluble the agent is, resulting in a faster onset of action; for example, lidocaine (pKa 7.9) has a faster onset than bupivacaine (pKa 8.1).

The duration of action is determined by protein binding at the site, the dose of the drug, the drugs inherent vasodilatation effects (e.g. lidocaine has a greater vasodilator effect therefore shorter action), and the local circulation (Table 3.19).

3.7.3 Adrenaline and local anaesthetics

Adrenaline can be added to local anaesthetic solutions decreasing the rate of vascular reabsorption and increasing the duration of action. It is commonly used with lidocaine but has little effect on the longer-acting drugs such as bupivacaine. The resulting vasoconstriction has the advantage of reducing bleeding at the site.

- Effective concentration of adrenaline is 5 mcg/ml or 1 in 200,000 (200 mcg maximum dose).
- Adrenaline should be avoided in blocks of terminal extremities (e.g. digits, pinna, nose, and penis) due to the risk of vascular compromise and ischaemia.
- Adrenaline should be avoided in or near flap lacerations due to the risk of vasoconstriction causing ischaemic necrosis.

Table 3.19 Local anaesthetic properties

Drug	Solution	Onset	Duration of action	Maximum dose	Uses
Lidocaine	0.5%	Rapid	30–60 min	3 mg/kg	Local infiltration.
	1%		90 min with adrenaline	7 mg/kg with adrenaline	Nerve blocks.
	2%				Topically.
Bupivacaine	0.25%	Slow	90–180 min	2 mg/kg with or without adrenaline	Nerve blocks.
	0.5%				Local infiltration (but slow onset).
	0.75%				Not suitable for IV anaesthesia due to level of cardiotoxicity.
Prilocaine	0.5%	Rapid	Similar to lidocaine	6 mg/kg 8 mg/kg with adrenaline	Agent of choice for IV anaesthesia.

- Adrenaline should be avoided in ischaemic heart disease, hypertension, peripheral vascular disease, phaeochromocytoma, and in patients taking β-blockers.

3.7.4 Topical local anaesthetic agents

Topical local anaesthetics are used most commonly in children, such as EMLA® cream ('eutetic mixture of local anaesthetics'), for venepuncture or venous cannulation.

EMLA® is a mixture of lidocaine 2.5% and prilocaine 2.5%. It must be applied for at least one hour before venepuncture to provide anaesthesia, which limits the use in the ED. It should not be used on broken skin, those <1 year, and cautiously in those with anaemia or methaemoglobinaemia. Side effects include blanching and vasoconstriction.

Tetracaine (amethocaine) gel (Ametop®) is similar to EMLA® but acts more quickly and causes vasodilatation aiding venous cannulation.

Lidocaine, adrenaline, tetracaine gel (LAT gel®) is being used more commonly as a topical local anaesthetic to facilitate cleaning and suturing of wounds. The gel should be applied for 30 minutes prior to the procedure. The maximum dose is 1.25 cm of gel on the body surface per kg.

EXAM TIP

Local anaesthetic calculations frequently appear in SAQs and often confuse candidates.

1% solution = 10 mg/ml

1:1000 = 1 g/L = 1000 mg/1000ml = 1 mg/ml.

Example question

A 60-kg female presents with multiple, deep lacerations to her forearm. What is the maximum dose of plain lidocaine she can receive (show your calculations)?

Answer: Maximum dose is 3mg/kg = 3×60 = 180 mg.

How much 1% lidocaine solution is this?

Answer: 1% lidocaine = 10 mg/ml

180 mg = 18ml of 1% lidocaine.

3.7.5 Complications of local anaesthesia

Previous MRCEM question

Local anaesthetic agents have well-recognized complications and the topic has appeared in previous SAQ papers. Complications can be subdivided into those related to technique and those related to the drugs used.

Technique-related complications:

- Direct neural trauma
- Bleeding and haematoma
- Intravascular injection
- Infection
- Damage to surrounding structures (e.g. artery, tendons, pneumothorax)

Drug-related complications:

- Toxicity by intravascular injection
- Toxicity by systemic absorption
- Anaphylactic reaction
- Methaemoglobinaemia (e.g. prilocaine)

3.7.6 Local anaesthetic toxicity

Systemic side effects arise when blood concentrations of local anaesthetic increase to toxic levels. This can result from accidental intravascular injection, rapid absorption from a highly vascular area, or an overdose of local anaesthetic.

Conditions that increase the risk of toxicity include:

- Elderly
- Small children
- Heart block
- Low cardiac output
- Epilepsy
- Myasthenia gravis
- Hepatic impairment
- Porphyria
- Anti-arrhythmic or β-blocker therapy (increased risk of myocardial depression)
- Cimetidine therapy (inhibits the metabolism of lidocaine)

Techniques to reduce the risk of toxicity include:

- Clear and accurate dose calculations
- Dose reduction in frail patients and those at the extremes of ages
- Local anaesthetic injected slowly and with regular aspiration (to avoid accidental intravenous injection)
- Use of adrenaline as a vasoconstrictor to reduce the systemic absorption of local anaesthetic
- Regional nerve blocks to anaesthetize large areas
- Use of ultrasound to facilitate nerve blocks
- Close monitoring

Clinical features of local anaesthetic toxicity

The progression of local anaesthetic toxicity correlates with ascending serum levels. Initially benign symptoms develop (blood concentration 5 mcg/ml) progressing ultimately to cardiac arrest (blood concentration >25 mcg/ml) (see Table 3.20). The speed of onset of symptoms

Table 3.20 Features of local anaesthetic toxicity

	CNS	Cardiovascular	Respiratory
Early (mild) features	Light headedness	Tachycardia and hypertension (with adrenaline)	
	Tinnitus		
	Circumoral/tongue numbness		
	Abnormal taste (metallic)		
	Confusion	Bradycardia	
	Drowsiness	Hypotension	
	Visual disturbance		
	Muscular twitching	Conduction blocks	Respiratory depression
	Convulsions		
	Reduced level of consciousness	Cardiovascular collapse (usually require 4–7 times the convulsant dose)	
Late (severe) features	Coma	Asystole ventricular arrhythmias	Respiratory arrest

depends on whether the toxicity is due to an accidental intravascular injection or absorption from a vascular site.

Management of local anaesthetic toxicity

The mainstay of treatment for local anaesthetic toxicity is supportive management following ALS principles. Patients with cardiovascular collapse or cardiac arrest may benefit from treatment with intravenous 20% lipid emulsion in addition to standard ALS management.

The management of severe local anaesthetic toxicity includes:

- Stopping the injection of local anaesthetic.
- Supportive management.
- High-flow oxygen and basic airway manoeuvres. Intubation should be performed if the conscious level is deteriorating or the patient is having recurrent seizures.
- Ventilatory support for respiratory failure. Mild hyperventilation may help because respiratory acidosis exacerbates local anaesthetic toxicity.
- Treating hypotension with IV fluids (followed by inotropes, if required).
- Arrhythmia management using ALS guidelines. (NB Lidocaine is not recommended as an anti-arrhythmic therapy.)
- Seizures treated with benzodiazepines.
- Standard ALS guidelines, if cardiac arrest develops (see Chapter 2). Prolonged resuscitation may be required because recovery from local anaesthetic-induced cardiac arrest may take longer than one hour.
- Intravenous lipid emulsion for cardiovascular collapse and cardiac arrest.

Guidance about the use of intravenous lipid emulsion comes from the Association of Anaesthetists of Great Britain and Ireland (AAGBI) and is included in the 2015 ALS guidance. Intravenous lipid emulsion is recommended in local anaesthetic-induced cardiac arrest and should be considered in cases of circulatory collapse.

Administering intravenous lipid emulsion:

- Give an initial intravenous bolus of 20% emulsion (1.5 ml/kg over one minute), followed by an infusion of 20% emulsion at 15 ml/kg/hour.
- Two repeat boluses (same dose), may be given at five-minute intervals, if cardiovascular stability has not been restored or an adequate circulation deteriorates.
- The infusion should be continued until the patient recovers or the maximum dose is reached (12 ml/kg).
- Propofol is not a suitable substitute for lipid emulsion.

Pancreatitis is a recognized complication of intravenous lipid emulsion and should be monitored for by regular clinical review, including daily amylase or lipase assays for two days. When local anaesthetic toxicity results in the need for intravenous lipid emulsion, it should be reported to the international registry for lipid use.

KEY POINTS

Maximum local anaesthetic doses:

- Lidocaine 3 mg/kg (with adrenaline 7 mg/kg)
- Bupivacaine 2 mg/kg (same with adrenaline)
- Prilocaine 6 mg/kg (with adrenaline 8 mg/kg)

$$1\% \text{ solution} = 10\,\text{mg per ml} \quad 1{:}100 = 1\text{g/L}.$$

Toxicity:

- Systemic toxicity of local anaesthetic involves the central nervous, respiratory, and cardiovascular systems. Severe agitation, loss of consciousness, with or without seizures, sinus bradycardia, conduction blocks, asystole, and ventricular tachyarrhythmias can all occur.
- Supportive management is the mainstay of treatment and ALS principles apply. Intravenous lipid emulsion should be given in the event of a cardiac arrest and considered in circulatory collapse.

3.8 Nerve blocks

3.8.1 Introduction

Nerve blocks are commonly performed in the ED and have advantages over local infiltration, including:

- Reduced dose of local anaesthetic
- Avoiding distortion of the anatomy to aid accurate closure of wounds (e.g. facial lacerations)
- Facilitating procedures otherwise not possible (e.g. penile nerve block for foreskin trapped in zip)
- Anaesthetizing inflamed or infected tissue where direct infiltration should not be undertaken.

The Royal College of Emergency Medicine curriculum includes knowledge of and the ability to perform the following nerve blocks:

- Digital
- Wrist (ulnar, median, radial)
- Femoral
- Facial (auricular, supratrochlear, supraorbital)
- Ankle

Contraindications to nerve blocks include:

- Contraindications to local anaesthetics (detailed in section 3.7)
- Bleeding disorders (where there is a risk of vascular puncture)
- Patients at risk of compartment syndrome where a nerve block may hinder clinical assessment

General measures that should be employed when performing a nerve block include:

- Lying the patient down (fainting is common).
- Warming the local anaesthetic to reduce the pain of injection.
- Considering the use of ultrasound guidance or other nerve locator devices.
- Sterile precautions and appropriate cleaning of the injection site.
- Using a narrow-gauge needle where possible to reduce the pain of injection.
- Aspirating frequently to avoid intravascular injection.
- Asking the patient about tingling in the distribution of the nerve. Paraesthesia is not the goal and if elicited, the needle should be withdrawn 2–3 mm before injecting.
- Injecting slowly and not forcing the syringe to reduce the pain of injection and avoid intra-axonal injection.
- Maintaining a conversation with the patient to detect early signs of toxicity.

3.8.2 Nerve blocks of the hand and wrist

Table 3.21 details the nerve blocks of the hand and wrist. Figure 3.9 details the nerve blocks at the wrist.

Table 3.21 Nerve blocks of the hand and wrist

Nerve	Anatomy	Technique	Volume/Dose
Digital nerve	Dorsal and palmar nerves run along each side of the digits. The nail bed is supplied by the dorsal digital nerves.	Inject at the base of the proximal phalanx through the dorsum to the palmar aspect; medial and lateral injections are required. Dorsal subcutaneous infiltration is also needed to block the dorsal digital nerves and their branches. The digital nerves can also be blocked by a metacarpal block.	2–3 ml of 1% lidocaine, prilocaine, or 0.25% bupivacaine.
Wrist			
Median nerve	The median nerve supplies sensation to the radial half of the palm, the thumb, index, and middle fingers, and the radial side of the ring finger. The median nerve lies under the flexor retinaculum on the volar aspect of the wrist. It lies between the tendons of palmaris longus and flexor carpi radialis.	Inject at the proximal wrist crease, between the tendons of flexor carpi radialis and palmaris longus to a depth of 1 cm. To block the palmar cutaneous branch infiltrate superficially, proximal to the flexor retinaculum. NB Carpal tunnel syndrome is a contraindication to a median nerve block.	3–5 ml at depth of 10–15 mm.

Table 3.21 Continued

Nerve	Anatomy	Technique	Volume/Dose
Ulnar nerve	The ulnar nerve supplies the ulnar side of the hand, the little finger, and the ulnar side of the ring finger. The ulnar nerve has two branches at the wrist: a palmar branch, which travels with the ulnar artery to supply the hypothenar eminence and palm; and a dorsal branch, which passes under flexor carpi ulnaris to supply the ulnar side of the dorsum of the hand.	Inject at the level of the ulnar styloid process between the ulnar artery and flexor carpi ulnaris. The dorsal branch can be blocked by subcutaneous infiltration of local anaesthetic from flexor carpi ulnaris around the ulnar border of the wrist.	3–5 ml at depth of 10–15 mm.
Radial nerve	The radial nerve supplies the dorsum of the radial side of the hand. The radial nerve lies subcutaneously on the dorsum of the radial side of the wrist.	Inject subcutaneously around the radial side and dorsum of the wrist from the tendon of flexor carpi radialis to the radioulnar joint. (NB The radial nerve block involves an infiltration technique and often has a shorter duration of action than other wrist blocks therefore adrenaline may be used to prolong the anaesthesia.)	5–8 ml with or without adrenaline.

3.8.3 Nerve blocks of the forehead

Table 3.22 details the nerve blocks of the forehead.

3.8.4 Nerve blocks of the ear

Table 3.23 details the nerve blocks of the ear. Figure 3.10 shows the nerve blocks of the forehead and the ear.

3.8.5 Nerve blocks of the lower limb

Table 3.24 details the nerve blocks of the lower limb. Figure 3.11 shows the nerve blocks at the ankle.

3.9 Intravenous regional anaesthesia (Bier's block)

Reduction of distal forearm fractures can be facilitated by intravenous regional anaesthesia (Bier's block). The Royal College of Emergency Medicine have produced guidance on this. It includes advice on how to perform the procedure and on the local clinical governance arrangements that

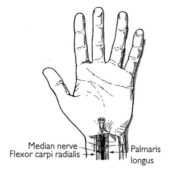

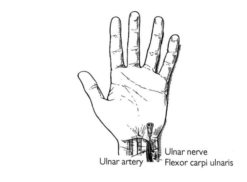

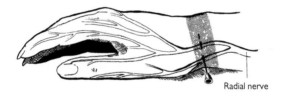

Figure 3.9 Nerve blocks at the wrist.

Reproduced from Jonathan P. Wyatt, Robin N. Illingworth, Colin A. Graham, Michael J. Clancy, Colin E. Robertson, *Oxford Handbook of Emergency Medicine*, 2006, 'Nerve blocks at the wrist' pages 295 and 297, with permission from Oxford University Press.

should be instituted. The full guideline is available via the Royal College of Emergency Medicine website.

3.9.1 Pre-procedure checks for a Bier's block

- The patient should receive a full explanation about the procedure and consent should be obtained.
- A pre-procedure assessment, appropriate for a general anaesthetic, should be performed.
- Ideally the patient should be fasted (four hours since last oral intake).
- The patient should have ECG, BP, and oxygen saturation monitoring.
- Intravenous access should be gained in both arms (on the fractured arm to administer prilocaine and on the unaffected arm in case resuscitative drugs/fluids are required).

Table 3.22 Nerve blocks of the forehead

Nerve	Anatomy	Technique	Volume/Dose
Supraorbital nerve	The supraorbital nerve supplies sensation to most of the forehead and the frontal region of the scalp. The supraorbital nerve divides into medial and lateral branches. Branches exit the orbit through. two holes in the superior orbital margin—2.5 cm from the midline.	Inject in the midline between the eyebrows, direct the needle laterally, and infiltrate subcutaneously along the upper margin of the eyebrow. Anaesthesia of the lateral part of the forehead may require local infiltration to block the zygomaticotemporal and auriculotemporal nerves. (NB If an injection is made at the supraorbital nerve foramen, local anaesthetic may enter the orbit, reaching the optic nerve and causing temporary blindness.)	5–10 ml with or without adrenaline.
Supratroch-lear nerve	The supratrochlear nerve supplies sensation to the medial part of the forehead. The supratrochlear nerve emerges from the upper medial corner of the orbit.		

- The double pneumatic tourniquet cuff should be checked for leaks by inflating and leaving it for five minutes.
- The patient should be weighed in kilograms.
- The dose of prilocaine should be calculated (3 ml/kg is the recommended dose; 0.5% or 1% solution without preservative is the recommended concentration). Prilocaine is the only licensed local anaesthetic agent for intravenous regional anaesthesia.
- A pre-procedure checklist should be completed.

Table 3.23 Nerve blocks of the ear

Nerve	Anatomy	Technique	Volume/Dose
Greater auricular nerve	Located inferior to the pinna.	Infiltrate 1 cm below the ear lobe, from the posterior border of the sternomastoid to the angle of mandible.	10 ml (total) in the appropriate areas or in a ring around the ear.
Lesser occipital nerve	Located posterior to the pinna.	Infiltrate behind the ear.	
Auriculotemporal nerve	Located anterosuperior to the pinna.	Infiltrate anterior to the external auditory meatus.	

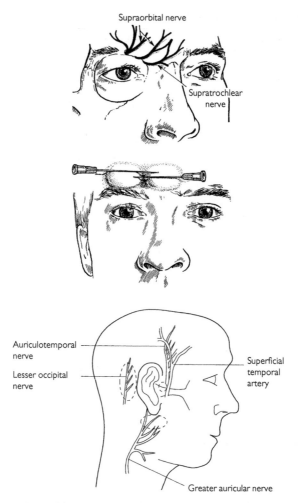

Figure 3.10 Nerve blocks of the forehead and ear.

Reproduced from Jonathan P. Wyatt, Robin N. Illingworth, Colin A. Graham, Michael J. Clancy, Colin E. Robertson, *Oxford Handbook of Emergency Medicine*, 2006, 'Nerve blocks of forehead and ear', p. 299, with permission from Oxford University Press.

3.9.2 The Bier's block procedure

- Exsanguinate the arm by elevating it for three minutes.
- Inflate the double-cuff tourniquet to greater than 100 mmHg above systolic BP or to 300 mmHg (whichever is higher). The time of cuff inflation should be recorded.
- Check for the absence of the radial pulse.
- Inject the prilocaine and record the time.
- Warn the patient about the mottled appearance of the arm and the hot/cold sensation.
- Check for anaesthesia. If it is not adequate after five minutes, flush the cannula with saline.
- Remove the cannula and perform the procedure.
- Perform a check X-ray.
- The cuff must remain inflated for a minimum of 20 minutes and a maximum of 45 minutes.

Table 3.24 Nerve blocks of the lower limb

Nerve	Anatomy	Technique	Volume/Dose
Femoral nerve	The femoral nerve supplies: the hip and knee joints; the skin of the medial and anterior aspects of the thigh; and quadriceps, sartorius, and pectineus muscles in the anterior compartment of the thigh It is useful for femoral shaft fractures and some advocate use for certain fractures of the neck of femur. The femoral nerve passes under the inguinal ligament where it lies laterally to the femoral artery.	Insert the needle 1 cm below the inguinal ligament and 1 cm lateral to the femoral artery to a depth 3–5 cm. Inject fanning out from this site (aspirating to guard against intravascular injection). Ultrasound guidance is increasingly used for this block. When a regional block needle is used, two 'pops' may be felt (fascia lata, fascia iliacus/pectineus).	10–15 ml of 1% lidocaine (0.5% bupivacaine or 1% prilocaine).
Ankle			
Superficial peroneal nerve	The superficial peroneal nerve supplies the front of the ankle and dorsum of the foot.	Infiltrate local anaesthetic subcutaneously above the ankle joint from the anterior border of the tibia to the lateral malleolus.	For each block use 5 ml of 1% lidocaine or 0.5% bupivacaine, (with or without adrenaline).
Deep peroneal nerve	The deep peroneal nerve supplies the lateral side of the great toe and medial side of the second toe.	Inject above the ankle joint between the tendons of tibialis anterior and extensor hallucis longus.	(NB For multiple blocks be careful to check the maximum dose.)
Saphenous nerve	The saphenous nerve supplies the medial side of ankle.	Infiltrate subcutaneously around the great saphenous vein, anterior and just proximal to the medial malleolus.	
Sural nerve	The sural nerve supplies the heel and lateral side of hind foot.	Infiltrate subcutaneously from lateral border of the Achilles tendon to the lateral malleolus.	
Tibial nerve	The tibial nerve forms the medial and lateral plantar nerves supplying the anterior half of the sole.	Inject medial to the Achilles tendon and level with the proximal edge of medial malleolus, just lateral to posterior tibial artery.	

- Deflate the cuff and record the time.
- Observe the patient and limb closely.
- Arrange follow-up and analgesia.
- In the event of problems, the cuff should be checked, supportive care commenced, and senior help requested. There should be ready access to Intralipid.

3.9.3 Contraindications to Bier's block

- Morbid obesity (cuff unreliable)
- Peripheral vascular disease

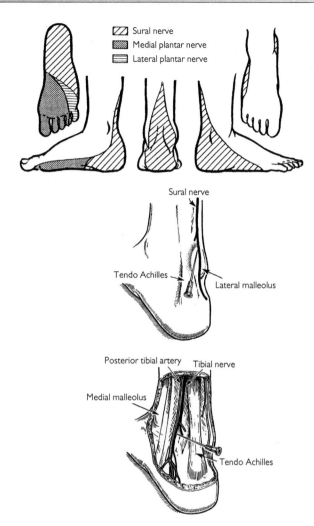

Sural nerve
Medial plantar nerve
Lateral plantar nerve

Sural nerve

Tendo Achilles

Lateral malleolus

Posterior tibial artery   Tibial nerve

Medial malleolus

Tendo Achilles

Figure 3.11 Nerve blocks at the ankle.

Reproduced from Jonathan P. Wyatt, Robin N. Illingworth, Colin A. Graham, Michael J. Clancy, Colin E. Robertson, *Oxford Handbook of Emergency Medicine*, 2006, 'Nerve blocks at the ankle' p. 305, with permission from Oxford University Press.

- Raynaud's disease
- Severe hypertension (> 200 mmHg)
- Scleroderma
- Epilepsy
- Sickle cell disease or trait
- Methaemoglobinaemia
- Monckeberg's calcinosis (visible arterial calcification on X-ray)
- Uncooperative or confused patient
- Procedures needed in both arms
- Allergy to local anaesthetic

- Infection in the limb
- Lymphoedema
- Children—consider on individual basis

3.10 Fascia iliaca block

Fascia iliaca block has similar indications to the traditional femoral nerve block; however, in addition to the femoral nerve it also blocks the lateral cutaneous nerve resulting in improved pain control. It is performed either guided by landmark technique or under ultrasound guidance, and is regarded as good practice in the provision for analgesia in patients with fractures of the femoral neck.

3.10.1 Anatomy

- The femoral and lateral femoral cutaneous nerves lie under the fascia iliaca in their intrapelvic course. The fascia iliaca lies anterior to the iliacus muscle within the pelvis and is bounded superolaterally by the iliac crest.
- The fascia iliaca compartment is a potential space bounded anteriorly by the posterior surface of the fascia iliaca and posteriorly by the anterior surface of the iliacus muscle and the psoas major muscle.

3.10.2 Procedure

- Supine position, with ideally the leg slightly externally rotated and the bed flattened.
- Find line joining anterior superior iliac spine and pubic tubercle: line of inguinal ligament and divide the line into three.
- Find and mark junction of lateral third and medial two-thirds and move 1-2 cm inferiorly (distal) from this point. The puncture site should be 3–4 cm lateral to the femoral artery (see Figure 3.12).

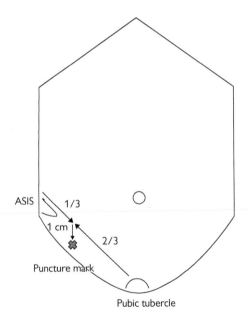

Figure 3.12 Fascia iliaca block landmarks.

- Palpate to ensure not close to the femoral artery.
- 0.5% chlorhexidine in 70% alcohol/povidone-iodine skin prep, sterile gloves, drape area.
- Raise bleb of 1% lidocaine (1–2 ml) at intended skin puncture site, 1–2 cm caudal from the junction of the lateral and middle thirds.
- Pierce skin with a large gauge needle.
- Change to a 22-gauge blunt ended or short-bevelled needle or a 18- or 20-gauge Tuohy-type needle connected via a short extension tube to syringe containing approximately 30–40 ml long-acting local anaesthetic such as bupivacaine (total dose should be calculated as per patients weight, maximum dose for bupivacaine 2 mg/kg).
- Pierce the skin at a right angle to its surface.
- Once through the skin, adjust the needle angle to about 60° directing the tip cranially.
- Keep the needle in the sagittal plane to avoid penetrating the major vessels (medially) and peritoneal cavity (cranially).
- Advance needle, aspirating intermittently, perpendicular to the skin. Two 'pops' will be felt, indicating penetration of the fascia lata followed by the fascia iliaca.
- Reangle needle and syringe to 30° cranially.
- Slowly inject local anaesthetic, aspirating after every 5 ml; there should be no resistance to injection.
- If subcutaneous tissues swell, needle placement is too superficial; resistance to injection indicates needle placement is too deep, within iliacus muscle.
- After injection, withdraw the needle and apply 30 seconds of pressure distal to the injection site to direct the local anaesthetic proximally.

3.10.3 Ultrasound guidance

- Transverse position of transducer: initial setting: depth 3–5 cm; frequency: 10–18 MHz; linear transducer), initially over femoral artery, distal to inguinal crease.
- Identify the femoral artery.
- Move transducer laterally to identify iliacus muscle, fascia iliaca, and fascia lata.
- The fascia iliaca should be identifiable as a bright, continuous, hyperechoic linear structure superficial to the iliopsoas muscle, which passes over the femoral nerve medially to form the lateral wall of the structure surrounding the femoral vessels.
- Raise a skin wheal with a 25 gauge needle.
- Insert the needle in-plane of the ultrasound beam, from the lateral side.
- Two fascial clicks are often perceived as the needle consecutively passes through fascia lata and fascia iliaca.
- After negative aspiration, inject 1–2 ml local anaesthetic to confirm the proper injection plane between the fascia and the iliopsoas muscle.
- A proper injection will result in the separation of the fascia iliaca by the local anaesthetic in the medial-lateral direction from the point of injection. Scanning further cranially after injection of the local anaesthetic shows cranial spread of the injectate within the fascia iliaca compartment.
- In an adult, between 30 to 40 ml of dilute local anaesthetic (0.25–0.375% bupivacaine) is usually required for successful blockade.
- Inject incrementally over 1 ½–2 minutes, aspirating after every 5 ml of administration.

3.10.4 Contraindications

- Patient refusal
- Anticoagulation
- Previous femoral bypass surgery
- Inflammation or infection over injection site
- Allergy to local anaesthetics

KEY POINTS

Nerve blocks are commonly performed in the ED and have advantages over local infiltration including:
- Reduced dose of local anaesthetic
- Avoiding distortion of the anatomy to aid accurate wound closure
- Facilitating procedures otherwise not possible
- Anaesthetizing inflamed or infected tissue where direct infiltration should not be undertaken

A good understanding of anatomy is required to perform nerve blocks and therefore such questions have appeared in previous SAQs because they test anatomy and require knowledge of local anaesthesia.

The Royal College of Emergency Medicine have produced guidance on intravenous regional anaesthesia, making it a possible exam question.

Prilocaine is the only licensed local anaesthetic agent for intravenous regional anaesthesia.

3.11 SAQs

3.11.1 Local anaesthesia

A 24-year-old man presents to the ED with a complex wound to his right index finger after punching a glass window. You decide the wound needs exploration.

a) (i) Describe the technique of a median nerve block. (4 marks)
   (ii) What would be the maximum volume of 1% lidocaine for this man assuming he is 85 kg? Show your calculations. (2 marks)
b) Give three symptoms and three signs of local anaesthetic toxicity? (½ mark per answer, 3 marks)
c) What specific drug should be considered in cases of severe local anaesthetic toxicity? (1 mark)

Suggested answer

a) (i) Describe the technique of a median nerve block. (4 marks)
   Consent and position patient.
   Clean the skin and use an aseptic technique.
   Identify the site of injection—the proximal wrist crease, between the tendons of flexor carpi radialis and palmaris longus.
   Inject 3–5 ml at depth of 10–15 mm using 25 G needle.
   Infiltrate superficially, proximal to the flexor retinaculum for the palmar cutaneous branch.
   Check the block and record the procedure in notes.
   (ii) What would be the maximum volume of 1% lidocaine for this man assuming he is 85 kg? Show your calculations. (2 marks)
   1% lidocaine = 10 mg/ml
   Maximum dose = 3 mg/kg × 85 kg = 255 mg
   Volume = 25.5 ml
   (Accept calculations of 7 mg/kg, if adrenaline used at not more than 1 in 80,000)
   (1 mark for calculation, 1 mark for volume)
b) Give three symptoms and three signs of local anaesthetic toxicity? (½ mark per answer; 3 marks)
   Symptoms:
   - Light headedness
   - Tongue numbness
   - Tinnitus
   - Visual disturbances
   - Circumoral numbness
   - Muscular twitching
   Signs:
   - Confusion
   - Reduced respiratory rate/effort or respiratory arrest
   - Convulsions
   - Cardiovascular collapse hypotension, bradycardia
   - Decreased GCS/coma
   - Tachycardia, if local anaesthetic given with adrenaline
c) What specific drug should be considered in cases of severe local anaesthetic toxicity? (1 mark)
   Intravenous lipid emulsion

3.11.2 Sedation

A 75-year-old woman is brought to the ED with a dislocated right hip prosthesis.
a) What further history should be sought before procedural sedation? (3 marks)
b) (i) Describe the components of the airway assessment that you would perform in any patient before sedation. (3 marks)
   (ii) Why should she be on a tilting trolley for the procedure? (1 mark)
   She is fully recovered from her sedation.
c) What advice should be given on discharge following sedation? (3 marks)

Suggested answer

a) What further history should be sought before procedural sedation? (3 marks)
   - Past medical history—cerebrovascular disease, heart disease, lung disease, renal disease, liver disease
   - Drug history
   - Allergies
   - Fasting status
   - Previous anaesthetics and adverse reactions
   - Use of alcohol/illicit drugs
   - Gastro-oesophageal reflux
b) (i) Describe the components of the airway assessment that you would perform in any patient before sedation. (3 marks)
   L = Look for signs indicative of difficult intubation or ventilation (e.g. abnormal face shape, edentulous, receding mandible, short neck, narrow mouth, obesity)
   E = Evaluate the 3–3–2 rule: three fingers between incisors, three hyoid to chin, two thyroid notch to floor of mouth.
   M = Mallampati—patient sits, mouth fully open, tongue protruding, use light to see how much of hypopharynx is visible.
   O = Obstructing lesions (e.g. tonsils, abscess).
   N = Neck mobility.
   (ii) Why should she be on a tilting trolley for the procedure? (1 mark)
   If she vomits the trolley can be tilted head down to avoid aspiration.
   (Tilt head down in event of hypotension.)
c) What advice should be given on discharge following sedation? (3 marks)
   Be accompanied by a responsible adult.
   Be advised not to drive/operate machinery.
   Be advised not to sign legally binding documents for 24 hours.
   Written advice about aftercare to accompanying adult.
   Avoid alcohol.

Further reading

Difficult Airway Society, 2015. DAS Guidelines. Available at: https://www.das.ac.uk.com [Online].
Mackway-Jones K, Manchester Triage Group. Emergency Triage, 2nd edn. London, UK: BMJ Publishing Group, 2005.
Royal College of Anaesthetists, 2012. Safe Sedation of Adults in the Emergency Department. Available at: https://www.rcoa.ac.uk [Online].

The Association of Anaesthetists of Great Britain and Ireland, 2010. AAGBI Safety Guidelines, 2010. Management of Severe Local Anaesthetic Toxicity. Available at: https://www.aagbi.org [Online].

The Royal College of Emergency Medicine, 2009. Clinical Effectiveness Committee Guideline for Ketamine Sedation of Children in Emergency Departments. Available at: https://www.rcem. ac.uk [Online].

The Royal College of Emergency Medicine, 2013. RCEM Best Practice Guideline: Management of Pain in Children. Available at: https://www.rcem.ac.uk [Online].

The Royal College of Emergency Medicine, 2014. Clinical Standards for Emergency Departments. Available at: https://www.rcem.ac.uk [Online].

The Royal College of Emergency Medicine, 2014. RCEM Best Practice Guideline: Intravenous Regional Analgesia for Distal Forearm Fractures (Bier's Block). Available at: https://www.rcem. ac.uk [Online].

The Royal College of Emergency Medicine, 2014. RCEM Best Practice Guideline: Assessment of Pain in Adults. Available at: https://www.rcem.ac.uk [Online].

World Health Organization. WHO's Pain Relief Ladder. Available at: https://www.who.int/can-cer/palliative/painladder/en/ [Online].

Major trauma

CONTENTS

4.1 Generic principles of trauma management

4.1.1 Introduction

Trauma is a major cause of morbidity and mortality worldwide. It is the leading cause of death in those aged 1–44 years of age.

Trauma management appears in the Royal College of Emergency Medicine curriculum as a 'major presentation' for both adults and children. A detailed knowledge of trauma guidelines, anatomy, and physiology may be assessed in the SAQ.

The same general principles and priorities for trauma management apply to adults and children. This chapter focuses on trauma in adults with the key differences in paediatric trauma covered in Chapter 19, section 19.5. Trauma in pregnancy is covered in Chapter 8, section 8.13.

4.1.2 Trimodal death distribution

The golden hour to definitive trauma care was described by Adams Cowley in 1975, followed by the trimodal distribution of death after trauma by Donald Trunkey in 1982. Death due to injury was felt to occur in one of three peaks: immediate, early, and late:

- First peak—occurs within seconds or minutes of the injury. Deaths are usually due to apnoea due to severe brain injury or high spinal cord injury, or rupture of heart, aorta, or other large vessels. The injuries sustained in this phase are rarely treatable. Only accident prevention can significantly reduce the mortality in this group.
- Second peak—occurs within minutes to several hours following injury. Deaths in this period are usually due to subdural or extradural haematomas, haemopneumothorax, splenic rupture, liver lacerations, pelvic fractures, and/or other multiple injuries associated with significant blood loss. These injuries may be treatable provided rapid assessment and resuscitation occurs.
- Third peak—occurs several days to weeks after the initial injury. Deaths are most often due to sepsis and multiorgan failure. Care provided during each of the preceding periods impacts on the outcome during this stage.

Improvements in trauma care have led to a more bimodal distribution of deaths after trauma, with a progressive flattening out of the late peak. Furthermore, the golden hour is no longer recognized as a fixed time interval but rather as a window of opportunity for reducing morbidity and mortality associated with trauma. The recognition that trauma care is time dependent, with the need for rapid assessment and resuscitation, continues to be emphasized. The concept of a 'platinum ten minutes' refers to the recommended time frame for on-scene stabilization prior to transfer to a trauma centre for definitive care.

4.1.3 Advanced trauma life support

The advanced trauma life support (ATLS) method is the internationally accepted approach to major trauma.

> **EXAM TIP**
>
> The underlying concepts of ATLS are:
>
> - Treat the greatest threat to life first.
> - The lack of a definitive diagnosis should never impede the application of an indicated treatment.
> - A detailed history is not essential to begin the evaluation of a patient with acute injuries.
>
> These concepts resulted in the development of the ABCDE approach. The mnemonic defines the specific, ordered evaluations, and interventions that should be followed in all injured patients:
>
> - **A**irway with cervical spine protection
> - **B**reathing and ventilation
> - **C**irculation with haemorrhage control
> - **D**isability: neurological status
> - **E**xposure/**E**nvironment control: completely undress the patient, but prevent hypothermia
>
> Trauma management consists of a rapid primary survey, resuscitation, a more detailed secondary survey, and, finally, the initiation of definitive care.

The primary survey

The ABCDE approach enables logical patient assessment and sequential treatment priorities to be established. During the primary survey, life-threatening conditions are identified, and management instigated simultaneously.

Candidates often find it difficult to answer trauma questions, not due to a lack of knowledge, but due to difficulty of knowing how to write the answer. The introduction to a question will often give information about interventions or treatments the patient has already received. There are no marks for repeating what you have already been told and writing 'ABCDE' as an answer is unlikely to gain marks. However, certain elements of the 'ABCDE' principle may be relevant to the answer and therefore it is important to read the introduction and question carefully.

A—adequacy of the airway should always be ensured and maintained. Patients should receive high-flow oxygen. Protection of the cervical spine must continue throughout resuscitation. Patients with severe head injuries who have an altered level of consciousness or a Glasgow coma scale score of 8 or less usually require the placement of a definitive airway. Drug-assisted rapid sequence induction (RSI) of anaesthesia and tracheal intubation is the definitive method of securing the airway in patients with major trauma who cannot maintain their airway and/or ventilation. If RSI fails, basic airway manoeuvres and adjuncts and/or a supraglottic airway device should be used until a surgical airway or assisted tracheal placement is performed.

B—ensure adequate oxygenation and ventilation. This may require intubation and ventilation. Life-threatening chest injuries should be identified and managed at this stage (see section 4.2). Chest decompression should only be performed before imaging in a patient with suspected tension pneumothorax if there is haemodynamic instability or severe respiratory compromise. Finger thoracostomy is preferred over needle decompression. In a patient with open pneumothorax, cover the open wound with a simple occlusive dressing and observe for the development of a tension pneumothorax. Immediate chest X-ray and or eFAST (extended focused assessment with sonography for trauma) should be considered as part of the primary survey to assess chest trauma in adults with severe respiratory compromise. Consider immediate computed tomography scanning (CT) for adults with suspected chest trauma without severe signs of respiratory compromise and those responding to resuscitation. In children, chest X-ray (CXR) or eFAST should be first-line imaging (CT is not recommended as first-line imaging in children with chest trauma).

C—priorities for the circulation include controlling obvious haemorrhage, obtaining adequate intravenous or intraosseous access, and assessing tissue perfusion. Rapid reversal of anticoagulation is necessary in patients with major trauma and haemorrhage, guided by haematological advice for those on anticoagulants other than vitamin K antagonists. Fluid resuscitation in trauma is a contentious issue and candidates are often uncertain how much fluid they should give in an answer. ATLS recommends 1–2 L (or 20 ml/kg in children) initial fluid bolus of warmed isotonic electrolyte solution (e.g. 0.9% sodium chloride or Hartmann's). In hospital settings, crystalloids should not be used for patients with active bleeding, instead using a fixed ratio of one unit of plasma to one unit of red cells until laboratory coagulation results are available. Volume resuscitation should be titrated to maintain central circulation until haemorrhage control is achieved. If major haemorrhage is present or suspected, 1G tranexamic acid should be administered as soon as possible. Tranexamic acid should not be used more than three hours after injury in patients with major trauma unless there is evidence of hyperfibrinolysis.

In the case of suspected major haemorrhage, NICE recommend limiting diagnostic imaging such as plain X-ray and eFAST to a minimum needed to direct intervention. In haemodynamically stable patients or those responding to resuscitation with suspected major haemorrhage, immediate CT should be considered.

D—neurological status should be assessed using AVPU and/or Glasgow coma scale (GCS). The prevention of secondary brain injury in head-injured patients is crucial and discussed further in the head injury (section 4.5). A basic neurological assessment should be carried out and documented before RSI wherever possible.

EXAM TIP

The concept of hypotensive fluid resuscitation or permissive hypotension is employed increasingly in trauma management but there is currently no national or international consensus on how much fluid should be given and what the target parameters for vital signs are. A target systolic blood pressure of 70–80 mmHg for penetrating trauma or 90 mmHg after blunt trauma, and an emphasis on blood product-based resuscitation and early definitive control of haemorrhage is suggested.

In the pre-hospital setting, NICE produced guidance in 2016 recommending that injured adults and older children should not be given fluid if a radial pulse is palpable (or, for penetrating torso injuries, if a central pulse can be felt). In the absence of a radial pulse, it is recommended that IV fluid should be administered in boluses of 250 ml until a radial pulse is palpable.

For the purposes of the exam, the ATLS approach to fluid resuscitation should be acceptable.

E—a full examination should be performed and the patient then covered up and kept warm. Hypothermic trauma patients do badly. Normoglycaemia should be maintained. Analgesia must be provided. Consideration for antibiotic and tetanus prophylaxis should occur at this point.

Resuscitation phase

During the resuscitation phase, treatment of life-threatening injuries identified in the primary survey continues. Practical procedures are performed, such as insertion of oro/nasogastric tubes, chest drains, and urinary catheters.

The secondary survey

The secondary survey does not begin until the primary survey is completed, resuscitative efforts are underway, and the normalization of vital functions has been demonstrated. It involves a head-to-toe examination, including a log roll, to identify other injuries. Log-rolling is contraindicated in the presence of a suspected unstable pelvic injury. A full history is obtained. The assessment is accompanied by relevant investigations (e.g. X-rays).

Any deterioration of the patient during the secondary survey necessitates a return to the primary survey and an ABCDE approach.

Repeated clinical assessment and a high index of suspicion are essential if occult injuries are not to be missed. If the secondary survey is not completed prior to the patient leaving the emergency department (ED) (e.g. for an emergency laparotomy), this information must be clearly documented in the notes and the admitting team made aware.

KEY POINTS

The sequence of priorities for assessment of a multiply injured patient is primary survey; resuscitation; adjuncts to the primary survey (e.g. ECG, urinary catheter, oro/nasogastric tube, and arterial blood gas); secondary survey; and definitive care.

The primary survey enables the rapid identification and initial management of life-threatening injuries.

NICE recommends limiting diagnostic imaging in the case if suspected haemorrhage and hemodynamic instability. It also recommends the use of whole body CT in adults with blunt injuries and suspected multiple injuries.

Always read the stem of the SAQ carefully to determine what assessment and treatment the patient has already received and what the next greatest threat to life is. This will enable you to determine the most important management priorities.

4.2 Chest trauma

4.2.1 Introduction

Chest trauma is a significant cause of mortality and common in the multiply injured patient. Hypoxia, hypercarbia, and acidosis often result from chest injuries. Tissue hypoxia results from inadequate delivery of oxygen to the tissues because of hypovolaemia (blood loss), pulmonary ventilation/perfusion mismatch (e.g. contusion, haematoma, and alveolar collapse), and changes in intrathoracic pressure (e.g. tension pneumothorax and open pneumothorax). Hypercarbia most often results from inadequate ventilation caused by changes in intrathoracic pressure relationships and decreased conscious level. Metabolic acidosis is caused by hypoperfusion of the tissues (shock).

4.2.2 Life-threatening chest injuries

Life-threatening chest injuries can be remembered by the mnemonic ATOM FC (see Table 4.1):

- **A**irway obstruction
- **T**ension pneumothorax
- **O**pen pneumothorax
- **M**assive haemothorax
- **F**lail chest and pulmonary contusion
- **C**ardiac tamponade

4.2.3 Other serious chest injuries

The following text includes other serious chest injuries that are included in the curriculum and therefore may appear in an SAQ.

Aortic injuries

- Most commonly caused by blunt deceleration trauma (e.g. RTC or fall from height).
- Any patient surviving to hospital will have a contained or partial aortic rupture.
- Identified by high index of suspicion.
- May have harsh systolic murmur, loss of pulses, differential blood pressures.
- CXR findings include: widened mediastinum; loss of aortic knuckle; altered aortic contour; deviation of trachea and/or nasogastric tube to the right; depression of the left main bronchus; left apical pleural cap; obscuration of the aortopulmonary window; fractures of the first or second rib or scapula.
- Investigation of choice is contrast-enhanced CT scanning of the chest. With a positive CT, the extent of the injury can be further defined with CT angiogram or aortography. Transoesophageal echocardiography is a useful and less invasive diagnostic tool.
- Management is to resuscitate and treat other life-threatening injuries, and refer to a cardiothoracic surgical unit for definitive treatment.

Diaphragmatic rupture

- Blunt trauma may produce a large diaphragmatic injury. Penetrating trauma may cause only a small perforation with the potential for delayed diagnosis.
- More often left-sided.
- Clinical signs and symptoms depend on the size of the defect. Small perforations may be clinically undetectable, large ruptures may produce severe cardiovascular and respiratory compromise. Auscultation may reveal bowel sounds in the thorax.
- CXR may show abdominal contents in the thorax, an elevated hemidiaphragm, or the nasogastric tube in the thorax. Missed diaphragmatic injuries are related to misinterpretations of the CXR as showing an elevated diaphragm, acute gastric dilatation, loculated haemopneumothorax, or subpulmonary haematoma.
- Management is operative repair.

Pulmonary contusion

- Usually the result of blunt trauma; likely to be present if there is a flail segment.
- Pulmonary contusions are commoner in children, with elastic chest walls.
- Presence or absence of associated rib fractures depends on chest wall compliance.
- Respiratory compromise and failure is the main concern.
- CXR changes can be subtle, patchy, and non-specific initially.
- Management is supportive, with intubation and ventilation in the presence of significant hypoxaemia.

Table 4.1 Life-threatening chest injuries

Condition	Causes	Clinical and radiological features	Management
Airway obstruction	Maxillofacial trauma Neck trauma Laryngeal trauma Reduced level of consciousness (e.g. head injury, hypercarbia, hypovolaemia, hypoglycaemia, and so on) Burns	Agitation Hoarseness Noisy breathing Tachypnoea or apnoea Use of accessory muscles/see-sawing of the chest and abdomen Evidence of maxillofacial, neck, or laryngeal trauma Hypoxia/cyanosis	Basic airway manoeuvres with cervical spine control (jaw thrust, suction) Airway adjuncts (oropharyngeal airway, nasopharyngeal airway) Advanced airway manoeuvres (endotracheal intubation) Surgical airway (needle cricothyroidotomy, surgical cricothyroidotomy) High-flow oxygen (Airway management is discussed in more detail in Chapter 3)
Tension pneumothorax	Blunt or penetrating chest trauma Iatrogenic—after central venous line insertion; or mechanical positive pressure ventilation Pathophysiology: a 'one-way valve' air leak occurs from the lung or through the chest wall. Air is forced into the thoracic cavity and is unable to escape, completely collapsing the affected lung The mediastinum is displaced to the opposite side, decreasing venous return, and compressing the other lung	Chest pain Tachypnoea/dyspnoea Hypoxia/cyanosis Hypotension Distended neck veins Surgical emphysema Deviated trachea (away) On the injured side: reduced air entry reduced chest wall movement hyper-resonance	Immediate needle decompression or finger thoracostomy Followed by chest drain insertion
Open pneumothorax	Penetrating chest trauma Blunt trauma with penetrating rib fractures Pathophysiology: when there is a defect in the chest wall >2/3, the diameter of the trachea air will preferentially pass through the defect because the resistance is lower. Effective ventilation is thereby impaired, leading to hypoxia and hypercarbia	Chest pain Tachypnoea/dyspnoea Hypoxia/cyanosis On the injured side: reduced air entry reduced chest wall movement hyper-resonance bubbling or sucking chest wound CXR findings: free lung edge visible hyperexpanded hemithorax	3-sided occlusive dressing over the wound to act as a one-way valve Followed by a chest drain (not through the existing wound)

Table 4.1 Continued

Condition	Causes	Clinical and radiological features	Management
Massive haemothorax (>1500 ml or >⅓ of circulating volume)	Blunt or penetrating chest trauma Pathophysiology: accumulation of blood in the hemithorax can result in hypovolaemia and shock Significant respiratory compromise can also occur due to blood compressing the lung and preventing adequate ventilation	Signs of hypovolaemic shock Chest findings as per open pneumothorax, except percussion note dull CXR findings: fluid level on an erect film on a supine film there is increased shadowing on the affected side (can be confused with pulmonary contusion)	Two large bore IV cannulae and cross match blood Fluid resuscitation as required Chest drain Refer to cardiothoracic team. (Operative intervention should be considered if: >1500 ml out of drain immediately; >200 ml/h for 2–4 hours; or ongoing blood transfusion requirements)
Flail chest	Blunt trauma resulting in two or more ribs being fractured in two or more places Pathophysiology: a segment of the chest wall does not have continuity with the rest of thoracic cage resulting in severe disruption of normal chest wall movement. This, combined with pulmonary contusion, can result in hypoventilation and hypoxia	Paradoxical movement of a section of chest wall (visible or palpable) Hypoxia (mainly due to underlying pulmonary contusion) Hypoventilation (due to pain and/or mechanical insufficiency of the chest wall) Palpable crepitus CXR findings: multiple rib fractures increased shadowing due to pulmonary contusion	Analgesia ± intercostal nerve block Monitor for development pneumo- or haemothorax May require mechanical ventilation for management of hypoxia
Cardiac tamponade	Most often from a penetrating injury Pathophysiology: rapid accumulation of blood in the pericardial sac restricts cardiac filling and contraction. Untreated pulseless electrical activity may ensue	Classic Beck's triad: distended neck veins, muffled heart sounds, and hypotension Kussmaul's sign = JVP elevation with inspiration (spontaneous ventilation) FAST scan or rapid transthoracic echocardiogram will show fluid in the pericardial sac	IV access and fluid resuscitation Pericardiocentesis as a temporizing emergency procedure, preferably with ultrasound guidance Resuscitative thoracotomy is required

Blunt myocardial injury

- Blunt cardiac trauma can result in myocardial contusion, cardiac chamber rupture, coronary artery dissection and/or thrombosis, or valvular disruption.
- Signs and symptoms include chest pain, hypotension, dysrhythmias, and ECG changes, and poor wall motility on echocardiogram. (NB ECG changes may suggest a myocardial infarction and this may have preceded the trauma.) The most common ECG changes are multiple premature ventricular contractions, unexplained sinus tachycardia, atrial fibrillation, bundle-branch block (usually right), and ST-segment changes.
- Cardiac troponins may help to diagnose a suspected myocardial infarction, but are not useful in evaluating blunt cardiac injury.
- Risk of serious dysrhythmia or cardiac failure. Patients with ECG abnormalities or clinical signs of concern should be admitted for cardiac monitoring for 24 hours.

Oesophageal rupture

- Caused by either direct penetration or blunt trauma causing forceful expulsion of gastric contents into the oesophagus.
- Clinical features include surgical emphysema in the neck, and chest/back/neck pain and shock, which are often more than anticipated from the apparent injury.
- The patient should have a normal ECG.
- CXR may show pneumomediastinum, left pleural effusion, or a left pneumothorax.
- Patients should be treated with broad-spectrum antibiotics and referred to a cardiothoracic surgeon for operative repair.

Tracheobronchial injury

- Usually the result of blunt trauma; patients often have severe associated injuries.
- Clinical features include haemoptysis, subcutaneous emphysema, and/or tension pneumothorax.
- Suspect if there is a pneumothorax with a persistent air leak after chest drain insertion.
- The diagnosis is confirmed by bronchoscopy.
- Operative repair is required.
- Interim measures may include selective intubation of the opposite main stem bronchus (although altered anatomy may make intubation very difficult), and the use of more than one chest tube to overcome massive air leak.

Rib fracture

- History of chest wall trauma, usually blunt.
- Chest wall tenderness over affected rib(s).
- Concerning features include multiple rib fractures, flail segment, respiratory compromise, pneumothorax, underlying respiratory disease, and signs of chest infection.
- Fractures of the first and second ribs may be associated with significant associated head, neck, spinal cord, lung, or great vessel injury.
- Fractures of the lower ribs (10 to 12) may be associated with injuries to the liver and spleen.
- Management will vary by patient.
- Discharge home with advice if patient is otherwise healthy with isolated fracture and no concerning features. Advise about the duration of symptoms (four to six weeks), analgesia, supporting the affected area to cough/sneeze, regular deep breaths, and when to seek further medical attention.
- Rib fractures with concerning features may require admission for analgesia, observation, and/or ventilatory support.

Sternal fracture

- Blunt trauma (e.g. from steering wheel in RTC).
- Risk of myocardial contusion, or injury to the great vessels.
- Diagnose clinically (chest pain, localized sternal tenderness with or without palpable step deformity) and with X-ray (chest and lateral sternum views).
- Perform an ECG to look for arrhythmias and ST changes. Consider echocardiogram if concerned about myocardial contusion.
- Only discharge if normal ECG, normal pre-morbid cardiovascular function, and no other injuries.

4.2.4 Imaging in chest trauma

Chest X-ray

CXR is the first-line investigation in the assessment of chest injuries and an adjunct to the primary survey. Ensure you have a system in practice to enable the identification of life-threatening and serious injuries. Some candidates find the ABCDE approach to CXR interpretation helpful:

- **A**—airway. Look at the position and integrity of the trachea and bronchi.
- **B**—breathing. Look at the lung fields for infiltrates that suggest pulmonary contusion, haematoma, aspiration, and so on. Look at the pleural space for abnormal collections of fluid or air.
- **C**—circulation. Look at the mediastinum and heart for evidence of injury. An enlarged cardiac silhouette may suggest a pneumo- or haemopericardium. Aortic rupture can be suggested by: a widened mediastinum; fractures of the first and second ribs; obliteration of the aortic knuckle; deviation of the trachea to the right; presence of a pleural cap; elevation and rightward shift of the right mainstem bronchus; depression of the left mainstem bronchus; obliteration of the space between the pulmonary artery and aorta; deviation of the oesophagus (nasogastric or NG tube) to the right.
- **D**—diaphragm. Look for evidence of elevation, disruption (stomach, bowel gas, or NG tube above the diaphragm), or poor identification (due to overlying fluid or soft tissue masses).
- **E**—everything else. Look at the bony thorax for evidence of fractures (e.g. ribs, sternum, clavicles, scapulae, humerus, and vertebrae). Look at the surrounding soft tissues for evidence of subcutaneous air. Look for evidence of tubes and lines (e.g. endotracheal tube, chest tubes, central venous lines, nasogastric tubes, and other monitoring).

Chest X-rays in trauma are often supine and portable, and the disadvantages of these approaches should be recognized (Table 4.2). If you are struggling to identify abnormalities, use the clinical scenario and mechanism of injury to guide you.

Table 4.2 Disadvantages of chest radiographs in trauma

Supine CXR	Portable CXR
Full inspiration not possible	Supine or semi-supine positioning
Blood flow in upper and lower lungs is equal	Inability to hold a breath, leading to expiratory films
The hemidiaphragms are elevated	
The mediastinum is widened	Artefacts such as bandages, ECG monitoring leads, ventilator tubing
Small pleural effusions lie in the posterior pleural space	Short tube-film distance
Small pneumothoraces move to the anterior pleural space	Lower power output
	Longer exposure times

Pericardial window of focused assessment with sonography in trauma

Focused assessment with sonography in trauma (FAST) is being used more commonly in the ED. FAST scanning is part of the Royal College of Emergency curriculum and is examined as part of higher specialist training, with attainment of level 1 standard a pre-requisite for obtaining a Certificate of Completion of Specialist Training.

Four locations are viewed, looking for the presence of free fluid, which appears black on ultrasound. The four views are:

- Morrison's pouch (between the liver and right kidney)
- Splenorenal angle (between the spleen and left kidney)
- Rectovesical pouch (men), or rectouterine pouch (pouch of Douglas) (women)
- Pericardial sac (a black rim of fluid around the heart suggests a pericardial effusion)

CT chest

Previous MRCEM question

Labelling and identification of abnormalities on a CT thorax has appeared in previous SAQ papers (Figure 4.1).

> **EXAM TIP**
>
> Candidates taking the FRCEM Intermediate exam are expected to be able to identify major traumatic injuries of the head, thorax, abdomen, and spine on CT.
>
> Prior to the exam, it is worth spending a few sessions with a radiologist reviewing such CT abnormalities.

4.2.5 Chest trauma management

The curriculum on chest trauma includes knowledge of needle thoracocentesis and chest drain insertion. These procedures are most likely to be examined in an objective structured clinical examination (OSCE) station but knowledge of the landmarks and complications could appear in a SAQ. Resuscitative thoracotomy is included in the curriculum for higher specialist training

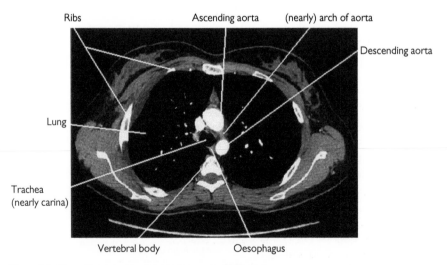

Figure 4.1 Normal chest computed tomography (CT) scan.

(ST4-6) but is not in the ACCS or ST3 curriculum and therefore should not appear in the FRCEM examination.

In the case of traumatic cardiac arrest, resuscitative thoracotomy should be considered for patients with penetrating chest trauma with less than 15 minutes of CPR or blunt trauma and less than 10 minutes CPR. These patients may benefit from release of cardiac tamponade, internal cardiac massage, and cross-clamping of the descending thoracic aorta.

Needle thoracocentesis

Landmarks for needle thoracocentesis:

- Second intercostal space (identified by tracing along from the angle of Louis on the sternum)
- Mid-clavicular line
- On the side of the pneumothorax

Procedure for needle thoracocentesis:

- Clean the skin and instil local anaesthetic if time permits and the patient is conscious.
- Insert a large bore cannula into the skin, direct the needle just above the rib, and into the intercostal space.
- Puncture the parietal pleura.
- Remove the needle, leaving the cannula in place and listen for the sudden escape of air which indicates the tension pneumothorax has been relieved.
- Reassess the patient, who should have improved clinically.
- Leave the cannula *in situ* and secure it in place.
- Insert a definitive chest drain.
- Perform a CXR.

Complications of needle thoracocentesis:

- Bleeding or local haematoma
- Damage to the neurovascular bundle (runs below each rib)
- Re-tension due to tube kinking, dislodging, or failure to progress to a definitive chest drain
- Creation of a pneumothorax
- Lung laceration

Chest drain

Landmarks for chest drain insertion:

- Fifth intercostal space on the side of the pneumothorax or haemothorax. To locate the fifth intercostal space, count down from the angle of Louis. The fifth intercostal space is often the nipple level, but this can be unreliable.
- Just anterior to the mid-axillary line.

Procedure for chest drain insertion:

- Clean and drape the area.
- Anaesthetize the skin, rib periosteum, and pleura.
- Make a transverse 2–3-cm skin incision just above the rib.
- Perform blunt dissection down to and through the parietal pleura.
- Perform a finger sweep to ensure the correct location, to avoid injuring other organs, and to clear any adhesions.
- Insert the thoracostomy tube (32–36 F) into the pleural space.
- Connect to an underwater seal.
- Suture and secure the tube in position.

- Confirm the correct location—tube fogging (may see blood draining in a haemothorax), underwater seal swinging, improvement of air entry on the affected side of the chest, clinical improvement, CXR.

Complications of chest drain insertion:

- Bleeding from intercostal vessels.
- Damage to intercostal nerves.
- Puncture of internal organs (lung or intra-abdominal organs if incorrectly placed).
- Incorrect tube placement.
- Tube dislodging, disconnecting, or kinking.
- Introduction of infection.
- Creation of a haemothorax.
- Subcutaneous emphysema.
- Persistence of the pneumothorax—either due to a poor seal around the tube at the skin, or a large primary leak (consider tracheobronchial disruption).

4.2.6 Indications for cardiothoracic referral

- Haemothorax with >1500 ml of blood initially from the chest drain or >200 ml/hour for 2–4 hours or ongoing blood transfusion requirements.
- Almost any penetrating chest injury.
- Cardiac tamponade.
- Tracheobronchial injury, suggested by massive subcutaneous emphysema and/ or persistent large air leak following chest tube placement.
- Oesophageal injury.

KEY POINTS

Life-threatening chest injuries are: airway obstruction; tension pneumothorax; open pneumothorax; massive haemothorax; flail segment; and cardiac tamponade.

Indications for cardiothoracic referral include: haemothorax >1500 ml of blood initially from the chest drain; or >200 ml/h for 2–4 h; or ongoing blood transfusion requirements; penetrating chest injuries; cardiac tamponade; and tracheobronchial injury.

Resuscitative thoracotomy should be considered in traumatic cardiac arrest in the presence of chest trauma

CXR is part of the trauma series and an adjunct to the primary survey. It should be performed on all multiply injured patients.

CT interpretation of thoracic injuries may appear in a SAQ.

4.3 Abdominal trauma

4.3.1 Introduction

Unrecognized abdominal injury continues to be a cause of preventable death after trauma. Evaluation of the abdomen is challenging and part of the assessment of circulation during the primary survey. Significant amounts of blood may be present in the abdominal cavity with no dramatic change in the appearance or dimensions, and with no obvious signs of peritoneal irritation. Any patient who has sustained significant blunt torso trauma from a direct blow, deceleration, or a penetrating torso injury must be considered to have an abdominal visceral or vascular injury until proven otherwise.

4.3.2 Anatomy of the abdomen

Anatomy questions will predominantly appear in the FRCEM primary exam, however elements of anatomy may be questioned in the Intermediate examination. This is not a complete guide to abdominal anatomy, but provides an overview of the external landmarks and internal anatomy. Such knowledge aids the abdominal assessment in trauma patients.

External anatomy

The anterior abdomen is defined as the area between the trans-nipple line superiorly, the inguinal ligaments and symphysis pubis inferiorly, and the anterior axillary lines laterally.

The flank is the area between the anterior and posterior axillary lines from the sixth intercostal space to the iliac crest.

The back is the area located posterior to the posterior axillary lines from the tip of the scapulae to the iliac crests.

The flanks and back have thick musculature, which acts as a partial barrier to penetrating wounds compared to the thin aponeurotic sheaths of the anterior abdomen.

Internal anatomy

The abdomen can be considered as three distinct regions: the peritoneal cavity; the retroperitoneal space; and the pelvic cavity (containing components of both the peritoneal cavity and retroperitoneal space).

The upper part of the peritoneal cavity is covered by the lower aspect of the bony thorax and contains the diaphragm, liver, spleen, stomach, and transverse colon. As the diaphragm rises to the fourth intercostal space during expiration, fractures of the lower ribs or penetrating wounds below the nipple line may injure abdominal viscera.

The lower part of the peritoneal cavity contains the small bowel, parts of the ascending and descending colons, the sigmoid colon, and, in females, the internal reproductive organs.

The retroperitoneal space contains the abdominal aorta; the inferior vena cava; the duodenum (except the first part); pancreas; kidneys and ureters; the posterior aspects of the ascending and descending colons; and the retroperitoneal components of the pelvic cavity. Injuries to the retroperitoneal visceral structures are difficult to identify clinically because the area is remote from physical examination.

The pelvic cavity, surrounded by the bony pelvis, is essentially the lower part of the retroperitoneal and intraperitoneal spaces. It contains the rectum, bladder, iliac vessels, and, in females, the internal reproductive organs. Examination of pelvic structures is compromised by overlying bones.

4.3.3 Mechanism of injury

Blunt trauma

The most common abdominal injuries in blunt trauma are:

- Spleen (40–55%)
- Liver (35–45%)
- Retroperitoneal haematoma (15%)
- Small bowel (5–10%)

Blunt abdominal trauma is usually caused by road traffic collisions. The mechanism of injury includes:

- Compression, shearing, and crush injuries to abdominal organs. Such forces deform solid and hollow organs leading to rupture, secondary haemorrhage, and peritoneal contamination by spill of visceral contents.
- Deceleration injuries, in which there is differential movement of fixed and non-fixed parts of the body, resulting in lacerations (e.g. the liver and spleen) are largely movable except at the sites of their supporting ligaments, where they are fixed.

Penetrating trauma

Low-velocity wounds

- Low-velocity penetrating trauma, such as stab wounds, cause tissue damage by lacerating and cutting in the track of the wound.
- Stab wounds traverse adjacent abdominal structures and most commonly involve the liver (40%), small bowel (30%), diaphragm (20%), and colon (15%).

High-velocity wounds

- High-velocity penetrating trauma, such as gunshot shot wounds, transfer large amounts of kinetic energy and cause temporary cavitation beyond the track of the missile, causing extensive damage.
- Gunshot wounds may cause additional intra-abdominal damage based on the length of the missile's path through the body, the greater kinetic energy, the possibility of ricochet off bony structures, and the possibility of fragmentation creating secondary missiles.
- Gunshot wounds most commonly involve the small bowel (50%), colon (40%), liver (30%), and abdominal vascular structures (25%).

4.3.4 Specific abdominal injuries

The curriculum includes specific knowledge of blunt splenic, hepatic, renal, pancreatic, hollow viscus, uretheral/bladder, and testicular trauma.

Splenic and hepatic injury

- Most often occur after blunt trauma (e.g. seatbelt injury, direct blow from an assault, or bicycle handlebars).
- If haemodynamically unstable (and unresponsive to initial resuscitation), then operative management is required.
- If haemodynamically normal, then many can be managed conservatively, but depends on each individual case.

Renal trauma

- Usually from direct blunt trauma.
- Loin pain and/or bruising on examination.
- If haemodynamically unstable, then emergency laparotomy is required.
- If haemodynamically stable but evidence of macroscopic haematuria, following blunt trauma, then renal imaging is required (CT is the gold standard).
- If haemodynamically stable and microscopic haematuria, following blunt trauma, patients can be managed conservatively. Urine should be re-checked at one week to ensure resolution. If microscopic haematuria persists, it may be an incidental finding and other causes should be investigated.
- Any haematuria in penetrating trauma requires further renal imaging.
- Haematuria may be absent if there is major anatomical disruption of the ureters or renal vasculature.

Pancreatic trauma

- Usually the result of blunt trauma to the epigastric area.
- Can be extremely difficult to detect.
- Amylase can be non-specific and normal, but a persistently high or rising amylase is suggestive of pancreatic injury. The amylase level can be elevated from non-pancreatic sources.
- Double-contrast CT can detect some, but not all of these injuries initially, but can be repeated after several hours if clinical concern remains.

Hollow viscus injury

- Suggested by clinical findings such as blood from the stomach or rectum, free air on abdominal imaging, and peritonism. The presence of abdominal wall bruising from a seat belt, or a lumbar distraction fracture (Chance fracture) on X-ray may indicate coexisting intestinal injury.
- Findings can be very subtle and diagnosis may therefore be delayed.
- Management depends on the site and size of the injury, as well as any coexistent injuries.

Bladder trauma

- Usually from a direct blow to the lower abdomen with a full bladder, or from pelvic fractures.
- Intraperitoneal bladder ruptures require operative repair.
- Extraperitoneal bladder ruptures may heal with catheter drainage (non-operative management).

Urethral trauma

- Urethral injuries can be classified as those above (posterior) or below (anterior) the urogenital diaphragm.
- Anterior urethral injuries can result from straddle impact to the perineum. Posterior urethral injuries coexist with pelvic fractures and multisystem trauma (e.g. fall astride).
- Suggested by blood or bruising around the urethral meatus.
- Rectal examination may reveal a high-riding prostate in men.
- If suspected, then avoid catheterization.
- Arrange a retrograde urethrogram—if normal, pass a catheter; if extravasation, call an urologist.
- If unable to catheterize, arrange for an ultrasound-guided suprapubic catheter (some urologists prefer this first line to a retrograde urethrogram). Alternatively, a suprapubic catheter can be inserted as an open surgical procedure.

Testicular trauma

- Usually the result of direct trauma to the scrotum.
- Ultrasound can help distinguish between scrotal haematoma, which can often be managed conservatively with good analgesia; and testicular rupture, which requires operative repair.

4.3.5 Investigating abdominal trauma

There are several different techniques to assist in the diagnosis and management of abdominal injuries. FAST scanning and CT both have advantages and disadvantages in the assessment of abdominal trauma, making it an ideal SAQ topic (Table 4.3).

4.3.6 Interpreting CT

As for the chest, CT scans of the abdomen have appeared in SAQs requiring the identification of normal anatomy and injuries. Preparation for this section of the exam is best achieved by looking through scans with a radiologist (Figure 4.2).

4.3.7 FAST scanning

- FAST is a rule-in diagnostic test looking for free fluid in the abdomen but cannot differentiate blood from other fluid and cannot definitively exclude the presence of free fluid.
- The principle behind FAST is that intraperitoneal fluid collects primarily in three dependent regions: peri-hepatic, peri-splenic, and pelvic.
- Free blood appears anechoic or dark. If clotted, it may be the same density as the liver and/or kidney.
- Free fluid usually has a triangular shape when it collects around bowel loops and a linear shape if between liver and kidney.

Table 4.3 Advantages and disadvantages of different abdominal imaging techniques

	FAST	CT
Indications	Blunt abdominal trauma and haemodynamic instability, especially if the patient's abdominal examination is unreliable (e.g. head injury, intoxication, spinal injury, injury to adjacent structures (lower ribs, pelvis), and general anaesthesia)	Haemodynamically normal patient with suspected intra-abdominal injury
Contraindications	Absolute: immediate indication for a laparotomy	Absolute: immediate indication for a laparotomy Allergy to contrast Relative: known renal failure, if contrast is used Uncooperative patient who cannot be safely sedated Haemodynamically unstable patient
Advantages	Non-invasive Can be performed in the resuscitation room No radiation Can be performed by non-radiologists Sensitivity 79–100%, specificity 95.6–100% Quick to perform Can be repeated Can identify pericardial fluid	Non-invasive Sensitivity 92–97.6%, specificity 98.7%. Can perform contrast scans if indicated Can assess the retroperitoneum and pelvis Provides information about specific organ injuries Can image the head, spine, and chest at the same time
Disadvantages	Does not exclude injury. Can only be used to rule-in intra-abdominal fluid, not rule out Requires a minimum amount of fluid (~200 ml) to be present for the scan to be positive Operator dependent Can be difficult in obese or gaseous patients Positive scan does not predict the need for surgery	Involves radiation ± contrast More time-consuming, and therefore less safe in haemodynamically unstable patients Patient has to be transferred out of the ED Can be difficult to identify hollow viscus, diaphragmatic, and pancreatic injuries

- Serial ultrasound examinations should be used to follow patients considered to be at high risk for intra-abdominal injury.
- False positive scans can be caused by fluid-filled structures (IVC, GB, intraluminal bowel fluid), fat (e.g. pericardial fat pad), ascites, and mirror artefact.

4.3.8 Indications for laparotomy

In individual patients, surgical judgement is required to determine the need for laparotomy. The following indications are commonly used to facilitate the decision-making process:

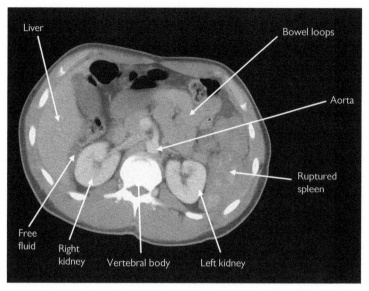

Figure 4.2 Abdominal CT scan showing splenic rupture and free fluid in Morrison's pouch.

- Haemodynamically unstable patient with suspicion of the abdomen as a source of blood loss
- Haemodynamically unstable patient with free fluid on FAST (or CT if they were previously stable)
- Free air on imaging
- Protruding bowel contents (cover with saline soak, do not replace into the abdomen)
- Penetrating abdominal trauma
- Peritonitis

The timing of laparotomy depends on haemodynamic stability and priority of any other injuries.

KEY POINTS

Evaluation of the abdomen is part of the assessment of circulation during the primary survey. Significant amounts of blood may be present in the abdominal cavity with no obvious clinical signs.

Maintain a high index of suspicion for any patient who has sustained significant blunt or penetrating torso trauma.

FAST scanning is used increasingly in the ED management of trauma patients. FAST scanning is indicated in patients who have suspected intra-abdominal injury. It is contraindicated if there is an immediate indication for laparotomy.

CT scanning should only be performed in those patients who do not have haemodynamic instability and do not have an indication for emergency laparotomy.

The indications for emergency laparotomy in trauma include:

- Haemodynamically unstable patient with suspicion of intra-abdominal injury as the source of blood loss
- Haemodynamically unstable patient with free fluid on FAST or CT
- Free air on imaging
- Evisceration
- Penetrating abdominal trauma
- Peritonitis

4.4 Pelvic trauma

4.4.1 Introduction

The pelvis is comprised of the sacrum and innominate bones (ilium, ischium, and pubis), along with many ligamentous complexes. Pelvic fractures are indicative of major forces that the patient has been subjected to. Many vessels lie close to the bones of the pelvis, so there is potential for major blood loss in areas that cannot be reached by direct compression. Pelvic fractures may damage the bladder, the bowel, and associated viscera.

4.4.2 Types of pelvic fracture

There are four patterns of force leading to pelvic fractures (Table 4.4).

4.4.3 Management of pelvic injuries

- Generic trauma management principles apply.
- Assessment of the pelvis occurs during 'C' assessment in the primary survey.
- A pelvic X-ray is part of the trauma series of X-rays and should be performed as an adjunct to the primary survey. Patients should be X-rayed in the resuscitation room to identify fractures.
- Manipulation of the pelvis to determine instability is not recommended.
- The log roll should be delayed until the pelvis has been 'cleared'. Excessive movement may disrupt clots that have formed.
- If a pelvic fracture is identified, the patient should be scooped for transfer and not log rolled.
- Pelvic splinting may be used for unstable fractures to close the increased volume of the pelvis. Specialized commercial splints are available (e.g. SAM sling™, T-POD™). If no splint is available, a sheet can be used as a temporary holding measure. The sheet should be wrapped around the pelvis at the level of the anterior superior iliac spines and the legs internally

Table 4.4 Types of pelvic injury

Type	Cause	Mechanism
Anterior–posterior compression (open book)	Pedestrian or cyclist hit by car Direct crush Fall from height	Disruption of symphysis pubis Pelvis opens anteriorly Sacral ligaments tear Haemorrhage from posterior venous complexes and/or the internal iliac artery
Lateral compression (commonest type)	RTCs (side impact)	Internal rotation of the hemi-pelvis Pubis driven into lower genitourinary tract Volume of the pelvis compressed Life-threatening haemorrhage not common
Vertical shear	High energy (e.g. fall from height)	Force applied in vertical plane across pelvis Sacral ligaments disrupted Major instability
Complex (combination) pattern	Any high-energy injury	Combination of compression and shear forces Combination injuries Very unstable Associated with major bleeding

rotated and secured in this position. The aim is to reduce the volume of the pelvis and allow tamponade of bleeding points.
- The patient should be referred early to the trauma surgeon.
- If the patient is haemodynamically unstable, a laparotomy as well as pelvic fixation may be required.
- Pelvic injuries may be managed operatively (internal or external fixation ± packing) or by interventional radiology (angiography ± embolization).

4.4.4 Sacral fractures

- Sacral fractures can be difficult to identify on X-ray, alignment of the sacral alar and the sacroiliac joints should be carefully assessed.
- Sacral nerve roots may be damaged, so check bladder and bowel function, saddle sensation, and lower limb function.

4.4.5 Acetabular fractures

- These are usually associated with traumatic posterior hip dislocation (e.g. from knees hitting the dashboard in a RTC).
- In major trauma, resuscitate and prioritize other injuries, as required.
- Longitudinal traction of the lower extremity may be useful.
- Massive haemorrhage may be a problem.
- Risk of damage to the sciatic nerve.
- Later problems with arthritis are likely.
- Once the patient is stable, dedicated Judet views (45° oblique) or CT of acetabulum will help guide operative management.

4.4.6 Coccygeal fractures

- May result from a heavy fall on to the bottom.
- Check for rectal tears/damage (refer if present).
- X-ray is rarely required, diagnosis is clinical.
- Majority are managed conservatively with advice (sit on ring cushion) and analgesia.
- If grossly displaced, may require manipulation (with anaesthetic) by orthopaedic team.

KEY POINTS

Pelvic fractures are indicative of a significant mechanism of injury.

Splint the pelvis early and avoid excessive movement or log-rolling to prevent haemodynamic instability.

The four patterns of force leading to pelvic fractures are: anterior–posterior (AP) compression; lateral compression; vertical shear; and complex pattern.

Consider interventional radiology as a treatment option in uncontrolled pelvic haemorrhage.

4.5 Head injury

4.5.1 Introduction

Head injuries are among the most common types of trauma seen in the ED. Although the incidence of head injury is high, the incidence of death from a head injury is low (6–10 per 100,000 population per annum). Of all patients sustaining a head injury, 90% will present with a minor or mild injury (GCS>12) but the majority of the fatal outcomes will be in the moderate (GCS 9–12) or severe (GCS≤8) head injury groups, which accounts for only 10% of attenders. Therefore, EDs are required to see large numbers of patients with minor head injuries and identify the very small number of these that will go on to have serious acute intracranial complications.

Falls (22–43%) and assaults (30–50%) are the most common cause of a minor head injury, followed by road traffic collisions (25%). Road traffic collisions account for a far greater proportion of moderate-to-severe head injuries. Alcohol may be involved in up to 65% of adult head injuries.

4.5.2 Anatomy of the scalp, skull, and brain

The curriculum includes knowledge of the anatomy of the scalp, skull, and brain.

The scalp

The scalp is composed of five layers, which can be remembered by the mnemonic SCALP (Figure 4.3):

Skin
Connective tissue
Aponeurosis
Loose areolar tissue
Periosteum

The skull

- The skull is composed of the cranial vault and the base.
- The skull is thin in the temporal regions, but cushioned by the temporalis muscle.
- The base of the skull is irregular, which may contribute to injury as the brain moves within the skull during acceleration and deceleration.
- The floor of the cranial cavity is divided into three regions: the anterior, middle, and posterior fossae. The tentorium cerebelli divides the head into supratentorial (comprising the anterior and middle fossae) and infratentorial compartments (containing the posterior fossa).
- The anterior fossa contains the frontal lobes.
- The middle fossa contains the temporal lobes.
- The posterior fossa contains the lower brainstem and the cerebellum.

The meninges

The meninges cover the brain and consist of three layers: the dura, arachnoid, and pia (Fig. 4.4). The dura is a tough, fibrous membrane that adheres to the internal surface of the skull. Between the dura and the skull are meningeal arteries; damage to these can result in an extradural haemorrhage. The dura also encloses large venous sinuses, which if damaged can result in an extradural haemorrhage.

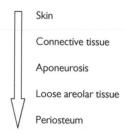

Skin

Connective tissue

Aponeurosis

Loose areolar tissue

Periosteum

Figure 4.3 Layers of the scalp.

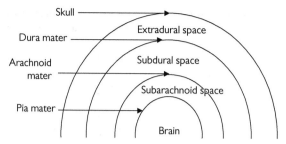

Figure 4.4 The meninges.

Beneath the dura is the arachnoid membrane. The two are not attached and are crossed by bridging veins. Damage to these veins can result in blood accumulating in the potential space between the dura and arachnoid, resulting in a subdural haemorrhage.

The pia is firmly attached to the surface of the brain. Cerebrospinal fluid (CSF) fills the space between the arachnoid and pia, which cushions the brain and spinal cord. Brain contusion or damage to major blood vessels at the base of the brain can result in subarachnoid haemorrhage.

The brain

The brain consists of the cerebrum, cerebellum, and the brainstem.

Cerebrum

- This is composed of right and left hemispheres that are separated by the falx cerebri (a downward dural reflection).
- The left hemisphere contains the language centres in virtually all right-handed people and more than 85% of left-handed people (dominant hemisphere).
- The frontal lobes control executive function, emotions, motor function, and expression of speech (on the dominant side).
- The parietal lobes direct sensory function and spatial orientation.
- The temporal lobes regulate certain memory functions.
- The left temporal lobe (in virtually all right-handed and most left-handed people) is responsible for speech reception and integration.
- The occipital lobe is responsible for vision.

Cerebellum

- Responsible for coordination and balance.

Brainstem

- Composed of midbrain, pons, and medulla.
- The midbrain and upper pons contain the reticular activating system.
- The medulla contains vital cardiorespiratory centres.

The ventricular system

- The ventricles are a system of CSF-filled spaces and aqueducts within the brain.
- The choroid plexus in the lateral and third ventricles produces CSF at a rate of 20 ml/hour.
- CSF circulates from the lateral ventricles through the foramen of Monro, the third ventricle, and the aqueduct of Sylvius into the fourth ventricle in the posterior fossa.

- CSF exits the ventricular system from the fourth ventricle into the subarachnoid space and the spinal cord. It is reabsorbed through arachnoid granulations that project into the superior sagittal sinus.
- Blood in the CSF may impair reabsorption, resulting in increased intracranial pressure (ICP) and enlarging ventricles (post-traumatic communicating hydrocephalus).
- Oedema and mass lesions may cause effacement of the usually symmetrical ventricles.

4.5.3 Physiology

Intracranial pressure

The skull is a rigid box, and its contents incompressible; therefore, the ICP depends on the volume of the intracranial contents: blood, CSF, and brain tissue. The ICP normally varies between 5 and 12 mmHg. Elevation of ICP may reduce cerebral perfusion and cause or exacerbate ischaemia.

The Monro–Kellie doctrine

The Monro–Kellie doctrine states that, because the volume of the skull is fixed, any increase in the volume of one of its contents (e.g. an expanding haematoma) has to be compensated for by a corresponding volume reduction of another of those contents, usually CSF in the first instance.

- 'Compensated' state—initially volumes of blood and CSF are able to be shunted out of intracranial cavity, so the ICP rises slowly.
- 'Decompensated' state—a critical point is reached when compensatory mechanisms are exhausted and an exponential rise in ICP occurs for minimal rises in volume.

Cerebral blood flow

The cerebral blood flow is autoregulated in healthy adults. This maintains a constant cerebral blood flow between mean arterial pressures (MAP) of 50–150 mmHg. In patients with chronic hypertension, these limits are raised.

The precapillary cerebral vasculature is able to reflexively constrict or dilate in response to changes in cerebral perfusion pressure (CPP); this is known as pressure autoregulation. There is also chemical autoregulation. Hypocapnia results in cerebral vasoconstriction and a reduction in cerebral blood flow. Hypercapnia increase cerebral blood flow by cerebral vasodilatation. The greatest effect is at normal $PaCO_2$ where a change of 1 kPa results in a 30% change in blood flow. Oxygen tension has minimal effect on cerebral blood flow until PaO_2 <6.7 kPa when cerebral vasodilatation occurs.

In severe traumatic brain injury, the normal autoregulation may be lost, and the CPP becomes proportional to the difference between the mean arterial pressure and the intracranial pressure (i.e. CPP ≈ MAP—ICP). In the presence of raised ICP, the MAP may increase in order to maintain CPP (Cushing's reflex).

CPP should ideally be maintained ≥70–80 mmHg, the critical level for cerebral ischaemia is thought to be 30–40 mmHg. To achieve this, most clinicians aim for a MAP≥90 mmHg and try to avoid unnecessary increases in ICP.

Clinical features of increased intracranial pressure

- Vomiting, headache, irritability.
- Seizures.
- Reducing GCS.
- Cushing's triad—hypertension, bradycardia, irregular respirations.
- Focal neurology.
- Dilated pupil and contralateral hemiparesis—uncal herniation causes compression of the third cranial nerve against the tentorium cerebelli, resulting in loss of parasympathetic supply to the

ipsilateral eye and unopposed sympathetic activity dilating the pupil; in addition, compression of the corticospinal tract in the midbrain results in contralateral weakness.

4.5.4 Imaging in head injuries

CT scanning is the recommended imaging in head-injured patients. NICE have produced guidance on when CT scanning is indicated. Plain X-rays of the skull are not recommended unless as part of a skeletal survey in children presenting with suspected non-accidental injury. Head injury in children is covered in Chapter 19, section 19.5.

Consideration should always be made about possible associated neck injuries. The management and investigation of suspected neck injuries is discussed in section 4.6.

NICE guidance 2014 on CT head scan in adults

Previous MRCEM question

Indications for a CT scan and result within one hour from request:

- GCS <13 on initial assessment in ED
- GCS <15 in ED at 2 hours post-injury
- Suspected open/depressed skull fracture
- Signs of base of skull fracture (haemotympanum, panda/racoon eyes, CSF leak from ears or nose, Battle's sign or mastoid bruising)
- Post-traumatic seizure
- Focal neurological deficit
- >1 episode of vomiting

A provisional written radiology report should be available within one hour of scan.

Scan within eight hours of injury for:

Adults with any of the following risk factors who have experienced some loss of consciousness or amnesia since the injury:

- Age ≥65
- History of bleeding or clotting disorder
- >30 minutes retrograde amnesia (for events before impact)
- Dangerous mechanism of injury (pedestrian or cyclist struck by a motor vehicle; occupant ejected from a motor vehicle; fall from >1 m or five stairs)
- Warfarin therapy (irrespective of INR)

A provisional written radiology report should be available within one hour of scan.

EXAM TIP

SIGN (http://www.sign.ac.uk) have also produced guidelines on head injury management in May 2009. They are similar, but not identical, to the NICE guidance. It is not necessary to know both guidelines, knowledge of one is sufficient for the exam.

4.5.5 CT head scan appearances

Candidates for the FRCEM Intermediate exam are expected to know the CT appearance of common head injuries (Table 4.5 and Figure 4.5):

- New blood on CT looks white.
- Older blood becomes a similar shade of grey to brain tissue.

Table 4.5 Types of intracranial injuries

Extradural haemorrhage (EDH)	Biconvex
	Cannot cross skull suture lines
	Commonly temporoparietal—usually middle meningeal artery
	Good prognosis with early treatment
	'Lucid' interval in one-third of patients—can be minutes or hours
Subdural haemorrhage (SDH)	Uniconvex
	Most common focal lesion
	Venous bleed (from bridging dural veins)
	Can be acute (RTC, NAI) or chronic (elderly, alcoholics, warfarin, i.e. frequent falls with cerebral atrophy and/ or increased bleeding potential)
	Acute-on-chronic: acute is whiter; chronic is nearly the same shade of grey as brain tissue. Often able to visualize a line demarcating the two ages of blood
Subarachnoid haemorrhage (SAH)	Blood in subarachnoid space (i.e. around the brain—blood conforms to sulci and gyri), and in ventricles (wherever CSF goes)
	Due to tearing of small leptomeningeal arteries and veins.
	Prognosis better in traumatic rather than spontaneous SAH
Pneumocephalus	Black 'spots' or patches around edge of the brain
	Indicates communication from outside to inside (i.e. fracture of either sinus or skull)
Intracerebral haematoma	Looks white when acute
	Size will often cause midline shift (mass effect)
	Location and size determines neurological signs and treatment
	If in posterior fossa, then evacuation more likely to be required
Cerebral contusion	Small bleeds = white spots on CT
	Can be subtle
	Often frontal/temporal due to impact of brain tissue with orbital plates or sphenoid ridge
	Often associated with SDH
Diffuse axonal injury	Often very little to see on scans initially. May be pinpoint haemorrhages in corpus callosum and lateral brainstem due to capillary rupture
	Widespread, severe white matter injury
	Shear strains in acceleration/deceleration injury causes severing of neuronal axons
	Commonest cause of a persistent vegetative state

- Air on a CT scan looks black and is the same density as whatever is around the outside of the skull.

Scheme for CT head scan interpretation:

- Adequacy: all slices included; correct windows; no head tilt
- Presence or absence of midline shift

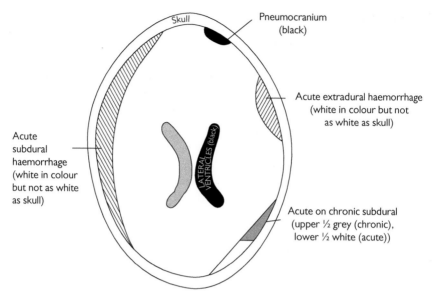

Figure 4.5 CT appearance of different intracranial injuries.

- Symmetry of the two halves of the cranium
- Cross-sectional anatomy
  Brain tissue: grey-white junction; parenchymal lesions or distortion
  CSF spaces: ventricles; sulci; fissures; basilar cisterns
  Skull and surrounding tissues: scalp swelling; fractures; fluid in sinuses, orbits
- Subdural windows: blood collections adjacent to skull
- Bone windows: calvarium; skull base; orbits and sinuses; intracranial air

Features of mass effect:

- Unilateral: midline shift; ipsilateral ventricular compression; contralateral ventricular dilatation
- Bilateral: effacement of the sulci; ventricular compression (ventricular size less than expected for age)

4.5.6 Management principles for preventing secondary brain injury

- Primary brain injury occurs during the initial trauma and results from the displacement of physical structures of the brain. The only way to significantly reduce such injuries is with accident prevention.
- Secondary brain injury occurs after the initial insult. Many factors are involved in secondary brain injury and are potentially preventable or treatable.
- Causes of secondary brain injury include: hypoxia; hypovolaemia and cerebral hypoperfusion; hypercapnia; intracranial haematoma with localized pressure effects and increased ICP; cerebral oedema; hyperthermia; seizures; and infection.
- The focus of ED management in head-injured patients is the prevention and treatment of secondary brain injury (Table 4.6).

In individuals with an acute neurological deterioration in the presence of head injury (dilated pupil, dropping GCS, hemiparesis). The use of mannitol or hypertonic saline should be considered to temporarily reduce ICP while awaiting definitive management.

Table 4.6 ABCDE approach to the prevention of secondary brain injury

A and B	Ensure adequate oxygenation (NICE recommend PaO_2>13 kPa)
	Aim for $PaCO_2$ in normal range (NICE recommend $PaCO_2$ 4.5–5 kPa)
	Intubate and ventilate as required to achieve these aims
	Tape the endotracheal tube in place rather than tie it (avoids increases in ICP)
	Avoid excessive intrathoracic pressures to avoid an increase in ICP
C	Maintain end organ perfusion (NICE recommend MAP≥80 mmHg)
	Use urine output as indicator of adequate renal perfusion
D	Maintain normoglycaemia
	Treat seizures (benzodiazepines, prophylactic phenytoin)
	Position—consider 30° head-up tilt to help reduce ICP
	Avoid cervical collars/compression if possible to avoid increased ICP
	Monitor for signs of neurological deterioration
	Neurosurgeons may insert an ICP bolt to measure pressures
	Consider mannitol on specialist advice
E	Pain management to avoid increases in ICP
	Temperature control (aim for normothermia)
	Infection control—wound management; consider need for tetanus booster/ immunoglobulin and antibiotics

A bolus of mannitol 1g/kg (usual strength 20%—20 g in 100 ml solution) should be administered over 10 minutes to euvolaemic individuals. Mannitol should not be given to hypotensive patients as it may exacerbate hypovolaemia and thus exacerbate cerebral ischaemia. Hypertonic (3%) saline is thus preferred in hypotensive patients.

4.5.7 Indications for referral to/discussion with neurosurgery

- 'New, surgically significant abnormalities on imaging' (NICE states that the exact definition of 'surgically significant' should be developed locally)
- Persisting coma (GCS ≤8) after initial resuscitation
- Unexplained confusion >4 hours
- Deterioration in GCS after admission
- Progressive focal neurological signs
- Seizure without full recovery
- Penetrating injury (definite or suspected)
- CSF leak

4.5.8 Admission criteria for head injuries (NICE)

- CT with clinically significant abnormalities
- GCS not returned to normal
- Awaiting scan
- Continued clinical concern (e.g. vomiting)
- Other ongoing concerns (e.g. intoxication, other injuries, suspected non-accidental injury (NAI), and so on)

Recommended observations of head-injured patients

The following observation should be recorded:

Table 4.7 The Glasgow coma scale

Eye opening (E)		Verbal response (V)		Best motor response (M)	
				6	Obeys commands
		5	Orientated	5	Localizes pain
4	Spontaneously	4	Confused	4	Withdraws from pain
3	To speech	3	Inappropriate words	3	Abnormal flexion
2	To pain	2	Incomprehensible sounds	2	Extension to pain
1	None	1	None	1	None

GCS score = (E + V + M); best possible score = 15; worst possible score = 3.

Reprinted from *The Lancet*, volume 304, issue 7872, Graham Teasdale, Bryan Jennett, *Asessment of coma and impaired consciousness*, A Practical Scale, pp.81–84, Copyright (1974), with permission from Elsevier

- GCS (see Table 4.7)
- Pupil size and reactivity
- Limb movements
- Respiratory rate
- Heart rate
- Blood pressure
- Temperature
  - Oxygen saturations

NICE recommend the following frequency of observations:

- Half-hourly until GCS 15
- Then half-hourly for two hours
- Then hourly for four hours
- Then two-hourly

4.5.9 Discharge advice for head injuries

Verbal and written advice should be given to all patients discharged following a head injury. Advice should be appropriate to the age and language of the patient/carer. If patients have had a CT scan, they should have follow-up arranged with their GP within one week.

Discharge advice should include symptoms that the patient/carer should observe for and return to the ED if they develop (Box 4.1). There should also be a section describing symptoms of post-concussional syndrome and where to get help if these are persistent.

KEY POINTS

Primary brain injury occurs at the time of the injury.

Secondary brain injury occurs later, due to various problems which commonly coexist.

ED management should focus on the early identification of significant brain injury and the prevention of secondary insults.

An ABCDE approach can be used to ensure adequate resuscitation of a brain injured patient to minimize secondary insults.

The NICE guideline details the indications for a CT head scan. These indications have appeared in several previous MRCEM examinations.

Box 4.1 Discharge advice for head-injured patients

Return to the ED if any of the following develop:

- Unconsciousness or lack of full consciousness
- Any confusion
- Any drowsiness that goes on for longer than one hour when you would normally be wide awake
- Any problems understanding or speaking
- Any loss of balance or problems walking
- Any weakness in one or both arms or legs
- Any problems with your eyesight
- Very painful headache that will not go away
- Any vomiting
- Any fits (collapsing or passing out suddenly)
- Clear fluid coming out of your ear or nose
- Bleeding from one or both ears
- New deafness in one or both ears

4.6 Spinal trauma

4.6.1 Introduction

Vertebral column injury, with or without neurological deficits, should always be considered in patients with multiple injuries. ATLS management involves cervical spine protection as part of the management of airway. As long as the patient's spine is protected, evaluation for spinal injury may be safely deferred, especially in the presence of systemic instability, such as hypotension and respiratory inadequacy.

Approximately 55% of spinal injuries occur in the cervical region, 15% in the thoracic region, 15% at the thoracolumbar junction, and 15% in the lumbosacral area. Approximately 10% of patients with a cervical spine fracture have a second, non-contiguous vertebral column fracture.

4.6.2 Anatomy of the spine

Spinal column
The spinal column consists of:

- Seven cervical vertebrae
- Twelve thoracic vertebrae
- Five lumbar vertebrae
- Sacrum
- Coccyx

Spinal cord anatomy
The spinal cord originates at the caudal end of the medulla oblongata at the foramen magnum. It ends around the level of L1 as the conus medullaris. Below this level is the cauda equina.

Three tracts in the spinal cord can be assessed clinically. These are: the corticospinal tract; the spinothalamic tract; and the posterior columns (Table 4.8 and Figure 4.6).

- Complete spinal cord injury—is the loss of all motor and sensory function below the level of the lesion. This diagnosis cannot be made acutely because of the possibility of spinal shock.

Table 4.8 Spinal cord tracts

	Corticospinal tract	Spinothalamic tract	Dorsal columns
Functions carried in the tract	Motor	Pain Temperature Light touch sensation	Vibration sense Proprioception Light touch sensation
Where it crosses the midline	Between the cord and brainstem	Immediately on entering the cord	Brainstem/medulla
Where it runs in the cord	Posterolaterally	Anterolaterally	Posteriorly
Result of spinal cord injury	Ipsilateral loss of motor function	Contralateral loss of pain and temperature sensation	Ipsilateral loss of vibration sense and proprioception

- Partial (incomplete) spinal cord injury—varies from near complete to near normal function. Initially, sparing of sensation in the perianal region (sacral sparing) may be the only sign of residual function.
- Neurological level—is the most caudal level with normal sensory and motor function (power 3/5 or greater) bilaterally.

4.6.3 Clinical features of spinal cord injury

Clinical signs of a spinal cord injury include:

- No movement/loss power
- Absent sensation
- Flaccid reflexes
- Lax anal sphincter
  - Priapism (early and short-lived)

Dermatomes and myotomes

Previous MRCEM question

Knowledge of the dermatomes and myotomes enables an initial assessment of the level of injury (Table 4.9). Such knowledge has been tested in previous part B and C examinations.

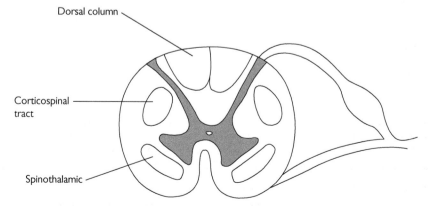

Figure 4.6 Anatomy of the spinal cord tracts.

Table 4.9 Nerve root values for assessing motor and sensory function, and reflexes

Motor		Sensory	
C5	Deltoid/shoulder abduction (elbow flexion)	C5	Deltoid
C6	Wrist extension	C6	Thumb
C7	Elbow extension	C7	Middle finger
C8	Finger flexion (middle finger FDP)	C8	Little finger
T1	Finger adduction	T4	Nipple
		T8	Xiphisternum
L2	Hip flexion	T10	Umbilicus
L3	Knee extension	T12	Symphisis pubis
L4	Ankle dorsiflexion	L1	Groin
L5	Great toe extension (EHL)	L2	Medial proximal thigh
S1	Ankle plantarflexion	L3	Knee
		L4	Medial shin/calf
		L5	Dorsum foot first web space
		S1	Around calcaneum
		S2	Posterior thigh
		S3	Ischial tuberosity
		S4/5	Perianal
			Kneel on L3
			Stand on S1
			Sit on S3

Reflexes	
C5/6	Biceps
C7/8	Triceps
L3/4	Knee
S1/2	Ankle

The sensory level is the lowest dermatome with normal sensory function and can often be different on the two sides of the body.

The motor level is defined as the lowest key muscle that has a power grade of at least 3/5. Each segmental nerve root innervates more than one muscle and most muscles are innervated by more than one nerve root. However, for assessment of myotomes, certain muscles are identified as representing a single spinal nerve segment.

Muscle power is graded on a six-point scale:

- 5 = normal power
- 4 = movement possible against gravity and some resistance
- 3 = movement possible against gravity
- 2 = movement possible when gravity excluded

Table 4.10 Spinal cord syndromes

Brown–Séquard syndrome	Caused by transection of the lateral half of the cord (e.g. bullet/stab wound)
	Ipsilateral upper motor neurone weakness
	Ipsilateral loss of vibration sense, proprioception, and joint position sense
	Contralateral loss of pain and temperature sensation, often 1–2 levels lower
Central cord syndrome	Most often seen in the older population, due to hyperextension injuries of the neck
	May not have a fracture on X-ray
	Thought to be caused by vascular compromise of the cord in the distribution of the anterior spinal artery (supplies the central cord)
	Motor weakness in the arms is greater than the legs (motor fibres of the arms lie more centrally in the cord)
	Variable sensory loss. Often described as suspended, 'cape-like'
	Upper limb areflexia
	Horner's syndrome
Anterior cord syndrome	Usually caused by vascular insufficiency (anterior spinal artery) due to disc herniation or tumour
	Paraparesis bilaterally
	Loss of pain and temperature bilaterally
	Preserved dorsal column function (proprioception and vibration)

- 1 = flicker of contraction possible
- 0 = complete paralysis*

Spinal cord syndromes

Certain characteristic patterns of neurological injury are frequently seen in patients with spinal cord injuries. Spinal cord syndromes are more common in exams than in real life (Table 4.10). They are easier to remember if you understand the anatomy of the tracts (see Table 4.8).

Neurogenic shock

Neurogenic shock is secondary to loss of sympathetic outflow (sympathetic chain originates from T1 to L2). Patients lose their vascular tone and become hypotensive resulting in end organ hypoperfusion.

Signs and symptoms of neurogenic shock include:

- Hypotension, bradycardia (or lack of appropriate tachycardia)—vagal tone dominates
- Flaccid paralysis
- Priapism
- Preserved anocutaneous and bulbocavernosus reflexes
    - Abdominal breathing if loss of diaphragmatic innervations (C3, 4, 5—phrenic nerve)

Patients with hypotension secondary to neurogenic shock may not respond to fluid resuscitation alone. Therefore, if active haemorrhage has been excluded and the patient is persistently hypotensive, despite 2 L of fluid, the possibility of neurogenic shock should be considered.

Overzealous fluid resuscitation may result in pulmonary oedema. Vasopressors may be required.

* Used with the permission of the Medical Research Council.

Spinal shock

Spinal shock refers to the flaccidity (loss of muscle tone) and absence of reflexes following a spinal cord injury. The 'shock' to the injured cord may make it appear completely non-functional, although all areas are not necessarily destroyed. It may last hours, days, or months, and can recover:

- Anocutaneous and bulbocavernosus reflexes are the first to return.
- Anocutaneous = scratch perianal skin ® anal contraction ('anal wink') (S4, 5 roots).
- Bulbocavernosus = squeeze glans penis ® bulbocavernosus contraction (S2, 3, 4 roots).

Autonomic dysreflexia

This is a medical emergency in patients with established spinal cord injuries. It is only seen in those with paraplegia higher than T6, or tetraplegia. It only occurs once reflexes begin to return.

A stimulus below the level of the spinal cord injury (e.g. noxious stimulus, blocked urinary catheter) causes imbalanced sympathetic discharge resulting in severe, sudden hypertension, headache, sweating, flushing, and/or mydriasis.

Management:

- Treat any identifiable stimulus, such as a blocked catheter, need for defecation, focal infection, or long-bone fracture.
  - Control blood pressure with nifedipine or nitrates (something with rapid onset and short duration).

4.6.4 Spinal imaging

There are well-recognized guidelines and clinical decision rules to assist in the imaging of the cervical spine. The same guidance does not exist for the thoracic and lumbar spine. Imaging of these regions should be based on knowledge of the mechanism of injury and the clinical assessment (back pain, bony tenderness, conscious level, associated injuries, and neurological findings).

Cervical spine imaging

There are several guidelines that are commonly used in EDs to guide imaging of patients with potential cervical spine injuries: the National Emergency X-Radiography Utilization Study (NEXUS) guidance; the Canadian C-spine rules; and the 2007 NICE clinical guidance.

In 2010, the Royal College of Emergency Medicine produced guidelines on the management of alert, adult patients with potential cervical spine injury. It includes guidance for those sustaining blunt or penetrating injuries, and recommends the type of imaging patients should have. The guidance incorporates elements of NEXUS, Canadian C-spine rules, and NICE guidance. Section 4.6.5 is based on the recommendations from the Royal College of Emergency Medicine.

4.6.5 NICE recommendations for cervical spine imaging

Blunt neck injury

Cervical spine imaging should be requested for the following patients that have been subjected to blunt trauma with a mechanism that may have injured the neck:

- GCS<13 on initial assessment in the ED
- Focal peripheral neurological deficit
- Paraesthesiae in upper or lower limbs
- Plain X-rays technically inadequate, or suspicious/definitely abnormal
- Urgent requirement to identify a cervical spine fracture (e.g. prior to surgery)
- Alert and stable patient:
  - aged 65 or greater
  - dangerous mechanism of injury
  - other body areas scanned for head injury or multiorgan trauma

Box 4.2 High-risk factors for a cervical spine injury (dangerous mechanisms of injury)

- A fall from greater than 1 m or five stairs
- An axial load to the head (e.g. diving)
- A high-speed motor vehicle collision (combined speed >60 mph)
- A rollover motor vehicle accident
- Ejection from a motor vehicle
- An accident involving motorized recreational vehicles
- A bicycle collision

Reproduced with kind permission of the Royal College of Emergency Medicine

If the patient has no high-risk factor and any of the low-risk factors (Box 4.3) then the collar can be removed and their range of movement assessed. If they can actively rotate their neck 45° to the left and right, then cervical spine imaging is not required because a 'significant' injury is excluded.

Patients unable to rotate their neck 45° in both directions, or those reporting severe pain (≥7/10 severity) on doing so, should have cervical spine imaging performed.

Penetrating neck injury

Neck immobilization is not required for patients with isolated gunshot wounds to the head, unless the bullet path traverses the neck.

Cervical spine immobilization is recommended for patients with gunshot wounds to the neck, given the association with direct spinal destruction in a proportion of patients. However, this should not take precedent over life-threatening airway and haemorrhage control.

Neck immobilization is not required for a patient with an isolated stab wound to the neck, even if a neurological deficit is identified. The fitting of a cervical collar in this setting may be associated with an increased mortality.

Primary imaging modality

CT should be used as the primary imaging modality for excluding cervical spine injury in adults following blunt trauma, if any of the following criteria are met:

- GCS below 13 on initial assessment
- Intubated patients
- Inadequate plain film series
- Suspicion or certainty of abnormality on plain film series
  - Patients being scanned for head injury or multiregion trauma

Box 4.3 Low-risk factors for a cervical spine injury

Low-risk factors for a cervical spine injury:

- Simple rear-end motor vehicle collision (but not if pushed into another vehicle, or if hit at high speed or by a large vehicle)
- Sitting position in ED
- Ambulatory at any time since injury
- Delayed onset of neck pain (i.e. not immediate)
- Absence of midline cervical spine tenderness

Reproduced with kind permission of the Royal College of Emergency Medicine

As a minimum, the CT should cover the area from the craniocervical junction to the thoracocervical junction, since selective scanning has been shown to miss injuries.

It is also recommended that CT be used as the primary imaging modality in the following settings:

- Patients with dementia (or a chronic disability precluding accurate clinical assessment)
- Patients with neurological signs and symptoms referable to the cervical spine
- Patients with severe neck pain (≥7/10 severity)
- Patients with a significantly reduced range of neck movement (i.e. unable to actively rotate the neck 45° in both directions)
  - Patients with known vertebral disease (e.g. ankylosing spondylitis, rheumatoid arthritis, spinal stenosis, or previous cervical surgery)

In the absence of an indication for CT, three-view plain radiographs (lateral, anteroposterior, and peg) should be used as the primary imaging modality for excluding cervical spine injury.

Advanced imaging

MRI should be used to exclude cervical spine injury in adults following blunt trauma if any of the following criteria are met:

- Neurological signs and symptoms referable to the cervical spine
  - Suspicion of vertebral artery injury (e.g. spinal column displacement, foramen transversarium or lateral process fracture, posterior circulation syndromes)

MRI should always be used in conjunction with another modality, preferably CT, in order not to miss bony injuries.

Flexion–extension views are not recommended because they cannot reliably exclude unstable cervical spine injuries in the acute setting.

Patients with injuries identified on MRI should be discussed with a spinal surgeon.

4.6.6 Interpreting cervical spine radiographs

ATLS recommend the ABCDs method of assessing cervical spine X-rays:

- Adequacy—ensure all seven of the cervical vertebrae and the superior aspect of T1 are visible.
- Alignment—four lines should be identified: the anterior vertebral line; the anterior spinal line; the posterior spinal line; and the spinous processes.
- Bones—each vertebra should be examined for height and integrity of the bony cortex. The facet joint and spinous processes should be examined.
- Cartilage—the disc spaces should examined for narrowing or widening.
- Dens—the peg should be assessed in all three views for symmetry and integrity of the bony cortex.
  - Soft tissues—the pre-vertebral soft tissues should be no wider than 7 mm at C3 (½ a vertebral body width) and no wider than 3 cm at C7 (a full vertebral body width).

Of patients with a spinal fracture or dislocation at one level, 10% have a non-concordant second fracture. Therefore, if one spinal injury is identified, the whole spine should be imaged.

Eponymous fractures

- Jefferson's = burst fracture of C1.
- Hangman's = fracture of the pedicles of C2.
- Clay shoveller's = avulsion of the tip of spinous process C7.
- Chance fracture = horizontal vertebral body fracture and its spinous process. Often occurs in the lumbar spine of a car passenger wearing only a lap-belt for restraint.

4.6.7 Emergency department management of spinal injuries

The main role of the ED in spinal injuries is a high index of suspicion of a potential injury and immobilization of the spine until an injury is excluded. Patients deemed at risk of a spinal injury should have their neck immobilized and be maintained in a neutral position; three-point immobilization of the neck is recommended (collar, head blocks, and tape). If a patient has pre-existing vertebral anatomical abnormalities (e.g. ankylosing spondylitis), they should have their necks immobilized in a position of comfort. In such cases, the use of a collar is not compulsory and may be detrimental.

If a patient is agitated and unable to cooperate with immobilization, then every effort should be made to relieve the cause of the agitation (e.g. pain management; correction of hypoxia, hypovolaemia, or hypoglycaemia; enabling the patient to pass urine). The patient should not be forcibly restrained by neck immobilization because this is likely to cause more harm. If necessary the patient may require sedation, intubation, and ventilation.

The use of a spinal board is for transport purposes only. Once the patient arrives in the ED, they should be removed from the board as soon as possible due to the risk of pressure sores developing. Patients should be log rolled for removal from the board and examination of the back. A log roll, in an adult, requires at least four people and the spine should be kept in neutral alignment.

Assessment of spinal immobilization is most likely to occur in the part C examination.

KEY POINTS

The three tracts in the spinal cord that can be assessed clinically are: the corticospinal tract; the spinothalamic tract; and the posterior columns.

The sensory level is the lowest dermatome with normal sensory function.

The motor level is the lowest muscle group that has a power grade of at least 3/5.

Neurogenic shock is secondary to loss of sympathetic outflow.

Spinal shock refers to the flaccidity and absence of reflexes following a spinal cord injury.

Of patients with a spinal fracture or dislocation at one level, 10% have a non-concordant second fracture, and therefore require imaging of the whole spine.

The Royal College of Emergency Medicine have produced guidance on the indications for cervical spine imaging in blunt and penetrating trauma.

Routine corticosteroids are not recommended in spinal cord injury.

4.7 Burns

4.7.1 Introduction

Burns are a major cause of morbidity and mortality. Burns cause coagulative destruction of skin and/or mucous membranes. The extent of destruction is related to the temperature and duration of contact.

Burns can be caused by:

- Thermal injury—dry heat (flame, hot metal) or moist heat (hot liquid or vapour)
- Electrical injury
- Chemical injury
- Radiation

4.7.2 Pathophysiology of burns

Burn injuries result in both local and systemic responses.

Local response

The classic description of the burn wound and surrounding tissues is a system of several circumferential zones radiating from primarily burned tissues, as follows:

- Zone of coagulation—this occurs at the point of maximum damage. In this zone there is irreversible tissue loss due to coagulation of the constituent proteins.
- Zone of stasis—the surrounding zone of stasis is characterized by decreased tissue perfusion. The tissue in this zone is potentially salvageable. The main aim of burns resuscitation is to increase tissue perfusion here and prevent any damage becoming irreversible. Additional insults such as prolonged hypotension, infection, or oedema can convert this zone into an area of complete tissue loss.
- Zone of hyperaemia—in this zone tissue perfusion is increased. The tissue will invariably recover unless there is secondary sepsis or prolonged hypoperfusion.

Systemic response

The release of cytokines and other inflammatory mediators at the site of injury has a systemic effect once the burn reaches 30% of total body surface area (BSA).

- Cardiovascular changes—capillary permeability is increased, leading to loss of intravascular proteins and fluids into the interstitial compartment. Peripheral and splanchnic vasoconstriction occurs. Myocardial contractility is decreased, possibly due to release of tumour necrosis factor. These changes, coupled with fluid loss from the burn wound, result in systemic hypotension, and end organ hypoperfusion.
- Respiratory changes—inflammatory mediators cause bronchoconstriction, and in severe burns adult respiratory distress syndrome can occur.
- Metabolic changes—the basal metabolic rate increases up to three times its original rate. This, coupled with splanchnic hypoperfusion, necessitates early and aggressive enteral feeding to decrease catabolism and maintain gut integrity.
- Immunological changes—non-specific down-regulation of the immune response occurs, affecting both cell mediated and humoral pathways.

4.7.3 Clinical assessment of burns

History

The history is extremely valuable in the assessment of a patient who has sustained burns. The history helps appreciate the nature of the insult and identify potential associated injuries (e.g. fractures or airway injury).

The history should include the following:

- Temperature/nature of agent (aids in determining the type and severity of injury)
- Time of burn (aids fluid resuscitation)
- Duration of contact/exposure (aids in determining the severity and predicting possible airway complications)
- Environment (risk of smoke inhalation and carbon monoxide poisoning if confined in an enclosed space)
- History of explosion (risk of associated trauma)
- Method of escape (risk of other injuries if the patient jumped or fell to escape)
- Past medical history
- Drug history and allergies
- Tetanus status

Estimating the size of a burn

There are several different methods for estimating the size of a burn. Size should only include those burns that are partial or full thickness; superficial burns are excluded from the estimation. Accurate estimation is important for managing fluid resuscitation and communicating with a burns centre.

Methods of size estimation:

- Rule of 9s (Table 4.11)
- Lund–Browder charts (Figure 4.7)
- Serial halves
- Patient's palm size (including the fingers) = approximately 1% BSA

Estimating the depth of a burn

The depth of burn is important in evaluating the severity of the burn, planning for wound care, and predicting functional and cosmetic results.

Superficial (first degree)

- Damage to the epidermis only
- Red and dry
- Blanch with pressure
- Very painful
- Heals within ~10 days
- No scarring

Partial thickness (second degree)

- Damage to epidermis and dermis (dermal involvement may be superficial or deep)
- Blisters and oedema
- Painful
- Healing occurs in 14 days
- Depigmentation may occur
- May require skin grafting

Table 4.11 Rule of 9's

Body area	Adult rule of 9's
Head	9%
Each arm	9%
Each leg	18%
Front of trunk	18%
Back of trunk	18%
Perineum	1%

Reprinted from The Lancet, volume 257, issue 6653, A.B. Wallace, The Exposure Treatment of Burns, pp.501–504, Copyright (1951), with permission from Elsevier

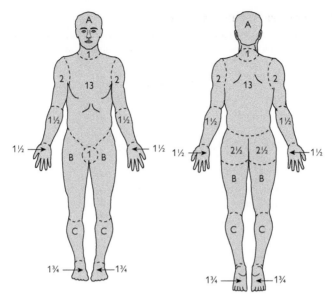

Figure 4.7 Lund–Browder charts.

Reproduced from Jonathan P. Wyatt, Robin N. Illingworth, Colin A. Graham, Michael J. Clancy, Colin E. Robertson, *Oxford Handbook of Emergency Medicine*, 2006, 'Assessing extent of burns—Lund and Browder charts', p. 389, with permission from Oxford University Press.

This article was published in *Surgery, Gynaecology, Obstetrics*, Vol 79, Lund C.C., Browder N.C., The estimation of areas of burns, pp.352–358, Copyright Elsevier 1944.

Full thickness (third degree)

- Loss of all layers of skin
- May appear dark and leathery or waxy-white
- Insensate (painless)
- No blanching
- Skin grafting required

Site of the burn

Burns at certain sites require specialist intervention and referral on to a burns' centre. These 'special' sites include:

- Face
- Eyes
- Ears
- Hands
- Feet
- Genitalia and perineum
- Overlying major joints

Circumferential burns must be identified because of the risk of a tourniquet effect. The neurovascular status of limbs should be assessed and if there is neurovascular compromise an escharotomy may be required.

4.7.4 Airway/breathing assessment

A high index of suspicion should be had for potential airway and inhalational injuries in patients sustaining burns. Although the larynx protects the subglottic airway from direct thermal injury, the airway is extremely susceptible to obstruction as a consequence of heat exposure.

Airway obstruction may not be obvious immediately. However, there are several well-recognized risk factors for potential airway obstruction, including:

- Facial or neck burns
- Singeing of eyebrows and nasal hairs
- Carbon deposits and acute inflammatory changes in oropharynx
- Carbonaceous sputum
- Hoarseness
- History of impaired conscious level
- History of confinement in a burning environment
- Explosion with burns to head and torso
- Carbon monoxide level >10% in a patient involved in a fire

Swelling can be subtle initially and progress/deteriorate rapidly. Early airway assessment and intubation can prevent later problems. In addition to direct thermal injury causing upper airway oedema, the patient may also suffer inhalation injury. The inhalation of products of combustion (carbon particles) and toxic fumes may lead to chemical tracheobronchitis, oedema, and pneumonia. The clinical manifestations of inhalational injury may be subtle, and frequently do not appear in the first 24 hours. Patients may require intubation and ventilation; if so, an endotracheal tube of sufficient size should be used in case subsequent bronchoscopy is required.

Patients may also suffer from carbon monoxide poisoning. The management of carbon monoxide poisoning is discussed further in Chapter 17, section 17.7.

4.7.5 Management of burns

- Generic trauma management principles should be followed.
- Potential airway injury should be considered and the patient intubated if there is concern.
- Early senior airway assessment should be sought.
- The burning process should be stopped—maximum of 20 minutes cooling.
- Hypothermia should be avoided by keeping the patient covered and warm.
- Careful fluid resuscitation is paramount (see 'Fluid resuscitation', next section).
- Intravenous opiates should be given for analgesia.
- The burns should be covered with sheets of cling film for pain relief.
- Any jewellery that may have a tourniquet effect on limbs or digits should be removed.
- Tetanus status should be determined and prophylaxis given, if necessary.
- Prophylactic antibiotics are not recommended.
- A nasogastric tube may be required due to gastric stasis.

Fluid resuscitation

Previous MRCEM question

Intravenous fluid resuscitation is required for any burn (partial and full thickness) >15% in an adult. There are several different equations available to calculate fluid requirements. ATLS use the Parkland formula (Box 4.4). Fluid calculations for burns have appeared in previous SAQ papers.

Fluids are calculated from the time of the burn and not the time of arrival in the ED. Therefore, if a patient arrives three hours after injury, the first volume of fluid should be given over five hours. If the patient is shocked, this should be treated first prior to calculating the burn fluid requirements.

Box 4.4 The Parkland formula for fluid calculation in burns

Parkland formula:

Percentage burn (partial and full) × weight (kg) × 4 = total fluid (ml).

This calculates the total volume required for the first 24 h of resuscitation.

Half should be given over the first 8 h and half over the next 16 h.

Data from Baxter CR, Shires T. 'Physiological response to crystalloid resuscitation of severe burns'.

Reproduced with permission from Charles R. Baxter, Tom Shires., Physiological Response To Crystalloid Resuscitation Of Severe Burns, *Annals of the New York Academy of Sciences*, Volume 150, pp. 874–894, Copyright © 1968 John Wiley and Sons

Burns rarely cause hypovolaemic shock acutely and, therefore, if the patient is haemodynamically compromised, another cause of fluid loss should be sought.

Fluid calculations are only an estimate and should be regularly reviewed based on ongoing assessment of the patient's haemodynamic and fluid-balance status (urine output >0.5 ml/kg/hr).

4.7.6 Complications of burns

- Infection
- Limb ischaemia
- Respiratory distress from inhalational injuries or circumferential burn
- Airway obstruction
- Burn scar contractures
- Hypertrophic scarring
- Rhabdomyolysis
- Compartment syndrome

4.7.7 Indications for transfer to burns centre

ATLS recommend the following patients require referral to a burns' centre:

- Partial/full thickness >10% BSA in patients <10 years or >50 years of age
- >20% BSA in all other age groups
- Burns to 'special areas'—face, ears, eyes, hands, feet, genitalia/perineum, and skin overlying major joints
- Full thickness >5% BSA
- Significant electrical and chemical burns
- Inhalation injury
- Burns in patients with pre-existing illness that could complicate treatment, prolong recovery, or affect mortality
- Patients with concomitant trauma that poses an increased risk of morbidity or mortality

4.7.8 Electrical injury

Electrical injuries can be high (>1000 V) or low (e.g. domestic 240 V) voltage. Both have the ability to cause fatal electrocution, but severe injury is more common with high voltage.

Current can be alternating (AC) or direct (DC):

- AC—is generally more dangerous because tetanic muscle contraction makes it difficult to release grip from the source.
    - DC—typically has a very short duration, with the victim thrown backwards (e.g. lightening).

Electrical injuries can cause damage in a variety of manners:

- Direct effect of current (e.g. arrhythmias, cardiac arrest, respiratory arrest).
- Direct thermal injury by acting as conductor of electrical energy or via flash burns (sudden vaporization of hot metal).
- Mechanical trauma (e.g. thrown back).
- Post-trauma sequelae (e.g. rhabdomyolysis).

The severity is determined by:

- Current
- Voltage
- Tissue resistance (reduced when wet, causing more severe burns)
- Duration of contact
- Point of entry and path of electricity to exit point (transthoracic is most dangerous)

Investigations for electrical burns

- ECG/cardiac monitoring
- Creatine kinase—looking for evidence of rhabdomyolysis
- Renal function—risk of renal failure
- Urine—looking for evidence of myoglobinuria (dipstick positive for blood)

Management of electrical burns

- Generic trauma management principles apply.
- Assess carefully for entry and exit wounds. The degree of external burns can severely underestimate the degree of tissue damage.
- Monitor for the development of compartment syndrome.
- Intravenous fluids to maintain urine output >100 ml/hour, if evidence of rhabdomyolysis.
- Mannitol and/or sodium bicarbonate, if urine remains positive for myoglobin despite fluid resuscitation.
- Analgesia.

Complications of electrical burns

- Musculoskeletal—fractures, dislocations, myonecrosis, compartment syndrome
- Neurological—seizures, coma, headache, transient paralysis, peripheral neuropathy
- Metabolic—rhabdomyolysis, renal failure
- Cardiac—arrhythmias, cardiac arrest, myocardial damage
- Ophthalmic—cataracts, glaucoma

Discharge criteria following electrical burns

- Asymptomatic
- Low voltage burns
- Normal ECG
- No history of arrhythmia (chest pain, palpitations, and so on)
- No myoglobinuria

4.7.9 Chemical injury

Chemical burns are usually the result of industrial or domestic accidents. Alkalis tend to produce more severe burns due to their ability to penetrate even after initial irrigation.

Most agents can be found on TOXBASE, which can advise on specific management (https://www.toxbase.org). General principles for removal of the chemical are to brush off any dry powder and wash thoroughly with running water.

Hydrofluoric acid

Hydrofluoric acid requires special attention because of the severity of burn it can cause and the systemic side effects.

- Used in glass etching, metal extracting, refining, and household rust removers.
- There may be a time delay (hours) before patients present because the burn may be painless initially, especially if due to lower concentration preparations.
- Causes liquefactive necrosis of tissues secondary to the formation of soluble salt. It is able to cross lipid membranes and penetrate deeply into tissues.
- Ongoing pain indicates ongoing tissue damage.
- Can result in eschar formation.
- Burns often difficult to heal.
- Absorbed fluoride ions chelate calcium, causing severe hypocalcaemia with subsequent myoclonus, tetany, convulsions, CNS depression, and ventricular fibrillation if untreated/ unrecognized.

Management of hydrofluoric acid burns:

- Remove any contaminated clothing.
- Thorough irrigation with water of the affected area (at least 20–30 minutes), even if initially it looks unremarkable.
- Check renal function, serum calcium, and magnesium.
- ECG and cardiac monitoring.
- Opiate analgesia.
- Antidote is 10% calcium gluconate. This can be applied as a gel to the burn, injected subcutaneously around the burn site, used intravenously in a Bier's block (continued until pain settles), or given intra-arterially in very severe cases.
- Intravenous calcium gluconate (10 ml of 10%) should be given if the patient is hypocalcaemic or symptomatic of probable hypocalcaemia (tetany, arrhythmias, prolonged QTc, seizures).

KEY POINTS

Burn injuries result in both local and systemic responses.

The rule of 9's can be used to estimate the size of the burn.

Immediate life-saving measures for patients with burns include the recognition of airway and inhalation injuries, with subsequent endotracheal intubation, and the rapid institution of intravenous fluid therapy.

The fluid requirements can be calculated using the Parkland formula. Percentage burn (partial and full) × weight (kg) × 4 = total fluid (ml over 24 h).

Previous MRCEM exams have included risk factors for potential airway injury.

4.8 SAQs

4.8.1 Head and neck injury

A 26-year-old man is brought into the emergency department following an alleged assault with a baseball bat. His friend tells you he has vomited once on the way in.

a) Give three signs (apart from vomiting) that you may find on examination that would suggest he has raised intracranial pressure? (3 marks)

b) He vomits again and you decide to arrange a CT of his head. His cervical spine is tender in the midline over C3. List two things that would indicate the need for a CT of his neck at the same time (according to CEM guidance). (2 marks)

He has a CT head scan (see Figure 4.8).

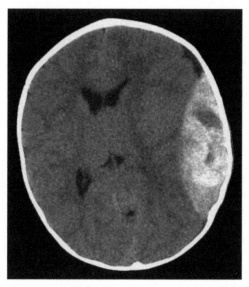

Figure 4.8 CT head scan.

Reproduced from Michael Nathanson, Iain K. Moppett, and Matt Wiles, *Oxford Specialist Handbook of Neuroanaesthesia*, 2011, Figure 7.1, p. 259, with permission from Oxford University Press.

c) Describe the abnormalities on this scan. (2 marks)

His friend has sustained a large scalp wound during the same altercation. The wound requires sutures. He weighs 60 kg.

d) How much local anaesthetic (1% lidocaine with 1:200,000 adrenaline) is it safe to use? Show your calculations, and give your answer as both mg and ml of 1% lidocaine with 1:200,000 adrenaline. (3 marks)

Suggested answer

a) Give three signs (apart from vomiting) that you may find on examination that would suggest he has raised intracranial pressure? (3 marks)

Any three of:

Hypertension

Bradycardia

Irregular respirations

Reduced level of consciousness/reduced GCS

Dilated pupil

Focal neurological abnormality

b) He vomits again and you decide to arrange a CT of his head. His cervical spine is tender in the midline over C3. List two things that would indicate the need for a CT of his neck at the same time (according to RCEM guidance). (2 marks)

Any two of:

GCS below 13 on initial assessment

Intubated patients

Inadequate plain film series

Suspicion or certainty of abnormality on plain film series

Patient being scanned for head injury or multiregion trauma

Neurological signs and symptoms referable to the cervical spine

Severe neck pain (≥7/10 severity)

Significantly reduced range of neck movement (i.e. unable to actively rotate the neck 45° in both directions)

Known vertebral disease (e.g. ankylosing spondylitis, rheumatoid arthritis, spinal stenosis, or previous cervical surgery)

c) Describe the abnormalities on this scan. (2 marks)

Left-sided, extradural haemorrhage/haematoma with midline shift to the right

d) How much local anaesthetic (1% lidocaine with 1:200,000 adrenaline) is it safe to use? Show your calculations, and give your answer as both mg and ml of 1% lidocaine with 1:200,000 adrenaline. (3 marks)

Maximum safe dose 7 mg/kg (1 mark)

= 7 mg × 60 kg= 420 mg lidocaine with adrenaline (1 mark)

420 mg = 42ml of 1% (1 mark)

4.8.2 Major trauma

An 84-year-old patient is brought in immobilized on a spinal board following a high-speed RTC. He is spontaneously ventilating with a respiratory rate of 24, but he is hypoxic with SpO_2 of 88% on high-flow O_2 (confirmed with an arterial blood gas). He is peripherally cool, with a pulse rate of 130 and a blood pressure of 70/40. He has two large bore cannulae *in situ*, and blood has already been sent for cross match.

His CXR is shown in Figure 4.9.

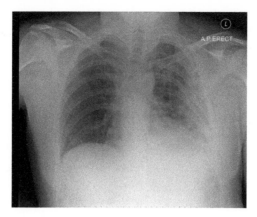

Figure 4.9 Chest X-ray.

a) (i)   Describe the abnormalities on his CXR. (2 marks)
   (ii) What are your next management steps? (2 marks)

His car did not have a head restraint on the seat, and he sustained a hyperextension injury to his neck during the RTC.

b) Give three clinical neurological findings which would lead you to suspect a central cord syndrome? (3 marks)

You have now been pre-alerted that the ambulance is bringing in a 40-year-old woman from a house fire. She arrives and has full thickness burns to 20% of her BSA.

c) Calculate her fluid requirements. Show all calculations, and state over what time period to give the fluids. You may assume she has arrived one hour post-injury and that she weighs 60 kg. (Do not include maintenance fluids) (3 marks)

Suggested answer

a) (i)   Describe the abnormalities on his CXR. (2 marks)
        Fractures of first to sixth ribs on left side
        Left-sided pulmonary contusion
        Left-sided haemothorax
        Subcutaneous emphysema on left

a) (ii) What are your next management steps? (2 marks)
        Commence fluid resuscitation with 20 ml/kg (or 1–2 L) bolus of IV crystalloid
        Insert left chest drain
        Plan for intubation and ventilation

b) Give three clinical neurological findings which would lead you to suspect a central cord syndrome? (3 marks)

Any three of:
Bilateral motor weakness—arms worse than legs
Dissociated/suspended/cape-like variable sensory loss
Upper limb areflexia

Horner's syndrome.

c) Calculate her fluid requirements. Show all calculations, and state over what time period to give the fluids. You may assume she has arrived one hour post-injury and that she weighs 60 kg. (Do not include maintenance fluids) (3 marks)

Fluid requirement (either formula acceptable):

$$\text{Parkland} = 4 \times \%\text{burn} \times \text{weight (kg)} = \text{total fluid (ml)}$$
$$4 \times 20 \times 60 = 4800 \text{ ml over 24 h.}$$

Half in first 7 hours, then half over 16 hours.

$$\text{Muir} - \text{Barclay} = \tfrac{1}{2} \times \%\text{burn} \times \text{weight (kg)} = \text{one aliquot of fluid}$$
$$\tfrac{1}{2} \times 20 \times 60 = 600 \text{ ml.}$$

Give 600 ml over 3 hours, then over 4, 4, 6, 6, and 12 hours.
(1 mark for correct formula, 1 mark for correct volume calculation, 1 mark for correct time periods)

Further reading

American College of Surgeons Committee on Trauma. 2012. *Advanced Trauma Life Support: Student Course Manual*, 9th edition. American Colledge of Surgeons.

Hoffman JR, Mower WR, Wolfson AB, et al. 2000. Validity of a set of clinical criteria to rule out injury to the cervical spine in patients with blunt trauma. National Emergency X-Radiography Utilization Study Group. *N Engl J Med* **343**(2):94–9.

National Institute for Health and Care Excellence, January 2014. NICE clinical guideline 176. Head injury: assessment and early management). Available at: https://www.nice.org.uk/Guidance/CG176 [Online].

National Institute for Health and Care Excellence, February 2016. NICE guideline 39. Major trauma: assessment and initial management. Available at: https://www.nice.org.uk/guidance/ng39 [Online]

Royal College of Emergency Medicine, November 2010. College of Emergency Medicine Clinical Effectiveness Committee. Guideline on the management of alert, adult patients with potential cervical spine injury in the Emergency Department. Available at: https://www.rcem.ac.uk [Online].

Scottish Intercollegiate Guideline Network, May 2009. SIGN guideline 110. Early management of patients with a head injury. Available at: http://www.sign.ac.uk/guidelines/fulltext/110/index.html[Online].

Stiell IG, Wells GA, Vandemheen KL, et al. 2001. The Canadian C-spine rule for radiography in alert and stable trauma patients. *JAMA* **286**(15):1841–8.

CHAPTER 5

Musculoskeletal and orthopaedic emergencies

CONTENTS

5.1 Musculoskeletal conditions: Introduction

Musculoskeletal conditions can appear in SAQs in the form of X-ray interpretation and subsequent management. Not every musculoskeletal injury will be covered in this chapter but those that have appeared in previous SAQs, or have particular features that make questions more likely, will be covered.

5.2 Long bone anatomy

Labelling diagrams sometimes appear in SAQs. Knowledge of long bone anatomy is ideal for this sort of question (Figure 5.1).

5.3 Fracture descriptions

Musculoskeletal X-ray interpretation commonly appears in SAQs although, perhaps surprisingly, is often poorly answered.

EXAM TIP

The quality of the image is the same for each candidate; therefore, if faced with a poor-quality X-ray, do not give up but make the best assessment of the image that you can. The question will indicate the number of marks available and this should guide your answer (e.g. if 3 marks are available, then give three descriptive terms).

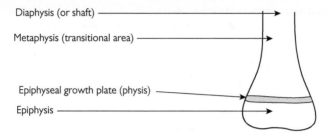

Diaphysis (or shaft)

Metaphysis (transitional area)

Epiphyseal growth plate (physis)

Epiphysis

Figure 5.1 Long bone anatomy.

State the side of the abnormality and the bone involved. Describe the location of the fracture within the bone (e.g. proximal, distal, supracondylar). Describe the nature of the fracture (e.g. transverse, oblique, comminuted, and so on). Mention if the fracture involves the articular surface. Note any associated dislocation or subluxation of related joints.

5.3.1 Checklist for evaluating plain films for fractures

- Check identity and date
- Minimum of two images AP and lateral, at right angles to each other
- Soft tissues
- Cortical outlines
- Medullary cavities
- Joint space width and congruity
- Correlate abnormal findings with site of symptoms

5.3.2 Fracture recognition

A fracture line is most visible when 90° to the X-ray beam
  Direct signs include:

- Fracture line: lucent or dense
- Cortical step/bulge
- Trabecular interruption

Indirect signs include:

- Soft tissue swelling at fracture site
- Joint effusion; intracapsular fat fluid level
- Fat pad sign
- Fat stripe obliteration or displacement
- Periosteal reaction
- Air in joint or tissue
- Fat fluid level with horizontal beam
- Widening of soft tissue shadows

5.3.3 Fracture description

- Anatomical site within bone (diaphysis/metaphysis/epiphysis)
- Alignment of fragments
- Displacement: distal fragment displaced anteriorly or posteriorly, medially or laterally
- Rotation: lateral or medial
- Angulation: anterior, posterior, varus, valgus

- Axial: impaction, distraction, overlapped (shortened)
- Direction of fracture line in relation to longitudinal axis of bone
- Normal/pathological bone
- Joint involvement

5.3.4 Descriptive terms for fractures

- Simple—fracture runs circumferentially around the bone with the formation of only two fragments.
- Comminuted—fractures involve more than two fragments.
- Transverse—fractures run at 90° to the long axis of the bone.
- Oblique—fractures run at an oblique angle of 30° or more.
- Spiral—fractures spiral around the bone and result from torsional forces.
- Wedge—fractures result from compression of the bone at one end.
- Crush—fractures result from compression of the bone resulting in loss of volume.
- Avulsion—fractures occur when a sudden muscular contraction avulses its bony attachment.
- Impacted—fractures occur when one fragment of bone is driven into the other.
- Displacement—describes how bone ends have shifted relative to one another. By convention, the direction of movement is described in terms of the distal fragment (e.g. in a Colles' fracture, the distal fragment displaces dorsally).
- Apposition—describes the degree of displacement. It can be expressed as the percentage of fracture surface still in contact (e.g. 50% bony apposition).
- Angulation—is described by the direction of the distal fragment (e.g. in a Colles' fracture the distal fragment is angulated dorsally). If possible, the degree of angulation should be measured.
- Rotation—occurs when one fracture fragment rotates on its long axis relative to the other fragment. To detect such rotation, the X-ray must include the joint above and the joint below. The rotation can be described as either internal or external, depending on which direction the distal part has moved.
- Greenstick—fractures occur in young bones. The bone bends and only partially breaks (one cortex remains intact).
- Buckle—fractures result from impaction causing a kinking of the cortex.

5.4 Open fractures

5.4.1 Introduction

Open (or compound) fractures occur when there is a breach of the skin overlying the fracture. They may result from sharp bone edges piercing the skin from inside out, or from trauma to the overlying skin and subcutaneous structures. Those that are open from 'outside in' are at greater infection risk and tend to have greater damage to other structures, such as muscle, nerves, and blood vessels.

5.4.2 Classification of open fractures

The Gustilo classification is a recognized system for classifying open fractures:

- Type I—open fracture with a wound <1 cm and clean.
- Type II—open fracture with a wound >1 cm and not associated with extensive soft tissue damage, avulsion, or flaps.
- Type IIIA—open fracture with adequate soft tissue coverage of bone despite extensive soft tissue damage or flaps; or any fracture where high-energy trauma has been responsible regardless of wound size.

- Type IIIB—open fracture with extensive soft tissue loss, with periosteal stripping, and exposure of bone.
- Type IIIC—open fracture associated with an arterial injury requiring repair.*

5.4.3 Management of open fractures

- Management should follow ATLS principles.
- Dramatic limb-threatening injuries must not distract from 'ABCDE' management.
- Haemorrhage control should be dealt with in 'C' by the use of direct pressure, elevation, and splinting. If this is unsuccessful, wound packing and/or indirect pressure at arterial pressure points (e.g. brachial artery) may be necessary. If these steps do not control haemorrhage, and the bleeding is life-threatening, a tourniquet may be required.
- Fluid resuscitation should be guided by the patient's haemodynamic status.
- Intravenous morphine should be provided for analgesia.
- A photograph should be taken of the wound to avoid repeated undressing and examination prior to surgery.
- Any obvious contamination (e.g. large lumps of debris) should be removed.
- The wound should be irrigated with saline and then covered with a sterile moist dressing.
- Distal pulses should be marked and their presence recorded in the notes. A Doppler ultrasound probe should be used if pulses are impalpable. Sensation should be assessed and documented. Neurovascular status should be reassessed frequently.
- The limb should be immobilized in plaster or an appropriate splint.
- Broad-spectrum intravenous antibiotics should be given.
- Tetanus status should be established and a booster/immunoglobulin given if indicated.

KEY POINTS

Open fractures occur when there is a breach of the skin overlying the fracture. They may result from sharp bone edges piercing the skin from inside out, or from trauma to the overlying skin and subcutaneous structures.

Repeated undressing of the wound, prior to theatre, should be avoided. A photograph should be taken of the wound and any obvious contamination removed. The wound should then be dressed with a sterile moist dressing.

Open fractures are tetanus-prone wounds. The patient's tetanus status should be assessed and prophylaxis given if indicated (section 5.22).

5.5 Compartment syndrome

5.5.1 Pathophysiology of compartment syndrome

Compartment syndrome develops when the pressure within an osteofascial compartment exceeds that of arterial pressure resulting in reduced or absent blood flow. The muscle becomes ischaemic and oedematous, further increasing compartment pressures. Ultimately, ischaemia can lead to muscle necrosis.

---

* Reproduced with permission from RB Gustilo, JT Anderson, Prevention of infection in the treatment of one thousand and twenty-five open fractures of long bones: retrospective and prospective analyses, *Journal of Bone & Joint Surgery*, Volume 58, Issue 4, pp.453-458, Copyright © 1976 Wolters Kluwer Health, Inc.

5.5.2 Causes of compartment syndrome

Compartment syndrome may be secondary to external compressive forces or internal expanding forces.

External compressive forces:

- Crush injuries due to entrapment or 'self-crushing' (unconscious patient lying on a hard surface)
- Circumferential burns
- Restrictive plasters, dressings, or splints

Internal expanding forces:

- Fractures, particularly of the tibia, resulting in haematoma and oedema
- Revascularization of an ischaemic extremity resulting in oedema
- Severe burns causing muscle oedema
- Prolonged exercise resulting in muscle oedema

The commonest sites for compartment syndrome are the lower leg, forearm, hands, and feet.

5.5.3 Clinical features of compartment syndrome

The six Ps of compartment syndrome

- Pain out of proportion to the injury and on passive stretch
- Paraesthesia (late sign)
- Pallor
- Paralysis (late sign)
- Pulseless (late sign)
- Poikilothermia

5.5.4 Investigations for compartment syndrome

- X-ray—if the mechanism of injury suggests a possible fracture.
- Urine—should be tested for myoglobin. Laboratory results can take several days, however myoglobin on a urinary dipstick tests positive for blood.
- CK and renal function—due to the high risk of rhabdomyolysis and renal failure.
- Coagulation screen—if disseminated intravascular coagulation is suspected.
- Intracompartmental pressure measurement—may be helpful if the diagnosis is uncertain. If the difference between the intracompartmental and diastolic pressure is <30 mmHg, then a fasciotomy is required.

5.5.5 Emergency department management of compartment syndrome

- High index of suspicion.
- Remove any restrictive dressings, casts, or splints.
- Intravenous morphine for analgesia.
- Avoid any nerve blocks which may mask symptoms.
- Urgent orthopaedic referral.

5.5.6 Definitive management for compartment syndrome

- Fasciotomy, excision of dead muscle tissue, and possible amputation

5.5.7 Complications of compartment syndrome

- Rhabdomyolysis (see Chapter 12, section 12.5)
- Renal failure
- Hyperkalaemia
- Hypocalcaemia
- Hypovolaemia secondary to bleeding and fluid shifts
- Local infection
- Ischaemic contractures (e.g. Volkmann's ischaemic contracture)
- Neurological deficit
- Limb amputation
- Death

KEY POINTS

A high index of suspicion is required to identify early compartment syndrome. The only initial feature may be pain out of proportion to the injury.

The pathophysiology of compartment syndrome includes:

- External compressive force or internal expanding force
- Osteofascial compartment pressure > arterial pressure
- Reduced or absent blood flow
- Muscle ischaemia and oedema
- Muscle necrosis, ischaemic contractures, neurological deficit, infection, rhabdomyolysis, renal failure, possible amputation, and death

---

5.6 Upper limb injuries

5.6.1 Introduction

There are certain upper limb musculoskeletal injuries that are more likely to appear in SAQs than others. These are often the conditions that are more difficult to interpret and therefore more discriminating between candidates in an exam.

5.6.2 Shoulder dislocations

Shoulder dislocations are a common injury presenting to the emergency department (ED). Anterior dislocations are the most common type, however shoulders can also dislocate posteriorly or inferiorly. Posterior dislocations are easily missed and therefore may appear in a SAQ.

Mechanism of injury:

- Anterior dislocation—forced external rotation/abduction of the shoulder.
- Posterior dislocation—blow to the anterior aspect of the shoulder; fall onto an internally rotated arm; strong muscular contractions during a seizure or electric shock.

X-ray appearance:

- Anterior dislocation—the humeral head lies below the coracoid on the AP view, the Y-view shows the humeral head anterior to the glenoid.
- Posterior dislocation—the humeral head may appear to have the contour of a 'light bulb' rather than a 'walking stick'. The Y-view shows the humeral head lying posteriorly.

There are numerous different techniques described to reduce dislocated shoulder and many clinicians use their own modified technique. The most widely used techniques include:

External rotation:

- With the patient supine, slowly adduct the dislocated arm against the patient's side.
- Flex the elbow to 90°.
- Hold the patient's wrist and slowly externally rotate the arm while held adduction and flexed at 90°.

Kocher's:

- Flex the elbow to 90° and apply downward traction in line with the humerus.
- Externally rotate the shoulder to bring the humeral head forward.
- Pull the elbow across the patient's body adducting the shoulder and then internally rotate the arm.

This manoeuvre has a higher rate of axillary nerve damage than other techniques.

Milch:

- With the patient supine, the arm is externally rotated and then abducted over the patients' head while maintaining external rotation.
- Gentle force can be applied over the humeral head by the operator's thumb in the axilla.

Stimpson's:

- The patient lies prone on a trolley with the affected arm hanging off the bed.
- Apply a weight to the wrist to provide slow traction.
- The patient is then left to allow gravity to reduce the dislocation.

The procedure may take up to 20 minutes, however sedation is not required.

Cunningham:

- The patient is in the sitting position with the clinician sitting opposite.
- Rest the patient's hand of the affected arm on the clinician's shoulder.
- The clinician rests one of their arms in the patient's antecubital fossa and gently massages the shoulder joint (bicep, deltoid, and trapezius) to promote relaxation.
- At the same time, the patient is encouraged to pull their shoulder blades together, thus moving their scapula out of the way and aiding reduction.

5.6.3 Monteggia and Galeazzi fracture dislocations

Monteggia fracture-dislocation

A Monteggia fracture-dislocation is a fracture of the shaft of the ulna associated with a dislocation of the radial head at the elbow (Figure 5.2). The radial head dislocation can be subtle. It is most easily detected by drawing a line along the centre of the shaft of the radius, which should normally pass through the capitellum (the radiocapitellar line). The radiocapitellar line can be drawn on an AP and lateral film.

The radiocapitellar line is also abnormal in elbow dislocations.

Galeazzi fracture-dislocation

A Galeazzi fracture-dislocation is a fracture of the radius associated with a dislocation of the distal radioulnar joint (Figure 5.3).

Both Monteggia and Galeazzi fracture dislocations will require open reduction and internal fixation.

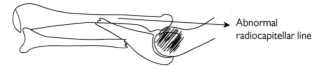

Abnormal
radiocapitellar line

Figure 5.2 Monteggia fracture-dislocation. The radiocapitellar line is abnormal and does not pass through the capitellum (shaded).

Reproduced from Jonathan P. Wyatt, Robin N. Illingworth, Colin A. Graham, Michael J. Clancy, Colin E. Robertson, *Oxford Handbook of Emergency Medicine*, 2006, 'Monteggia fracture-dislocation', p. 447, with permission from Oxford University Press.

EXAM TIP

In any patient with a forearm shaft fracture, the elbow and wrist must be imaged to assess for associated dislocations. A fracture of one bone may be associated with a fracture or dislocation involving the other bone.

5.6.4 Fractures of the distal radius

Colles' fracture

A Colles' fracture involves the distal radius with dorsal angulation. The X-ray appearances include:

- Posterior and radial displacement of the distal fragment.
- Dorsal angulation of the distal fragment (normally the articular surface of the distal radius has a 5° volar tilt on the lateral view).
- Radial angulation of the distal fragment (normally the articular surface of the distal radius has a 22° tilt in the ulnar direction on the AP view).
- Impaction, resulting in shortening of the radius relative to the ulna.

Such injuries are usually reduced in the ED under a haematoma block or Bier's block.

Smith's fracture

A Smith's fracture is a fracture of the distal radius with volar displacement and angulation. This is an unstable injury which usually requires operative fixation.

Barton's fracture

A Barton's fracture is an intra-articular fracture involving only the volar portion of the distal radius. The fracture fragment tends to displace in a volar direction and is unstable. Operative reduction and fixation is required.

Dislocation of radio-ulnar joint

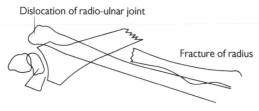

Fracture of radius

Figure 5.3 Galeazzi fracture-dislocation.

Reproduced from Jonathan P. Wyatt, Robin N. Illingworth, Colin A. Graham, Michael J. Clancy, Colin E. Robertson, *Oxford Handbook of Emergency Medicine*, 2006, 'Galeazzi fracture-dislocation', p. 446, with permission from Oxford University Press.

5.6.5 Scaphoid fractures

Scaphoid fractures can appear normal on initial X-rays, so a high degree of clinical suspicion is required. Clinical signs to suggest a scaphoid injury include:

- Tenderness in the anatomical snuffbox
- Swelling around the anatomical snuffbox
- Tenderness of the scaphoid tuberosity (palmar surface)
- Tenderness over the dorsum of the scaphoid
- Pain on telescoping the thumb
- Pain on flexion and ulna deviation of the wrist

If a fracture is identified, the patient should be immobilized in a scaphoid plaster and referred to the orthopaedic clinic. If the fracture is displaced, patients should be considered for acute operative fixation.

If the initial X-ray appears normal, the patient should be treated with a wrist splint or plaster and followed up in 10–14 days. Further imaging of suspected scaphoid injuries varies between hospitals but may include repeat X-rays, bone scanning, or MRI.

The complications of undiagnosed scaphoid fractures are avascular necrosis, non-union, malunion, and increased risk of arthritis. These complications are due to the anatomy of the blood supply to the scaphoid. The scaphoid can be divided into proximal, middle (the waist), and distal thirds. The majority of the blood supply enters the scaphoid distally. The proximal part has no direct blood supply instead depending on supply from the vessels that enter at the waist. Fractures of the waist are the most common type (60–80%) and impair blood flow to the proximal pole in approximately a third of cases. This can result in avascular necrosis of the proximal pole of the scaphoid. Fractures involving the proximal pole itself almost always lead to avascular necrosis.

5.6.6 Lunate and peri-lunate dislocations

The most common injury of the carpal bones is scaphoid fractures (90%). Dislocations of the carpus are rare, but often missed and have typical X-ray appearances.

Lunate dislocations

A fall onto an outstretched hand can result in a lunate dislocation, which clinically appears as pain and swelling over the volar aspect of the wrist. There may also be median nerve paraesthesia.

The important X-ray to detect a dislocation is the lateral wrist view (Figure 5.4). The distal radius, lunate, and capitate articulate with each other and lie in a straight line on the lateral wrist view.

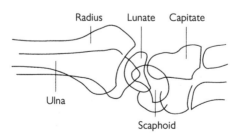

Figure 5.4 Normal lateral wrist view.

Reproduced from Jonathan P. Wyatt, Robin N. Illingworth, Colin A. Graham, Michael J. Clancy, Colin E. Robertson, *Oxford Handbook of Emergency Medicine,* 2006, 'Wrist: normal lateral', p. 441, with permission from Oxford University Press.

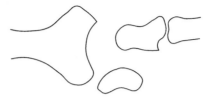

Figure 5.5 Lunate dislocation.

Reproduced from Jonathan P. Wyatt, Robin N. Illingworth, Colin A. Graham, Michael J. Clancy, Colin E. Robertson, *Oxford Handbook of Emergency Medicine*, 2006, 'Lunate dislocation', p. 441, with permission from Oxford University Press.

In a lunate dislocation (Figure 5.5), the radiological features are:

- Lunate dislocates anteriorly.
- The concavity of the lunate is empty on the lateral view.
- The radius and capitate remain in a straight line on the lateral view.
- The lunate appears 'triangular' on the AP view.

Patients must be referred immediately for manipulation under anaesthesia. Complications include median nerve injury, avascular necrosis, and complex regional pain syndrome.

Peri-lunate dislocations

The whole of the carpus (except for the lunate) is displaced posteriorly. Clinically the hand is very swollen. The lateral view shows mal-alignment of the carpal bones and an empty lunate concavity (Figure 5.6). The scaphoid is often fractured, known as a trans-scaphoid peri-lunate dislocation.

5.6.7 Bennett's fracture-dislocation

A Bennett's fracture-dislocation typically follows a fall onto the thumb or from a blow onto a closed fist around the thumb (Figure 5.7). The resulting fracture is through the base of the thumb metacarpal. The metacarpal may subluxe radially due to the pull of the abductor pollicis longus. Operative fixation is required if there is any displacement.

KEY POINTS

The key radiographic lines in upper limb injuries are:
- Anterior humeral line—supracondylar fractures.
- Radiocapitellar line—dislocation of the radial head.
- Radius, lunate, and capitate line—lunate and peri-lunate dislocations.

The clinical features of a scaphoid fracture include:
- Tenderness in the anatomical snuff box.
- Swelling around the anatomical snuffbox.
- Tenderness of the scaphoid tuberosity (palmar surface).
- Tenderness over the dorsum of the scaphoid.
- Pain on telescoping the thumb.
- Pain on flexion and ulna deviation of the wrist.

The blood supply to the scaphoid enters distally leading to possible avascular necrosis following fractures of the waist and proximal pole.

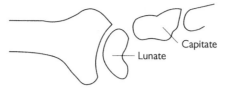

Figure 5.6 Peri-lunate dislocation.

Reproduced from Jonathan P. Wyatt, Robin N. Illingworth, Colin A. Graham, Michael J. Clancy, Colin E. Robertson, *Oxford Handbook of Emergency Medicine*, 2006, 'Perilunate dislocation', p. 441, with permission from Oxford University Press.

5.7 Lower limb injuries

5.7.1 Introduction

Certain lower limb conditions are more likely to appear in SAQs than others. Where there is national guidance (e.g. SIGN management of hip fractures), or well-recognized clinical decision rules (e.g. Ottawa knee and ankle rules), questions are more common. Injuries such as calcaneal fractures and Lisfranc fractures can be subtle and have specific radiological signs making them ideal for SAQs.

5.7.2 Hip fractures

Neck of femur fractures are a common injury in the elderly, often resulting from low-energy falls in patients with pre-existing osteoporosis. Fractures in younger patients are usually the result of high-energy injuries.

The blood supply to the femoral head is derived principally from an arterial ring at the base of the neck. Fractures of the neck of femur may lead to avascular necrosis of the femoral head, especially if they are intracapsular.

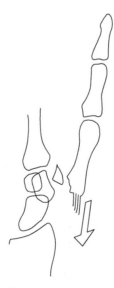

Figure 5.7 Bennett's fracture-dislocation.

Reproduced from Jonathan P. Wyatt, Robin N. Illingworth, Colin A. Graham, Michael J. Clancy, Colin E. Robertson, *Oxford Handbook of Emergency Medicine*, 2006, 'Bennett's fracture-dislocation', p. 437, with permission from Oxford University Press.

Level of fracture:

- Intracapsular
- Subcapital
- Transcervical
- Extracapsular
- Basicervical/intertrochanteric
- Pertrochanteric

The Garden classification

The Garden classification is used to describe the degree of displacement of the fracture and to assist in deciding the most appropriate operative management, for example reduction and internal fixation, hemiarthroplasty, or total hip replacement (Figure 5.8).

- Garden I—the inferior cortex is not completely broken but the trabecular are angulated. No significant displacement.
- Garden II—the fracture line is complete and the inferior cortex is broken. The trabecular lines are interrupted but not angulated. No significant displacement.

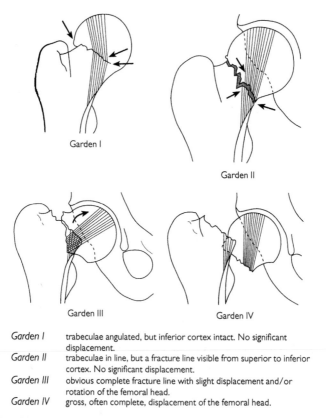

Garden I

Garden II

Garden III

Garden IV

Garden I	trabeculae angulated, but inferior cortex intact. No significant displacement.
Garden II	trabeculae in line, but a fracture line visible from superior to inferior cortex. No significant displacement.
Garden III	obvious complete fracture line with slight displacement and/or rotation of the femoral head.
Garden IV	gross, often complete, displacement of the femoral head.

Figure 5.8 The Garden classification.

Reproduced from Jonathan P. Wyatt, Robin N. Illingworth, Colin A. Graham, Michael J. Clancy, Colin E. Robertson, *Oxford Handbook of Emergency Medicine*, 2006, 'The Garden classification', p. 469, with permission from Oxford University Press.

Reproduced with permission and copyright © of the British Editorial Society of Bone and Joint Surgery Garden RS. Low-angle fixation in fractures of the femoral neck. *The Journal of Bone & Joint Surgery*, 1961;43-B:647–663.

- Garden III—obvious complete fracture with slight displacement and/or rotation of the femoral head.
- Garden IV—fracture fully displaced.*

SIGN and NICE guidance—management of hip fractures

SIGN and NICE have produced guidance on the management of hip fractures in the elderly with a specific section on ED management. The pertinent points are summarized here.

Early assessment, in the ED or on the ward, should include a formal recording of:

- Pressure sore risk
- Hydration and nutrition
- Fluid balance
- Pain
- Temperature
- Continence
- Co-existing medical problems
- Mental state
- Previous mobility
- Previous functional ability
- Social circumstances and whether the patient has a carer

Patients attending the ED with a suspected hip fracture should have the following management instigated:

- Adequate pain relief.
- Consideration of nerve block (such as fascia iliaca) if pain is poorly controlled with paracetamol and opioid analgesia (see Chapter 3, section 3.10).
  - Early radiology. If there is doubt regarding the diagnosis, MRI is the investigation of choice, although CT is a more readily available alternative.
- Fluid and electrolyte abnormalities measured and corrected.
- Anaemia identified and corrected.
- Any co-existing medical conditions optimized (e.g. uncontrolled diabetes, uncontrolled heart failure, acute chest infection, exacerbation of chronic chest condition, correctable arrhythmias, or ischaemia).
- Pressure sore prevention. Use of soft surfaces to protect the heels and sacrum. Those judged to be at very high risk should be nursed on an alternating-pressure air mattress.

Fast tracking:

- Patients should be transferred to the ward within two hours of their arrival in the ED.

Patients should be offered a multidisciplinary orthogeriatric assessment on the ward to optimize the patient for surgery and to facilitate rehabilitation.

Royal College of Emergency Medicine clinical standards

Neck of femur management is one of the conditions included in the Royal College of Emergency Medicine clinical standards. The standards set by the College for patients with a fractured neck of femur are:

- Early pain scoring, analgesia, and reassessment (as per the College's pain guidance—see Chapter 3)

*Reproduced with permission from RB Gustilo, JT Anderson, Prevention of infection in the treatment of one thousand and twenty-five open fractures of long bones: retrospective and prospective analyses, *Journal of Bone & Joint Surgery*, Volume 58, Issue 4, pp.453-458, Copyright © 1976 Wolters Kluwer Health, Inc.

- Early X-ray (90% within 60 minutes of arrival)
- Early referral (75% confirmed NOF# within 120 minutes or arrival)
- Prompt admission to the ward (within four hours)

> **EXAM TIP**
>
> The Royal College of Emergency Medicine Clinical Effectiveness Committee produce and publish clinical standards, which form the basis of regular College-led audits. These standards are reviewed annually and are available via the College website http://www.rcem.ac.uk/. Prior to the exam, it is worth looking through these standards for any recent updates.

5.7.3 Ottawa knee and ankle rules

The Ottawa knee and ankle rules are well-recognized clinical decision rules used in the ED to determine which injuries require an X-ray. They have been extensively validated and been shown to be applicable to children.

Ottawa knee rules

A knee X-ray series is only required for patients with knee injuries and any of the following findings:

- Age 55 years or older
- Isolated patella tenderness
- Tenderness of the head of fibula
- Inability to weight bear both immediately and in the ED (4 steps)

Ottawa ankle rules

An ankle X-ray series is only required if there pain in the malleolar zone and any of the following findings:

- Bone tenderness over the posterior margin of the distal 6 cm of the lateral malleolus
- Bone tenderness over the posterior margin of the distal 6 cm of the medial malleolus
- Inability to weight bear both immediately and in the ED (4 steps)

A foot X-ray series is only required if there is pain in the mid-foot zone and any of the following findings:

- Bone tenderness at the base of the fifth metatarsal
- Bone tenderness over the navicular
- Inability to weight bear both immediately and in the ED (4 steps)*

5.7.4 Calcaneal fractures

Calcaneal fractures most commonly result following a fall from a height. Associated injuries of the cervical spine, lumbar spine, pelvis, hips, and knees should be examined for.

If a calcaneal fracture is suspected, an axial view of the calcaneum should be requested in addition to standard ankle views. Most fractures will be visible on the lateral view, however some will only be detected when Böhler's angle is assessed (Figure 5.9). It is measured by drawing a line from the posterior aspect of the calcaneum to its highest midpoint. A second line is drawn from this point to the highest anterior point. The normal angle is 35–45°.

---

* Reprinted from *Annals of Emergency Medicine*, volume 21, issue 4, Ian G Stiell, Gary H Greenberg, R Douglas McKnight, Rama C Nair, I McDowell, James R Worthington, A study to develop clinical decision rules for the use of radiography in acute ankle injuries, pp.384-390, Copyright (1992), with permission from Elsevier.

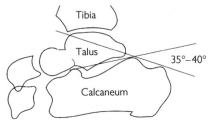

Figure 5.9 Böhler's angle.

Reproduced with permission from Lorenz Böhler, diagnosis, pathology, and treatment of fractures of the oscalcis, *Journal of Bone & Joint Surgery*, Volume 13, Issue 1, pp.75–89, Copyright © 1931, Wolters Kluwer Health, Inc.

Reproduced from Jonathan P. Wyatt, Robin N. Illingworth, Colin A. Graham, Michael J. Clancy, Colin E. Robertson, *Oxford Handbook of Emergency Medicine*, 2006, 'Böhler's angle (normally 35–45°)', p. 486, with permission from Oxford University Press.

Calcaneal fractures should be referred to orthopaedics acutely and most require admission for elevation, analgesia, and in certain cases, operative fixation.

KEY POINTS

The important radiographic lines for lower limb injuries include:
- Trethowan's line (superior border of femoral neck)—SUFE (see Chapter 19, section 19.23)
- Böhler's angle—calcaneal fracture
- Metatarsal alignment with the cuneiforms—Lisfranc fracture

The Royal College of Emergency Medicine's Clinical Effectiveness Committee have produced standards for the management of patients with neck of femur fractures:
- Early pain scoring, analgesia, and reassessment (as per the College's pain guidance)
- Early X-ray (90% within 60 min of arrival)
- Prompt admission to the ward (within 4 h)

5.7.5 Tarso-metatarsal dislocation (Lisfranc injury)

Tarso-metatarsal dislocations are rare and result from severe trauma, for example a vehicle running over the foot or a heavy object dropped on to the foot (Figure 5.10). They can be easily missed on foot X-rays, especially if the normal alignment of the metatarsals is unfamiliar. To detect such injuries, two questions should be asked:
- On the AP view, does the medial margin of the second metatarsal align with the medial margin of the middle cuneiform?
- On the oblique view, does the medial margin of the third metatarsal align with the medial margin of the lateral cuneiform?

If either of these alignments are lost, it suggests a dislocation at the tarso-metatarsal joint. Urgent orthopaedic referral is required for operative reduction and fixation.

5.8 Rheumatology: Introduction

Patients frequently present to the ED with an acutely painful joint without a history of trauma. The possibility of septic arthritis should always be considered and actively ruled out. There are many other causes of monoarthritis, and knowledge of these and how to differentiate between causes

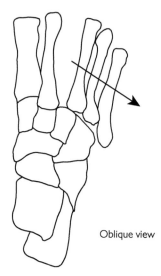

Oblique view

Figure 5.10 Lisfranc injury (tarso-metatarsal dislocation). The medial margin of the third metatarsal is not in alignment with the medial margin of the lateral cuneiform due to subluxation of the third, fourth, and fifth metatarsals.

is essential for the part B exam. Polyarthritis is a less common presentation to the ED, but may appear in a SAQ paper.

Acute lower back pain is a common ED presentation, which may have a number of sinister causes that actively need excluding. Knowledge of the 'red flags' in back pain could be examined in a SAQ.

5.9 Monoarthritis

Causes of acute inflammatory monoarthritis (red hot joint)—septic until proven otherwise:

- Septic arthritis
- Crystal synovitis: gout, pseudogout (calcium pyrophosphate arthropathy); calcific periarthritis
- Osteoarthritis
- Neuropathic arthropathy(Charcot's joint)
- Haemarthroses
- Reactive arthritis: signs of systemic illness; enthesopathy; conjunctivitis; skin and mucosal lesions; triad of seronegative arthropathy, urethritis, and conjunctivitis
- Enteropathic arthritis; systemic autoimmune disease (e.g. systemic lupus erythematosus, sarcoidosis); infective endocarditis foreign body synovitis (e.g. plant thorn)
- Synovial disease: pigmented villondular synovitis; synovial osteochondromatosis
- Monoarticular presentation of polyarthropathy: rheumatoid arthritis; seronegative spondyloarthropathy (psoriatic arthropathy; ankylosing spondylitis)

5.10 Polyarthritis

Causes of polyarthritis include:

- Rheumatoid arthritis
- Ankylosing spondylitis

- Psoriatic arthritis
- Reactive arthritis
- Rheumatic fever
- Gonococcal arthritis
- Viral arthritis
- Gout

5.11 Septic arthritis

5.11.1 Introduction

Septic arthritis should be the first consideration when a patient presents with an acutely painful joint in the absence of trauma. Delayed detection can result in joint destruction, sepsis, and even death.

5.11.2 Causes of septic arthritis

Organisms may invade the joint via three main routes:

- Haematogenous spread (commonest)
- Contiguous spread from infected peri-articular tissue (osteomyelitis, cellulitis)
- Direct inoculation (external skin puncture)

Joints that are chronically arthritic (e.g. rheumatoid arthritis) are more susceptible to infection, as are joints that have been instrumented (e.g. arthroscopy), or had prostheses inserted (e.g. total knee replacement). Superimposed infection is possible in a patient with underlying gout or pseudogout; therefore, the presence of crystals in the synovial fluid does not exclude septic arthritis.

Infective agents

The most likely causative agent of septic arthritis depends on the age of the patient, any underlying joint disease, and the presence of risk factors (e.g. IVDU, steroid use, joint prosthesis).
    Causes include:

- *Staphylococcus aureus* (commonest cause overall)
- *Haemophilus* (commonest cause age 6–24 months)
- *Neisseria gonorrhoea* (commonest cause in the younger sexually active patient)
- *Streptococcus viridians* or *pneumoniae*
- *Group B streptococci*
- Aerobic gram-negative rods (*Pseudomonas, Enterobacter*)

5.11.3 Clinical features of septic arthritis

A painful, hot, swollen, red joint is the classic presentation. Usually only one joint is affected. Only very limited movement of the joint is possible and it is usually held slightly flexed. The patient may be systemically unwell with fever and rigors. The use of analgesics, steroids, or antibiotics may obscure some of the clinical features.

    The commonest joint affected is the knee (50%), followed by the hip (20%), shoulder (8%), ankle (7%), and wrist (7%). Detection of septic arthritis in the hip can be very difficult owing to the lack of obvious external findings due to its deep location. Patients who are intravenous drug users may have involvement of atypical joints (e.g. vertebral, sacroiliac, or sternoclavicular joints).

5.11.4 Investigations for septic arthritis

- Joint aspiration and synovial fluid analysis is the most important diagnostic test. Fluid should be sent for gram stain, cultures, crystal examination, and cell count. Aspiration should not be performed in the ED if a patient has a joint prosthesis or metal work *in situ*.
- FBC, ESR, and CRP are all supportive of septic arthritis if positive but do not have a high enough sensitivity to rule it out.
- Blood cultures are useful in identifying the organism but do not help confirm or exclude the diagnosis in the ED.
- X-ray—initially may be normal but is a useful baseline. Later X-rays may show bone destruction.

5.11.5 Emergency department management

- Intravenous antibiotics (e.g. flucloxacillin and benzylpenicillin)
- Analgesia—consider splintage in addition to pharmacological treatment
- Urgent orthopaedic referral—for joint irrigation/drainage

KEY POINTS

Septic arthritis should be the first consideration in any patient presenting with an acutely hot, painful, and red joint.

The commonest cause of septic arthritis is *Staphylococcus aureus*.

The most useful investigation in septic arthritis is a joint aspirate.

5.12 Gonococcal arthritis

Neisseria gonococcus can cause a localized septic arthritis or an arthritis–dermatitis syndrome. Septic arthritis caused by *gonococcus* is commonest in young, sexually active patients. It should be managed as any other septic arthritis, with joint irrigation and antibiotics. Investigations should include swabs of the urethra, cervix, throat, and rectum to help identify the causative agent.

Arthritis–dermatitis syndrome is caused by a disseminated gonococcal infection; the classic triad is dermatitis (small papular or pustular lesions), tenosynovitis, and migratory polyarthritis. Investigations are the same as septic arthritis, including mucosal swabs to identify the cause. Treatment is with broad-spectrum antibiotics until the causative agent is identified. Cephalosporins are appropriate once gonococcus is confirmed. Open drainage of affected joints is rarely required. Patients should be advised that they and their partner(s) require a full sexual health screen.

KEY POINTS

Gonococcus may cause two types of arthritis:

- A localized septic arthritis affecting one joint
- An arthritis–dermatitis syndrome (classic triad is dermatitis, tenosynovitis, and migratory polyarthritis)

Gonococcus is the commonest cause of septic arthritis in young sexually active patients.

5.13 Crystal arthropathies

5.13.1 Gout

Previous MRCEM question

Gout is a disorder of purine metabolism characterized by a raised uric acid level in the blood and the deposition of urate crystals in the joints and other tissues, such as soft connective tissues or the urinary tract. The first metatarsophalangeal joint (MTPJ) and knee are the most commonly affected joints.

Pathogenesis of gout

Uric acid is the end product of purine breakdown. Two-thirds of uric acid is excreted via the kidneys and one-third via the gastrointestinal tract. Hyperuricaemia may be caused by increased production of uric acid or decreased excretion (Table 5.1).

   The duration and magnitude of hyperuricaemia is directly correlated with the likelihood of developing gouty arthritis, uric acid kidney stones, and the age of onset of clinical manifestations. However, gout can occur in people with normal plasma urate levels and many people with hyperuricaemia never develop gout.

   Gout tends to attack joints in the extremities because temperatures are cooler, which encourages urate to precipitate out from plasma. Similarly, tophi typically form in the helix of the ear, finger tips, and olecranon bursae, where temperatures are cooler.

   When urate crystals precipitate in the joint or soft tissues they cause a local immune-mediated inflammatory reaction. Triggers for urate to precipitate out include cool temperatures, sudden changes in uric acid levels (e.g. secondary to trauma, surgery, chemotherapy, diuretics, or starting/stopping allopurinol), and acidosis.

Clinical features of gout

- Acutely painful, hot, red, swollen joint (most commonly first MTPJ or knee)
- Tophi—ear, fingers, toes, elbows

Investigations for gout

- Synovial fluid analysis—reveals negatively birefringent crystals. Gram stain and culture should also be performed to exclude superimposed septic arthritis.
- X-ray—may show soft tissue swelling initially and later punched out lesions in peri-articular bone.

Table 5.1 Causes of hyperuricaemia

Increased production of uric acid	Decreased excretion of uric acid (90% of cases)
Myeloproliferative disorders	Idiopathic (commonest)
High-purine diet (e.g. beer, meat)	Enzyme defect (Lesch–Nyhan syndrome)
Cytotoxic drugs	Drugs (e.g. diuretics, low dose aspirin)
Trauma	Renal failure
Exercise	
Alcoholism	

- Plasma urate level—not useful acutely. Urate levels may be normal in an acute flare, even in hyperuricaemic patients, and some patients with hyperuricaemia never develop gout. Therefore a raised or normal urate level does not aid in the acute diagnosis.

Emergency department management of gout

If a diagnosis of gout is made and septic arthritis is excluded, then patients can be treated with rest and non-steroidal anti-inflammatory drugs (NSAIDs). If NSAIDs are contraindicated, colchicine can be used. If both NSAIDs and colchicine are contraindicated, corticosteroids can be prescribed.

Allopurinol is a xanthine oxidase inhibitor that reduces uric acid production. It can rapidly reduce the level of uric acid, which can conversely exacerbate a flare of gout so should not be started acutely in the ED.

5.13.2 Pseudogout

Pseudogout is caused by the deposition of calcium pyrophosphate crystals in the joints. It typically affects the knees, wrists, or hips. It is a disease of the elderly precipitated by illness, surgery, or trauma.

Risk factors include:

- Hyperparathyroidism
- Haemachromatosis
- Hypomagnesaemia
- Hypophosphataemia
- Hypothyroidism
- Acromegaly
- Diabetes
- Any underlying arthritis (e.g. rheumatoid, osteoarthritis)

Synovial fluid analysis shows weakly positive birefringent crystals. X-ray may show destructive changes like osteoarthritis (e.g. loss of joint space, subchondral sclerosis and cysts, marginal osteophytes) in addition to chondrocalcinosis (calcification in the joint, menisci, tendons, and ligaments).

Treatment is symptomatic with NSAIDs.

KEY POINTS

Gout is a disorder of purine metabolism characterized by raised uric acid levels and the deposition of urate crystals in the joints and other tissues.

Hyperuricaemia may be caused by increased production of uric acid or decreased excretion.

Urate levels are not a useful ED investigation because they may be normal in an acute flare, even in hyperuricaemic patients, and some patients with hyperuricaemia never develop gout.

Treatment options in gout are rest, splintage, NSAIDs, colchicine, and/or steroids. Allopurinol should not be given acutely.

Pseudogout is caused by the deposition of calcium pyrophosphate crystals in the joints. It is a disease of the elderly precipitated by illness, surgery, or trauma.

5.14 Seronegative spondyloarthropathies

The seronegative spondyloarthropathies are a group of related disorders. They have the following common features:

- Involvement of the axial skeleton (spine and sacroiliac joints)
- Inflammation of tendon insertions (enthesitis)
- Peripheral inflammatory arthropathy
- Rheumatoid factor negative
- Linked to HLA-B27 serotype

The group includes:

- Ankylosing spondylitis
- Reactive arthritis
- Psoriatic arthritis
- Enteropathic arthritis (associated with inflammatory bowel disease)
- Undifferentiated spondyloarthropathy

5.14.1 Ankylosing spondylitis

Ankylosing spondylitis usually presents with chronic low back pain in men aged 15–30 years. Progressive spinal fusion ultimately results in a fixed kyphotic spine (bamboo spine), hyperextended neck, and restricted respiration. Extra-articular manifestations include uveitis, lung fibrosis, aortitis, plantar fasciitis, and Achilles' tendonitis.

Treatment is multifactorial with physical therapy and medications. Patients should be under the care of rheumatologist. Patients may present to the ED with spinal fractures after relatively minor trauma due to the fixed nature of their spine. They may also present with complications such uveitis or aortic regurgitation.

5.14.2 Reactive arthritis

Reactive arthritis, previously known as Reiter's syndrome, is an autoimmune condition that develops in response to an infection elsewhere in the body. The classic triad is:

- Urethritis
- Conjunctivitis
- Arthritis

Reactive arthritis is triggered following enteric or urogenital infections. It is associated with the HLA-B27 sero-type.

Bacterial infections associated with reactive arthritis include:

- *Chlamydia*
- *Shigella*
- *Salmonella*
- *Campylobacter*
- *Yersinia*

Clinical features of reactive arthritis

The symptoms of reactive arthritis generally appear one to three weeks after the enteric or urogenital infection. The initial infection may be asymptomatic in the case of urogenital infections.

Clinical features include:

- Urethritis—dysuria, frequency, urgency, uretheral discharge, circinate balanitis
- Arthritis—asymmetric arthralgia and joint swelling, typically affecting the knees, ankles, and feet
- Conjunctivitis and uveitis—redness, eye pain/irritation, watering, photophobia
- Keratoderma blenorrhagicum (small, hard nodules on the soles and palms)

- Mouth ulcers
- Cardiac—aortic regurgitation, myocarditis

Investigations for reactive arthritis

There are no specific tests for reactive arthritis. Investigations are mainly directed at excluding other causes. Identification of the HLA-B27 serotype can be helpful in the diagnosis but is not a useful ED investigation.

- Joint aspiration reveals inflammatory cells with a negative culture
- WCC, ESR, and CRP are likely to be raised
- Swabs of the urethra, cervix, and throat may identify the causative organism

Ultimately the diagnosis is based on the history of a preceding illness with features suggestive of reactive arthritis.

Management of reactive arthritis

If an infective cause is identified it should be treated with appropriate antibiotics. Symptomatic relief with NSAIDs is the mainstay of treatment in the ED, with referral on to rheumatology.

KEY POINTS

The seronegative spondyloarthropathies have the following common features:
- Involvement of the axial skeleton (spine and sacroiliac joints)
- Inflammation of tendon insertions (enthesitis)
- Peripheral inflammatory arthropathy
- Rheumatoid factor negative
- Linked to HLA-B27 serotype

Patients with ankylosing spondylitis may present to the ED with spinal fractures after relatively minor trauma due to the fixed nature of their spine. They may also present with complications such as uveitis or aortic regurgitation.

Reactive arthritis is an autoimmune condition that develops in response to an infection (enteric or urogenital) elsewhere in the body. The classic triad is:
- Urethritis
- Conjunctivitis
- Arthritis

5.15 Rheumatoid arthritis

5.15.1 Introduction

Rheumatoid arthritis is a chronic, systemic, inflammatory disorder that may affect many tissues and organs, but principally synovial joints. The cause of rheumatoid arthritis is unknown. Approximately 70% of patients have a positive rheumatoid factor.

5.15.2 Clinical features of rheumatoid arthritis

Clinical manifestations of rheumatoid arthritis include:

- Joints—most commonly the small joints of the hands and feet, with pain and stiffness worse in the morning. Clinical signs include: metacarpophalangeal joint (MCPJ) and proximal

interphalangeal joint (PIPJ) swelling; ulnar deviation and volar subluxation at the MCPJs; Boutonnière and 'swan-neck' deformities of fingers; and 'Z thumbs'.
- Neck—degeneration of the transverse ligament of the Peg results in an increased risk of subluxation and cord damage.
- Skin—manifestations include rheumatoid nodules (subcutaneous nodules usually found over bony prominences, e.g. olecranon, MCPJs); nail fold infarcts; or livedo reticularis due to vasculitis.
- Lung—complications include pulmonary fibrosis and pleurisy.
- Cardiovascular—effects include pericarditis and endocarditis.
- Other—effects include anaemia, splenomegaly, and scleritis.

5.15.3 Emergency department presentations of rheumatoid arthritis

Patients with rheumatoid arthritis may present to the ED due to complications of the disease or drugs used to treat the disease.

Possible ED presentations:

- Septic arthritis—increased risk in rheumatoid arthritis
- Cervical myelopathy—'glove and stocking' numbness, weakness, and neck pain
- Myocardial infarction or stroke—patients are more prone to atherosclerosis
- Pericarditis/endocarditis
- Scleritis
- Gastrointestinal bleed—due to long-term NSAID use
- Blood dyscrasias (leucopenia, neutropenia, thrombocytopenia)—due to disease modifying agents (sulfasalazine, methotrexate, ciclosporin, gold, penicillamine)
- Deranged liver function or renal failure—due to disease modifying agents
- Skin rashes—due to disease modifying agents

5.16 Acute back pain

Acute back pain is a very common ED presentation and the commonest cause of lost work days in the United Kingdom. The commonest cause is simple, mechanical back pain but there are a number of serious pathologies that can present with back pain. The initial history and examination should be directed at identifying 'red flags' that suggest serious pathology (Table 5.2).

If any red flags are present, further investigation (according to the suspected underlying pathology) is required to exclude a serious underlying condition. These include blood tests (blood counts, inflammatory markers, metabolic bone screen, myeloma screen), plain film radiology, and MRI scanning, dependent on the likely diagnosis.

5.16.1 Cauda equina syndrome

Cauda equina syndrome is compression of the nerve roots below the termination of the spinal cord (conus medullaris). The cauda equina contains nerve roots from L1-5 and S1-5.

Causes of cauda equina syndrome include:

- Central disc prolapse
- Tumour
- Spinal stenosis (e.g. osteoarthritis, ankylosing spondylitis)
- Epidural haematoma (e.g. post-spinal anaesthesia or lumbar puncture)
- Trauma (blunt or penetrating)
- Spinal epidural abscess

Table 5.2 Red flags for back pain

Possible diagnosis	Red flags
Vertebral fracture	History of trauma (this may be minimal in the elderly or those with osteoporosis)
	Prolonged steroid use
Tumour	Age <20 or >50
	History of malignancy
	Non-mechanical pain
	Thoracic pain
	Systemically unwell
	Weight loss
Spinal infection	Fever
	Systemically unwell
	IVDU
	Immunosuppression
	HIV
	Recent bacterial infection
	Non-mechanical pain
	Pain worse at night
Cauda equina syndrome	Saddle anaesthesia
	Bladder or bowel dysfunction
	Gait disturbance
	Widespread or progressive motor weakness
	Bilateral sciatica
AAA	Systemically unwell
	Cardiovascular compromise
	Pulsatile abdominal mass
Inflammatory rheumatic disease (e.g. ankylosing spondylitis)	Age <20
	Structural deformity of the spine
	Systemically unwell

Clinical features of cauda equina syndrome

- Weakness/numbness in the distribution supplied by the compressed nerve roots:
  - L1—sensation to groin
  - L2—sensation to medial proximal thigh; hip flexion
  - L3—sensation to knee; knee extension; knee jerk
  - L4—sensation to medial lower leg; ankle dorsi-flexion; knee jerk
  - L5—sensation to lateral lower leg and great toe; great toe extension
  - S1—sensation to little toe and lateral foot; ankle plantar-flexion; ankle jerk
  - S2—sensation to posterior thigh
  - S3, 4, 5—sensation to ischial tuberosity and perianal region (saddle anaesthesia)

- Bladder disturbance (S2, 3, 4)—urinary retention, incontinence, hesitancy, decreased urethral sensation
- Bowel disturbance (S2, 3, 4)—constipation, incontinence, loss of anal tone and sensation

Emergency department management of cauda equina syndrome

Patients with suspected cauda equina syndrome need an urgent MRI of their spine and specialist referral for surgical decompression.

5.16.2 Nerve root pain/simple back pain

If there are no 'red flags', then urgent investigation and referral is not usually required. Patients may have nerve root pain/radicular pain or non-specific low back pain. The patient's pain distribution and clinical examination should indicate whether it originates from a nerve root.

Clinical features suggesting nerve root pain:

- Pain radiates down to the foot or toes
- Numbness in the distribution of a nerve root
- Straight leg raise reproduces the pain
- Localized neurology at one nerve root

If there are no features suggesting nerve root pain, then the term 'non-specific low back pain' is appropriate. Pain is not attributable to pathology or neurological encroachment in about 85% of people. Psychosocial yellow flags can further help identify patients at risk from chronicity and long-term disability, and are determined by attitudes, beliefs, compensation, diagnosis, emotions, family, and work-related issues.

Treatment includes simple analgesia and advice to remain active; bed rest is not recommended. Patients should be advised to return if they develop any 'red flag' symptoms or rapidly progressing neurology. Acute low back pain is usually self-limiting and approximately 90% of people recover within six weeks.

KEY POINTS

Sinister causes for back pain include:

- Vertebral fractures
- Tumour
- Spinal infection
- Cauda equina syndrome
- AAA
- Inflammatory rheumatic disease

Red flags for back pain include:

- Thoracic pain
- Fever
- Unexplained weight loss
- Bladder or bowel dysfunction
- History of carcinoma
- Systemically unwell
- Progressive neurological deficit
- Disturbed gait, saddle anaesthesia
- Age <20 years or >50 years

5.17 Wound management: Introduction

The curriculum includes a detailed knowledge of functional anatomy of the hand and wrist. The ability to accurately describe hand injuries is essential for clinical practice and the exam. Knowledge is required of 'special wounds' (e.g. bites, puncture wounds, degloving injuries, and accidental digital adrenaline injection). Tetanus prophylaxis is an area with clear guidance, which has previously appeared in SAQs and is likely to again.

5.18 Describing wounds and hand injuries

Describing hand injuries accurately is very important to avoid misinterpretation both clinically and in the exam.

The following rules should be followed when recording findings:

- Fingers should be named (little, ring, middle, index, and thumb) and not numbered.
- Metacarpals should be referred to by the name of the finger.
- Phalanges should be termed proximal, middle, and distal.
- The side of the hand should be referred to as ulnar or radial, and not medial or lateral.
- The surfaces of the hand should be referred to as dorsal or volar (palmar), and not anterior or posterior.

Wound descriptions are often incorrect with candidates calling every breach in the skin a laceration. The following is a list of commonly occurring injuries and the correct terminology:

- Incised or cut wound—injury caused by a sharp object (e.g. knife or glass). Wound edges are clean-cut.
- Laceration—caused by blunt injury causing the skin to tear. Wound edges are irregular.
- Puncture—usually from a sharp object, although a blunt object with sufficient force can also penetrate the skin.
- Abrasion—injury caused by blunt force applied tangentially.
- Bruise—blunt injury causing damage to blood vessels within the tissues.
- Haematoma—injury causing a collection of localized bleeding.

Special features in the history:

- Mechanism of injury
- Time of injury: relevant for replants and open fractures
- Potential for foreign bodies
- Position of hand at time of injury
- Age
- Hand dominance
- Occupation
- Recreation; hobbies requiring dexterity or strength
- Prior hand function
- Prior hand injuries
- Co-morbidity: diabetes mellitus
- Tetanus immunization

Initial assessment:

- ABC
- Remove all rings
- Note normal resting cascade of fingers (progressive flexion of digits from index to little finger)
- Wounds

- Tissue loss
- Rotational mal-alignment: make a fist
- Sensation: two-point tactile discrimination (2–5 mm at fingertips normally); skin sweating (stroke digit with a smooth object; less resistance owing to loss of sweating over denervated area)
- Capillary refill (normally less than two seconds)
- Ulnar and radial arteries; Allen test
- Draw a picture or photograph the wounds to avoid repeated dressing changes

5.19 Hand and wrist anatomy

The anatomy of the hand and wrist allows a complex range of movements. The hand is a person's most direct means of interacting with the environment and injury can have major consequences for their profession, hobbies, and self-care.

5.19.1 The bones of the hand and wrist

There are eight carpal bones arranged in two rows. The scaphoid runs across the proximal and distal carpal rows and hence is prone to fracture. Each finger has a metacarpal and three phalanges, the proximal, middle, and distal. The thumb has one metacarpal and two phalanges, the proximal and distal (Figure 5.11).

5.19.2 Muscles and tendons of the hand and wrist

Long extensors

The tendons on the dorsum of the hand are known as the long extensors and extend the fingers at the MCPJs. At the level of the fingers, these tendons flatten into an extensor expansion. They are joined by the tendons of the intrinsic hand muscles (lumbricals). The PIPJs are extended by the central slip which inserts on the base of the middle phalanx, and the distal phalanx is extended by the terminal slip which inserts on the base of the distal phalanx (Figure 5.12).

The extensor tendons lie superficially and are covered by a thin layer of skin, so can be easily damaged by wounds to the dorsum of the hand. The extensor expansion is quite thin and can be damaged by relatively minor trauma leading to a Boutonnière deformity (central slip division) at the PIPJ or a mallet finger at the distal interphalangeal joint (DIPJ) (Figure 5.13).

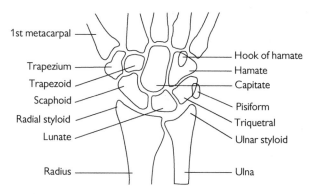

1st metacarpal

Trapezium
Trapezoid
Scaphoid
Radial styloid
Lunate

Radius

Hook of hamate
Hamate
Capitate
Pisiform
Triquetral
Ulnar styloid

Ulna

Figure 5.11 Bones of the wrist.

Reproduced from Jonathan P. Wyatt, Robin N. Illingworth, Colin A. Graham, Michael J. Clancy, Colin E. Robertson, *Oxford Handbook of Emergency Medicine*, 2006, 'AP view of normal wrist', p. 428, with permission from Oxford University Press.

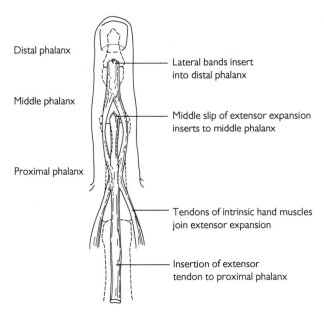

Distal phalanx

Lateral bands insert
into distal phalanx

Middle phalanx

Middle slip of extensor expansion
inserts to middle phalanx

Proximal phalanx

Tendons of intrinsic hand muscles
join extensor expansion

Insertion of extensor
tendon to proximal phalanx

Figure 5.12 Anatomy of finger extensor tendons.

Reproduced from Jonathan P. Wyatt, Robin N. Illingworth, Colin A. Graham, Michael J. Clancy, Colin E. Robertson, *Oxford Handbook of Emergency Medicine*, 2006, 'Anatomy of finger extensor tendon', p. 429, with permission from Oxford University Press.

The extensors of the thumb are extensor pollicis longus and brevis, and abductor pollicis longus. Extensor pollicis longus inserts on the base of the distal phalanx and extends the interphalangeal joint (IPJ). Extensor pollicis brevis and abductor pollicis longus insert on the base of the proximal phalanx and extend and abduct the thumb at the carpometacarpal joint and MCPJ. These tendons form borders of the anatomical snuff box.

The borders of the anatomical snuff box are:

- Ulnar border—extensor pollicis longus
- Radial border—extensor pollicis brevis and abductor pollicis longus
- Proximal border—radial styloid process
- Distal border—base of the thumb metacarpal
- Floor—scaphoid and trapezium

Within the anatomical snuff box is the radial artery.

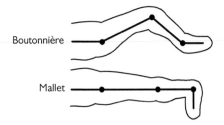

Boutonnière

Mallet

Figure 5.13 Extensor tendon injuries.

Reproduced from Jonathan P. Wyatt, Robin N. Illingworth, Colin A. Graham, Michael J. Clancy, Colin E. Robertson, *Oxford Handbook of Emergency Medicine*, 2006, 'Finger deformities (Boutonnière and Mallet)', p. 431, with permission from Oxford University Press.

Long flexors

There are two flexor tendons to each finger and one for the thumb (Figure 5.14). Each finger has a flexor digitorum superficialis (FDS), which inserts on the base of the middle phalanx and flexes the PIPJ. The flexor digitorum profundus (FDP) lies deep to the FDS in the palm but comes to lie superficially in the finger and inserts on the base of the distal phalanx flexing the DIPJ. The thumb is flexed at its IPJ by the flexor pollicis longus which inserts on the base of distal phalanx.

A laceration or cut in the forearm or proximal part of the palm would divide the FDS first but a cut in the finger would divide FDP first.

Intrinsic muscles of the hand

The intrinsic muscle groups are the interossei, the lumbricals, the thenar muscles, and the hypothenar muscles.

There are four dorsal and three palmar interossei, innervated by the ulnar nerve. The dorsal interossei primarily flex the MCPJs and extend the IPJs, thus assisting the lumbricals. In addition, the dorsal interossei abduct the fingers. The palmar interossei adduct the fingers. This can be remembered by the mnemonic 'DAB and PAD':

- **D**orsal **AB**ducts
- **P**almar **AD**ducts

There are four lumbricals, which flex the MCPJs and extend the IPJs. The first and second lumbricals (those on the radial side) are innervated by the median nerve. The third and fourth lumbricals (those on the ulnar side) are innervated by the ulnar nerve.

The thenar muscles control movements of the thumb and consist of the abductor pollicis brevis, flexor pollicis brevis, opponens pollicis, and adductor pollicis. They are innervated by the median nerve except for the adductor pollicis, which is innervated by the ulnar nerve.

The hypothenar muscles control movements of the little finger and consist of abductor digiti minimi, flexor digiti minimi, and opponens digiti minimi. They are innervated by the ulnar nerve.

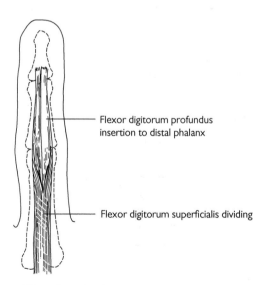

Flexor digitorum profundus insertion to distal phalanx

Flexor digitorum superficialis dividing

Figure 5.14 Anatomy of finger flexor tendons.

Reproduced from Jonathan P. Wyatt, Robin N. Illingworth, Colin A. Graham, Michael J. Clancy, Colin E. Robertson, *Oxford Handbook of Emergency Medicine*, 2006, 'Anatomy of finger flexor tendon', p. 429, with permission from Oxford University Press.

5.19.3 Carpal tunnel

At the level of the wrist the muscles of the forearm are tendons and lie grouped together in the carpal tunnel before dispersing to each finger. The carpal tunnel is a fibro-osseous tunnel on the palmar side of the wrist (Figure 5.15). The borders of the tunnel are formed by the carpal bones and the flexor retinaculum. The flexor retinaculum runs between the hamate and pisiform on the ulnar border to the scaphoid and trapezium on the radial border.

Nine flexor tendons and the median nerve pass through the carpal tunnel:

* FDP (four tendons)
* FDS (four tendons)
* Flexor pollicis longus (one tendon)

Superficial to the carpal tunnel and flexor retinaculum is the ulnar tunnel (or Guyon's canal) which contains the ulnar artery and ulnar nerve.

EXAM TIP

Sections of the basic sciences curriculum (e.g. hand anatomy) may be questioned in the Intermediate FRCEM SAQs. Look through your part primary FRCEM revision notes prior to Intermediate FRCEM to refresh your memory.

Know the anatomy of the carpal tunnel and anatomical snuff box. These make ideal SAQs.

5.19.4 Nerves of the hand and wrist

The hand and wrist are innervated by the median, ulnar, and radial nerves.

The median nerve enters the palm through the carpal tunnel except for the palmar cutaneous branch, which supplies the skin over the thenar eminence and may be spared in carpal tunnel syndrome. The median nerve in the hand supplies sensation to the radial 3½ fingers on the palmar surface. Motor branches supply the thenar eminence (except the adductor pollicis), and the first and second lumbricals. In the forearm, the median nerve supplies all the flexors except the flexor carpi ulnaris and FDP to the little and ring fingers.

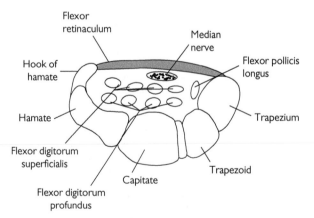

Figure 5.15 The carpal tunnel.

Reproduced from Gavin Bowden, Martin McNally, Simon Thomas, and Alexander Gibson, *Oxford Handbook of Orthopaedics and Trauma*, 2010, Figure 8.10, p. 309, with permission from Oxford University Press.

KEY POINTS

The borders of the anatomical snuff box are:

- Ulnar border—extensor pollicis longus
- Radial border—extensor pollicis brevis and abductor pollicis longus
- Proximal border—radial styloid process
- Distal border—base of the thumb metacarpal
- Floor—scaphoid and trapezium

The borders of the carpal tunnel are:

- Dorsal border—the carpal bones
- Volar border—the flexor retinaculum
- Ulnar border—hamate and pisiform
- Radial border—scaphoid and trapezium

Within the carpal tunnel passes:

- Median nerve
- FDP (four tendons)
- FDS (four tendons)
- Flexor pollicis longus (one tendon)

The ulnar nerve enters the palm through the ulnar tunnel. It supplies sensation to the little and ulnar half of the ring finger, and the hypothenar eminence. Motor branches supply the hypothenar muscles, the third and fourth lumbricals, the interossei, and adductor pollicis. In the forearm, the ulnar nerve supplies the flexor carpi ulnaris and FDP to the little and ring fingers.

The radial nerve innervates the wrist extensors and provides sensation to the dorsum of the hand on the radial aspect and the dorsum of the thumb.

Table 5.3 summarizes nerve injuries to the hand and wrist.

Table 5.3 Nerve injuries in the hand and wrist

Nerve	Clinical features of injury
Median nerve injury—at the wrist Median nerve injury—in the proximal forearm	• Loss of sensation to radial 3½ fingers on the palmar surface (sensation to the thenar eminence may be spared because the palmar cutaneous branch does not travel through the carpal tunnel). • Weakness of thenar muscles—unable to abduct or oppose thumb against resistance. In addition there is: • Weakness of wrist flexion and pronation. • Loss of flexion at the PIPJs of all fingers, except the little finger (due to flexor digiti minimi innervated by the ulnar nerve). • Loss of flexion at the DIPJs of the index and middle fingers. • If the patient tries to make a fist, the index and middle finger remain extended at MCPJs, PIPJs, and DIPJs ('hand of benediction').

(continued)

Table 5.3 Continued

Nerve	Clinical features of injury
Ulnar nerve injury—at the wrist Ulnar nerve injury—in the forearm	• Loss of sensation to the ulnar 1½ fingers on the palmar and dorsal surface. • Weakness of the hypothenar muscles—unable to abduct, flex, or oppose the little finger. • Weakness of the interossei muscles—unable to abduct and adduct fingers. Unable to cross index and middle fingers. • Weakness of the third and fourth lumbricals. The little and ring finger are hyperextended at the MCPJs and flexed at the IPJs ('claw hand'). • In a more proximal injury, the 'claw hand' is less obvious because there is loss of the innervation of the FDP to the little and ring fingers. The flexion at the IPJs is weakened and the 'claw-like' appearance is diminished. This is known as the 'ulnar paradox' because one would normally expect a more debilitating injury to result in a more deformed appearance.
Radial nerve injury	• Loss of sensation to the dorsum of the hand (the first web space is the most reliable site). • There are no motor branches in the hand but a more proximal injury results in weakness of the wrist extension.

5.20 Hand infections

5.20.1 Introduction

The hand consists of multiple compartments and planes, which can act as potential spaces for infection. The main compartments are:

• Paronychium (lateral nail fold).
• Felon (pulp).
• Thenar space.
• Hypothenar space.
• Mid-palmar space (potential space between the middle, ring, and little finger flexor tendons and palmar interossei).
• Flexor tendon sheaths.
• Radial bursa.
• Ulnar bursa.

5.20.2 Causes of hand infections

Infections are usually due to untreated minor wounds or bites, particularly human bites. Causes of infection vary according to the type of wound (Table 5.4).

Admission is required for elevation, parenteral antibiotics, and operative debridement and washout.

5.20.3 Flexor tendon sheath infections

Tendon sheaths in the ring, middle, and index fingers run from the metacarpal neck to the insertion of the FDP distally. The little finger and thumb tendon sheaths are continuous with the ulnar and

Table 5.4 Bacterial causes of hand infections

Contaminated open wound	*Staphylococcus aureus* (responsible for most hand infections)
	Streptococcus viridians
	β-haemolytic streptococci
	Anaerobes (especially in IVDU or diabetes)
Human bites	*Staphylococcus aureus*
	Streptococcus epidermidis
	α and *β-haemolytic streptococci*
	Eikenella corrodens (anaerobe that is part of normal human oral flora)
	Anaerobes
Animal bites	*Pasteurella multocida*
	As for human bites

radial bursae in the palm, respectively, and therefore infections in these sheaths can spread to the carpal tunnel.

Once bacteria have gained entry to the tendon sheath, pus can accumulate, and the pressure increases because the sheath is a closed space. The increasing pressure can lead to compartment syndrome. The process has the ability to rapidly destroy a finger's functional capacity and is an orthopaedic emergency.

The four cardinal clinical signs (Kanavel's signs) are:

- Tenderness along the course of the flexor tendon
- Symmetrical oedema of the finger
- Pain on passive extension of the finger
- Flexed resting posture of the finger

Treatment is intravenous broad-spectrum antibiotics, elevation, and urgent orthopaedic referral for operative drainage and washout.

5.20.4 Bites

Bite wounds to the hand may cause cellulitis and abscesses. Human bites are particularly virulent because of the high concentration of gram-positive and anaerobic bacteria present in the mouth.

'Fight-bites' are particularly problematic when sustained on the teeth of the punched opponent. Frequently patients will deny the mechanism of injury and any wounds over or near the MCPJs should be considered potentially contaminated and penetrating the joint. At the time of injury, the fingers are flexed in a fist and a tooth can penetrate the skin, extensor tendon, and joint capsule of the MCPJ or IPJs. When the hand is examined with the fingers in extension, the skin and tendon injuries migrate proximally, and therefore the injury can be missed.

X-rays should be obtained if there is a risk of fracture, joint penetration (air in the joint), or a radio-opaque foreign body (tooth).

Wounds should be anaesthetized, explored, and thoroughly irrigated. Wounds over joints, involving tendons, or with large amounts of devitalized tissue, should be referred for operative exploration and debridement. Primary closure should be avoided in the ED unless significant cosmetic implications (e.g. facial wounds). Antibiotic cover should be provided and tetanus prophylaxis given, if indicated.

Human bites should be assessed for the risk of hepatitis B, C, and HIV. Patients should be risk-assessed and treated as for needlestick injuries (see Chapter 15, section 15.6).

KEY POINTS

The commonest bacterial cause of hand infections is *Staphylococcus aureus*.

The four cardinal clinical signs of a flexor tendon sheath infection are:

- Tenderness along the course of the flexor tendon
- Symmetrical oedema of the finger
- Pain on passive extension of the finger
- Flexed resting posture of the finger

Patients sustaining human bites are at risk of hepatitis B, C, and HIV. Patients should be risk-assessed and may require post-exposure prophylaxis.

5.21 Special hand injuries

The curriculum specifically states knowledge of certain hand injuries and these may appear in SAQs.

5.21.1 Amputation

Patients with partial or complete digital amputation with bony loss should be referred to a hand surgeon for consideration of reimplantation. The ultimate procedure, reimplantation or terminalization, will depend on the location of the amputation and the condition of the amputated part.

The digit and amputated part should be X-rayed. The wound should be dressed with a non-adherent dressing and elevated. Tetanus prophylaxis should be provided and broad-spectrum antibiotics given. The amputated part should be wrapped gently in moist saline swabs and placed in a sealed plastic bag surrounded by a mixture of ice and water. The part should not be allowed to freeze or get waterlogged.

5.21.2 High-pressure injection

A variety of industrial equipment contains liquids at high pressure (e.g. paint sprays, grease guns, and hydraulics). Leakage through small holes in pipes, cables, or nozzles can drive the material through intact skin. Initially the wound may appear trivial but the underlying injury can be devastating with the risk of permanent stiffness and tissue loss.

X-rays may help identify the extent of foreign material. All high-pressure injuries should be referred immediately to a hand surgeon for exploration and debridement.

5.21.3 Adrenaline digital injection

Accidental digital injection of adrenaline may occur from an autoinjector used for anaphylaxis. This can result in severe vasoconstriction and the risk of digital ischaemia. There are various treatment options, including immersing the digit in warm water, topical or systemic glyceryl trinitrate, and local infiltration of phentolamine (a short acting α-blocker).

5.21.4 Degloving injuries

Degloving injuries are a type of avulsion injury where the skin is completely torn off the underlying tissues and thereby deprived of its blood supply. In the hand, such injuries can occur when a ring gets avulsed off a finger, or a hand gets caught between an overturned car and the road.

Degloving injuries require immediate referral to a hand surgeon.

5.22 Tetanus

Tetanus is an acute disease caused by the action of tetanus toxin released following infection by *Clostridium tetani*. Tetanus spores are present in soil or manure and may be introduced into the

Box 5.1 Tetanus immunization schedule

Primary immunizations

The primary tetanus immunizations are given with diphtheria, pertussis, polio, and Hib vaccines at the following intervals:

- Two months old
- Three months old
- Four months old

Reinforcing immunizations

Tetanus boosters are combined with diptheria, pertussis, and polio vaccines. The timing of the boosters is as follows:

- First booster—between ages 3½ to 5 years (ideally three years after completion of primary course)
- Second booster—between ages 13 and 18 years (ideally 10 years after the first booster)

Data from Immunisations against infectious disease—'The Green Book' (2010 update). www.dh.gov.uk/greenbook.

body through a puncture wound, burn, or scratch. The bacteria grow anaerobically at the site of the injury and have an incubation period of 4–21 days.

The following information is based on the Department of Health document on immunizations against infectious disease—'The Green Book' (see Further reading).

Tetanus immunization has been provided nationally in the United Kingdom since 1961. The vaccine is a cell-free toxin extract from a strain of *C. tetani*. The immunization schedule for tetanus involves five doses of vaccine at appropriate age intervals (Box 5.1).

5.22.1 Tetanus-prone wounds

Previous MRCEM question

Knowledge of the management of tetanus-prone wounds is important for all parts of the FRCEM examination and often appears (Table 5.5).

Table 5.5 Tetanus immunization required for wounds

Immunization status	Clean wound	Tetanus-prone wound	High-risk wound
Fully immunized	Nil required	Nil required	Immunoglobulin
Primary immunizations complete	Nil required	Nil required	Immunoglobulin
Primary immunizations incomplete or boosters not up to date	Tetanus booster and advise completion at GP	Tetanus booster and immunoglobulin	Tetanus booster and immunoglobulin
Not immunized	Give first dose of vaccine and advise completion at GP	Give first dose of vaccine and immunoglobulin	Give first dose of vaccine and immunoglobulin

Reproduced from Immunisations against infectious disease—'The Green Book' (2010 update). www.dh.gov.uk/greenbook.

Tetanus-prone wounds include:

- Wounds or burns that require surgical intervention that is delayed for more than six hours
- Wounds or burns that show a significant degree of devitalized tissue or a puncture-type injury, particularly where there has been contact with soil or manure
- Wounds containing foreign bodies
- Compound fractures
- Wounds or burns in patients who have systemic sepsis*

High-risk tetanus-prone wounds are those heavily contaminated with material likely to contain tetanus spores and/or extensive devitalized tissue. If the patient has a high-risk tetanus-prone wound, they should receive human tetanus immunoglobulin, regardless of their immunization history.

Tetanus vaccine given at the time of a tetanus-prone injury may not boost immunity early enough to give additional protection within the incubation period of tetanus. Therefore, tetanus vaccine is not considered adequate for treating a tetanus-prone wound. However, this provides an opportunity to ensure that the individual is protected against future exposure.

Patients who are immunosuppressed may not be adequately protected against tetanus, despite having been fully immunized. They should be managed as if they were incompletely immunized. For those whose immunization status is uncertain, and individuals born before 1961 who may not have been immunized in infancy, a full course of immunization is likely to be required.

Injecting drug users may be at risk from tetanus-contaminated illicit drugs, especially when they have sites of focal infection, such as skin abscesses, that may promote growth of anaerobic organisms. Every opportunity should be taken to ensure that they are fully protected against tetanus. Booster doses should be given if there is any doubt about their immunization status.

Dosage of human tetanus immunoglobulin

The dose of tetanus immunoglobulin is 250 IU intramuscularly, or 500 IU if more than 24 hours have elapsed since the injury; or there is a risk of heavy contamination; or following burns. The immunoglobulin injection must be given at a different site to the tetanus booster.

5.22.2 Tetanus infection

Tetanus is a notifiable disease and infections are now rare in the United Kingdom, there being only seven recorded cases in England and Wales in 2013. It cannot be completely eradicated, as spores are commonly present in the environment, including soil. Clostridium tetani produces an exotoxin that blocks inhibitory neurons in the central nervous system. The disease is characterized by generalized rigidity and spasm of skeletal muscle. The muscle stiffness usually involves the jaw (lockjaw) and neck, and then becomes generalized. In severe cases, muscle spasms affect breathing and swallowing. Autonomic disturbance causes profuse sweating, tachycardia, and hypertension, alternating with bradycardia and hypotension.

Management of tetanus infection

- Supportive—paralysis and intubation may be required if breathing becomes inadequate.
- Diazepam—to control muscle spasms.
- Wounds—cleaned and debrided.
- Broad-spectrum antibiotic cover.
- Human tetanus immunoglobulin—5000–10,000 IU as an intravenous infusion.

---

* Reproduced from *Immunisations against infectious disease*—'The Green Book' (2010 update). www.dh.gov.uk/greenbook.

KEY POINTS

Wounds can be categorized as: clean; tetanus-prone; or high-risk tetanus-prone. The wound category and the patient's immunization status determine what prophylaxis is required.

Tetanus-prone wounds include:

- Wounds or burns that require surgical intervention that is delayed for more than six hours
- Wounds or burns that show a significant degree of devitalized tissue or a puncture-type injury, particularly where there has been contact with soil or manure
- Wounds containing foreign bodies
- Compound fractures
- Wounds or burns in patients who have systemic sepsis

High-risk tetanus-prone wounds are those heavily contaminated with material likely to contain tetanus spores and/or extensive devitalized tissue.

If the patient has a high-risk tetanus-prone wound, they should receive human tetanus immunoglobulin, regardless of their immunization history.

Patients who are immunosuppressed should be considered as incompletely immunized, regardless of their previous vaccination history.

In addition to providing tetanus prophylaxis, it is essential that wounds are thoroughly cleaned.

5.23 SAQs

5.23.1 'Fight bite'

A 21-year-old man presents to the ED on Monday morning having injured his hand on Saturday night when he punched a wall. He has a 1-cm ragged laceration just proximal to the MCPJ of the middle finger.

a) (i)   What underlying structures could have been damaged given the location of the injury? (3 marks)

a) (ii) Why is the wound not directly over the MCPJ? (1 mark)

a) (iii) Give three indications for X-raying the hand in this patient. (3 marks)

The case is discussed with the orthopaedic registrar who plans to take the patient for operative wound exploration and debridement.

b) What are the most important ED management steps that need to occur prior to surgery? (3 marks)

Suggested answer

a) (i)   What underlying structures could have been damaged given the location of the injury? (3 marks)

- Extensor tendon.
- Joint capsule of MCPJ.
- Bone (head of metacarpal and/or base of proximal phalanx).
- (Not skin because question asks for underlying structures.)

a) (ii) Why is the wound not directly over the MCPJ? (1 mark)

- During a punch the fist is clenched, but as the finger is extended the skin and tendon migrate proximally.

a) (iii) Give three indications for X-raying the hand in this patient. (3 marks)

- Possible fracture
- To identify air in the joint
- To identify any radio-opaque foreign body (e.g. tooth)

b) What are the most important ED management steps that need to occur prior to surgery? (3 marks)

- Antibiotics to cover typical oral flora (e.g. co-amoxiclav or erythromycin).
- Ensure appropriate tetanus prophylaxis.
- Risk assess for transmission of hepatitis B, C, and HIV. Take blood for serum save and start accelerated hepatitis B vaccination course.

5.23.2 Gout

A 58-year-old gentleman presents with an acutely painful, hot, and red first MTPJ. He has a history of gout and thinks he is having a flare.

a) Describe the pathophysiology of gout. (2 marks)

b) The F2 has taken a blood sample from the patient and asks if you want a urate level adding? Justify your answer. (½ mark answer, ½ mark reason)

c) (i)   What pharmacological treatment options are available to him and what is their mechanism of action? (6 marks)

   (ii) Why should he not be started on allopurinol in the ED? (1 mark)

Suggested answer

a) Describe the pathophysiology of gout. (2 marks)

Disorder of purine metabolism (increased production or decreased excretion of uric acid).
Raised uric acid levels.
Urate crystals precipitate out into joints, resulting in a localized inflammatory reaction.
(2 marks for any two)

b) The F2 has taken a blood sample from the patient and asks if you want a urate level adding?
Justify your answer. (½ mark answer, ½ mark reason)

No.
Urate levels may be normal in an acute flare, even in hyperuricaemic patients, and some
patients with hyperuricaemia never develop gout.

c) (i)   What pharmacological treatment options are available to him and what is their
mechanism of action? (6 marks)

NSAIDs—cyclo-oxygenase inhibitor. Reduces production of prostaglandins and therefore
acts as an anti-inflammatory and analgesic.
Colchicine—the exact mechanism of action is unknown. It is thought to reduce urate
crystal deposition and reduce the inflammatory response to urate crystals.
Prednisolone—anti-inflammatory.
(1 mark for drug, 1 mark for mechanism of action)

(ii)   Why should he not be started on allopurinol in the ED? (1 mark)

Allopurinol is a xanthine oxidase inhibitor which reduces uric acid production. It can rapidly reduce
the level of uric acid, which can conversely exacerbate a flare of gout.

Further reading

Coakley G, Mathews C, Field M, et al. 2006. Guidelines for management of the hot swollen joint in
adults. Rheumatology (Oxford) **45**(8):1039–41.

Cunningham N. 2003. A new drug-free technique for reducing anterior shoulder dislocations.
Emerg Med (Fremantle) **15**(5-6):521–4.

Department of Health, 2006. Immunizations Against Infectious Disease—'The Green Book' (updated
edn). The Stationary Office under license from the Department of Health. Available at: https://
www.dh.gov.uk/greenbook [Online].

National Institute for Health and Care Excellence, May 2009. NICE clinical guideline 88. Low
back pain in adults: early management. Available at: https://www.nice.org.uk/guidance/CG88
[Online].

National Institute for Health and Care Excellence, June 2011. NICE clinical guideline 124. Hip fracture: the management of hip fractures in adults. Available at: https://www.nice.org.uk/guid-
ance/CG124 [Online].

Royal College of Emergency Medicine, September 2013. College of Emergency Medicine Clinical
Effectiveness Committee. Clinical Standards for the management of fractured neck of femur.
Available at: https://www.RCEM.ac.uk [Online].

Scottish Intercollegiate Guideline Network, June 2009. SIGN guideline 111, Management of hip
fracture in older people. Available at: http://www.sign.ac.uk/guidelines/fulltext/111/ [Online].

CHAPTER 6

Surgery

CONTENTS

6.1 The acute abdomen

6.1.1 Introduction

A patient presenting acutely unwell, with signs and symptoms predominantly related to the abdomen has an acute abdomen. An acute abdomen is not in itself a diagnosis and the list of causes is extensive.

A short-answer question (SAQ) on acute abdominal pain is unlikely to ask for a long differential list of causes but may ask for the 'most likely' cause based on the age, sex, or particular presentation of a patient. Questions may focus on specific investigations that help differentiate between causes of abdominal pain.

6.1.2 Causes of abdominal pain

The following paragraphs focus on causes of acute abdominal pain based on the site of pain, specific clinical features, and age of the patient (Figure 6.1, Tables 6.1 and 6.2). An abrupt onset of pain may be associated with hollow viscus perforation or vascular causes, such as leaking abdominal aortic aneurysm and mesenteric ischaemia.

Associated symptoms of nausea, vomiting, anorexia, and fever are present for many causes of abdominal pain and usually do not help differentiate between causes. A gynaecological history should be sought in female patients because of the additional differential causes, for example ectopic pregnancy, ovarian torsion, ovarian cyst rupture, pelvic inflammatory disease, endometriosis, Mittelschmerz, and so on (see Chapter 8, section 8.1). It is worth remembering medical causes of acute abdominal pain (Table 6.3)

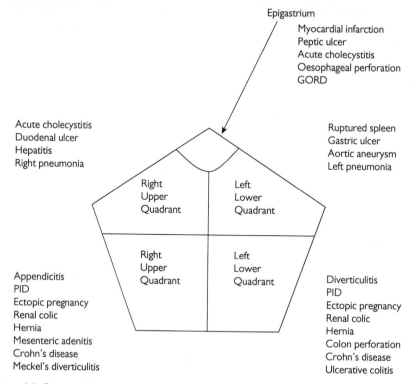

Epigastrium
- Myocardial infarction
- Peptic ulcer
- Acute cholecystitis
- Oesophageal perforation
- GORD

Acute cholecystitis
Duodenal ulcer
Hepatitis
Right pneumonia

Ruptured spleen
Gastric ulcer
Aortic aneurysm
Left pneumonia

Right Upper Quadrant

Left Lower Quadrant

Right Upper Quadrant

Left Lower Quadrant

Appendicitis
PID
Ectopic pregnancy
Renal colic
Hernia
Mesenteric adenitis
Crohn's disease
Meckel's diverticulitis

Diverticulitis
PID
Ectopic pregnancy
Renal colic
Hernia
Colon perforation
Crohn's disease
Ulcerative colitis

Figure 6.1 Causes of abdominal pain, based on location.

Table 6.1 Clinical features suggesting particular causes of abdominal pain

Clinical features	Differential diagnosis
Abdominal pain out of proportion to clinical findings	Leaking aortic aneurysm
	Mesenteric infarction
	Renal colic
Abdominal pain in patients with atherosclerotic disease/AF	Aortic aneurysm
	Mesenteric infarction (embolic or thrombotic)
Severe abdominal pain radiating through to back	Aortic aneurysm
	Acute cholecystitis
	Ascending cholangitis
	Acute pancreatitis
	Peptic ulcer disease
Flank pain radiating to the groin	Renal colic
	Pyelonephritis
	Testicular torsion
	Aortic aneurysm

Table 6.1 Continued

Clinical features	Differential diagnosis
Abdominal pain with collapse or signs of shock	Aortic aneurysm
	Ectopic pregnancy
	Massive GI bleed
	Myocardial infarction
Abdominal pain associated with shoulder tip pain (due to diaphragmatic irritation)	Ectopic pregnancy
	Acute pancreatitis
	Acute cholecystitis
	Ascending cholangitis
	Aortic aneurysm
	Bowel perforation
Abdominal distension	Bowel obstruction
	Pregnancy
	Ascites
	Cancer
Abdominal bruising	Trauma
	Aortic aneurysm
	Acute pancreatitis—haemorrhagic fluid collecting in the paracolic gutters (Grey Turner's sign) or around umbilicus (Cullen's sign)
Evidence of GI bleeding (haematemesis or melena)	Peptic ulcer
	Diverticular disease
	Malignancy
	Varices
	Angiodysplasia
Constipation	Bowel obstruction
	Bowel ischaemia
	Diverticular disease

6.1.3 Investigations for abdominal pain

There is an extensive list of investigations that may be performed on a patient with an acutely painful abdomen. Blood tests such as a white cell count and C-reactive protein (CRP) do not help differentiate between causes and may be normal even in patients with significant intra-abdominal pathology, especially in the early stages.

In female patients of child-bearing age, a urinary pregnancy test (+/- serum BHCG) should always be performed.

This chapter will highlight the clinical features and investigations that help identify particular conditions or grade severity.

Table 6.2 Differential diagnosis based on age group

Age	Differential diagnosis
Infants	Meconium ileus
	Hypertrophic pyloric stenosis
	Intussusception
	Appendicitis
	Hernia
	Volvulus
	Testicular torsion
Adolescents	Appendicitis
	Testicular torsion
	Epididymo-orchitis
	Ectopic pregnancy
Elderly	Aortic aneurysm
	Urinary retention
	Mesenteric infarction
	Acute cholecystitis
	Bowel obstruction
	Acute pancreatitis
	Diverticular disease
	Malignancy
	Hernia

Table 6.3 Medical causes for acute abdomen

Aetiology	Differential diagnosis
Cardiorespiratory	Inferior ST-elevation myocardial infarction
	Pericarditis
	Lower lobe pneumonia
	Pulmonary embolism
Metabolic/Endocrine	Diabetic ketoacidosis
	Acute adrenocortical insufficiency
	Acute intermittent porphyria
	Hyperlipidaemia
	Familial mediterranean fever
Drug induced	Opioid withdrawal
	Lead poisoning
Haematological	Sickle cell crisis
	Acute leukaemia
Central nervous system:	Herpes zoster
	Nerve root compression

KEY POINTS

SAQs are unlikely to ask for a long differential list of causes but may want to know the 'most likely' cause(s) based on the information given in the question. Read the question carefully to avoid jumping to the wrong answer.

Investigations should be directed at differentiating between causes of abdominal pain or grading severity, and not simply 'routine bloods'. If an SAQ asks what investigations you want, think carefully about the answer. Some questions will ask you to justify your reason(s) for the investigation.

6.2 Biliary tract disorders

6.2.1 Introduction

The commonest biliary tract disorder presenting to the emergency department (ED) is gallstones. Gallstones are precipitants of bile that form in the gallbladder. Bile contains cholesterol, bile pigments (from haemoglobin breakdown), and phospholipids. The varying concentrations of these components results in three main types of stone:

- Cholesterol—large, often solitary stones that account for the majority of UK gallstone disease. Risk factors include increasing age, female sex, obesity, family history, hyperlipidaemia, diabetes, and cystic fibrosis.
- Pigmented—small, dark stones composed of bilirubin and calcium salts. Risk factors for pigmented stones include haemolytic anaemias, such as sickle cell disease.
- Mixed—contain varying amounts of cholesterol, calcium salts, and bilirubin. The calcium salts allow the stones to be seen radiographically. Approximately 10% of gallstones are radio-opaque.

6.2.2 Biliary colic

Biliary colic occurs when a gallstone lodges in the neck of the gallbladder, the cystic duct, or common bile duct. The blockage causes increased intraluminal pressure and distension of the gallbladder. The gallstone then dislodges and passes out of the biliary tract.

The patient experiences abdominal pain, often located in the right-upper quadrant, associated with nausea and vomiting. The symptoms resolve when the stone passes.

Patients may suffer recurrent episodes of biliary colic when further stones pass and therefore are diagnosed with chronic cholecystitis.

An ultrasound scan is indicated to confirm the presence of gallstones, which appear as mobile echogenic objects with distal acoustic shadowing. Blood tests are normal. If symptoms settle, then outpatient management is appropriate, pending a cholecystectomy.

6.2.3 Acute cholecystitis

In 95% of acute cholecystitis, a gallstone or biliary sludge becomes impacted at the neck of the gallbladder. Only 5% of patients have no stone; these are usually patients that have been admitted for trauma, burns, or have diabetes. Acalculous acute cholecystitis has a worse prognosis than those with gallstones.

The obstructed gallbladder becomes distended, inflamed, and ischaemic. Bacteria are able to penetrate the gallbladder wall causing infection. Prolonged obstruction may result in a gallbladder empyema.

Clinical features of acute cholecystitis

- Abdominal pain—typically located in the right-upper quadrant. Pain is often dull and poorly localized initially due to distension of the gallbladder and stimulation of the visceral peritoneum. As the inflammatory process progresses, inflammatory fluid leaks out stimulating the local parietal peritoneum, which is innervated by intercostal nerves and felt as a sharp, well-localized pain.
- Murphy's sign—this is an indication of local peritonism. Deep palpation in the right-upper quadrant, during inspiration, causes pain as the inflamed gallbladder impinges on the palpating hand. This causes a sudden inspiratory arrest. The test is only positive if repetition in the left-upper quadrant doesn't cause pain.
- Jaundice—may occur if the stone moves and obstructs the common bile duct, or if the gallbladder causes compression of the common hepatic duct (Mirizzi's syndrome).

Specific investigations for acute cholecystitis

- Ultrasound scan—is the most useful investigation for confirming the diagnosis. It may show gallbladder wall thickening, a dilated gall bladder, peri-cholecystic fluid, gas in the gall bladder wall, and an impacted gallstone.
  - Amylase or lipase should be sent to exclude pancreatitis.
  - Urinary pregnancy test.
  - Electrocardiogram (ECG)—to exclude a MI or ACS.
- Chest X-ray (CXR)—to exclude pneumonia and look for evidence of air under the diaphragm in a suspected perforation.

Management of acute cholecystitis

- Fluid resuscitation—if the patient has signs of sepsis or dehydration.
  - Analgesia—intravenous morphine titrated to effect.
  - Antibiotics—usually a third-generation cephalosporin but local antibiotic policy should be followed.
  - Nil by mouth.
- Urgent surgical review—surgical options depend on the severity of illness ranging from medical therapy, to endoscopic retrograde cholangiopancreatography (ERCP), to cholecystectomy (open or laparoscopic).

6.2.4 Common bile duct stones

Choledocholithiasis

Choledocholithiasis is when a gallstone becomes stuck in the common bile duct resulting in jaundice and hepatic damage. Investigations are the same as acute cholecystitis. Treatment is removal of the stone via ERCP.

Ascending cholangitis

Obstruction of the common bile duct leads to biliary stasis and a predisposition to bacterial infection ascending from the duodenal ampulla.

The classic presentation of ascending cholangitis is Charcot's triad:

- Abdominal pain
- Jaundice
- Fever

Ascending cholangitis is a life-threatening emergency with a high mortality. Patients should be aggressively resuscitated with intravenous fluids and broad-spectrum antibiotics. Urgent surgical input is required.

Obstructive jaundice

A gallstone in the common bile duct is a cause of post-hepatic jaundice. The patient will have dark urine and pale stools. Cholangio-/pancreatic carcinomas may present in a similar manner but are usually not painful. If the gallbladder is palpable, a pancreatic carcinoma is the more likely diagnosis (Courvoisier's law: 'In the presence of jaundice, if the gallbladder is palpable, the cause is unlikely to be a stone').

Gallstone ileus

Prolonged obstruction and inflammation of the gallbladder may result in a fistula developing between the gallbladder and the duodenum. The gallstone can then enter the GI tract and obstruct the terminal ileum. An abdominal X-ray may show air in the biliary tree and evidence of small bowel obstruction.

Patients should be resuscitated and referred urgently for surgical review.

KEY POINTS

Approximately 10% of gallstones are radio-opaque.

Murphy's sign is an indication of local peritonism due to gallbladder inflammation. Deep palpation in the right-upper quadrant, during inspiration, causes pain as the inflamed gallbladder impinges on the palpating hand.

Choledocholithiasis is when a gallstone becomes stuck in the common bile duct resulting in jaundice and hepatic damage.

The classic presentation of ascending cholangitis is Charcot's triad:

- Abdominal pain
- Jaundice
- Fever

Courvoisier's law: 'In the presence of jaundice, if the gallbladder is palpable, the cause is unlikely to be a stone'.

6.3 Acute pancreatitis

6.3.1 Introduction

Acute pancreatitis is sudden inflammation of the pancreas, associated with acinar cell injury. Inappropriately activated pancreatic enzymes, such as proteases and lipases, result in autodigestion of the pancreas.

6.3.2 Causes of acute pancreatitis

Causes of acute pancreatitis can be remembered using the mnemonic 'GET SMASHED'.

- **G**allstones—account for approximately 50% of cases in the United Kingdom.
- **E**thanol—accounts for 20–25% of cases.
- **T**rauma.
- **S**teroids.
- **M**umps—other viruses include cytomegalovirus and Epstein–Barr virus.
- **A**utoimmune.
- **S**corpion venom (do not use this as an answer in the exam because it is very rare and is likely to be marked as incorrect).
- **H**yperlipidaemia, hypercalcaemia, hypothermia.

- **E**RCP.
- **D**rugs (oestrogens, azathioprine, thiazide diuretics, and valproate).
- **I**diopathic.
- **P**regnancy.

6.3.3 Specific investigations for pancreatitis

- Amylase or lipase—lipase if available is the preferred pancreatic enzyme because it has greater sensitivity and specificity. Serum amylase should be three times the upper limit of laboratory normal or >1000 units/litre to be diagnostic, although lower levels can be expected in relapsing acute pancreatitis, related to loss of pancreatic exocrine cell mass. A normal serum amylase level does not exclude pancreatitis.
- Ultrasound—is helpful in identifying gallstones. Diffuse enlargement of the pancreas, with blurred irregular margins, dilatation of pancreatic duct > 2 mm, and fluid collections (hypoechoic areas) in lesser sac, anterior and posterior pararenal spaces, splenic hilum, and transverse mesocolon may be seen.
- CT abdomen (with contrast)—diffuse or focal (segmental) enlargement of gland up to three times the normal size, with decreased density, and ill-defined margins may be seen. There may be abnormal (heterogeneous) enhancement of gland, and thickening of peri-pancreatic tissue planes.

6.3.4 Severity scoring in acute pancreatitis

Several different severity scores exist to try and predict the prognosis of patients with acute pancreatitis. The 'UK guidelines for the management of acute pancreatitis' recommend the following prognostic features to predict complications:

- Clinical impression of severity:
  - Obesity
  - APACHE II score >8 in the first 24 hours
  - CRP >150 mg/L
  - Glasgow score ≥3
- Persisting organ failure after 48 hours in hospital.

APACHE II (Acute Physiology and Chronic Health Evaluation) is a severity of disease classification system used most commonly in intensive care patients (Table 6.4). A score from 0 to 71 is possible and is calculated by computer, based on physiological measurements, blood test results, age, and previous health status. Higher scores imply more severe disease and a higher risk of death.

The Glasgow scoring system can be applied when the patient first presents but will not be complete until 48 hours (Table 6.5). It has been validated in the UK population and an initial score of three or more suggests severe disease.

The Ranson criteria provide another scoring system that can be used on admission and at 48 hours but are not recommended by the 'UK Working Party on Acute Pancreatitis'.

6.3.5 Emergency department management of acute pancreatitis

- Fluid resuscitation—adequate fluid resuscitation is essential for the prevention of systemic complications. A urine output >0.5 ml/kg/h should be maintained. In severe pancreatitis, fluid resuscitation should be guided by central venous pressure monitoring.
- Oxygen—should be given to maintain saturations above 95%.
- Analgesia and anti-emetics—intravenous opiates should be titrated to pain.
- Antibiotics—there is no consensus on whether prophylactic antibiotics against pancreatic necrosis should be given or not.

Table 6.4 Components of the APACHE II score

Physiological measurements	Temperature
	Mean arterial blood pressure
	Heart rate
	Respiratory rate
	GCS
Blood tests	PaO_2
	Arterial pH
	Serum sodium
	Serum potassium
	Serum creatinine
	Haematocrit
	White cell count
Age	
Previous health status	

Data from Knaus WA, Draper EA, Wagner DP, et al (1985). 'APACHE II: a severity of disease classification system'. Critical Care Medicine 13 (10): 818–29

- Nil by mouth—the aim is to rest the bowel and reduce pancreatic enzyme release. Once patients are admitted, they may be started on enteral feeding via a nasogastric or nasojejunal tube if nutritional support is required.
- Surgical referral—patients with gallstone pancreatitis should have an urgent ERCP and sphincterotomy within the first 72 hours of admission. Ideally a cholecystectomy should be performed in the same admission.

Table 6.5 Glasgow scoring system for acute pancreatitis

Age	>55 years
White cell count	>15 × 10^9/L
Glucose	>10 mmol/L
Urea	>16 mmol/L
PaO_2	<8 kPa
Corrected calcium	<2 mmol/L
Albumin	<32 g/L
Lactate dehydrogenase	>600 units/L
Asparate/alanine aminotransferase	>100 units/L

Data from Blamey SL, Imrie CW, O'Neill J, et al (1984). 'Prognostic factors in acute pancreatitis'. Gut;25(12):1340–6

Table 6.6 Complications of acute pancreatitis

Local complications	Systemic complications
Pancreatic necrosis	Hypocalcaemia
Pseudocyst	Hyperglycaemia
Pancreatic abscess	Disseminated intravascular coagulation
Ascites	
Biliary tract obstruction	Acute kidney injury
Portal vein thrombosis	Acute respiratory distress syndrome
Paralytic ileus	Sepsis
GI haemorrhage	Multiorgan failure
	Death

Table 6.6 summarizes the complications of acute pancreatitis.

KEY POINTS

Lipase is the most sensitive and specific blood test in suspected pancreatitis.

A normal serum amylase does not exclude pancreatitis.

Causes of acute pancreatitis can be remembered using the mnemonic 'GET SMASHED'.

The 'UK guidelines for the management of acute pancreatitis' recommend the following prognostic features to predict complications:

- Clinical impression of severity
- Obesity
- APACHE II score >8 in the first 24 h
- CRP >150 mg/L
- Glasgow score ≥3
- Persisting organ failure after 48 hours in hospital

6.4 Appendicitis

6.4.1 Introduction

Appendicitis is one of the commonest surgical presentations to the ED. Appendicitis results from obstruction of the lumen of the appendix, due to a faecolith, lymphoid tissue, or adhesions. This increases intraluminal pressure and the appendix distends. As the pressure rises, the appendix wall ulcerates allowing bacterial invasion and ultimately gangrene. If left untreated, the appendix may perforate causing general peritonitis.

6.4.2 Clinical features of appendicitis

- Abdominal pain—initially central and poorly localized due to stimulation of autonomic nerves in the appendix wall. Eventually the inflamed appendix irritates the parietal peritoneum resulting in a well-localized, sharp pain in the right iliac fossa.
- Rovsing's sign—palpation in the left iliac fossa causes pain in the right iliac fossa.
- Other symptoms—nausea, vomiting, anorexia, constipation, fever.

6.4.3 Investigations for appendicitis

- Diagnosis is clinical.
- Urine should be checked to exclude pregnancy or a urinary tract infections (UTI) as the cause of pain. However, 30–40% of patients will have an abnormal urinalysis in appendicitis.
- White cell count and CRP may be elevated, but can be normal.
- Ultrasound scan can be useful as a rule-in test for appendicitis but a normal ultrasound does not rule it out. Ultrasound may also identify other pathologies as the cause of pain (e.g. ectopic pregnancy, ovarian torsion).
- The Alvarado score may be used as a diagnostic aid (Table 6.7) in suspected acute pancreatitis. A popular mnemonic used to remember the scoring system is MANTRELS.

  Alvarado scores:

- 5 or 6: Compatible with the diagnosis of acute appendicitis
- 7 or 8: Probable appendicitis
- 9 or 10: Very probable acute appendicitis

6.4.4 Emergency department management of appendicitis

- Fluid resuscitation—as required by the patient's haemodynamic status
- Analgesia (there is no evidence that opiates mask signs of peritonism)
- Nil by mouth
- Surgical referral

KEY POINTS

Appendicitis is a clinical diagnosis.

Rovsing's sign is when palpation in the left iliac fossa causes pain in the right iliac fossa.

Alvarado (Mantrels) scoring system can be used to aid diagnosis

Table 6.7 The Alvarodo scoring system (aka Mantrels)

Variable	Score
Symptoms	1
Migration of pain to right lower quadrant	1
Anorexia	1
Nausea and vomiting	1
SIGNS	1
Tenderness in RIF	1
Rebound tenderness	2
Elevated temperature (>37.3°C)	1
Laboratory tests	Total 10
Leucocytosis (>10,000/μL)	
Left shift leucocytosis	

6.5 Bowel obstruction

Bowel obstruction is mechanical or functional obstruction of the gastrointestinal tract (Table 6.8).

Classic symptoms are abdominal pain, distension, vomiting, and absolute constipation. The exact nature of the symptoms depends upon the cause and site of obstruction.

6.5.1 Specific investigations for bowel obstruction

Abdominal X-ray—this is one of the few acute abdominal presentations where an abdominal X-ray may be helpful. Films are initially performed supine, but may be repeated erect if the film is inconclusive when looking for evidence of multiple fluid levels in the bowel.

- Small bowel obstruction—dilated loops of small bowel are seen centrally. The valvulae conniventes should be visible across the whole width of the dilated bowel wall. Small bowel loops greater than 3 cm in diameter are abnormal. The sensitivity of an abdominal X-ray for small bowel obstruction is approximately 70%.
- Large bowel obstruction—peripheral, loops of bowel greater than 5 cm suggest large bowel obstruction. The haustra do not cross the full diameter of the bowel. Unless the ileocaecal valve is incompetent, the dilatation should not extend into the small bowel. Sensitivity is approximately 90%.
- Functional bowel obstruction—typically air is seen in both the small and large bowel.

There is no evidence of a 'cut-off' as it is bowel peristalsis, not the obstruction that is the problem.

- Volvulus—a sigmoid volvulus results in an extremely dilated loop of sigmoid colon on which appears as an inverted U-shaped loop. In a caecal volvulus, the caecum is markedly distended, elevated, and displaced to the left-upper quadrant and is seen as one large, dilated loop. Distal to the volvulus, the large bowel is empty.

CT is the gold standard investigation for identifying bowel obstruction because it has a greater sensitivity that X-ray and is often able to identify the cause. CT scanning identifies dilated bowel with a transition point beyond which the bowel diameter is normal or collapsed. The characteristics of the transition point may provide clues to the aetiology of the obstruction (e.g. a solitary eccentric notch may suggest the presence of adhesions). Bowel wall oedema and absence of wall perfusion suggest coexisting bowel ischaemia.

Table 6.8 Causes of bowel obstruction

Small bowel obstruction	Large bowel obstruction	Functional bowel obstruction (due to reduced bowel motility)
Adhesions	Volvulus	Hypokalaemia
Hernias	Hernias	Hyponatraemia
Crohn's disease	Adhesions	Hypomagnesaemia
Gallstone ileus	Inflammatory bowel disease	Intestinal ischaemia
Tumour	Tumour	Intra-abdominal infection
Intussusception	Faecal impaction	Trauma
Foreign bodies	Diverticulitis	Pseudo-obstruction (chronic impairment of GI motility often exacerbated by drugs, e.g. tricyclic antidepressants)

6.5.2 Emergency department management of bowel obstruction

- Fluid resuscitation.
- Intravenous analgesia and anti-emetic.
- Nasogastric tube.
- An enema may be given after discussion with the surgical team.
- Surgical referral for further management, either conservative or surgical.

KEY POINTS

There are only a few indications for abdominal X-ray: suspected obstruction; suspected oesophageal foreign body; suspected ingestion of a sharp or poisonous foreign body. Abdominal X-ray has approximately 70% sensitivity for small bowel obstruction. The small bowel can be identified by the central location and valvulae conniventes, which cross the whole width of the bowel wall. Small bowel loops greater than 3 cm in diameter are abnormal. Abdominal X-ray has approximately 90% sensitivity for large bowel obstruction. The large bowel can be identified by the peripheral location and haustra which do not cross the full diameter of the bowel. Loops of bowel greater than 5 cm suggest large bowel obstruction.

6.6 Bowel perforation

Bowel perforation is a life-threatening surgical emergency. Perforations may affect any part of the GI tract.

6.6.1 Causes of bowel perforation

- Peptic ulcer
- Appendicitis
- Diverticulitis
- Colonic carcinoma
- Trauma
- Toxic megacolon
- Prolonged strangulated bowel

6.6.2 Specific investigations for bowel perforation

- **Erect CXR**—aims to identify free intraperitoneal gas under the diaphragm due to hollow viscus perforation. Patients should be sat upright for at least 10 minutes before the CXR. Figures vary but an erect CXR identifies 70–80% of pneumoperitoniums, so can be used as a rule-in but a not rule-out test. A lateral CXR has better sensitivity than an anteroposterior film for free air, but in clinical practice is rarely performed.
- **Ultrasound**—in trained hands this has a greater sensitivity for free intraperitoneal air than CXR and has the advantage that it can be performed in the resuscitation room.
- **CT abdomen with contrast**—is the most sensitive investigation and is very useful in patients where there is diagnostic uncertainty.

6.6.3 Emergency department management of bowel perforation

- Fluid resuscitation
- Intravenous analgesia and anti-emetic
- Intravenous broad-spectrum antibiotics
- Nil by mouth
- Urgent surgical referral

KEY POINTS

An erect CXR has a sensitivity of approximately 70–80% for free intraperitoneal air.

6.7 Bowel ischaemia/infarction

6.7.1 Mesenteric infarction

Acute mesenteric infarction may result from an embolus or thrombosis. It can also be secondary to profound hypotension or mesenteric venous thrombosis. The superior mesenteric artery is most commonly affected by emboli due to the small take-off angle from the aorta and higher flow rate.

Clinically the patient develops acute severe abdominal pain but often the clinical signs are minimal. There may be a history of chronic mesenteric ischaemia ('abdominal angina') with pain after eating, fear of food, and weight loss. The patient may be a known arteriopath.

Investigations for mesenteric infarction

There is no specific ED investigation to diagnose mesenteric infarction. Serum lactate is usually elevated with a metabolic acidosis, indicating inadequate perfusion. An ECG should be performed looking for evidence of atrial fibrillation (AF) and an echocardiogram for a mural thrombus. CT scan of the abdomen may identify another cause for the pain. CT angiography is the most useful test in diagnosing mesenteric infarction.

6.7.2 Ischaemic colitis

Chronic arterial insufficiency typically occurs at the splenic flexure because it is a watershed territory supplied by the superior and inferior mesenteric arteries. Patients report abdominal pain, classically in the left iliac fossa, associated with loose, bloody stools. The patient may have a history of cardiovascular disease and report recurrent episodes of similar pain.

Patients should be referred to the surgical team for further investigation and management. A barium enema may show evidence of 'thum printing' due to submucosal swelling. Complications include stricture formation and gangrenous ischaemic colitis.

KEY POINTS

If a patient has pain out of proportion to clinical findings, think of mesenteric infarction.

An ECG can be a useful investigation to identify AF and indicate the source of a possible embolus.

Lactate is usually elevated in bowel infarction due to hypoperfusion. An elevated lactate is a non-specific finding and is raised in many causes of acute abdomen. However, a raised lactate gives an indication of the severity of disease.

6.8 Abdominal aortic aneurysm

6.8.1 Introduction

An abdominal aortic aneurysm (AAA) is an abnormal dilatation of the aorta. The majority are saccular and occur infrarenally. Patients over the age of 50, presenting with acute abdominal pain, should always have an abdominal aortic aneurysm considered in their differential diagnosis. Rupture usually leads to haemorrhage into the retroperitoneal space.

6.8.2 Clinical features of abdominal aortic aneurysm

The classic presentation is central abdominal and back pain in a patient with a known aneurysm. However, presentation may vary from a pulseless electrical activity (PEA) arrest to painless, sudden collapse. Patients may be mistaken as having renal colic due to the presence of haematuria caused by irritation of the ureter or rupture into the renal artery. The classical triad of acute hypotension, back or abdominal pain, and a palpable abdominal mass is often not seen.

Examination may reveal a tender pulsatile mass. One or both femoral pulses may be absent. In the obese or elderly, the diagnosis can be particularly challenging and a high index of suspicion should be maintained.

6.8.3 Investigations for abdominal aortic aneurysm

Diagnosis is largely clinical, supplemented by the use of emergency ultrasound. Ultrasound is now considered a core skill of emergency medicine trainees and one of the main indications is the diagnosis of AAA. USS is a useful rule-in test for identifying an aneurysm but poor for detecting a leak. Ultrasound is user-dependent and if there is ongoing clinical suspicion of an AAA, further imaging is required.

Normal maximum aortic diameters are:

- Level of diaphragm 2.5 cm
- Level of renal arteries 2 cm
- Bifurcation 1.5-2 cm
- Iliac arteries just distal to the bifurcation 1 cm

Abdominal aortic aneurysm is dilatation of the aorta greater than 3 cm or 1.5 times the normal diameter for that person.

CT scanning is useful in the stable patient to confirm the diagnosis and determine the extent of the aneurysm.

KEY POINTS

Any patient over the age of 50 with an acute abdomen should have an AAA consider in their differential diagnosis.

Ultrasound scanning in the resuscitation room is the most commonly used investigation to rule-in an AAA.

Patients with leaking AAA should be given minimal IV fluid in the ED. The aim is for the patient to be conscious and/or have systolic BP >90 mmHg.

6.8.4 Emergency department management of abdominal aortic aneurysm

- Cautious fluid resuscitation—should be instituted, aiming for a systolic BP of around 90 mmHg. Aggressive fluid resuscitation has been shown to worsen outcome in patients with leaking AAA. Therefore, if the patient is conscious and passing urine, minimal fluid should be given until the aorta is cross-clamped in theatre. The blood bank should be informed and 10 units of blood and 2 units of platelets should be cross-matched.
- ABC management—should be instituted as for any surgical emergency.

6.9 Aortic dissection

6.9.1 Introduction

Aortic dissection occurs following a tear in the intima, allowing a column of blood to split the aortic media.

The dissection may spread in a variety of directions:

- Proximally—possibly resulting in aortic incompetence, coronary artery blockage, or cardiac tamponade.
- Distally—possibly involving the origin of various arteries.
- Internally—rupturing back into the aortic lumen.
- Externally—rupturing into the mediastinum, resulting in rapid exsanguination.

6.9.2 Classification of aortic dissection

The two commonest classification systems used for aortic dissections are Stanford and DeBakey (Table 6.9).

6.9.3 Risk factors for an aortic dissection

- Hypertension—more than 70% of patients have a history of hypertension
- Connective tissue disorders (e.g. Ehlers–Danlos syndrome, Marfans syndrome)
- Bicuspid aortic valve
- Coarctation of the aorta
- Cocaine abuse
- Giant cell arteritis
- Iatrogenic—following angiography or cardiac surgery

6.9.4 Consequences of aortic dissection

The clinical consequence of an aortic dissection depend on the origin, compression, or dissection of branch vessels, and if and where it ruptures (Table 6.10).

6.9.5 Clinical features of aortic dissection

- Pain is the most common symptom and is usually of abrupt onset. The pain is typically sharp, maximal at the onset, and usually located in the anterior chest or back. The classically described tearing interscapular pain occurs in only about half of patients. Migration of the pain may reflect extension of the dissection.
- Haemopericardium—should be examined for (e.g. quiet heart sounds, pulsus paradoxus, and distended neck veins).
- Aortic regurgitation murmur.
- Pulse deficits are present in approximately 20% of patients. Asymmetry of pulses or a difference of >20 mmHg between arms is considered significant. Signs and symptoms of lower limb ischaemia should be elucidated.
- New neurological signs, related to spinal cord ischaemia.

Table 6.9 Classification of aortic dissections

Stanford classification	DeBakey classification
Type A—involves the ascending aorta and/or arch.	Type I—originates in the ascending aorta and propagates to involve the whole aorta.
	Type II—originates and is confined to the ascending aorta/arch.
Type B—involves only the descending aorta and arises distal to the origin of the left subclavian artery.	Type III—involves only the descending aorta.

Table 6.10 Consequences of aortic dissection

Origin of dissection	Consequences
Ascending aorta	Cardiac tamponade
	Aortic valve incompetence
	Coronary vessel occlusion
	Right haemothorax
Arch of the aorta	Mediastinal haematoma
	Compression of the pulmonary trunk/artery
	Carotid artery occlusion leading to a stroke
	Subclavian artery occlusion leading to acute limb ischaemia
Descending aorta	Left haemothorax
	Aortic-oesophageal fistula
Abdominal aorta	Retroperitoneal haemorrhage
	Coeliac/mesenteric artery occlusion leading to ischaemic bowel
	Renal artery occlusion leading haematuria and renal failure
	Spinal artery occlusion leading to paralysis

6.9.6 Investigations for aortic dissection

CXR—may identify a widened mediastinum or provide another diagnosis. However, a patient may have entirely normal CXR and still have a dissection.

There are several radiological signs that may suggest a thoracic dissection on CXR:

- Widened or abnormal mediastinum
- Obliteration of the aortic knuckle
- Pleural cap
- Pleural effusion
- Trachea or nasogastric tube deviated to the right
- Left mainstem bronchus pushed inferiorly
- Calcium sign—separation of two parts of the calcified aortic wall
- Globular heart—suggestive of a haemopericardium

ECG—is normal in approximately 30% of patients but may show evidence of an ST-elevation myocardial infarction (STEMI), non-ST-elevation myocardial infarction (NSTEMI), or left ventricular hypertrophy (LVH). Such changes can be the consequence of the dissection and should not be assumed to indicate an alternative diagnosis.

Echocardiogram—should ideally be transoesophageal and has a sensitivity of 90–98%.

Transoesophageal echocardiography can demonstrate an aortic intimal flap that divides the aorta into true and false lumina, intramural haematoma, ulcerated plaques, and blood flow between the true and false lumina (entry site). An intimal flap is seen as a mobile, linear echo within the vascular lumen. A thickening of the aortic wall in excess of 15 mm is also used as a sign.

CT angiogram is the definitive investigation, allowing for visualization of the intimal flap, differentiation of true and false lumina, recognition of the extent of dissection, rupture, and involvement of branch vessels and infarction of organs.

6.9.7 Emergency department management of aortic dissection

- Intravenous opiates are important to treat pain and reduce the sympathetic response, which can cause progression of the dissection.
- Blood pressure should be actively reduced if the systolic BP >120 mmHg. Intravenous labetalol is the agent of choice, having both α and β blocking properties. Invasive blood pressure monitoring should guide the infusion dose.
- Definitive treatment:

  Type A dissections: require urgent cardiothoracic surgery due to the risk of rupturing into the pericardium.

  Type B dissections: are usually managed medically unless complications develop (e.g. rapidly expanding aorta, mediastinal haematoma, malperfusion of branch vessels, or intractable pain).

KEY POINTS

Aortic dissection can be a difficult diagnosis to make because the presentation can mimic other conditions (e.g. MI. A high index of suspicion is required).

The absence of supportive clinical signs (e.g. pulse deficits) cannot exclude an aortic dissection; if clinical suspicion remains a CT angiogram is required.

CXR signs of an aortic dissection include: a widened mediastinum; obliteration of the aortic knuckle; pleural cap; pleural effusion; trachea or nasogastric tube deviated to right; depression of the left mainstem bronchus; calcium sign; and a globular heart.

6.10 Acute limb ischaemia

6.10.1 Introduction

Acute limb ischaemia results from a sudden interruption of arterial blood flow in a limb and is a surgical emergency. Irreversible muscle and nerve damage can occur within six hours.

There are three main groups of patients with acute limb ischaemia:

- Acute limb ischaemia—due to thromboembolism in a non-diseased arterial tree, or secondary to arterial trauma. In this group of patients, pain can be very severe and the onset of critical ischaemia very fast due to a lack of collateral circulation.
- Acute on chronic limb ischaemia—due to *in situ* thrombosis of an atherosclerotic plaque. Often there is a preceding history of limb claudication.
- Acute limb ischaemia after revascularization—due to acute graft occlusion.

6.10.2 Clinical features of acute limb ischaemia

The six Ps are the cardinal features of acute limb ischaemia:

- **P**ain
- **P**allor
- **P**araesthesia
- **P**ulselessness
- **P**aralysis
- **P**erishingly cold

Examination should focus on identifying a potential embolic source and evidence of atherosclerotic disease.

- Arrhythmias
- Carotid bruits
- Heart murmurs or prosthetic valves
- Aneurysms
- Peripheral pulses (Doppler examination should be performed to detect pulses that are impalpable and, if possible, to record an ankle-brachial pressure index.)

6.10.3 Investigations for acute limb ischaemia

Acute limb ischaemia is a clinical diagnosis. Investigations should be directed at determining any underlying cause and preparing the patient for theatre.

Angiography is the gold standard investigation to determine the level, extent, and type of arterial compromise. It may enable radiological treatment of the thromboembolic event or provide information regarding distal vasculature should a bypass graft be necessary.

6.10.4 Management of acute limb ischaemia

Emergency department:

- Urgent vascular referral
- Intravenous opiates for pain

Definitive treatment options include:

- Intravenous heparin—to reduce propagation of the thrombus and promote distal reperfusion
- Intra-arterial thrombolysis
- Angioplasty
- Surgical thromboembolectomy
- Surgical bypass grafting

KEY POINTS

Pain is one of the earliest signs of acute limb ischaemia; paraesthesia, paralysis, and pulselessness are late signs.

Examination should focus on identifying a potential embolic source and evidence of atherosclerotic disease.

6.11 Haematuria

6.11.1 Introduction

Haematuria can be divided into two groups:

- Macroscopic haematuria—visible blood in the urine
- Microscopic haematuria—positive urine dipstick for 1 + or greater of blood

6.11.2 Causes of haematuria

Table 6.11 summarizes the possible causes of haematuria.
    Paediatric causes of haematuria include:

- UTI
- Glomerulonephritis
- Trauma
- Wilm's tumour

Table 6.11 Causes of haematuria

Pre-renal	Renal	Ureteric	Bladder	Urethral
Sickle cell disease	Glomerulonephritis	Calculus	Malignancy (bladder or prostate)	Malignancy
Leukaemia	Malignancy	Carcinoma	Benign prostatic hypertrophy	Calculus
Anticoagulants	Trauma	Schistosomiasis		Foreign body
Exercise-induced	Calculus		Calculus	
Infective endocarditis	Polycystic disease		UTI	
	Pyelonephritis		Schistosomiasis	
	Ruptured AAA		Trauma	

- Bleeding diathesis
- Urinary tract stones
- Exercise
- Foreign bodies
- Factitious

Other causes of coloured urine include:

- Myoglobin
- Porphyria
- Beetroot
- Rifampicin
- Doxorubicin

6.11.3 ED investigations for haematuria

- Urine dipstick/MSU—if a UTI is diagnosed (positive nitrites and leucocytes) the patient can be discharged with appropriate antibiotics. GP follow-up should be arranged following completion of the antibiotics to ensure resolution of the haematuria.
- Renal function—urea, electrolytes, creatinine, and glomerular filtration rate.
- FBC and clotting—should be checked to look for evidence of bleeding diathesis/coagulopathies.
- Cross-match blood—if significant, frank haematuria.
- Renal tract imaging—if a calculus is suspected. The imaging modalities used vary between hospitals and are discussed further in section 6.12.
- Further investigations may be necessary for the patient (e.g. renal ultrasound, protein:creatinine ratios, and so on) but do not assist ED management.

6.11.4 Indications for admission

- Clot retention—until the clot is removed the patient will be unable to pass urine and will continue to bleed. A 3-way catheter should be inserted and bladder irrigation started.
- Uncontrolled pain.
- Evidence of secondary infection.
- Urinary tract obstruction.
- Symptomatic anaemia.
- Acute kidney injury.

6.11.5 Indications for outpatient urology referral

If a transient cause of haematuria has been excluded (e.g. simple UTI, exercise-induced haematuria, menstruation) and the patient has no indication for emergency admission, follow-up should be arranged in a urology clinic.

In patients under the age of 40 with an intercurrent illness (e.g. upper respiratory tract infection), a nephrology referral may be more appropriate to investigate for glomerulonephritis.

KEY POINTS

The causes of haematuria can be more easily remembered when divided into the components of the renal tract: pre-renal, renal, ureteric, bladder, and urethral.

Patients with haematuria require admission if they have:
- Clot retention
- Uncontrolled pain
- Evidence of secondary infection
- Urinary tract obstruction
- Symptomatic anaemia
- Acute renal impairment

6.12 Renal colic

6.12.1 Causes of renal colic

Calculi or blood clots may cause renal colic. Ureteric obstruction causes increased intraluminal pressure and muscle spasm.

Types of renal calculi

- Calcium oxalate—accounts for 80% of stones. It may be due to underlying metabolic disease such as hyperparathyroidism, renal tubular acidosis, and hyperoxaluria.
- Calcium phosphate—associated with hyperparathyroidism and renal tubular acidosis.
- Magnesium ammonium phosphate—associated with UTIs caused by urea-splitting organisms such as Proteus.
- Urate—associated with gout.
- Cystine.

6.12.2 Clinical features of renal colic

- Pain—is classically severe, radiating from loin to groin. The patient is often rolling around in agony and unable to get comfortable.
- Nausea and vomiting.
- Abdominal examination is often unremarkable but the presence of an AAA should be actively sought in patients >50 years old.

6.12.3 Investigations for renal colic

- Urinalysis/MSU—haematuria is present in the majority of patients but a negative result does not exclude renal colic.
- Renal function—may be abnormal due to urinary tract obstruction.

- Calcium, phosphate, and urate levels—may help identify the type of causative stone.
- FBC—may indicate a secondary infection if the white cell count is elevated.
- KUB (kidney, ureters, and bladder) X-ray—is occasionally used as the first-line radiological investigation. Around 90% of stones are radio-opaque but the sensitivity of a KUB is less than this (60–70%) because of the size, artefacts, and location of stones. Serial KUBs are useful to monitor the passage of radio-opaque stones at follow-up.
- CT KUB is increasingly being used as a definitive first-line investigation. A ureteric calculus is visualized as an oval high attenuation focus within the ureter, with its long axis parallel to the ureter. Secondary signs include peri-renal and peri-ureteric stranding, ureteric and pelvicalyceal system dilatation, and hydronephrosis.
- Renal ultrasound—may be used preferentially in pregnancy, young women, and children.

> **EXAM TIP**
>
> CT KUB and ultrasound have different advantages and disadvantages for investigating renal colic (Table 6.12). These differences make them a potential SAQ.

6.12.4 ED management of renal colic

- Analgesia—NSAIDs are the mainstay of treatment either rectally or parenterally (e.g. rectal or intramuscular diclofenac, or intravenous ketorolac).
- Anti-emetic.
- Medical expulsive therapy can be associated with increased stone expulsion rate; reduced expulsion time; and reduced need for hospitalization and endoscopic procedures. It is indicated in the presence of adequate renal functional reserve, a newly diagnosed distal ureteric stone (< 10 mm), symptoms that are controlled, and no clinical evidence of sepsis. Drugs of choice include:
  - Alpha 1 blockers: Tamsulosin 400 mcg daily (short term-10 days; off-label use)
  - Calcium channel blockers: Nifedipine XL 30 mg daily
- Stone removal—may be necessary depending on the size, site, and shape of the stone on presentation, and is indicated with persistent obstruction, failure of stone progression, and increasing or unremitting colic. This decision will be made by the urology team.

6.12.5 Indications for admission with renal colic

Not all patients with renal colic require admission. Outpatient urology follow-up should be arranged for those who are discharged from the ED, along with instructions on when to return.

Table 6.12 Advantages and disadvantages of different imaging techniques in renal colic

	CT KUB	Ultrasound
Advantages	• Greatest sensitivity and specificity. • No contrast required. • Will identify non-radio-opaque stones. • Will identify other pathologies. • Quick	• Non-invasive • No radiation • Useful in pregnancy and children • May identify other causes of pain (e.g. gynaecological) • Can identify hydronephrosis
Disadvantages	• No indication of renal function • Higher radiation dose • More difficult to interpret by non-radiologist • Less likely to be available out of hours	• Less sensitive and specific than CT KUB • Operator dependent • Will miss small stones and ureteric stones

Patients that require admission include those with:

- Uncontrolled pain or recurrence of severe pain
- Inability to tolerate oral fluids due to vomiting
- Acute kidney injury
- Evidence of obstructed kidney
- Evidence of systemic infection
- Increased risk from loss of renal function (e.g. solitary or transplanted kidney, pre-existing renal impairment)
- Unclear diagnosis

KEY POINTS

Haematuria is present in the majority of patients with renal colic but a negative result does not exclude it.

Around 90% of stones are radio-opaque but the sensitivity of a KUB is less than this (60–70%) because of the size, artefacts, and location of stones. CT KUB is the preferred diagnostic investigation.

NSAIDs are very effective for pain relief in renal colic.

Alpha blockers (e.g. tamsulosin) have been shown to facilitate stone clearance in patients with a small (<10 mm), distal calculus.

6.13 Urinary tract infections

6.13.1 Lower urinary tract infections

Uncomplicated versus complicated urinary tract infections

Acute, uncomplicated UTIs in adults include episodes of acute cystitis and acute pyelonephritis occurring in otherwise healthy individuals. These UTIs are seen mostly in women who have no risk factors (i.e. no structural or functional abnormalities within the urinary tract and the kidneys and no underlying disease known to increase the risks of acquiring infection or of failing therapy). Uncomplicated UTIs are extremely common infections. Approximately 25–35% of women between the ages of 20 and 40 years have had an uncomplicated UTI.

Uncomplicated lower tract urinary infections are usually dealt with in primary care and managed with a short course of antibiotics.

The distinction between an uncomplicated and a complicated UTI is important because of implications with regard to pre- and post-treatment evaluation, the type and duration of antimicrobial regimens, and the extent of the evaluation of the urinary tract. In contrast to an uncomplicated UTI, a complicated UTI is an infection associated with a condition that increases the risks of acquiring an infection or of failing therapy.

Factors that suggest a potential complicated UTI include:

- Male sex
- Elderly
- Hospital-acquired infection
- Pregnancy
- Indwelling urinary catheter
- Recent urinary tract intervention
- Functional or anatomical abnormality of the urinary tract

- Recent antimicrobial use
- Symptoms for > 7 days at presentation
- Diabetes mellitus
- Immunosuppression

Indications for urology follow-up

Indications for urology follow-up after a lower UTI vary for men and women.
Indications for follow-up in women include:

- Failure to respond to two courses of antibiotics shown by urine culture to be appropriate treatment
- Two or more episodes of acute pyelonephritis
- Suspected urological cancer

Indications for men include:

- Failure to respond to appropriate antibiotic treatment
- First episode of acute pyelonephritis
- Suspected urological cancer
- Underlying cause for the UTI (e.g. prostatic enlargement)
- Frequent UTIs
- History of pyelonephritis, calculi, or previous genitourinary tract surgery

6.13.2 Acute pyelonephritis

Acute pyelonephritis is diagnosed in a patient with a proven urinary tract infection who has loin pain and/or fever. There are no clinical features or routine investigations that conclusively distinguish acute pyelonephritis from cystitis.

Causes of acute pyelonephritis

- *E. coli*
- *Proteus*
- *Klebsiella*
- *Enterobacteria*
- *Staphylococcus*

Indications for admission with acute pyelonephritis

- Dehydrated or unable to take oral fluids
- Evidence of sepsis
- Pregnancy
- Elderly
- Failure to improve after 24 hours of antibiotics
- Abnormal renal tract anatomy or function
- Pre-existing renal impairment
- Evidence of renal stones
- Immunocompromized
- Diabetes
- Nephrostomy or ureteric catheters

Emergency department management of acute pyelonephritis

- Antibiotics—ciprofloxacin or co-amoxiclav (guided by local antibiotic policy)
- Fluid rehydration—orally or intravenously
- Analgesia

6.13.3 Acute prostatitis

Bacterial prostatitis is a disease entity diagnosed clinically and by evidence of inflammation and infection localized to the prostate. According to the duration of symptoms, bacterial prostatitis is described as either acute or chronic when symptoms persist for at least three months. Acute bacterial prostatitis can be a serious infection.

Clinical features of acute prostatitis

- Fever
- Dysuria, frequency, and/or urgency
- Acute urinary retention
- Suprapubic/perineal pain
- Tender prostate

Investigations for acute prostatitis

- Urinalysis and culture.
- Analysis of prostatic secretions is not recommended because prostatic massage may precipitate an abscess or septicaemia.

Management of acute prostatitis

- Antibiotics—a quinolone for 28 days is recommended.
- Analgesia.
- Laxatives if defecation is painful.
- Suprapubic catheterization if in urinary retention (uretheral catheterization is not recommended due to the risk of disseminating the infection).

6.13.4 Epididymo-orchitis

Definitions of epididymitis and orchitis

Epididymitis is inflammation of the epididymis causing pain and swelling, which is almost always unilateral and relatively acute in onset. In some cases, the testis is involved in the inflammatory process (epididymo-orchitis). Bacteria spread from the urethra or bladder, and the likely cause depends on the age of the patient. Patients under the age of 35 are more likely to have infection secondary to *Chlamydia* or *Gonococcus*. More elderly patients usually develop epididymitis secondary to a UTI and may have underlying urinary tract pathology.

Orchitis is inflammation of the testicle and more commonly the result of a viral infection (e.g. mumps-orchitis). Secondary inflammation of the epididymis is common.

Clinical features of epididymo-orchitis

- Progressive testicular ache and swelling of the epididymis and testis
- Low lying testis
- Tender epididymis
- Urethral discharge
- Fever

Investigations for epididymo-orchitis

- Urinalysis and culture
- Chlamydia testing—urethral swab or urinary

Management of epididymo-orchitis

- Antibiotics—quinolone (e.g. ciprofloxacin for 10 days), add in doxycyline if *Chlamydia* is suspected (or as per local guidelines).

- Patients should be followed up by urology or genitourinary medicine, if a sexually transmitted cause is suspected.

KEY POINTS

An uncomplicated UTI is an episode of acute cystitis or acute pyelonephritis occurring in an otherwise healthy individual.

A complicated UTI is an infection associated with a condition that increases the risks of acquiring an infection or of failing therapy.

The likely cause of epididymo-orchitis depends on the age of the patient. Patients under the age of 35 are more likely to have a sexually transmitted infection (e.g. *Chlamydia* or *Gonococcus*). More elderly patients are likely to develop epididymitis secondary to a UTI.

Testicular torsion should always be considered in a young patient presenting with testicular pain.

6.14 Testicular torsion

6.14.1 Introduction

Testicular torsion is a urological emergency most commonly presenting around puberty. Patients with a high attachment of the tunica vaginalis on the testis are more prone to torsion because the testis can rotate on the spermatic cord and obstruct the blood supply.

6.14.2 Clinical features of testicular torsion

- Sudden scrotal pain and swelling
- Vomiting
- Abdominal pain
- Elevated, swollen, tender testis
- Horizontally lying testis
- Loss of cremasteric reflex

6.14.3 Investigations for testicular torsion

Testicular torsion is a clinical diagnosis and unnecessary investigation delays definitive surgical treatment. The urology team may occasionally arrange a Doppler ultrasound to assess blood flow if the diagnosis is equivocal.

6.14.4 Emergency department management of testicular torsion

This should be directed at urgently informing the urology team of the patient and providing symptomatic relief with analgesia and anti-emetics if required.

6.14.5 Differential of an acutely painful scrotum

- Testicular torsion.
- Torsion of the hydatid of Morgagni—this is a remnant of the paramesonephric duct on the superior aspect of the testis. Necrosis of the appendage may be visible as a blue dot and is virtually diagnostic of the condition. However, if testicular torsion is suspected then surgical exploration is warranted.
- Epididymitis.
- Orchitis.

- Trauma.
- Incarcerated hernia.

KEY POINTS

Testicular torsion is a clinical diagnosis and unnecessary investigation should not delay theatre.

6.15 Priapism

6.15.1 Introduction

Priapism is a persistent erection that continues hours beyond, or is unrelated to, sexual stimulation. There are two types of priapism: low flow and high flow. Low flow is the commonest type and is due to veno-occlusion, where venous stasis and deoxygenated blood pools within the cavernous tissue. High-flow priapism is usually secondary to trauma where the cavernous artery ruptures and allows unregulated flow into the lacunar spaces.

6.15.2 Causes of priapism

- Iatrogenic—following intracavernosal injection of drugs for impotence (e.g. papaverine, alprostadil)
- Haematological conditions (e.g. sickle cell anaemia, myeloma, and leukaemia)
- Pelvic trauma
- Spinal cord injury
- Bladder or prostate malignancy
- Medications (e.g. antipsychotics (chlorpromazine), antidepressants (fluoxetine), heparin used in dialysis)
- Recreational drugs (e.g. cocaine)
- Idiopathic—40% of cases

6.15.3 Management of priapism

- Urgent urology referral
- Analgesia
- Ice packs
- Exercise
- Intravenous fluids for hydration in haematological causes
- Oral pseudoephedrine (α-agonist) or oral terbutaline (β-agonist)
- Aspiration of the corpus cavernosum and injection of phenylephrine in low flow priapism
- Embolization or surgical ligation may be required in high-flow priapism

---

6.16 Fournier's gangrene

Fournier's gangrene is necrotizing fasciitis of the external genitalia and perineum. It is due to polymicrobial, synergistic infection of the subcutaneous tissues. Predisposing factors include diabetes, immunosuppression, trauma, peri-anal disease, alcohol excess, obesity, uretheral stricture, and peripheral vascular disease.

The classic triad is severe pain, swelling, and fever. Pain may be out of proportion to clinical findings initially. Plain X-ray may show a soft-tissue gas collection. Ultrasound may show scrotal wall thicken, subcutaneous air, and free fluid.

Mortality ranges from 3 to 40%. Patients should be given high-flow oxygen, broad-spectrum antibiotics, and fluid resuscitation as for severe sepsis (Chapter 15, section 15.1). Urgent surgical debridement is required.

KEY POINTS

Fournier's gangrene is necrotizing fasciitis of the external genitalia and perineum.

It is due to polymicrobial, synergistic infection of the subcutaneous tissues.

The classic triad is:

- Severe pain
- Swelling
- Fever

6.17 SAQs

6.17.1 Bowel obstruction and pancreatitis

A 37-year-old woman presents with a short history of abdominal pain and vomiting. She cannot recall when her bowels were last open and she hasn't passed flatus. Her only medical history of note is an appendicectomy aged eight.

a) (i) Give four features on abdominal X-ray that distinguish small from large bowel obstruction. (2 marks)

a (ii) Give four likely causes of bowel obstruction in this patient. (2 marks)

A 45-year-old man presents with a history suggestive of pancreatitis.

b) (i) Which ED investigation is most sensitive and specific to confirm the diagnosis? (1 mark)

b) (ii) Name a recommended scoring system used in the assessment of this disease and give two of its components. (3 marks)

c) List four systemic complications of pancreatitis. (2 marks)

Suggested answer

a) (i) Give four features on abdominal X-ray that distinguish small from large bowel obstruction. (2 marks)

Location of bowel loops—small bowel is central, large bowel is peripheral.
Haustra (large bowel) versus valvulae conniventes (small bowel).
Size of bowel loops—small bowel >3 cm is dilated, large >5 cm is dilated.
The large bowel is empty in small bowel obstruction.
If the ileocaecal valve is competent, then the small bowel is not dilated in large bowel obstruction.
(½ mark per answer)

(ii) Give four likely causes of bowel obstruction in this patient. (2 marks)
Adhesions
Strangulated hernia
Inflammatory bowel disease
Malignancy
Caecal volvulus
(½ mark per answer)

b) (i) Which ED investigation is most sensitive and specific to confirm the diagnosis? (1 mark)
Lipase

(ii) Name a recommended scoring system used in the assessment of this disease and give two of its components. (3 marks)

Table 6.13 lists the severity scoring systems for acute pancreatitis

c) List four systemic complications of pancreatitis. (2 marks)
Hypocalcaemia
Hyperglycaemia
Disseminated intravascular coagulation
Acute kidney injury
Acute respiratory distress syndrome
Sepsis
Multiorgan failure
Death
(½ mark per answer)

Table 6.13 Severity scoring systems for acute pancreatitis

APACHE II	Glasgow
Temperature	Age
Mean arterial blood pressure	White cell count
Heart rate	Glucose
Respiratory rate	Urea
GCS	PaO2
PaO$_2$	Corrected calcium
Arterial pH	Albumin
Serum sodium	Lactate dehydrogenase
Serum potassium	Asparate/alanine aminotransferase
Serum creatinine	
Haematocrit	
White cell count	
Age previous health status	
Age	

6.17.2 Aortic dissection

A 69-year-old man presents to the ED with excruciating interscapular pain. His ECG shows evidence of anterolateral ST-elevation. You are concerned the patient may be having an aortic dissection.

a) Name a classification system for aortic dissection and describe its components. (3 marks)
b) (i) You arrange a CXR in the resuscitation room. List four abnormalities that would support a diagnosis of aortic dissection. (2 marks)
    (ii) The CXR is normal. What definitive investigation does this patient require? (1 mark)
c) The investigation confirms a dissection of the descending aorta. What are the two most important treatments to start in the ED and what drugs would you use? (2 marks)
d) Suspected aortic dissection is a contraindication to thrombolysis in a suspected MI. List four other contraindications to thrombolysis. (2 marks)

Suggested answer

a) Name a classification system for aortic dissection and describe its components. (3 marks)
    Table 6.14 lists the classification systems for aortic dissection
    (1 mark for the classification system, 2 marks for the components)

Table 6.14 Classification systems for aortic dissection

Stanford classification	DeBakey classification
Type A—involves the ascending aorta and/or arch	Type I—originates in the ascending aorta and propagates to involve the whole aorta
	Type II—originates and is confined to the ascending aorta/arch
Type B—involves only the descending aorta and arises distal to the origin of the left subclavian artery	Type III—involves only the descending aorta

b) (i) You arrange a CXR in the resuscitation room. List four abnormalities that would support a diagnosis of aortic dissection. (2 marks)

Widened mediastinum—Obliteration of the aortic knuckle

Pleural cap—Pleural effusion

Calcium sign—Globular heart

Trachea or nasogastric tube deviated to the right

Left mainstem bronchus pushed inferiorly

(½ mark per answer)

   (ii) The CXR is normal. What definitive investigation does this patient require? (1 mark)

CT aorta

c) The investigation confirms a dissection of the descending aorta. What are the two most important treatments to start in the ED and what drugs would you use? (2 marks)

Analgesia—intravenous opiates

Blood pressure control—intravenous labetalol

d) Suspected aortic dissection is a contraindication to thrombolysis in a suspected MI. List four other contraindications to thrombolysis. (2 marks)

Haemorrhagic stroke—Ischaemic stroke in last six months

Bleeding disorder—GI bleed in last one month

CNS neoplasm

Recent major surgery/trauma/head injury (last three weeks)

(Based on the European Society of Cardiology guidance)

(½ mark per answer)

Further reading

European Association of Urology, 2015. Guidelines on urological infections. Available at: https://uroweb.org [Online].

Renal Association and British Association of Urological Surgeons, July 2008. Joint Consensus statement on the Initial Assessment of Haematuria. Available at: https://www.renal.org [Online].

UK Working Party on Acute Pancreatitis. 2005. UK guidelines for the management of acute pancreatitis. *Gut* **54**:1–9.

CHAPTER 7

Surgical sub-specialties

CONTENTS

7.1 Ear infections

7.1.1 Otitis externa

Otitis externa is an infection of the external auditory canal usually due to *Pseudomonas, Staph. aureus*, or *Strep. pneumoniae*. It is more common in swimmers and after minor trauma. Presentation is usually with pain, pruritus, and discharge. Hearing may be reduced in the affected ear.

On examination the external canal is inflamed, oedematous, and may contain debris, obscuring the tympanic membrane. Palpation over the tragus and movement of the pinna is uncomfortable.

Management of otitis externa

- Keep the ear dry and advise against inserting anything into the ear.
- Simple analgesia.
- Topical ear drops (e.g. combined corticosteroid and antibiotic. An aminoglycoside is contraindicated if the tympanic membrane is perforated).
- Aural toilet ± wick insertion if extensive debris.
- If there is evidence of 'malignant' otitis externa (associated osteomyelitis of the temporal bone), the patient should be started on intravenous antibiotics and urgently referred to ENT.

7.1.2 Otitis media

Otitis media is an infection of the middle ear. The most common bacterial pathogens are *Strep. pneumoniae* and *Haemophilus influenzae*. Viral pathogens are usually respiratory syncytial virus and rhinovirus; 75% of cases occur in those under age 10.

Clinical features of otitis media

- Earache and deafness (older children).
- Non-specific symptoms—fever, lethargy, irritability, poor feeding (younger children).
- Tympanic membrane—is red, inflamed, and bulging with loss of the light reflex. It may also be perforated with purulent discharge present in the external canal.

Management of otitis media

Treatment should be aimed at symptomatic relief with simple analgesia and anti-pyretics. The indications for antibiotics (e.g. amoxicillin) have been clarified by the NICE guideline on respiratory tract infections published in 2008. The guideline advocates three antibiotic strategies: no prescribing, delayed prescribing, and immediate prescribing (Table 7.1).

7.1.3 Mastoiditis

Mastoiditis is an infection of the mastoid process of the temporal bone. It is fortunately an uncommon complication of acute otitis media but can lead to intracranial infection.

Clinical features that help identify mastoiditis

- Erythema, swelling, and tenderness over the mastoid process
- Displacement of the pinna forwards and outwards
- Narrowing of the external auditory canal
- Failure of treatment in acute otitis media

Management of mastoiditis

- Intravenous broad-spectrum antibiotics
- Urgent ENT referral

7.1.4 Cholesteatoma

Cholesteatoma is an erosive disorder of the middle ear and mastoid, which can lead to life-threatening intracranial infection. It can be caused by a tear or retraction of the tympanic membrane.

Patients may present with recurrent otorrhoea, which is offensive plus conductive hearing loss, vertigo, headache, tinnitus, and/or facial nerve palsy. Granulation tissue and a discharge may be seen on examination. Patients should be referred to ENT.

Table 7.1 Antibiotic prescribing in otitis media

No/delayed antibiotic prescribing	Immediate antibiotic prescribing
- Suitable for most cases - Reassure that antibiotics are not needed immediately because they make little difference to symptoms and may cause side effects - Advise patient that symptoms usually resolve in 4 days - Advise to return/start delayed prescription if symptoms get significantly worse or persist beyond 4 days	- Systemically very unwell - Evidence of complications (e.g. mastoiditis) - Co-morbidity increasing risk of complications (e.g. significant heart, lung, renal, liver or neuromuscular disease, immunosuppression, cystic fibrosis, premature children) Also consider immediate prescribing in: - Under 2s with bilateral acute otitis media - Children with otorrhoea and acute otitis media

Data from the NICE guidance on antibiotic prescribing in self-limiting respiratory tract infections: Prescribing of antibiotics for self-limiting respiratory tract infections in adults and children in primary care (July 2008). NICE clinical guideline 69. www.nice.org.uk/CG69.

KEY POINTS

Otitis externa is an infection of the external auditory canal usually due to *Pseudomonas, Staph. aureus*, or *Strep. pneumoniae*.

'Malignant' otitis externa is infection associated osteomyelitis of the temporal bone. It requires intravenous antibiotics and urgent ENT referral.

Otitis media is an infection of the middle ear. The most common causes are *Strep. pneumoniae, H. influenza*, respiratory syncytial virus, and rhinovirus.

Most patients with otitis media do not need antibiotics, just symptomatic treatment.

NICE have produced guidance on when to prescribe immediate antibiotics in otitis media:

- Systemically very unwell
- Evidence of complications (e.g. mastoiditis)
- Co-morbidity increasing risk of complications

Immediate prescribing should also be considered in:

- Under twos with bilateral acute otitis media
- Children with otorrhoea and acute otitis media

Clinical features of mastoiditis include:

- Erythema, swelling, and tenderness over the mastoid process
- Displacement of the pinna forwards and outwards
- Narrowing of the external auditory canal

An offensive smelling discharge is the hallmark of a cholesteatoma.

7.2 Ear injuries

7.2.1 Tympanic perforation

Traumatic tympanic perforation may be caused by barotrauma, direct penetrating injury (e.g. cotton bud), or following a base of skull fracture. The patient experiences pain, reduced hearing, and sometimes a bloody discharge.

Most perforations will heal spontaneously and the patient should be advised to keep the ear clean and dry. They should not put anything into the auditory canal. GP follow-up should be arranged to ensure adequate healing.

7.2.2 Traumatic auricular haematoma ('cauliflower ear')

Blunt trauma to the external ear can result in a haematoma forming under the perichondrium. This separates the cartilage, which is avascular, from the perichondrium, which supplies it, resulting in necrosis. The haematoma should be aspirated acutely and a firm dressing applied over the ear and around the head. ENT follow-up should be arranged.

7.3 Epistaxis

Previous MRCEM question

7.3.1 Introduction

Epistaxis is a common emergency department (ED) presentation and has appeared in previous part B SAQs. Due to the number of arterial anastomoses between branches of the internal and external carotid arteries, 95% of epistaxis originates anteriorly. The area is known as Kiesselbach's plexus or Little's area. Its anterior location makes it susceptible to trauma and thus bleeding. Posterior epistaxis is less common and more likely to present in the elderly population.

7.3.2 Risk factors for epistaxis

- Hypertension
- Bleeding disorders
- Anticoagulants
- Previous epistaxis/cauterization
- History of recent trauma to nose
- Recent upper respiratory tract infection or rhinitis
- Nasal foreign body (consider in children)
- Cocaine use (intranasal)

7.3.3 Investigations for epistaxis

- Full blood count (FBC) and clotting—should be checked if the patient has a history of coagulopathy or anticoagulant use. They should also be checked in patients with haemodynamic compromise.
- Group and Save—should be taken in those with haemodynamic compromise, or a history of coagulopathy/anticoagulant use.

7.3.4 Management of epistaxis

- ABC assessment—ensure a clear airway, and fluid resuscitate as dictated by the patients haemodynamic status.
- If there is haemodynamic compromise the patient will need fluid resuscitation and epistaxis control simultaneously.
- Epistaxis management should proceed in a step-wise manner, as detailed in Figure 7.1.
- If the patient is on warfarin and has torrential epistaxis, prothrombin complex may be required to reverse the warfarin.

KEY POINTS

Have a logical step-wise progression on management of epistaxis:

- First-aid measure –pinch tip of nose for 15 minutes, apply ice pack to the back of the neck.
- Remove any clot and insert pledget soaked with adrenaline (1:1000) and lidocaine.
- Attempt cauterization of anterior bleeding points under local anaesthesia and Otrivine-Antistin® (antazoline sulfate 0.5%, xylometazoline hydrochloride 0.05%), using silver nitrate sticks. Avoid contact with skin—the upper lip can be protected with petroleum jelly. A hot wire or electrocautery may also be used. Thereafter, topical Naseptin® (chlorhexidine and neomycin) cream is advised four times daily for ten days, or mupirocin thrice daily for seven days (if allergic to neomycin, peanut, or soya).
- Anterior nasal pack: pack with a nasal tampon (Merocel® pack), lubricated with water soluble jelly, inflatable pack (Rapid Rhino®), or ribbon gauze impregnated with white soft paraffin or bismuth-iodoform-paraffin paste, along nasal floor, parallel to the palate, leaving no residual pack outside the nostril.
- Bilateral anterior nasal packs.
- Posterior nasal packing and contact ENT urgently. Posterior bleeds can be controlled with a Rapid Rhino®. If this is unsuccessful, a Brighton balloon (with anterior and posterior balloons), or a Foley catheter in the post-nasal space with a BIPP (bismuth iodine paraffin paste-impregnated ribbon gauze) pack anteriorly may be useful. Balloon inflation with air carries the risk of spontaneous rupture and deflation and inflation with water that of aspiration.

Ongoing bleeding   **Bleeding stopped**

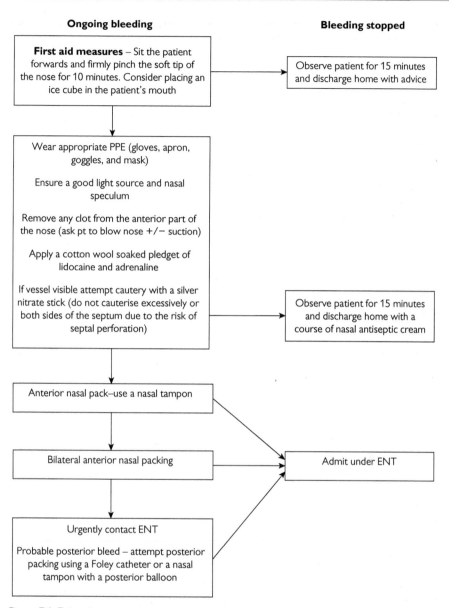

First aid measures – Sit the patient forwards and firmly pinch the soft tip of the nose for 10 minutes. Consider placing an ice cube in the patient's mouth

Observe patient for 15 minutes and discharge home with advice

Wear appropriate PPE (gloves, apron, goggles, and mask)

Ensure a good light source and nasal speculum

Remove any clot from the anterior part of the nose (ask pt to blow nose +/− suction)

Apply a cotton wool soaked pledget of lidocaine and adrenaline

If vessel visible attempt cautery with a silver nitrate stick (do not cauterise excessively or both sides of the septum due to the risk of septal perforation)

Observe patient for 15 minutes and discharge home with a course of nasal antiseptic cream

Anterior nasal pack–use a nasal tampon

Bilateral anterior nasal packing

Admit under ENT

Urgently contact ENT

Probable posterior bleed – attempt posterior packing using a Foley catheter or a nasal tampon with a posterior balloon

Figure 7.1 Epistaxis management.

7.4 Throat infections

7.4.1 Tonsillitis

Acute pharyngotonsillitis is the commonest cause of a sore throat and can have a viral or bacterial aetiology.

- Viral: Epstein–Barr virus (EBV), herpes simplex virus, adenoviruses
- Bacterial: group A β-haemolytic streptococcus, mycoplasma, *Corynebacterium diptheriae*

Clinical features are typically a sore throat, fever, headache, and mild dysphagia. On examination the tonsils appear enlarged, inflamed, and may have a suppurative exudate.

Investigations for tonsillitis

- Most patients require no investigations.
- Consider a throat swab and anti-streptolysin O titre in severe infection.
- Monospot or Paul–Bunnell test in suspected EBV.

Management of tonsillitis

Symptom control is the mainstay of treatment (e.g. paracetamol or aspirin).

Antibiotic use is guided by the NICE guidance on respiratory tract infections published in 2008 (Table 7.2). The antibiotic of choice is phenoxymethylpenicillin. Amoxicillin and ampicillin should be avoided due to the risk of a rash if the cause is EBV.

> **EXAM TIP**
>
> Learn the NICE guidance on antibiotic prescribing in acute otitis media and acute pharyngotonsillitis.

Complications of tonsillitis

ENT complications:

- Otitis media
- Peri-tonsillar abscess
- Retropharyngeal abscess
- Sinusitis

Systemic complications (mainly secondary to group A β-haemolytic streptococcus):

- Scarlet fever
- Rheumatic fever

Table 7.2 Antibiotic prescribing in acute pharyngotonsillitis

No/Delayed antibiotic prescribing	Immediate antibiotic prescribing
• Suitable for most cases • Reassure that antibiotics are not needed immediately because they make little difference to symptoms and may cause side effects • Advise symptoms usually resolve in one week • Advise to return/start delayed prescription if symptoms do not settle or get significantly worse	• Systemically very unwell • Evidence of complications (e.g. peri-tonsillar abscess/cellulitis) • Co-morbidity increasing risk of complications (e.g. significant heart, lung, renal, liver or neuromuscular disease, immunosuppression, cystic fibrosis, premature children) Also consider immediate prescribing in patients with acute pharyngotonsillitis and three or more 'Centor criteria': • Presence of tonsillar exudates • Tender anterior cervical lymphadenopathy • History of fever • Absence of cough

Data from the NICE guidance on antibiotic prescribing in self-limiting respiratory tract infections: Prescribing of antibiotics for self-limiting respiratory tract infections in adults and children in primary care (July 2008). NICE clinical guideline 69. www.nice.org.uk/CG69.

- Post-streptococcal glomerulonephritis
- Infectious mononucleosis (secondary to EBV)

7.4.2 Peri-tonsillar abscess (quinsy)

Development of a peri-tonsillar abscess is often heralded by a high fever, unilateral throat pain, and increasing dysphagia. Any inspection of the oropharynx should be performed cautiously due to the potential for airway obstruction, and may be limited by trismus.

Patients with potential or partial airway obstruction indicated by stridor, inability to swallow, and holding a tripod position should be managed in the resuscitation room and a senior anaesthetist and ENT surgeon contacted urgently.

Patients without airway compromise can be managed with intravenous benzylpenicillin and referred to ENT for aspiration and drainage.

7.4.3 Epiglottitis

Following the introduction of the Hib vaccination, epiglottitis is an infection rarely seen in children, although it may still present in young unvaccinated adults. Symptoms develop rapidly, resulting in a systemically unwell patient with high fever and impending airway obstruction. The patient often sits very still and tripods, they may have little or no stridor, and their voice may be inaudible.

Patients with suspected epiglottitis should be disturbed as little as possible. The priority of treatment is securing a definitive airway followed by broad-spectrum antibiotics (cephalosporin and metronidazole). Nebulized adrenaline may 'buy time' while preparing for intubation.

7.4.4 Retropharyngeal abscess

A retropharyngeal abscess is a rare condition. Indicators suggesting the diagnosis are a sore throat, fever, neck stiffness, and stridor. The posterior pharynx may appear oedematous. Clinically it is difficult to distinguish from epiglottitis and should be managed in the same manner. Lateral cervical spine X-rays (performed in the resuscitation room) may show soft-tissue swelling.

7.4.5 Post-tonsillectomy bleeds

Post-tonsillectomy bleeding is either reactionary or delayed. Reactionary bleeding usually occurs within 24 hours of the operation and delayed bleeding can occur up to 14 days postoperatively.

Presentation is often a complaint of spitting blood and sometimes difficulty or pain on swallowing. The degree of bleeding can vary from blood tinged saliva to torrential haemorrhage. Bleeding may be occult in children because they often swallow the blood and the extent of haemorrhage may only become evident once they vomit.

Management of post-tonsillectomy bleeding

- Use an ABC approach and ensure a clear airway.
- Gain intravenous access and send blood for FBC, clotting and 'group and save'.
- Fluid resuscitate if there is haemodynamic compromise.
- Gently suction any blood from the mouth.
- Give the patient diluted hydrogen peroxide in water (1:1) to gargle.
- In adults, soak a cotton-wool pledget with hydrogen peroxide or topical adrenaline, hold with forceps, and press against the bleeding tonsillar fossa.
- Consider cauterization with a silver nitrate stick.
- Start intravenous antibiotics.
- Refer to ENT.

KEY POINTS

Complications of tonsillitis can be divided into ENT and systemic:

- ENT complications include: otitis media; peri-tonsillar abscess; retropharyngeal abscess; and sinusitis.
- Systemic complications include: scarlet fever; rheumatic fever; post-streptococcal glomerulonephritis; infectious mononucleosis (secondary to EBV).

Epiglottis and peri-tonsillar abscesses are ENT emergencies that can potentially obstruct the airway. Patients should be managed in the resuscitation room and require urgent ENT review.

7.5 Foreign bodies

ENT foreign bodies are most commonly found in children. Therefore, a foreign body in either the nose or ear should prompt the search for a second ENT foreign body.

7.5.1 Ear foreign bodies

All manner of foreign bodies become lodged in the external auditory canal. The patient may present acutely or more delayed with pain, deafness, or discharge. There are a variety of techniques for removal including the use of wax hooks, drowning in lidocaine, fine-bore suctioning, and syringing. In children, one well-planned attempt should be made in the ED and, if unsuccessful, the patient should then be referred to ENT.

7.5.2 Nasal foreign bodies

There may be a history of insertion or the development of an offensive unilateral nasal discharge. Techniques for removal include nose blowing, 'mother's kiss', suction, and forceps. Good lighting and nasal speculum are essential for success. If the patient is uncooperative or the foreign body is not easily accessible, the patient should be referred to ENT.

7.5.3 Throat foreign bodies

The most common foreign body to get stuck in the throat is a fishbone in the piriform fossa. Direct visualization with a good light and tongue depressor/laryngoscope may reveal the foreign body, which can then be removed with forceps. If no foreign body is seen, a lateral soft-tissue neck X-ray may aid the diagnosis. X-ray may show pre-vertebral soft-tissue swelling and the bone (if radio-opaque). Referral to ENT is required for nasoendoscopy to locate and remove the foreign body.

7.5.4 Oesophageal foreign bodies

Usually a lump of poorly masticated meat lodges in the oesophagus. In complete obstruction, the patient is unable to swallow even saliva. Patients are often given a trial of fizzy drinks or muscle relaxants (e.g. hyoscine or diazepam) but their efficacy is questionable. Ultimately the patient requires referral to ENT for a rigid oesophagoscopy.

7.5.5 Inhaled/ingested foreign bodies

Determining whether a child has swallowed or inhaled a foreign body can sometimes be difficult. Respiratory symptoms such as persistent coughing or wheeze suggest inhalation but often the patient is asymptomatic.

If the object is radio-opaque, a chest X-ray (CXR) including the neck should be performed. If the foreign body is seen below the diaphragm, it excludes inhalation, and suggests that the object is likely to pass without incident. A metal detector may also be used for metallic objects to determine if they have reached the stomach.

If the object is not radio-opaque, a CXR may still be useful by revealing an area of distal pulmonary collapse or hyperinflation on an expiratory film (the foreign body may act as a one-way valve in the bronchial tree leading to an area of hyperinflation).

If inhalation is confirmed or strongly suspected, referral for bronchoscopy is required.

Patients who have ingested foreign bodies usually pass it from the gastrointestinal (GI) tract without complication and can be discharged. More careful monitoring is required of patients who have swallowed batteries, razor blades, or open safety pins. Removal of these items is necessary if the patient becomes symptomatic or the object fails to pass. Therefore, these patients should be followed up at three to four days and have a repeat X-ray if the object was not beyond the pylorus on the original imaging.

KEY POINTS

'Dangerous' foreign bodies, such as button batteries, require urgent removal if they are placed in the nose/ear due to the risk of corrosive damage (septal burns, perforation, and necrosis).

Swallowed objects do not usually require follow-up X-rays if they are below the diaphragm. However, patients who have swallowed button batteries should be monitored carefully for adverse symptoms and have a repeat abdominal X-ray in three to four days if the object was not beyond the pylorus on the original imaging.

TOXBASE (www.toxbase.org) provides advice on the management of various different types of batteries that may be ingested/lodged.

7.6 Facial pain

7.6.1 Introduction

There is a large differential for the cause of facial pain including:

- Trigeminal neuralgia
- Post-herpetic neuralgia
- Temporal arteritis (see section 7.17)
- Dental pathology
- Sinusitis
- Trauma

7.6.2 Trigeminal neuralgia

Trigeminal neuralgia is a neuropathic disorder of the maxillary branch of the fifth cranial nerve. It results in recurrent paroxysms of excruciating, unilateral, stabbing pain. The pathophysiology of the condition is poorly understood. Treatment is mainly with anticonvulsants, such as carbamazepine or gabapentin. The pain can be so debilitating that the patient cannot eat or drink, in which case admission is required. In less severe cases, referral to the pain team may be beneficial.

7.6.3 Post-herpetic neuralgia

Following a herpes zoster infection (shingles), a neuropathic pain develops that can become chronic and intractable. Anti-virals within the first 72 hours of developing shingles may reduce the incidence and duration of post-herpetic neuralgia. Once established, treatment involves anti-epileptics (gabapentin) and/or tricyclic antidepressants (amitriptyline) for pain control.

7.7 Facial nerve palsy

7.7.1 Facial nerve course

Facial nerve palsy has multiple causes and an understanding of its course aids in diagnosing the cause. The facial nerve originates from its nucleus in the pons and travels past the cerebellopontine angle, through the petrous temporal bone with the chorda tympani, to emerge from the stylomastoid foramen and pass through the parotid gland where it divides.

It is important to understand the difference between upper (above the facial nucleus in the pons) and lower motor neuron facial nerve palsy.

7.7.2 Upper motor neuron

Above the facial nucleus in the pons, the facial nerve is an upper motor neuron (UMN).

UMN facial nerve palsy results in facial weakness with sparing of the forehead due to bilateral UMN innervation of the frontalis muscle.

The cause is usually a stroke.

7.7.3 Lower motor neuron

Below the nucleus in the pons the facial nerve is a lower motor neuron (LMN).

LMN facial nerve palsy results in weakness of the entire half of the face. Causes include:

- Bell's palsy
- Pontine tumours
- Acoustic neuromas at the cerebellopontine angle
- Ramsay–Hunt syndrome
- Trauma (fractures of the base of skull or face)
- Middle ear infections and cholesteatoma
- Sarcoidosis
- Parotid gland tumours

Bell's palsy

Bell's palsy is the commonest cause of isolated LMN facial nerve weakness. The cause is unclear but may be secondary to a viral infection that causes swelling of the nerve within the temporal bone. Due to the anatomy of the canal in the petrous temporal bone, there may also be loss of taste to the anterior two-thirds of the tongue (chorda tympani) and hyperacusis (stapedius).

Treatment includes:

- Prednisolone in tapering dose: 60 mg daily for 5 days, followed by a daily reduction in dose of 10 mg for a total treatment time of 10 days, especially for presentation in the first 72 hours, or 25 mg bd for 10 days.
- Ophthalmic care: taping/eye patch at night and lubricant eye drops. Corneal exposure after attempted eyelid closure indicates the need for urgent ophthalmic care.
- Anti-viral treatment is not recommended.

Eighty-five per cent (85%) of people make a full recovery within nine months.

Ramsay–Hunt syndrome

This is due to a herpes zoster infection of the geniculate ganglion. The patient has a LMN facial nerve weakness and vesicles in external auditory meatus. Treatment with aciclovir and prednisolone is most commonly used but this has not been demonstrated to be more effective than prednisolone alone. Patients should be referred to ENT.

KEY POINTS

UMN facial nerve palsy results from a lesion above the facial nucleus in the pons. It causes unilateral facial weakness, with sparing of the forehead due to bilateral UMN innervation. The cause is usually a stroke.

LMN facial nerve palsy results in weakness of the entire half of the face. The commonest cause is Bell's palsy.

Prednisolone has been shown to be effective in reducing the severity and duration of Bell's palsy if given in the first 72 hours after symptom onset.

7.8 Vertigo

7.8.1 Introduction

Vertigo is the illusion of rotatory movement when there is none. It should be differentiated from 'dizziness', which can have a multitude of meanings and thus causes. Vertigo implies a dysfunction of the vestibular system.

7.8.2 Pathophysiology of vertigo

The vestibular system enables the body to maintain a position of equilibrium. The vestibular nucleus receives information from the eyes, ears (labyrinths), and joints. It integrates this information and produces an output to drive the vestibulo-ocular reflex and the vestibulospinal reflex. Constant readjustment of these reflexes occurs and is mediated predominantly by the cerebellum. Disease of any part of this system can result in vertigo.

It is important to try and differentiate peripheral from central vertigo (Table 7.3). Generally, peripheral vertigo can be managed as an outpatient but central vertigo requires in patient investigation and management.

Table 7.3 Differences between peripheral and central vertigo

	Peripheral	Central
Onset	Sudden	Gradual (e.g. space occupying lesions)
		Very sudden (e.g. stroke/TIA)
Duration	Usually resolves <48 h	Persists >48 h (except TIA)
Nausea and vomiting	Severe	Often mild
Auditory symptoms	May have: Aural fullness Tinnitus Hearing loss	Usually absent (exception acoustic neuromas)
Triggers	Often exacerbated by head movement	Little effect from head movement.
Neurological symptoms	None	Usually present (e.g. dysarthria, diplopia, dysphagia, dysdiadochokinesia, dysmetria, hemiparesis)
Past history/risk factors	Previous history of paroxysmal vertigo Recent ear infection	Atrial fibrillation Hypertension Cardiac disease Previous stroke

Table 7.4 Differences between peripheral and central nystagmus

	Peripheral nystagmus	Central nystagmus
Effect of fixation	Decreases with fixation	Persists with fixation
Direction	Horizontal	Any (vertical, horizontal, rotational)
Effect of gaze	Nystagmus remains the same direction regardless of direction of gaze	Nystagmus may change direction with direction of gaze
Fatigability	Fatigues	Does not fatigue

7.8.3 Nystagmus

Nystagmus is involuntary movement of the eyes. It is an important clinical sign, which may help identify if vertigo is peripheral or central. The eye drifts slowly in one direction (slow phase) and then rapidly jerks back (fast phase). By convention, the direction of the nystagmus is named by the direction of the fast phase.

Certain features of the nystagmus enable differentiation between peripheral and central (Table 7.4).

7.8.4 Causes of vertigo

Table 7.5 lists the peripheral and central causes of vertigo.

7.8.5 Investigations for vertigo

The most useful investigation in suspected central vertigo is a CT or MRI brain. Other investigations are aimed at looking for risk factors or excluding other causes of dizziness (e.g. ECG, postural BPs, and echocardiography).

Peripheral vertigo requires very little investigation but arranging formal audiological testing, via ENT, may be useful.

7.8.6 Symptomatic treatment options for vertigo

- Vestibular suppressants (e.g. diazepam, lorazepam)
- Antihistamines with anti-cholinergic properties (e.g. cinnarizine, cyclizine)
- Anti-emetics (e.g. prochlorperazine, metoclopramide)
- Intravenous fluids

Table 7.5 Peripheral and central causes of vertigo

Peripheral	Central
• Benign paroxysmal positional vertigo	• Stroke
• Ménière's disease	• TIA
• Vestibular neuritis	• Acoustic neuroma
• Acute labyrinthitis	• Cerebellopontine tumours
• Otitis media	
• Cholesteatoma	

7.8.7 Benign paroxysmal positional vertigo

Debris (otoconia) collects in the semi-circular canals, which can cause vertigo on head movements. It is seen most commonly in the over 60s due to the formation of debris (calcium carbonate) but can occur in younger age groups following head injuries.

Sudden changes in head position result in short paroxysms of vertigo. Diagnosis is confirmed by the Hallpike test and can be treated by Epley's manoeuvre.

Hallpike test

Sit the patient on the bed and turn the head 45° laterally, then quickly place the patient in the supine position and extend the head 20° backwards (i.e. head over the edge of the bed). Ensure the patient keeps their eyes open and focuses forwards (e.g. on the examiner's nose). Hold the position for 30 seconds, looking for the development of nystagmus. Then sit the patient up and return the head to neutral, again look for nystagmus for 30 seconds. Repeat on the opposite side. The test is positive in benign paroxysmal positional vertigo (BPPV) when the affected ear is down.

BPPV can be treated with a canalith repositioning procedure which moves the canaliths from the posterior semi-circular canal back to the saccule (Epley's manoeuvre) and with Cawthorne and Cooksey exercises.

7.8.8 Ménière's disease

Ménière's disease is also known as endolympahtic hydrops and is due to excess endolymph production resulting in increased pressure in the semi-circular canals. Patients experience aural fullness, tinnitus, fluctuating hearing loss, and peripheral vertigo.

ED treatment is symptomatic. Longer term treatments include a low-salt diet, diuretics (acetazolamide, amiloride), betahistine, calcium-channel blockers (verapamil), or surgery.

7.8.9 Vestibular neuritis

Inflammation of the vestibular nerve, thought to be secondary to a viral infection, results in acute peripheral vertigo and vomiting. Symptoms are exacerbated by head movements. There is no disturbance of hearing and no other neurological deficits. Treatment is symptomatic, although steroids may be beneficial. Dysfunction of the vestibular system can be diagnosed with the head thrust or head impulse test. The test involves the ocular vestibular reflex. In the sitting position and facing each other, the patient fixates on the examiner's nose. The examiner rapidly turns the patient's head to one side, if the vestibular system is intact, the patient will be able to fixate on the examiner's nose. In vestibular neuritis, the patient's eyes will briefly deviate laterally and then back to the examiner's nose. This is called corrective saccade and indicates a positive test, diagnosing a vestibular apparatus problem.

7.8.10 Acute labyrinthitis

Acute and chronic ear infections can result in inflammation of the labyrinth. The patient presents with acute peripheral vertigo, usually associated with ear pain, fever, headache, and hearing loss. Otoscopy must be performed to look for evidence of infection.

7.8.11 Acoustic neuroma (vestibular schwannoma)

This is a benign tumour of the myelin sheath surrounding the vestibulocochlear nerve. They are usually located at the cerebellopontine angle and can impinge upon other cranial nerves (V, VI, and VIII). Unlike other central cause of vertigo, acoustic neuromas can result in gradual hearing loss and tinnitus.

KEY POINTS

Vertigo is the illusion of rotatory movement when there is none. It implies a dysfunction of the vestibular system.

Vertigo may have a peripheral or central cause.

The question stem in an SAQ may give details that suggest either a peripheral or central cause (e.g. a patient with risk factors for atherosclerosis and other neurological signs is far more likely to have a central cause).

ED management focuses on identifying the cause and symptomatic relief (e.g. anti-emetics, antihistamines).

7.9 Anatomy of the eye

Ophthalmology questions can appear, often involving a picture in the question stem.

Knowledge of the anatomy of the eye is useful for understanding the various pathologies that can affect it (Figure 7.2).

- *Conjunctiva* is the thin, transparent layer covering the anterior aspect of the eye, including the sclera, and the inner aspect of the eyelids.
- *Sclera* is the white, tough external covering of the eye. The sclera is avascular.
- *Cornea* is a continuation of the external covering of the eye. It is transparent and avascular. It refracts the light entering the eye onto the lens.
- *Choroid* is the middle layer of the eye between the retina and the sclera. It is heavily pigmented to absorb excess light, thereby preventing blurring of vision. It is vascular and supplies the adjacent layers of sclera and retina.

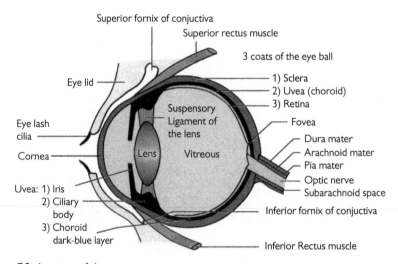

Figure 7.2 Anatomy of the eye.

Reproduced from Judith Collier, Murray Longmore, Tom Turmezei, and Ahmad Mafi, *Oxford Handbook of Clinical Specialties*, 2009, Figure 2, p. 433, with permission from Oxford University Press.

- *Ciliary body* is the part of the eye that connects the choroid to the iris. The ciliary body produces aqueous humour. The ciliary muscle is connected to the suspensory ligaments, which hold the lens in place, and facilitate accommodation.
- *Iris* is anterior to the lens and regulates the amount of light that enters the eye. The iris controls dilation and constriction of the pupil.
- *Anterior chamber* is the space between the cornea anteriorly and the iris posteriorly.
- *Posterior chamber* is the space between the iris anteriorly and the lens posteriorly.
- *Aqueous humour* is produced by the ciliary body and fills the anterior and posterior chambers. It passes through the pupil from the posterior to the anterior chambers and is drained off through the trabecular meshwork at the iridocorneal angle. It provides nutrients for the avascular cornea and lens.
- *Lens* is a biconvex, transparent structure situated behind the pupil of the eye. It is avascular and is held in place by the suspensory ligaments. It refracts light and focuses it onto the retina.
- *Retina* is a light-sensitive layer that lines the interior of the eye. It is composed of approximately 125 million rods and 6–7 million cones.
- *Macula* is the yellow spot on the retina at the back of the eye, which surrounds the fovea. The fovea is the area with the greatest concentration of cone cells, and the area of most acute vision.

7.10 Red eye

7.10.1 Clinical assessment of the red eye

A thorough history and examination are essential in the management of all eye conditions. Key features in the history of a patient with an acutely red eye are:

- Nature of the discharge.
- Contact lens use—risk of corneal ulceration and keratitis.
- 'Deep' pain and/or photophobia—suggests glaucoma, uveitis, or scleritis.
- Visual disturbance—may indicate corneal ulcer, glaucoma, or uveitis.
- Symptoms suggestive of inflammatory bowel or joint disease.
- Drug history—certain drugs can precipitate acute angle-closure glaucoma (e.g. adrenergic agonists (salbutamol), anticholinergics (ipratropium, atropine), antidepressants (SSRIs), and antihistamines).

Key features in the examination of a patient with an acutely red eye are:

- Visual acuity
- Patterns of redness:
  Maximal redness in fornices: conjunctivitis
  Segmental: episcleritis
  Segmental, maximal near limbus: focal keratitis
  Limbal and circumferential(ie, ciliary): iritis; glaucoma
  Brawny red: scleritis(mostly segmental)
  Interpalpebral: dry eyes
  Deep crimson red and confluent: subconjunctival haemorrhage
- Conjunctival oedema or inflammation
- Corneal opacification—may be seen in glaucoma and uveitis
- Pus in the anterior chamber resulting in a cloudy appearance or a hypopyon
- Pupillary size and reaction

- Fluorescein staining, assessing for deficiencies in the epithelial surface of the cornea due to abrasions, ulcers, or keratitis
- Intraocular pressure using a tonometer

7.10.2 Differential diagnosis of the acutely red eye

- Conjunctivitis
- Corneal abrasions
- Foreign bodies
- Ocular burns
- Corneal ulcers
- Keratitis
- Acute angle-closure glaucoma
- Anterior uveitis (iritis)
- Scleritis/episcleritis
- Cellulitis (orbital and pre-orbital)
- Subconjunctival haemorrhage

7.11 Conjunctivitis

7.11.1 Introduction

Conjunctivitis can be bacterial, viral, or allergic:

Bacterial causes are most commonly *Strep. pneumoniae, H. Influenzae,* or *Staph. aureus.* However, *Chlamydia* and *Gonococcus* should be considered in adults with urogenital symptoms, neonates, or those failing to respond to treatment.

Viral conjunctivitis is usually adenovirus and is highly contagious, so may affect several family members.

Allergic conjunctivitis is usually seasonal and associated with other atopic diseases. Treatment is with oral or topical antihistamines.

7.11.2 Management of infective conjunctivitis

- Eye swabs—should be performed if *Chlamydia* is suspected or in patients who are not improving with treatment.
- Topical antibiotics (chloramphenicol or fusidic acid).
- Patients should dispose of their current contact lenses and not restart wearing contact lenses until their symptoms have resolved.
- Patients should be advised not to share towels or pillows and to return if symptoms have not settled in 5 days.

KEY POINTS

Conjunctivitis can be bacterial, viral, or allergic.
Chlamydia and *Gonococcus* should be considered in adults with urogenital symptoms, neonates, or those failing to respond to treatment.

7.12 Corneal trauma and infections

7.12.1 Corneal trauma

Injuries to the cornea are common, usually due to foreign bodies that get blown or flicked into the eye. Such foreign bodies may become lodged on the cornea or under the upper eyelid. Foreign bodies travelling at high velocity may penetrate the orbit and an intraocular injury should always be considered.

A thorough eye examination should be performed. The upper lid should be everted, looking for subtarsal foreign bodies. Fluorescein should be instilled to assess for a corneal abrasion or a corneal foreign body.

A penetrating injury can be very subtle and the eye should be carefully inspected with a slit lamp for a corneoscleral wound. Other signs include reduced visual acuity, pupil irregularity, hyphaema (bleeding into the anterior chamber), and/or vitreous haemorrhage.

Management of corneal trauma: non-penetrating trauma

- Foreign body removal—local anaesthetic drops should be instilled and the foreign body removed with a cotton bud. If this is unsuccessful, a 23 G needle can be used, with a slit lamp. If removal is incomplete, referral to ophthalmology is required.
- Topical antibiotics.
- Dilation of the pupil with cyclopentolate can ease the pain from iris spasm.
- Oral analgesics.
- Eye pad (only required for patient comfort).
- Advise the patient not to drive until their vision has returned to normal.

Management of corneal trauma: penetrating trauma

- Orbital X-ray (eyes up, eyes down) to look for a radio-opaque foreign body.
- Apply an eye shield (an eye pad should not be used because the pressure on the eye may exacerbate the injury).
- Analgesia.
- Ensure adequate tetanus prophylaxis.
- Urgent ophthalmology referral.

7.12.2 Ocular burns

The most serious chemical burns to the eyes are due to acid and alkali substances. Alkali burns are often more severe due to their ability to penetrate deeper.

The pH of both eyes should be checked and copious irrigation with 0.9% sodium chloride should be performed (local anaesthetic drops may be required to enable this). Irrigation should continue until the pH has returned to normal (pH 7.4). Once irrigation is complete, the eye should be examined with a slit lamp and fluorescein staining. If the pH will not return to normal or a burn is visible on the cornea, the patient should be referred to ophthalmology.

7.12.3 Keratitis and corneal ulcers

Keratitis is a breach of the corneal epithelium, which may be due to infection or trauma. It is characterized by corneal ulceration which may be punctate, rounded, or dendritic (suggestive of herpes simplex). Patients have a unilateral, painful, photophobic, and injected eye. Vision may be affected depending on the location of the ulcer.

All patients with keratitis or corneal ulcers should be referred urgently to an ophthalmologist.

Superficial keratitis (arc eye/'snow blindness') is less serious than keratitis. It occurs following exposure to UV light, often in welders, skiers, and sunbed users without adequate eye protection. Patients present with pain, watering, and blepharospasm. Fluorescein reveals multiple punctate corneal lesions. Treatment includes NSAID eye drops, cyclopentolate, oral analgesia, and an eye pad. Arc eye usually resolves within 24 hours.

KEY POINTS

The possibility of a penetrating eye injury should always be considered when a patient reports a foreign body going into their eye, especially if the mechanism involves high velocity (e.g. grinding, hammering, and chiselling).

Examination of the eye should involve eversion of the upper lid to look for subtarsal foreign bodies.

The pH of the eye should always be checked when there is the possibility that a chemical has entered it (e.g. cement dust, detergents, and so on).

Keratitis is a breach of the corneal epithelium, which may be due to infection or trauma.

Superficial keratitis (arc eye/'snow blindness') occurs following exposure to UV light resulting in multiple punctate corneal lesions.

7.13 Acute angle-closure glaucoma

Previous MRCEM question

7.13.1 Pathophysiology

Acute angle-closure glaucoma develops when drainage of aqueous humour is compromised and intraocular pressure increases.

Aqueous humour is produced by the ciliary body and fills the anterior and posterior chambers. It passes through the pupil from the posterior into the anterior chamber and is drained off through the trabecular meshwork at the iridocorneal angle into the canal of Schlemm.

Three main factors are involved in the pathogenesis of acute angle-closure glaucoma:

- Shallow anterior chamber—the lens is positioned relatively anteriorly in the eye, often associated with hypermetropia (long-sightedness).
- Lens growth—the lens thickens throughout life and so encroaches on the anterior chamber.
- Pupillary dilatation—whether physiological (e.g. low-light conditions) or pharmacological (e.g. sympathomimetics, anti-cholinergics) may block the flow of aqueous humour. The iris contracts and is pushed anteriorly against the trabecular meshwork. Aqueous reabsorption is impeded resulting in an acute increase in intraocular pressure.

7.13.2 Clinical features of acute angle-closure glaucoma

- History of blurred vision or haloes around lights due to corneal oedema
- Headache
- Eye pain
- Abdominal pain
- Nausea and vomiting
- Decreased visual acuity
- Mid-dilated and unreactive pupil
- Hazy oedematous cornea
- Circumcorneal erythema
- Raised intraocular pressure

7.13.3 ED management of acute angle-closure glaucoma

- Pilocarpine 2% eye drops—applied every 15 minutes. Pilocarpine acts by constricting the pupil, which opens the angle, and improves drainage of aqueous humour. Prophylactic drops should be applied to the other eye.

- Analgesia—intravenous morphine plus an anti-emetic.
- Acetazolamide—500 mg intravenously followed by 500 mg orally. Acetazolamide is a carbonic-anhydrase inhibitor, which reduces aqueous humour production, thereby reducing intraocular pressure. It also causes a weak diuresis.
- Mannitol 20% (up to 500 ml)—causes an osmotic diuresis reducing intraocular pressure.
- Timolol (beta-blocker) eye drops—reduce aqueous humour production and thereby intraocular pressure.
- Urgent ophthalmology referral.
- Definitive treatment is a laser iridotomy or iridectomy.

KEY POINTS

Acute angle-closure glaucoma develops when drainage of aqueous humour is compromised and intraocular pressure increases.

Patients who have shallow anterior chambers (e.g. long-sighted) and thick lenses (e.g. elderly) are predisposed to getting acute angle-closure glaucoma.

ED treatment of acute angle-closure glaucoma includes:

- Pilocarpine eye drops, which constrict the pupil, open the iridocorneal angle, and improve drainage of aqueous humour.
- Acetazolamide—a carbonic-anhydrase inhibitor that reduces aqueous humour production.
- Mannitol—an osmotic diuretic that reduces intraocular pressure.
- Timolol eye drops—a beta-blocker that reduces aqueous humour production.

7.14 Anterior uveitis (iritis)

The terms iritis and anterior uveitis are used interchangeably and can sometimes cause confusion. A knowledge of the anatomy of the uveal tract aids in the understanding of this disease (see Figure 7.2). The uveal tract is made up of the choroid, ciliary body, and iris. The choroid forms the posterior uveal tract. The ciliary body and iris form the anterior uveal tract.

Iritis is most commonly associated with autoimmune conditions (e.g. ankylosing spondylitis, ulcerative colitis, sarcoid) and is strongly associated with the HLA-B27 serotype. However, it can also occur following trauma, ocular surgery, or keratitis.

Patients present with a photophobic, painful eye. The pain is often described as feeling 'deep' and is exacerbated by accommodation (due to iris constriction). Photophobia may be consensual, where light shone in the unaffected eye causes pain due to pupillary constriction.

On examination there may be circumcorneal erythema and the pupil may be irregular due to the formation of posterior synechiae (adhesions formed between the iris and lens). Slit lamp examination may show inflammatory cells in anterior chamber and a foggy appearance due to 'flare' from protein which has leaked from inflamed blood vessels.

Patients should be urgently referred to ophthalmology.

7.15 Scleritis/episcleritis

7.15.1 Introduction

The sclera forms a tough protective shell for the eye. The sclera is avascular and receives its blood supply from the choroid inside the eye and a deep vascular plexus lying in the episclera. On the outer surface of the sclera are three layers: the episclera, Tenon's capsule, and conjunctiva.

7.15.2 Scleritis

Scleritis is an inflammatory process that involves the deep episcleral vascular plexus. There is an association with rheumatological disorders, particularly rheumatoid arthritis and Wegner's granulomatosis.

Clinical features of scleritis

- Localized or generalized bluish discoloration of the sclera
- Deep, dull ache in the eye
- Painful eye movements (the extraocular muscles insert into the sclera)
- Visual acuity may be reduced
- Palpation of the orbit is painful

The inflammation may ultimately lead to thinning of the sclera and perforation of the globe.
   Urgent ophthalmology referral is required.

7.15.3 Episcleritis

Episcleritis is a self-limiting condition involving the superficial episcleral vascular plexus. There is localized inflammation of the superficial plexus and patients tend to report irritation rather than pain. Treatment with topical or oral NSAIDs may ease discomfort.

KEY POINTS

The sclera forms a tough protective shell for the eye.

The episclera is one of three layers (episclera, Tenon's capsule, and conjunctiva) on the outer surface of the sclera.

Scleritis is an inflammatory process that involves the deep episcleral vascular plexus. The inflammation may ultimately lead to thinning of the sclera and perforation of the globe.

Episcleritis is a self-limiting condition involving the superficial episcleral vascular plexus.

7.16 Cellulitis (orbital and peri-orbital)

Previous MRCEM question

7.16.1 Introduction

The distinction between orbital and peri-orbital (preseptal) cellulitis is very important clinically. Orbital cellulitis is an ophthalmological emergency and requires admission for intravenous antibiotics and possible surgical drainage. Peri-orbital cellulitis is less severe and can usually be treated as an outpatient with oral antibiotics.

   The orbital septum extends from the orbital rims to the eyelids and provides the anatomical barrier between these two conditions.

7.16.2 Orbital cellulitis

Orbital cellulitis is an infection of the tissues posterior to the orbital septum. It may arise from direct extension from peri-orbital structures, direct inoculation of the eye from trauma or surgery, or via haematogenous spread. The most common causative organisms are *Strep. pneumoniae* or *pyogenes*, *Staph. aureus*, and *H. influenzae*.

   Signs that distinguish orbital from peri-orbital cellulitis are:

- Loss of vision/red desaturation (due to optic nerve compression)
- Ophthalmoplegia

- Painful eye movements
- Proptosis
- Chemosis
- Conjunctival oedema

Management of orbital cellulitis

- Broad-spectrum intravenous antibiotics.
- Urgent ophthalmology referral.
- A CT scan may be performed to look for evidence of abscess formation.
- Surgical drainage may be necessary if visual acuity reduces, an afferent pupillary defect develops, or if antibiotics fail to improve symptoms.

Complications of orbital cellulitis

- Visual loss
- Death
- Septicaemia
- Cavernous sinus thrombosis
- Central retinal artery occlusion
- Secondary glaucoma
- Optic neuritis
- Osteomyelitis
- Meningitis
- Orbital abscess
- Endophthalmitis

7.16.3 Peri-orbital cellulitis

Peri-orbital cellulitis tends to be a less severe disease than orbital cellulitis. It involves the eyelids and soft tissues anterior to the orbital septum. Infection usually starts following an upper respiratory tract infection, external ocular infection, or following trauma to the eyelids. The most common organisms are Staphylococci and Streptococci.

Treatment is with co-amoxiclav or a cephalosporin, which may be given orally initially. Intravenous antibiotics may be required if the patient is a child, if there is inadequate response to oral antibiotics, or if there is concern that the cellulitis may be orbital.

KEY POINTS

Orbital cellulitis is an ophthalmological emergency and requires admission for intravenous antibiotics and possible surgical drainage.

Peri-orbital cellulitis is less severe and can usually be treated as an outpatient with oral antibiotics.

Signs that distinguish orbital from peri-orbital cellulitis are:

- Loss of vision/red desaturation
- Ophthalmoplegia
- Painful eye movements
- Proptosis
- Chemosis
- Conjunctival oedema

7.17 Sudden visual loss

7.17.1 Classification of visual loss

Sudden visual loss can have multiple causes. It can be transient or permanent, painless or painful, monocular or binocular (see Table 7.6).

7.17.2 Central retinal artery occlusion

The central retinal artery is an end artery and occlusion is usually embolic (Figure 7.3).

On examination, the direct pupillary reaction is sluggish or absent but the consensual response is intact. Fundoscopy shows a pale retina with a 'cherry red spot'. The 'cherry red spot' is at the fovea where the choroidal circulation, which is normal, is visible due to the thinness of the retina in this area.

Management of central retinal artery occlusion

- Rebreathe CO_2—to vasodilate the retinal artery
- Timolol eye drops—to reduce intraocular pressure
- Acetazolamide 500 mg IV—to reduce the production of aqueous humour and intraocular pressure
- Massage the globe—aiming to dislodge the embolus
- Sublingual GTN—to vasodilate the central retinal artery

7.17.3 Central retinal vein occlusion

Central retinal vein occlusion (CRVO) is more common than central retinal artery occlusion (CRAO) (Figure 7.4). The patient presents with severely decreased visual acuity and an afferent

Table 7.6 Different classifications of visual loss

Transient visual loss	Permanent visual loss
Transient ischaemic attack	Retinal detachment
Migraine	Retinal vascular occlusions (untreated)
Vitreous haemorrhage	Drug related (methanol or quinine poisoning)
	Stroke
Painless visual loss	**Painful visual loss**
Central retinal artery occlusion	Optic neuritis
Central retinal vein occlusion	Temporal arteritis
Retinal detachment	Glaucoma
	Migraine
Monocular visual loss	**Binocular visual loss**
Central retinal artery occlusion	Migraine
Central retinal vein occlusion	Papilloedema
Retinal detachment	Transient ischaemic attack/stroke
Vitreous haemorrhage	

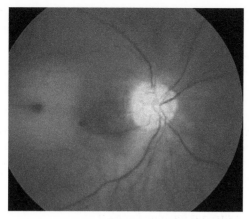

Figure 7.3 Central retinal artery occlusion.

Reproduced from Venki Sundaram, Allon Barsam, Amar Alwitry, and Peng Khaw, *Training in Ophthalmology*, 2009, Figure 4.27, p. 169, with permission from Oxford University Press

pupillary defect. Fundoscopy reveals a 'stormy sunset' appearance: tortuous dilated veins, flame haemorrhages, hyperaemia, and cotton-wool spots.

Treatment is aimed at the management of risk factors, to try and preserve the other eye. Risk factors include old age, chronic glaucoma, atherosclerosis, hypertension, and polycythaemia.

7.17.4 Vitreous haemorrhage and retinal tears

The vitreous body represents 80% of the eye and is 99% water and 1% hyaluronic acid/collagen. It fills the space between the lens and the retina. It is adherent to the retina in three places: anteriorly at the border of the retina, at the macula, and at the optic nerve.

With increasing age, the vitreous may liquefy and the collagen fibres clump together, causing the vitreous to collapse. The pockets left by the collapsed vitreous are often seen as 'floaters'.

Vitreous haemorrhage can occur due to rupture of abnormal blood vessels or due to stress on normal vessels.

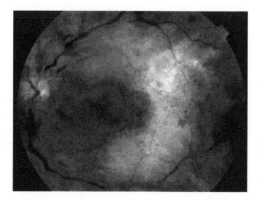

Figure 7.4 Central retinal vein occlusion.

Reproduced from Venki Sundaram, Allon Barsam, Amar Alwitry, and Peng Khaw, *Training in Ophthalmology*, 2009, Figure 4.23, p. 165, with permission from Oxford University Press.

- Abnormal vessels—are typically the result of neovascularization due to ischaemia, most commonly from diabetic retinopathy or coagulopathies (e.g. sickle cell anaemia). The new vessels are fragile and more prone to rupture.
- Normal vessel rupture—can occur when sufficient mechanical force is applied. If the vitreous detaches posteriorly, it may pull on these vessels resulting in rupture. The force may also cause the retina to tear or detach. Blunt or penetrating trauma can damage intact vessels and is the leading cause in patients younger than 40 years old.

Clinical features of vitreous haemorrhage

- Early or mild haemorrhage may present as floaters, cobwebs, haze, shadows, or a red hue.
- In large bleeds, visual acuity may be severely reduced.
- Loss of red reflex.
- Retina is difficult to visualize on fundoscopy.

ED management of vitreous haemorrhage

- Sit the patient head up to allow blood to collect inferiorly.
- Refer to ophthalmology. Urgent assessment is required to assess for an associated retinal tear.

7.17.5 Retinal detachment

Retinal detachment is an ophthalmological emergency. It occurs most commonly in the elderly, diabetics, myopes, and following trauma. It is more common in severe myopes due to the longer eye causing the retina to stretch thinly. In diabetics, neovascularization can cause a tractional retinal detachment.

Patients often report premonitory flashing lights and increased floaters before a 'curtain' develops across their vision. On examination there is loss of the red reflex and the retina may be difficult to visualize or appear dark and opalescent. Visual acuity may be reduced if there is macular involvement or there may be a visual field defect.

Patients should be referred urgently for surgery and reattachment.

7.17.6 Optic neuritis

Optic neuritis is inflammation of the optic nerve that may cause partial or complete visual loss. It presents subacutely over a few days. It is associated with an ache behind the eye and pain on eye movements. Prior to visual loss the patient may have red desaturation (red colour appears less vivid in affected eye).

On examination there is a relative afferent pupillary defect and the optic disc may be swollen. Most recover untreated but there is an association with multiple sclerosis. It is the initial presenting symptom in 20–30% of multiple sclerosis cases.

7.17.7 Temporal arteritis

Temporal arteritis, also known as giant cell arteritis, is a relatively common vasculopathy affecting patients over 50 years of age. It is strongly associated with polymyalgia rheumatica (PMR) and they are thought to be slightly different manifestations of the same disease process.

Inflammation of the temporal artery results in temporal lobe headaches. Involvement of the ophthalmic, posterior ciliary, and central retinal artery can cause irreversible visual impairment, and ischaemic optic neuritis.

Clinical features of temporal arteritis

- Headache (temporal region) + scalp/forehead tenderness
- Jaw claudication
- Relative afferent pupillary defect

- Red desaturation
- Unilateral visual loss (progressing to bilateral in up to 30%)
- Pale and swollen optic disc
- Symptoms of PMR—malaise, myalgia in the shoulders and pelvic region, weight loss

Investigations for temporal arteritis

- ESR and CRP
- A temporal artery biopsy will be required but is usually arranged by the admitting team

Management of temporal arteritis

- Start steroids empirically (e.g. prednisolone 60 mg daily)
- Refer jointly to ophthalmology and rheumatology

7.17.8 Amaurosis fugax

Amaurosis fugax is not a diagnosis but describes a transient monocular visual loss. The visual loss is sudden and usually lasts 5–20 minutes. The reason is a temporary arterial obstruction, which can be due to different causes: embolic, atheromatous disease; temporal arteritis; acute angle-closure glaucoma; increased intracranial pressure; or hypercoagulability. Amaurosis fugax as a consequence of an embolus indicates a significant subsequent stroke risk and requires immediate investigation.

KEY POINTS

Sudden visual loss can have multiple causes. It can be transient or permanent, painless or painful, monocular or binocular.

CRAO and CRVO make good picture questions in SAQs.

In CRAO, the retina is pale except for the 'cherry red spot' of the fovea.

In CRVO, the retina has a 'stormy sunset' appearance: tortuous dilated veins, flame haemorrhages, hyperaemia, and cotton-wool spots.

Red desaturation is a sign of optic nerve or chiasmal disease (e.g. optic neuritis, compression of the chiasm (e.g. pituitary tumour), orbital cellulitis)

7.18 Facial trauma

7.18.1 Introduction

Questions on facial trauma are usually presented with photographs or X-rays. The most important initial consideration is airway management. It is important to read the question carefully to determine if the airway is adequate and maintained; if not, it needs addressing in any answer to a management-type question. Consideration must also be given to associated injuries to the head and neck.

7.18.2 Clinical features of a facial fracture

Key clinical features that suggest a facial fracture include:

- Flattened cheek (depressed zygomatic fracture).
- 'Dish face' deformity or elongated face (mid-face fractures).
- Saddle deformity of the nose (nasoethmoidal fracture).
- Uneven pupils/diplopia (orbital floor fracture).
- CSF rhinorrhoea (base of skull fracture).
- Subconjunctival haemorrhage without a posterior border (orbital wall fracture).

- Hypoesthesia (orbital floor fractures damaging the infraorbital nerve ® numbness of the cheek, side of nose, and upper lip/teeth. Mandibular fractures damaging the inferior dental nerve ® numbness of the lower teeth and lip).
- Subcutaneous emphysema.
- Dental malocclusion.
- Sublingual haematomas or gum lacerations (mandibular fractures).

7.18.3 Investigations for facial trauma

- Occipitomental views are required in two planes (10° and 30°).
- Mandibular view and an orthopantomogram (OPG) are required for mandibular injuries.
- Nasal X-rays are not indicated.
- Imaging of the head and neck may be required depending on the clinical scenario.
- CT scanning may be required to plan surgical intervention but is best organized by the maxillofacial team.

7.18.4 Management of facial fractures

- Resuscitate and establish a clear airway (ATLS principles).
- Treat any epistaxis.
- Analgesia.
- Ensure appropriate tetanus prophylaxis.
- Avoid nose blowing (risk of surgical emphysema).
- Prophylactic antibiotics (e.g. co-amoxiclav).
- Clean and cover facial lacerations, but do not close them if there is an associated fracture because they can provide access for surgical reduction.
- Refer to maxillofacial surgery.

7.18.5 Types of facial fracture

Mid-face fractures

Much of the understanding of mid-face fractures originates from the work of Le Fort in the early 1900s. He subjected cadaveric skulls to a variety of blunt forces and found three predominant patterns of fracture (Figure 7.5):

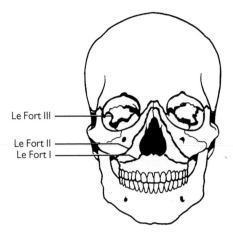

Le Fort III

Le Fort II
Le Fort I

Figure 7.5 Le Fort classification of facial fractures.

Reproduced from Jonathan P. Wyatt, Robin N. Illingworth, Colin A. Graham, Michael J. Clancy, Colin E. Robertson, *Oxford Handbook of Emergency Medicine*, 2006, 'Le Fort classification of facial features', p. 371, with permission from Oxford University Press.

- Le Fort I—fracture involving the tooth-bearing portion of the maxilla. There may be an associated split in the hard palate, a haematoma of the soft palate, and malocclusion.
- Le Fort II—fracture involving the maxilla, nasal bones, and the medial aspect of the orbit. The maxilla may be 'floating' and cause potential airway obstruction.
- Le Fort III—fracture involving the maxilla, zygoma, nasal bones, ethmoid, and base of skull.

Patients may have different types of Le Fort fractures on either side of their face.

Nasoethmoidal fractures result in splaying of the nasal complex and a 'saddle-shaped' deformity. There is significant peri-orbital bruising and may be associated with supraorbital or supratrochlear hypoesthesia.

Zygomatic fractures

These are usually due to a direct blow. These may involve just the zygomatic arch or the zygoma and associated structures. 'Tripod fractures' involve the zygomatico-temporal and zygomatico-frontal sutures, and the infraorbital foramen.

Orbital fractures

A direct blow to the globe may result in a fracture of the orbital floor and herniation of the intraocular contents into the maxillary sinus. There may be an associated globe rupture. Patients may have uneven pupils due to herniation and diplopia due to entrapment of the inferior rectus.

On X-ray, the herniation may be seen as a 'tear-drop' sign from the soft tissue protruding through the roof of the maxillary sinus. X-ray may also show the 'eyebrow' sign due to air tracking superiorly around the orbit from a fracture of the maxillary sinus.

Mandibular fractures

The mandible should be considered a ring. Greater than 50% of mandibular fractures involve two or more breaks. Therefore, identification of one fracture should prompt the search for a second.

Knowledge of the anatomy of the mandible aids in the description of fractures (Figure 7.6).

Nasal fractures

Nasal fractures are the most common facial fracture. The diagnosis is clinical and an X-ray is not required.

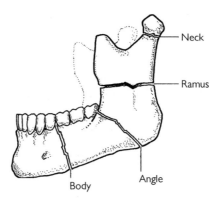

Figure 7.6 Common fracture sites of the mandible.

Reproduced from Jonathan P. Wyatt, Robin N. Illingworth, Colin A. Graham, Michael J. Clancy, Colin E. Robertson, *Oxford Handbook of Emergency Medicine*, 2006, 'Common fracture sites of the mandible', p. 375, with permission from Oxford University Press.

A septal haematoma should always be assessed for and, if present, the patient should be urgently referred for incision and drainage to avoid septal necrosis.

ENT follow-up at five to seven days allows assessment once the swelling has subsided, in case manipulation is required.

7.18.6 Other facial injuries

Temporomandibular joint dislocation

Temporomandibular joint (TMJ) dislocations are usually sustained by a direct blow to an open jaw or following yawning/eating in patients with lax joint capsules/ligaments. An anterior dislocation is the most common type; however, they can occur in any direction when associated with fractures of the mandible or base of skull.

Reduction of anterior dislocations can usually be achieved in the ED with the aid of analgesia and sedation. Following reduction the patient should have a soft diet and be advised not to open their mouth widely for two weeks. They should be referred for outpatient maxillofacial follow-up.

KEY POINTS

Always ensure appropriate airway management in any patient with facial trauma.

Spend time getting used to interpreting facial X-rays prior to the exam.

Non-radiological signs of a facial fracture include:
- Flattened cheek (depressed zygomatic fracture).
- 'Dish face' deformity or elongated face (mid-face fractures).
- Saddle deformity of the nose (nasoethmoidal fracture).
- Uneven pupils/diplopia (orbital floor fracture).
- CSF rhinorrhoea (base of skull fracture).
- Subconjunctival haemorrhage without a posterior border (orbital wall fracture).
- Hypoesthesia (orbital floor fractures damaging the infraorbital nerve ® numbness of the cheek, side of nose, and upper lip/teeth. Mandibular fractures damaging the inferior dental nerve ® numbness of the lower teeth and lip).
- Subcutaneous emphysema.
- Dental malocclusion.
- Sublingual haematomas or gum lacerations (mandibular fractures).

Discharge advice for patients with facial fractures includes:
- No nose blowing
- Antibiotic prophylaxis
- Tetanus prophylaxis
- Head injury advice
- Epistaxis advice
- Maxillofacial follow-up

7.19 Dental emergencies

7.19.1 Dentition

The primary (deciduous) set of teeth erupts between six months and two years. Twenty teeth make up the primary dentition and, by convention, the four quadrants of teeth are labelled A (first incisor) to E (second molar).

Secondary (permanent) dentition starts to erupt from age six years. The permanent dentition comprise 32 teeth, divided into four quadrants and notated 1 (first incisor) to 8 (third molar).

7.19.2 Dental fractures

Dental fractures can be classified into four groups: enamel only; enamel and dentine; enamel, dentine, and pulp; root fracture. All of these can be managed by a dentist. Fractures involving the root, or those that are mobile should be referred acutely.

7.19.3 Avulsed teeth

Previous MRCEM question

Avulsed primary teeth are not suitable for reimplantation but avulsed permanent teeth are.

A major concern with chipped or avulsed teeth is the risk of aspiration, especially in the obtunded or pre-verbal patient. If the whole tooth is not seen, a CXR should be obtained to exclude aspiration.

Emergency department management of avulsed teeth

- If the tooth needs to be transported, it should be placed in milk or in the buccal fold of the patient.
- The tooth should be handled as little as possible and cleaned gently in normal saline. The root should not be handled or scrubbed.
- The earlier the tooth is reimplanted, the greater the success rate.
- The tooth should be correctly orientated before insertion into the socket.
- The tooth should be temporarily secured using foil (e.g. from a suture pack) or a mouth guard.
- Tetanus status should be confirmed and prophylaxis given, if indicated.
- Prophylactic antibiotics (e.g. co-amoxiclav) should be prescribed.
- The patient should be referred to a dentist for stabilization.

7.19.4 Dental abscess

Dental abscesses can usually be managed with oral analgesia and antibiotics, with follow-up by a dentist. Inpatient referral for intravenous antibiotics and possible surgical drainage should be prompted by associated facial swelling, Ludwig's angina (infection of the floor of the mouth), trismus, dysphagia, or systemic symptoms of infection.

7.19.5 Bleeding socket

Haemorrhage post-extraction usually responds to simple first-aid measures. It is important to ensure removal of any ineffective blood clot from the socket first and then get the patient to bite down on rolled-up gauze. If this fails, the gauze can be soaked in 1:1000 adrenaline or a mattress suture inserted under local anaesthetic (lidocaine with adrenaline).

KEY POINTS

There are 20 deciduous teeth (first incisor to second molar), which erupt between six months and two years of age.

The permanent dentition comprises 32 teeth (first incisor to third molar), which erupt from the age of six years.

A major concern with chipped or avulsed teeth is the risk of aspiration. If the whole tooth is not seen in the ED, a CXR should be obtained.

Avulsed deciduous teeth are not suitable for reimplantation, but avulsed permanent teeth are.

7.20 Neck trauma

7.20.1 Zones of the neck

The neck is divided into three zones to aid in the evaluation of injuries.

- Zone 1—covers the area from the clavicles to the cricoid cartilage. Structures at risk are the great vessels (subclavian vessels, brachiocephalic veins, common carotid arteries, aortic arch, and jugular veins), trachea, lung apices, cervical spine, spinal cord, and cervical nerve roots.
- Zone 2—covers the area from the cricoid cartilage to the angle of mandible. Important structures in this region include the carotid and vertebral arteries, jugular veins, pharynx, larynx, trachea, oesophagus, cervical spine, and spinal cord.
- Zone 3—covers the area from the angle of the mandible to the skull base. Injuries in this zone include the salivary and parotid glands, oesophagus, trachea, vertebral bodies, carotid arteries, jugular veins, and cranial nerves IX–XII.

7.20.2 Life-threatening neck injuries

Life-threatening injuries from penetrating neck trauma include:

- Direct airway injury (e.g. transected trachea)
- Tension pneumothorax
- Massive haemothorax
- Massive external haemorrhage

7.20.3 Management of neck injuries

Management of penetrating neck injuries should follow ATLS principles (see Chapter 4).

The Royal College of Emergency Medicine (2010) have produced guidelines on the management of alert, adult patients with potential cervical spine injury, including those sustaining penetrating injuries. Their guidance states:

- Cervical spine immobilization is recommended for patients with gunshot wounds to the neck given the association with direct spinal destruction in a proportion of patients. However, this should not take precedent over life-threatening airway and haemorrhage control.
- Neck immobilization is not required for a patient with an isolated stab wound to the neck, even if a neurological deficit is identified. The fitting of a cervical collar in this setting may be associated with an increased mortality.

Indications for immediate surgical exploration include:

- Persistent major bleeding
- Breach of platysma
- Evidence of vascular injury
- Surgical emphysema (indicating laryngeal or oesophageal injury requiring repair)*

---

* Reproduced with kind permission of the Royal College of Emergency Medicine

Patients who are haemodynamically stable may undergo angiography and oesophagoscopy to determine the extent of the injuries prior to surgery.

KEY POINTS

The neck is divided into three zones to aid in the evaluation of injuries.

Management of penetrating neck injuries should follow ATLS principles.

Indications for immediate surgical exploration include:

- Persistent major bleeding
- Breach of platysma
- Evidence of vascular injury
- Surgical emphysema (indicating laryngeal or oesophageal injury requiring repair)

7.21 SAQs

7.21.1 Orbital cellulitis

A 14-year-old boy attends the ED with a red, painful left eye. He has recently had an upper respiratory tract infection (URTI), but is otherwise fit and well.

a) Give three signs or symptoms that distinguish orbital from peri-orbital cellulitis. (3 marks)
b) Describe three routes of contracting orbital cellulitis. (3 marks)
c) (i) What are the two most common causative organisms of orbital cellulitis? (2 marks)
   (ii) List two complications of orbital cellulitis. (2 marks)

Suggested answer

a) Give three signs or symptoms that distinguish orbital from peri-orbital cellulitis. (3 marks)
   Loss of vision/red desaturation
   Ophthalmoplegia
   Painful eye movements
   Proptosis
   Chemosis
   Conjunctival oedema
b) Describe three routes of contracting orbital cellulitis. (3 marks)
   Extension from peri-orbital structures (e.g. sinuses, face, globe, lacrimal sac)
   Direct inoculation of orbit from trauma or surgery
   Haematogenous spread
   (Not post-URTI because this is usually from local extension)
c) (i) What are the two most common causative organisms of orbital cellulitis? (2 marks)
       Streptococcus pneumoniae or pyogenes
       Staph. aureus
       Haemophilus influenzae
   (ii) List two complications of orbital cellulitis. (2 marks)
       Visual loss
       Sinusitis
       Death
       Septicaemia
       Cavernous sinus thrombosis
       Osteomyelitis
       Meningitis
       Orbital abscess

7.21.2 Epistaxis and otitis media

A 42-year-old man attends the ED with a nosebleed, which started spontaneously (Figure 7.7). He is catching the drips in a bowl. His wife tells you that he is on warfarin, his international normalized ratio (INR) last week was 2.5. Observations: HR 80 bpm, BP 120/74 mmHg, RR 14/min, SpO_2 100% in air.

a) (i) List four factors you should ask about in the past history of any patient presenting with a nosebleed apart from medication? (2 marks)
   (ii) What is the name of the anatomical area that is most often the source of epistaxis in younger patients? (1 mark)
b) (i) While you take a history from him he applies direct pressure to his nose. Where should he press? (1 mark)
   (ii) However, his nose continues to bleed, and you are unable to see a bleeding point to cauterize, what would be your next three steps in treating the epistaxis? (3 marks)

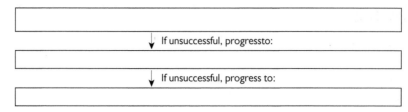

Figure 7.7 Nosebleed—next steps.

A four-year-old patient presents with a painful left ear. You diagnose otitis media.

c)   According to the NICE guidance, what are three possible indications for immediate antibiotic prescribing in acute otitis media? (3 marks)

Suggested answer

a)   (i)   List four factors you should ask about in the past history of any patient presenting with a nosebleed apart from medication? (2 marks)

Hypertension
Previous nasal problems
Bleeding disorders
History of recent trauma to nose
Previous epistaxis/cauterization
Rhinitis/tumours
Nasal foreign body
Cocaine use
(½ mark each)

a)   (ii)   What is the name of the anatomical area that is most often the source of epistaxis in younger patients? (1 mark)

Little's area/Kiesselbach's plexus or area

b)   (i)   While you take a history from him, he applies direct pressure to his nose. Where should he press? (1 mark)

Soft part/end/tip of nose

(ii)   However, his nose continues to bleed, and you are unable to see a bleeding point to cauterize, what would be your next three steps in treating the epistaxis? (3 marks)

Any three in a logical progression:
Remove clot and insert a pledget soaked with adrenaline (1:1000) and lidocaine
Re-attempt cauterization
Anterior nasal pack
Bilateral anterior nasal packs
Posterior nasal packing
ENT referral

c)   According to the NICE guidance, what are three possible indications for immediate antibiotic prescribing in acute otitis media? (3 marks)

Systemically very unwell
Evidence of complications (e.g. mastoiditis)
Co-morbidity increasing risk of complications (e.g. significant heart, lung, renal, liver or neuromuscular disease, immunosuppression, cystic fibrosis, premature children)
Under 2s with bilateral acute otitis media
Children with otorrhoea and acute otitis media

Further reading

National Institute for Health and Care Excellence, July 2008. NICE clinical guideline 69. Respiratory tract infections (self-limiting): prescribing antibiotics. Available at: https://www.nice.org.uk/CG69 [Online].

CHAPTER 8

Obstetrics and gynaecology

CONTENTS

8.1 Abdominal pain in women

Women presenting with abdominal pain have a wide differential of gynaecological and surgical causes (see Chapter 6, section 6.1). The most important investigation to undertake in any woman of childbearing age is a urinary pregnancy test, which will aid in the exclusion of an ectopic pregnancy.

The differential for gynaecological causes of abdominal pain includes:

- Ectopic pregnancy
- Endometriosis
- Ovarian cysts/torsion
- Pelvic inflammatory disease
- Dysmenorrhoea
- Fibroids
- Corpus luteum rupture
- Mittelschmerz

It is necessary to have an appreciation of all the potential causes but the most important to understand, from a clinical and exam point of view, is ectopic pregnancy.

KEY POINTS

All female patients of childbearing age must have a urinary pregnancy test when presenting with abdominal pain.

EXAM TIP

The Royal College of Obstetricians and Gynaecologists (https://www.rcog.org.uk/) produce Green-top Guidelines, which have useful information on the management of certain conditions, including: pelvic inflammatory disease; pre-eclampsia; thromboembolic disease in pregnancy; use of anti-D immunoglobulin; post-partum haemorrhage. The relevant points for emergency department (ED) management are summarized in this chapter.

8.2 Ectopic pregnancy

8.2.1 Introduction

An ectopic pregnancy is one that is not within the uterus. The incidence of ectopic has remained static in recent years and affects approximately 1 in 100 pregnancies. The majority of these pregnancies occur in the Fallopian tube but can occur in the abdominal cavity, ovary, or cervix. The risk of a heterotopic pregnancy (combined intrauterine and ectopic) is estimated to be between 1 in 4000 and 1 in 8000.

Ectopic pregnancy is the commonest cause of maternal death in the first trimester. As the gestation enlarges, there is increased potential for organ rupture, resulting in massive haemorrhage, infertility, and death.

Implantation of the gestational sac in the Fallopian tube may have three results:

- Extrusion (tubal abortion) into the peritoneal cavity
- Spontaneous involution of the pregnancy
- Rupture through the tube causing pain and bleeding

8.2.2 Risk factors for an ectopic pregnancy

Any condition that delays or limits normal transit of the fertilized ovum to the uterus increases the risk of an ectopic pregnancy.

Risk factors include:

- Previous ectopic pregnancy
- Pelvic inflammatory disease
- History of tubal surgery or other pelvic surgery
- Endometriosis
- Assisted fertilization
- Use of an intrauterine contraceptive device (IUCD)
- Progesterone-only pill
- Congenital genital anatomical variants
- Ovarian or uterine cysts/tumours

8.2.3 Clinical features of ectopic pregnancy

- Amenorrhoea or missed period
- Abdominal or pelvic pain (often unilateral)
- Abnormal vaginal bleeding, with or without clots, in the first trimester
- Shoulder tip pain (due to diaphragmatic irritation)
- Dizziness, faintness, or syncope
- Breast tenderness
- Gastrointestinal symptoms
- Urinary symptoms

- Pelvic or abdominal tenderness
- Adnexal tenderness +/- mass
- Cervical motion tenderness
- Abdominal distension
- Shock; orthostatic hypotension

8.2.4 Investigations in suspected ectopic pregnancy

- Urinary pregnancy test—should be performed on every female of childbearing age with abdominal pain.
- Ultrasound scan—may confirm an extrauterine pregnancy (mass) or show free fluid in the pouch of Douglas. Often a transvaginal scan is required in early pregnancy because transabdominal scanning may not be sensitive enough.
- Rhesus status—should be checked because as anti-D immunoglobulin (section 8.10) may be required.
- Serial β HCG and progesterone levels—are useful if no sac is visualized on ultrasound. With a normal intrauterine pregnancy, the β HCG level doubles every 48 hours. In an ectopic pregnancy, the level will fail to rise.
- Clotting—due to the risk of disseminated intravascular coagulation (DIC).

8.2.5 Emergency department management of ectopic pregnancy

- Two large intravenous cannulae and cross-match blood (6 units).
- Fluid resuscitate with intravenous crystalloid, as required.
- Give anti-D immunoglobulin if the patient is rhesus negative.
- Urgently refer to the gynaecology team.

8.2.6 Definitive management of ectopic pregnancy

This guidance is based on the recommendations in the Green-top Guideline on the management of tubal pregnancies produced by the Royal College of Obstetricians and Gynaecologists.

Surgical management

If the patient is haemodynamically unstable, there should be no delay between diagnosis and operative intervention. The patient will usually require a laparotomy and salpingotomy or salpingectomy. If the patient is haemodynamically stable, then a laparoscopic approach may be used.

Medical management

Medical treatment with methotrexate may be offered to women with minimal symptoms and a β HCG lower than 3000 IU/L.

Expectant management is an option for clinically stable women with minimal symptoms and a pregnancy of unknown location. They can be monitored with serial β HCG and ultrasound scans.

KEY POINTS

Ectopic pregnancy is the commonest cause of maternal death in the first trimester.

- Any condition that delays or limits normal transit of the fertilized ovum to the uterus increases the risk of an ectopic pregnancy.
- Implantation of the gestational sac in the Fallopian tube may have three outcomes:
  - Extrusion (tubal abortion) into the peritoneal cavity.
  - Spontaneous involution of the pregnancy.
  - Rupture through the tube causing pain and bleeding.

A high index of suspicion is required for ectopic pregnancy in any woman of childbearing age, presenting with abdominal pain, or vaginal bleeding.

ED management should focus on early diagnosis, resuscitation, and urgent gynaecology referral.

8.3 Pelvic inflammatory disease

8.3.1 Introduction

The following is based on the British Association for Sexual Health and HIV (BASHH) UK National Guideline for the Management of Pelvic Inflammatory Disease 2011 (https://www.bashh.org/documents/3572.pdf).

Pelvic inflammatory disease (PID) is usually the result of infection ascending from the endocervix causing endometritis, salpingitis, oophoritis, tubo-ovarian abscess, and/or peritonitis.

8.3.2 Causes of pelvic inflammatory disease

- Sexually transmitted (90%)—*Chlamydia, Gonorrhoea, Mycoplasma genitalium*
- Non-sexually transmitted (10%, often post-surgical instrumentation)—*E. Coli*, Group B Strep, *Bacteroides, Gardenella*

8.3.3 Clinical features of pelvic inflammatory disease

- Lower abdominal pain and tenderness, typically bilateral
- Abnormal vaginal or cervical discharge
- Fever (>38°C)
- Abnormal vaginal bleeding (intermenstrual, menorrhagia, post-coital, or 'breakthrough')
- Deep dyspareunia
- Cervical excitation (cervical motion tenderness on bimanual vaginal examination)
- Adnexal tenderness ± mass
- Fitz-Hugh Curtis syndrome (right-upper quadrant pain associated with perihepatitis)

8.3.4 Investigations in pelvic inflammatory disease

- Endocervical swabs for *Chlamydia* and *Gonorrhoea:* negative swabs do not exclude PID.
- Urinary pregnancy test.
- Bloods—ESR, CRP, and WCC are supportive but not specific.
- Testing for gonorrhoea and chlamydia in the lower genital tract is recommended, along with screening for HIV.
- Transvaginal ultrasound may demonstrate inflamed/dilated Fallopian tubes or a tubo-ovarian abscess.

8.3.5 Management of pelvic inflammatory disease

- Empirical treatment—a low threshold is recommended for empirical broad spectrum antimicrobial treatment because of the lack of definitive clinical diagnostic criteria and the potential significant consequences of not treating PID. Delayed treatment increases the risk of complications, such as ectopic pregnancy, subfertility, and chronic pelvic pain.
- Those presenting with mild to moderate PID can be treated as an outpatient with oral ofloxacin 400 mg bd and oral metronidazole 400 mg bd, both for 14 days. An alternative regimen, which is particularly applicable if the risk of gonococcal infection is high, involves a single intramuscular injection of ceftriaxone 500 mg, followed by oral doxycycline 100 mg bd and oral metronidazole 400 mg bd, both for 14 days.
- Inpatient management is indicated in the following circumstances:
    - Clinically severe disease, with severe symptoms (nausea and vomiting).

- Fever greater than 38°C.
- Tubo-ovarian abscess.
- Signs of pelvic peritonitis.
- PID in pregnancy, when intravenous antimicrobial therapy is indicated to reduce the risk of maternal and foetal morbidity and pre-term delivery.
- Intolerance or lack of response to oral therapy.
- Surgical emergency not excluded.

- Inpatient antibiotic therapy may include intravenous ceftriaxone and doxycycline.
- Surgical drainage may be required for tubo-ovarian abscesses.
- Consideration should be given to removing an IUCD in patients presenting with PID, especially if symptoms have not resolved within 72 hours.
- After treatment, further screening for sexually transmitted infections is indicated.
- Sexual partners from the previous six months should be contacted and offered screening via the genitourinary medicine clinic.

8.3.6 Complications of pelvic inflammatory disease

- Infertility
- Ectopic pregnancy (fivefold increased risk)
- Chronic pelvic pain
- Peritonitis
- Abscess formation

KEY POINTS

PID is usually the result of infection ascending from the endocervix causing endometritis, salpingitis, oophoritis, tubo-ovarian abscess, and/or peritonitis.

Clinical features include lower abdominal pain, vaginal discharge, nausea/vomiting, fever, lower abdominal tenderness, cervical excitation, and adnexal tenderness.

A low threshold is recommended for empirical treatment because of the lack of definitive clinical diagnostic criteria and the potential significant consequences of not treating PID.

Patients who have had PID have a fivefold increased risk of ectopic pregnancy.

8.4 Other gynaecological causes of abdominal pain

8.4.1 Endometriosis

Endometriosis is the presence of endometrial tissue outside the uterus. The disease may consist of only a few lesions, to large cystic lesions causing fibrosis and formation of adhesions.

Symptoms include:

- Severe dysmenorrhoea
- Deep dyspareunia
- Chronic pelvic pain
- Ovulation pain
- Infertility
- Cyclical, premenstrual symptoms

ED treatment consists of symptomatic relief with NSAIDs and exclusion of an ectopic pregnancy. Patients should be referred to the gynaecology team as an outpatient. Diagnosis is made via laparoscopy and direct visualization of the pelvis with positive histology.

8.4.2 Ovarian cyst rupture/torsion

Ruptured cysts

Patients may develop abdominal pain when ovarian cysts rupture because the contents can cause peritoneal irritation and localized tenderness. Treatment is symptomatic and referral to the gynaecology team.

Ovarian torsion

Ovarian torsion causes sudden, unilateral, lower abdominal pain. The ovary is usually enlarged from a cyst or neoplasm and twists around the pedicle. Abdominal and adnexal tenderness may be present.

The torsion may resolve spontaneously or progress to ovarian infarction.

Diagnosis is difficult and may be made by transvaginal ultrasound or laparoscopy.

Patients with a suspected ovarian torsion should be managed symptomatically (e.g. analgesia, fluids, and so on) and referred to gynaecology as an inpatient.

8.4.3 Dysmenorrhoea

Dysmenorrhoea (pain during menstruation) may be primary, without underlying organ pathology, or secondary to uterine pathologies such as endometriosis, PID, or fibroids.

Primary dysmenorrhoea is worse in the first few days of menstruation. Excess prostaglandins cause painful uterine contractions. Treatment with prostaglandin inhibitors, such as mefenamic acid or NSAIDs, helps control symptoms. Patients should be referred to their GP for further management.

8.4.4 Fibroids

Fibroids are nodules of smooth muscle cells and fibrous connective tissue that develop within the wall of the uterus. Symptoms include menorrhagia, dysmenorrhoea, and deep dyspareunia.

Fibroids may undergo torsion resulting in sudden, severe, colicky pain, or they may infarct ('red degeneration'), particularly during pregnancy.

Patients require referral to gynaecology for further investigation.

8.4.5 Corpus luteum cyst rupture

The corpus luteum is formed when a mature ovarian follicle ruptures and releases an ovum.

Rupture of a corpus luteum cyst may cause frank haemorrhage into the peritoneum. Patients present during the second half of their menstrual cycle with abdominal pain and occasionally syncope.

Fluid resuscitation and admission may be required if significant haemorrhage has occurred.

8.4.6 Mittelschmerz

This is mid-cycle pain due to the leakage of prostaglandin-containing follicular fluid at the time of ovulation.

Treatment is symptomatic and patients can usually be discharged from the ED.

KEY POINTS

Women presenting with abdominal pain have a wide differential of gynaecological and surgical causes.

Clues in the history to suggest a gynaecological cause include radiation of pain to the back or legs, vaginal discharge, vaginal bleeding, or missed menstruation.

Indications for admission include suspected ectopic pregnancy, suspected ovarian torsion, uncontrolled pain, and/or haemodynamic compromise.

8.5 Abnormal vaginal bleeding

8.5.1 Introduction

There is a large differential diagnosis in women with abnormal vaginal bleeding. A careful menstrual history should be taken, including any history of post-coital or intermenstrual bleeding. Quantifying the volume of bleeding can be difficult but the presence of clots and rate of tampon use are helpful pointers.

A pregnancy test must always be performed, regardless of whether the patient has missed a period or not.

The causes of bleeding in pregnancy are discussed in section 8.7.

8.5.2 Menorrhagia

Menorrhagia is excessive menstrual blood loss. The differential includes:

- Dysfunctional uterine bleeding—heavy or irregular periods without obvious pelvic pathology. Often seen around menarche due to hormonal imbalance. Symptomatic relief with NSAIDs (e.g. mefenamic acid) are the mainstay of treatment.
- Fibroids.
- Endometriosis.
- Pelvic inflammatory disease.
- IUCD.
- Polyps.
- Hypothyroidism.

8.5.3 Post-menopausal bleeding

Post-menopausal bleeding is one of the most common presentations to a gynaecology clinic. The differential includes:

- Atrophic vaginitis
- Endometrial polyps
- Fibroids
- Endometrial hyperplasia
- Endometrial carcinoma
- Cervical carcinoma
- Vaginal carcinoma
- Bleeding from non-gynaecological sites (e.g. urethra, bladder, or lower GI tract)

An abdominal examination, speculum, and bimanual vaginal examination should be performed to look for evidence of tenderness or masses. Patients should be referred to gynaecology as an out-patient for further investigation.

8.5.4 Vaginal bleeding unrelated to menstruation or pregnancy

- Trauma.
- IUCD insertion.
- Post-gynaecological operations.
- Cervical erosions—occur when the stratified squamous epithelium is replaced by columnar epithelium. The cervix appears red and the patient may experience post-coital or intermenstrual bleeding.
- Cervical polyp.
- Cervical cancer—90% are squamous carcinoma. Speculum examination may reveal nodules, ulcers, or erosions, which may bleed on contact.
- Endometrial cancer.

- Fibroids.
- Genital ulcers.
- PID.
- Bleeding diathesis (e.g. thrombocytopenia, haemophilia).
- Anticoagulant medication.
- Oral contraceptive problems—breakthrough bleeding due to endometrial hyperplasia.

Most patients with vaginal bleeding can be managed as outpatients with GP or gynaecology follow-up. Patients with evidence of severe bleeding or hypovolaemia should be resuscitated and admitted. Patients with suspected genital tract malignancy should be referred urgently for gynaecological follow-up.

KEY POINTS

There are many causes of abnormal vaginal bleeding. The differential diagnosis varies according to whether the bleeding is menstrual, intermenstrual, post-menopausal, pregnancy-related, or post-coital.

The initial priority in the ED is to exclude an ectopic pregnancy or threatened miscarriage.

Follow-up should be arranged urgently if there is a possibility that the bleeding is caused by a genital tract carcinoma.

8.6 Emergency contraception

8.6.1 Introduction

Emergency contraception is intervention aimed at preventing pregnancy after unprotected intercourse or contraceptive failure. Two methods of emergency contraception are available in the United Kingdom:

- Oral emergency contraception: levonorgestrel or ulipristal acetate
- The copper intrauterine contraceptive device (cIUCD)

EXAM TIP

Emergency contraception makes an ideal SAQ topic because there are two possible treatment options, both with advantages and disadvantages (Table 8.1).

8.6.2 Levonorgestrel

Levonorgestrel is taken as a single dose (1.5 mg) up to 72 hours after unprotected sexual intercourse. If taken within 24 hours, it prevents 95% of pregnancies but this diminishes with time to 58% at 72 hours. The mechanism of action is believed to be inhibition of ovulation for 5–7 days.

8.6.3 Ulipristal acetate

Ulipristal is taken as a single oral dose or 30 mg. It acts as a progesterone receptor modulator and is thought to inhibit or delay ovulation. It can be taken up to 120 hours after unprotected sexual intercourse and is the only oral emergency contraceptive licensed for use between 72 and 120 hours.

Table 8.1 Advantages and disadvantages of different forms of emergency contraception

Method of contraception	Advantages	Disadvantages
Oral emergency contraceptive	Readily available.	High failure rate if taken >72 h for levonorgestrel or >120 h for uliprista acetate after unprotected intercourse.
	Available without prescription to women >16 years of age.	
	Single dose.	A repeat dose is required if vomiting occurs within 2 h.
	No limit to the number of times it can be taken.	Does not provide long-term contraception.
		Side effects—spotting, mild bleeding, change in menstrual cycle length.
		Less effective in women taking enzyme-inducing medications (require double dose).
		Contraindications—severe liver disease, porphyria, migraine, severe malabsorption syndromes, pregnancy.
Copper IUCD	More effective than oral medication	Less readily available.
	Can be used up to 5 days after unprotected intercourse.	Requires trained professional to insert.
		Insertion may result in abdominal pain.
	Provides long-term contraception.	Some women experience heavier and longer periods with an IUCD.
	Unaffected by other medications being taken.	If a pregnancy occurs there is a higher risk of ectopic pregnancy.
		Rarely, it can be expelled without the woman noticing.
		Risk of uterine perforation (very rare).
		Risk of PID.

8.6.4 Copper IUCD

This is the most effective method of emergency contraception. It prevents 98% of expected pregnancies and can be inserted up to five days after unprotected sexual intercourse. The mechanism of action is via direct toxic effects on sperm and the inhibition of implantation.

Women should be risk assessed for sexually transmitted infections and offered screening. If the risk of an infection is felt to be high then prophylactic azithromycin should be given on insertion.

8.6.5 Emergency contraception aftercare advice

Patients should be given the following advice after receiving emergency contraception:

- A repeat dose of oral medication is required if vomiting occurs within two hours of taking it.
- The next menstruation may be early or late.
- A pregnancy test should be performed if menstruation is five to seven days late, if bleeding is lighter or heavier than usual, or if the patient feels she might be pregnant.
- Medical attention should be sought if lower abdominal pain occurs because this could signify an ectopic pregnancy.
- Women continuing to use hormonal contraception are advised to use additional methods of contraception for seven days post levonogestrel or 14 days post uliprista actetate.

8.6.6 Under 16s and emergency contraception

Knowledge of the law regarding contraceptive advice and treatment could appear in an SAQ on emergency contraception.

Consent to sexual activity

- The legal age of consent to sexual activity is 16 years in Scotland, England, and Wales.
- Sexual activity under the age of consent is an offence, even if consensual.
- Offences are considered more serious (statutory rape) when the person is less than 13 years old.

Consent to medical treatment

In the United Kingdom, people over the age of 16 years are presumed to be competent to consent to medical treatment. Under the age of 16 years, competency to consent to medical treatment must be demonstrated.

In England and Wales, it is lawful to provide contraceptive advice and treatment to young people without parental consent, provided that the practitioner is satisfied that the Fraser criteria for competence are met. The criteria are that:

- The young person understands the practitioner's advice.
- The young person cannot be persuaded to inform their parents, or will not allow the practitioner to inform the parents, that contraceptive advice has been sought.
- The young person is likely to begin or to continue having intercourse with or without contraceptive treatment.
- Unless she receives contraceptive advice or treatment, the young person's physical or mental health (or both) is likely to suffer.
- The young person's best interest requires the practitioner to give contraceptive advice or treatment (or both) without parental consent.

KEY POINTS

Two methods of emergency contraception are available in the United Kingdom:
- Emergency oral contraception: levonorgestrel or ulipristal actetate
- The copper intrauterine contraceptive device (IUCD)

Levonorgestrel is taken as a single dose (1.5 mg) up to 72 h after unprotected sexual intercourse. Ulpristal acetate is taken as a single dose of 30 mg and is the only licensed medication for use from 72–120 hours after unprotected sexual intercourse

Copper IUCD is the most effective method of emergency contraception. It prevents 98% of expected pregnancies and can be inserted up to five days after unprotected sexual intercourse. The mechanism of action is via direct toxic effects on sperm and the inhibition of implantation.

8.7 Bleeding in pregnancy

8.7.1 Introduction

The causes of pregnancy-related vaginal bleeding vary according to the gestation (Table 8.2).

Table 8.2 Causes of pregnancy-related vaginal bleeding

1st trimester	Spontaneous miscarriage
	Ectopic pregnancy (section 8.2)
	Trophoblastic disease
2nd trimester	Spontaneous miscarriage
	Trophoblastic disease
	Placental abruption
	Placenta praevia
3rd trimester	Placental abruption
	Placenta praevia
	Vasa praevia
	'Show' of pregnancy

8.7.2 Spontaneous miscarriage

Miscarriage is the loss of a pregnancy before 24 weeks gestation. It occurs in approximately one in five pregnancies. Most women present in the first 12 weeks with vaginal bleeding and/or abdominal pain.

There are a variety of terms used to describe different types of miscarriage:

- Threatened miscarriage—is vaginal bleeding through a closed cervical os—50% proceed to miscarriage.
- Inevitable miscarriage—is vaginal bleeding through an open cervical os or passage of some products of conception.
- Incomplete miscarriage—is vaginal bleeding but not all products of conception have passed.
- Missed miscarriage—occurs when failure of the pregnancy is 'silent' and is often first noticed on ultrasound.
- Miscarriage with infection—occurs when retained products become infected.
- Complete miscarriage—is once all the products of conception have passed.

Clinical features of spontaneous miscarriage

- Vaginal bleeding—varies from light spotting to heavy bleeding with clots.
- Abdominal pain—is usually lower abdomen and crampy. Unilateral pain or shoulder tip pain (diaphragmatic irritation) suggests an ectopic pregnancy.
- Cervical shock—is when the products of conception become stuck in the cervical os, resulting in profound vagal stimulation (hypotension and bradycardia) and severe abdominal pain.
- Vaginal examination—may reveal an open os indicating an inevitable miscarriage. Cervical or adnexal tenderness indicates a possible ectopic pregnancy or infection.

Investigations for spontaneous miscarriage

- Urinary pregnancy test—should be performed. A positive test does not necessarily indicate a viable pregnancy because it may remain positive for several days after foetal death.
- Urine dipstick—should be tested to look for evidence of infection which may account for the lower abdominal pain.
- Serum β-HCG—can be helpful for subsequent serial monitoring. In a miscarriage levels would be expected to fall on serial testing.

- Ultrasound scan—should be arranged. The earliest a gestation sac can be seen via transabdominal scanning is at seven weeks and five to six weeks via transvaginal. Referral to an early pregnancy diagnostic unit is appropriate, and this service should be available seven days a week.
- Rhesus status—should be checked in case anti-D is required (see section 8.10).
- Full blood count (FBC), clotting, and cross-match—should be performed if the patient is shocked.

ED management of spontaneous miscarriage

- Fluid resuscitation as required by the patient's haemodynamic status.
- Analgesia.
- Removal of the products of conception from the os if the patient has cervical shock.
- Ergometrine (500 mcg intramuscularly) should be considered if the patient has severe bleeding.
- Urgent referral to gynaecology, if the patient is haemodynamically compromised or an ectopic pregnancy is suspected.
- Referral to the early pregnancy assessment unit, as an outpatient, if the patient is stable. Expectant management for 7–14 days is the first-line management strategy for most cases of spontaneous miscarriage.

8.7.3 Gestational trophoblastic disease

Occasionally, a fertilized ovum may form abnormal trophoblastic tissue but no foetus. The disease encompasses a spectrum that can be benign (hydatidiform mole) or malignant (choriocarcinoma).

There is excessive production of β HCG from abnormal placental tissue, which may cause exaggerated symptoms of early pregnancy. Around 50% patients develop vaginal bleeding at 12–16 weeks gestation, which may be heavy and include the passage of molar tissue that resembles frog spawn.

Ultrasound shows a 'snowstorm' and no foetus. The serum β-HCG is grossly elevated.

ED management involves intravenous fluids, analgesia, and prompt referral to gynaecology for evacuation of the uterus.

8.7.4 Antepartum haemorrhage

Antepartum haemorrhage is bleeding after 24 weeks gestation, it occurs in approximately 2.5% of pregnancies. The causes of antepartum haemorrhage include:

- Placental abruption
- Placenta praevia
- Vasa praevia
- Uterine rupture
- Bleeding from the lower genital tract (e.g. cervicitis, cervical cancer or polyp, vaginal cancer)
- Bleeding that may be confused with vaginal bleeding, e.g. haemorrhoids, inflammatory bowel disease, urinary tract infection (UTI)

Placental abruption

Placental abruption is premature separation of part of the placenta from the uterus. The outcome depends on the degree of separation and amount of blood loss.

Risk factors for placental abruption:

- Pre-eclampsia
- Previous placental abruption
- Trauma

- Smoking
- Multiparity

Clinical features of placental abruption include:

- Vaginal bleeding—the amount depends on the location and degree of separation. Sometimes the bleeding is limited to the confines of the uterus resulting in a 'concealed haemorrhage'.
- Abdominal pain and tenderness.
- Premature labour.
- Haemodynamic compromise, which may be out of proportion to the degree of visible blood loss.
- DIC or absent foetal heart sounds, in large bleeds.

Placenta praevia

Placenta praevia exists when the placenta is inserted wholly or partially in the lower segment of the uterus. If it lies over the cervical os it is considered a major praevia, if not a minor praevia.
Risk factors for placenta praevia include:

- Maternal age >35 years old
- High parity
- Previous placenta praevia
- Twin pregnancy
- Uterine abnormalities (e.g. previous caesarean section, fibroids)

Clinical features of placenta praevia include:

- Bright red, painless, vaginal bleeding in the third trimester
- Labour (presentation in 15%)

Vasa praevia

Vasa praevia is a rare condition where foetal blood vessels grow within the membranes and over the internal os. Haemorrhage may occur when the membranes rupture resulting in foetal exsanguination.

Investigations for antepartum haemorrhage

- FBC, clotting, fibrinogen—risk of DIC
- Cross-match blood (6 units)
- Rhesus status—anti-D may be required (see section 8.10)
- Kleihauer test—to determine the degree of foetal–maternal haemorrhage

Emergency department management of antepartum haemorrhage

- Manage the patient in the resuscitation room.
- Call an obstetrician immediately.
- Insert two large-bore cannulae and fluid resuscitate.
- Transfuse blood as required.
- Give anti-D immunoglobulin if the patient is rhesus negative.

KEY POINTS

Miscarriage is the loss of a pregnancy before 24 weeks gestation. It occurs in approximately one in five pregnancies. Most women present in the first 12 weeks with vaginal bleeding and/ or abdominal pain.

Cervical shock is when the products of conception become stuck in the cervical os, resulting in profound vagal stimulation (hypotension and bradycardia) and severe abdominal pain. Patients require speculum examination and removal of products from the os, in addition to fluid resuscitation.

Gestational trophoblastic disease occurs when a fertilized ovum forms abnormal trophoblastic tissue, but no foetus.

Antepartum haemorrhage is bleeding after 24 weeks gestation.

Antepartum haemorrhage should be managed in the resuscitation room. Patients should be aggressively fluid resuscitated and given anti-D immunoglobulin if rhesus negative. The obstetrician should be called urgently to see the patient in the resuscitation room.

Patients with antepartum haemorrhage are at risk of massive haemorrhage and DIC. A FBC, clotting, fibrinogen, and cross-match (6 units) should be sent urgently.

8.8 Hyperemesis gravidarum

8.8.1 Introduction

Hyperemesis gravidarum is unrelenting, excessive pregnancy-related nausea and/or vomiting that prevents adequate intake of food or fluids. Hyperemesis is rare (1 in 1000) but lesser degrees of nausea and vomiting ('morning sickness') are common.

8.8.2 Investigations for hyperemesis gravidarum

- Renal function—risk of hyponatraemia, hypokalaemia, and renal failure.
- Bicarbonate and chloride—risk of hypochloraemic metabolic alkalosis.
- FBC—increased mean cell volume (MCV) due to dehydration.
- LFTs—ALT, AST, and bilirubin may be increased.
- Urine dipstick—to look for evidence of an UTI and increased specific gravity as a marker of dehydration.
- Ultrasound scan—to exclude twins or hydatidiform mole.

8.8.3 Emergency department management of hyperemesis gravidarum

- Admit the patient if they are unable to maintain adequate hydration and nutrition.
- Intravenous fluids.
- Thiamine—to prevent Wernicke's encephalopathy.
- Anti-emetics (no anti-emetic is licensed for use in pregnancy but promethazine and cyclizine have proven safety records).
- TED stockings and low molecular weight heparin—due to the risk of venous thromboembolism.
- Consider a proton-pump inhibitor.

8.8.4 Complications of hyperemesis gravidarum

- Mallory–Weiss tear
- Wernicke's encephalopathy
- Hyponatraemia
- Central pontine myelinosis (if sodium is corrected too quickly)
- B12 and B6 deficiency
- Foetal intrauterine growth retardation
- Venous thromboembolism

KEY POINTS

Hyperemesis gravidarum is unrelenting, excessive pregnancy-related nausea and/or vomiting that prevents adequate intake of food or fluids. Hyperemesis is rare (1 in 1000) but lesser degrees of nausea and vomiting ('morning sickness') are common.

Patients with hyperemesis gravidarum are at risk of thiamine deficiency. Ensure supplemental thiamine is given.

8.9 Pre-eclampsia and eclampsia

Previous MRCEM question

Pre-eclampsia affects approximately 6% of pregnancies. It is classically defined as a triad of:

- Hypertension (systolic >140 mmHg or diastolic >90 mmHg, or a rise above booking BP of systolic >30 mmHg or diastolic >15 mmHg)
- Proteinuria (>0.3g/24 hours)
- Oedem

More modern definitions concentrate on the rise in BP and proteinuria, excluding oedema which is a non-specific finding. Onset is usually after 20 weeks gestation.

Eclampsia occurs in approximately 1–2% of pre-eclamptic pregnancies. It is heralded by the occurrence of one or more convulsions.

8.9.1 Risk factors for pre-eclampsia

- Nulliparity
- Multiple pregnancy
- Hydatidiform mole
- Age <20 years old or >40 years old
- Previous pre-eclampsia
- Family history of pre-eclampsia
- Pre-existing hypertension
- Diabetes or insulin resistance
- Pre-existing vascular or renal disease
- High body mass index of 35 kg/m² or more
- Anti-phospholipid syndrome
- Long interval between pregnancies (>10 years)

8.9.2 Clinical features of pre-eclampsia

- Malaise
- Right-upper quadrant and epigastric pain—due to liver oedema and haemorrhage
- Headache, visual disturbance (blurring or flashing before the eyes), and papilloedema—due to cerebral oedema
- Occipital lobe blindness
- Hyperreflexia, clonus
- Convulsions—due to cerebral oedema (heralds the onset of eclampsia)

8.9.3 Investigations for pre-eclampsia

- FBC—risk of thrombocytopenia and haemoconcentration.
- Blood film—should be checked because the patient may develop microangiopathic haemolytic anaemia.

- Clotting screen—should be checked if the patient is thrombocytopenic.
- Renal function—risk of renal failure.
- LFTS—elevated transaminases in haemolysis, elevated liver enzymes, and low platelets (HELLP) syndrome.
- Urinary dipstick—≥2 + protein indicates significant proteinuria and the need for 24-hour urine collection.
- Foetal monitoring via ultrasound and cardiotocography.

8.9.4 Emergency department management of pre-eclampsia

- Contact the obstetricians early.
- Manage the patient in the resuscitation room with full monitoring.
- Consider positioning the patient left lateral.
- Control hypertension with oral labetalol.
- Careful fluid management is required. Fluid overload is a significant cause of maternal death due to pulmonary oedema. Limit fluids to approximately 1ml/kg/hr. Urine output should be monitored.
- Magnesium should be considered in women with severe pre-eclampsia (systolic BP ≥170 mmHg or diastolic BP ≥110 mmHg plus significant proteinuria, >1g/L).
- Delivery is the definitive treatment for pre-eclampsia. However, 44% of eclampsia occurs post-partum.

8.9.5 Emergency department management of eclampsia

- Airway and breathing adequacy should be assessed. High-flow supplemental oxygen should be given. Ventilation should be assisted if inadequate. Intubation should be considered early due to the increased risks of aspiration and ventilatory inadequacy in pregnancy.
- Magnesium is the therapy of choice to control seizures. A loading dose of 4 g intravenously should be given over 5–10 minutes followed by maintenance of 1 g/hour for 24 hours. A further bolus of 2 g can be given if the patient has recurrent seizures.

8.9.6 Complications of pre-eclampsia and eclampsia

See Box 8.1 for the complications of pre-eclampsia and eclampsia.

KEY POINTS

Pre-eclampsia is defined as:

- Hypertension (systolic >140 mmHg or diastolic >90 mmHg, or a rise above booking BP of systolic >30 mmHg or diastolic >15 mmHg)
- Proteinuria (>0.3 g/24 h) ±
- Oedema

Eclampsia is heralded by the occurrence of one or more convulsions.

Magnesium is the therapy of choice to treat eclampsia. The initial dose is 4 g IV.

Delivery is the definitive treatment for pre-eclampsia; however 44% of eclampsia occurs post-partum.

HELLP (haemolysis, elevated liver enzymes, and low platelets) syndrome is a severe variant of pre-eclampsia.

Box 8.1 Complications of pre-eclampsia and eclampsia

Central nervous system

- Intracerebral haemorrhage
- Cerebral oedema
- Cortical blindness
- Retinal oedema and blindness

Liver

- HELLP—haemolysis, elevated liver enzymes, and low platelets
- Intra-abdominal haemorrhage (hepatic rupture)
- Jaundice

Respiratory

- Pulmonary oedema
  Cardiac
- Cardiac failure

Renal

- Renal cortical necrosis
- Renal tubular necrosis

Coagulation

- Disseminated intravascular coagulation
- Microangiopathic haemolysis
- Venous thromboembolism

Placental

- Placental abruption
- Placental infarction

Foetal

- Intrauterine growth retardation
- Premature delivery
- Perinatal death (15% in eclampsia)

8.10 Rhesus prophylaxis—anti-D immunoglobulin

8.10.1 Introduction

The following guidance is based on the British Committee for Standards in Haematology (BCSH) Guideline on anti-D administration in pregnancy (http://www.b-s-h.org.uk/guidelines/).

8.10.2 Pathophysiology

A rhesus D negative mother exposed to the blood of a rhesus D positive foetus may develop anti-D antibodies. These antibodies are IgG and are not usually a problem in the initial pregnancy because they do not have time to develop before delivery. However, in a subsequent pregnancy, with a rhesus D positive foetus, the antibodies are formed and can cross the placenta. The antibodies attack and destroy red blood cells of the foetus resulting in haemolytic disease of the newborn.

8.10.3 Sensitizing episodes before delivery

The BCSH guideline recommends prophylactic anti-D immunoglobulin for pregnant women who are D negative in the following circumstances:

- Closed abdominal injury/fall (particularly in the third trimester)
- Antepartum haemorrhage
- Intrauterine death
- Invasive prenatal diagnostic or therapeutic intervention (amniocentesis, chorionic villus sampling, intrauterine transfusion)
- Ectopic pregnancy
- Spontaneous miscarriage (all pregnancies >12/40; <12/40 if intervention is required to evacuate the uterus)
- Threatened miscarriage (all pregnancies >12/40; <12/40 if heavy or repeated bleeding, or associated with abdominal pain)
- Therapeutic termination of pregnancy
- External cephalic version

The guidance for spontaneous and threatened miscarriage depends on the gestation. Beyond 12 weeks gestation, anti-D immunoglobulin is indicated. Below 12 weeks gestation, the evidence is scant. The Royal College of Obstetricians and Gynaecologists guidance is that in a spontaneous miscarriage <12 weeks gestation, anti-D immunoglobulin is only required if there is instrumentation to evacuate the products of conception. In a threatened miscarriage it is recommended that anti-D immunoglobulin is only administered when the bleeding is heavy, or repeated, or where there is associated abdominal pain, particularly if these events occur as gestation approaches 12 weeks.

8.10.4 Anti-D immunoglobulin doses

Routine antenatal prophylaxis

- 500 IU should be given at 28 weeks and 34 weeks gestation.

Prophylactic administration following a sensitizing episode

- 250 IU up to 20/40 gestation.
- 500 IU after 20/40 gestation, plus a Kleihauer test to detect large feto-maternal haemorrhage and direct further doses as required.

Following delivery

- 500 iu, plus a Kleihauer test to detect large feto-maternal haemorrhage and direct further doses as required.

Anti-D immunoglobulin is given intramuscularly and should be given as soon as possible and definitely within 72 hours of the sensitizing episode.

KEY POINTS

The development of anti-D antibodies results from feto-maternal haemorrhages occurring in rhesus D negative women who carry a rhesus D positive foetus.

Anti-D IgG antibodies attack and destroy red blood cells of the foetus resulting in haemolytic disease of the newborn.

Sensitizing events likely to be encountered in the ED include:

- Closed abdominal injury (particularly in the third trimester)
- Antepartum haemorrhage
- Intrauterine death
- Ectopic pregnancy
- Spontaneous miscarriage (all pregnancies >12/40; <12/40 if intervention is required to evacuate the uterus)
- Threatened miscarriage (all pregnancies >12/40; <12/40 if heavy or repeated bleeding, or associated with abdominal pain)

Anti-D immunoglobulin is given intramuscularly and should be given as soon as possible and definitely within 72 h of the sensitizing episode.

8.11 Emergency delivery

In the ED the 'occiput anterior' presentation is the only one that is likely to proceed so fast that delivery occurs before specialist help arrives.

8.11.1 Stages of labour

- First stage—onset of labour until the cervix is fully dilated (10 cm).
- Second stage—full dilatation until the baby is born.
- Third stage—placenta and membranes deliver and uterus retracts.

8.11.2 Complications of delivery

- Cord prolapse—this is an emergency because of potential cord compression and foetal asphyxia. ED intervention aims to prevent the presenting part from occluding the cord:
  - Displace the presenting part by putting a hand in the vagina and pushing it back up.
  - Use gravity by positioning the woman head down or knee-elbow position.
  - Infuse 500 ml saline into the bladder through a catheter.
  - Keep the cord in the vagina and do not handle it, to prevent spasm.
- Shoulder dystocia—this is the inability to deliver the shoulders after the head has been delivered. Place the woman in the lithotomy position to increase the pelvic outlet. Perform an episiotomy. Apply firm suprapubic pressure and gently bend the baby's head towards the mother's anus to free the anterior shoulder.
- Perineal tear—this can be minimized by a controlled delivery. If a tear is imminent, perform an episiotomy.
- The following complications usually present to labour ward rather than the ED:
  - Retained placenta.
  - Uterine inversion.
  - Amniotic fluid embolus.

8.12 Post-partum haemorrhage

8.12.1 Introduction

Primary post-partum haemorrhage—is blood loss of greater than 500 ml in the first 24 hours post-delivery. Primary post-partum haemorrhage can be minor (500–1000 ml) or major (>1000 ml).

Secondary post-partum haemorrhage—is excessive blood loss from the genital tract between 24 hours and 12 weeks postnatally.

8.12.2 Risk factors for post-partum haemorrhage

- Placental abruption
- Placenta praevia
- Placenta accreta (abnormally adherent placenta)
- Multiple pregnancy
- Pre-eclampsia/gestational hypertension
- Previous post-partum haemorrhage
- Haemophilia
- Anticoagulant use

8.12.3 Causes of post-partum haemorrhage

Causes of primary post-partum haemorrhage include:

- Uterine atony (commonest cause)
- Retained placenta
- Genital tract trauma (e.g. vaginal or cervical lacerations, uterine rupture)
- DIC

Causes of secondary post-partum haemorrhage include:

- Retained products of conception
- Intrauterine infection
- Genital tract trauma
- Trophoblastic disease
- DIC

8.12.4 Emergency department management of post-partum haemorrhage

Primary post-partum haemorrhage

- Call the obstetric team immediately.
- Manage the patient in the resuscitation room.
- Airway and breathing should be assessed, maintained, and assisted if required. High-flow oxygen should be given.
- Two large-bore cannulae should be inserted. Blood should be sent for FBC, clotting, and fibrinogen.
- A cross-match sample (4 units minimum) should be sent urgently and the transfusion department alerted that a massive transfusion may be required.
- Large amounts of fluid resuscitation are likely to be required, initially crystalloid, and then cross-matched blood as soon as it is available. If cross-matched blood is not available in a timely fashion, type-specific or O-negative blood may have to be given. The patient may require blood products (e.g. platelets, fresh frozen plasma, and cryoprecipitate).

- Uterine atony is the commonest cause of primary post-partum haemorrhage. Stimulation of uterine contraction may reduce bleeding. This can be achieved by bimanual uterine compression (rubbing up the fundus) and/or pharmacologically with oxytocin and ergometrine IV.
- Ultimately the patient may require surgical control of bleeding.

Secondary post-partum haemorrhage

Secondary post-partum haemorrhage is most commonly due to retained products of conception and often associated with infection.

- Airway and breathing should be assessed and managed as for a primary post-partum haemorrhage.
- Fluid resuscitation should be directed by the patient's haemodynamic status.
- IV antibiotics (e.g. ampicillin and metronidazole) should be given if infection is suspected. Prior to antibiotics a low vaginal swab and blood cultures should be sent.
- Patients should be referred to the obstetric team for further management.

KEY POINTS

Primary post-partum haemorrhage is blood loss of greater than 500 ml in the first 24 h post-delivery.

Secondary post-partum haemorrhage is excessive blood loss from the genital tract between 24 h and 12 weeks postnatally.

The commonest cause of primary post-partum haemorrhage is uterine atony.

The commonest cause of secondary post-partum haemorrhage is retained products of conception.

Patients with post-partum haemorrhage may require a massive blood transfusion.

8.13 Pregnancy and trauma

8.13.1 Introduction

The advanced trauma life support (ATLS) principles (see Chapter 4) are the same for the pregnant patient; however, there are anatomical and physiological considerations that make the management of pregnant patients challenging.

8.13.2 Anatomical considerations for trauma in pregnancy

- The enlarged uterus is more prone to injury once it is outside the pelvis (>12/40 gestation) and makes abdominal assessment difficult.
- The bony pelvis is less prone to fracture but retroperitoneal haemorrhage may be massive due to increased vascularity.
- Inferior vena cava (IVC) compression occurs when the patient is supine resulting in hypotension and potential for increased bleeding from lower limb injuries due to increased venous pressure. Decompress the IVC by manual displacement of the uterus or using a 'Cardiff wedge' to achieve the left lateral position.
- The diaphragm is higher resulting in decreased residual volume.
- The airway is difficult to control (large breasts, full dentition, neck oedema, and obesity).
- The pituitary is twice its normal size and at risk of infarction if hypovolaemia occurs (Sheehan's syndrome).

8.13.3 Physiological considerations for trauma in pregnancy

- Pregnant patients can tolerate up to 35% blood loss before showing signs of hypovolaemia. However, the foetus maybe compromised prior to such signs developing.
- The functional residual capacity is reduced and oxygen requirements are increased, resulting in hypoxia developing more quickly.
- Increased risk of aspiration (decreased oesophageal pressure, increased gastric pressure, and prolonged gastric emptying).
- Coagulation can become rapidly deranged especially following an amniotic fluid embolus.

KEY POINTS

The ATLS principles are the same for the pregnant patient.

If possible, position the patient in the left lateral position or manually displace the uterus to the left to decompress the IVC and improve venous return.

8.14 SAQs

8.14.1 Pelvic inflammatory disease

A 30-year-old woman presents to the ED with lower abdominal pain, deep dyspareunia, and fever. You make a diagnosis of pelvic inflammatory disease.

a) List two sexually transmitted causes and one non-sexually transmitted cause of PID. (3 marks)
b) Give four indications for admission with PID. (2 marks)
c) You decide your patient can be discharged and prescribe her antibiotics. Which two antibiotics would you prescribe? (2 marks)
d) List three complications of PID. (3 marks)

Suggested answer

a) List two sexually transmitted causes and one non-sexually transmitted cause of PID. (3 marks)

Sexually transmitted—*Chlamydia, Gonorrhoea, Mycoplasma genitalium*

Non-sexually transmitted—*E. Coli*, Group B Strep, *Bacteriodes, Gardenella, Ureaplasma*

b) Give four indications for admission with PID. (2 marks)

Clinically severe disease
Tubo-ovarian abscess
PID in pregnancy
Intolerance or lack of response to oral therapy
Surgical emergency not excluded

c) You decide your patient can be discharged and prescribe her antibiotics. Which two antibiotics would you prescribe? (2 marks)

Ofloxacin 400 mg bd and metronidazole 400 mg bd for 14 days.

d) List three complications of PID. (3 marks)

Infertility
Ectopic pregnancy
Chronic pelvic pain
Peritonitis
Abscess formation

8.14.2 Ectopic pregnancy

A 25-year-old woman has presented to the ED with isolated left iliac fossa pain. Her last menstrual period was six weeks ago. Her urine pregnancy test performed in the ED is positive. The triage nurse thinks the patient may have an ectopic pregnancy. Her initial observations are: HR 90 bpm, BP 110/50 mmHg, RR 18/min, T 36.8°C, CRT 1 s.

a) List three additional features in this patient's past medical history that would increase her risk of ectopic pregnancy. (3 marks)
b) (i) List four key features in the examination of this patient that may indicate an ectopic pregnancy. (2 marks)
b) (ii) List the four most likely alternative gynaecological diagnoses of left iliac fossa pain in this patient. (2 marks)

She is known to be rhesus D negative and has a confirmed ectopic pregnancy on transvaginal ultrasound.

c) Apart from an ectopic pregnancy, give three other sensitizing episodes where anti-D immunoglobulin would be indicated? (3 marks)

Suggested answer

a) List three additional features in this patient's past medical history that would increase her risk of ectopic pregnancy. (3 marks)

IUCD/coil
PID/STI
Previous ectopic
Previous gynaecological surgery
Progesterone-only pill
Endometriosis
IVF
Congenital genital anatomical variants
Ovarian and uterine cysts/tumours

b) (i) List four key features in the examination of this patient that may indicate an ectopic pregnancy. (2 marks)

Peritonism/rebound tenderness/guarding
Adnexal tenderness
Cervical excitation
Pallor
Hypotension/shock
LIF mass

b) (ii) List the four most likely alternative gynaecological diagnoses of left iliac fossa pain in this patient. (2 marks)

Threatened miscarriage
Ovarian cyst torsion
Ovarian cyst rupture/haemorrhage
Corpus luteum cyst rupture
STI/PID
Red degeneration of fibroid

c) Apart from an ectopic pregnancy, give three other sensitizing episodes where anti-D immunoglobulin would be indicated? (3 marks)

Closed abdominal injury
Antepartum haemorrhage
Intrauterine death
Invasive prenatal diagnostics
Therapeutic termination
Spontaneous miscarriage (all pregnancies >12/40; <12/40 if intervention is required to evacuate the uterus)
Threatened miscarriage (all pregnancies >12/40; <12/40 if heavy or repeated bleeding, or associated with abdominal pain)

Further reading

British Association for Sexual Health and HIV (BASHH) UK National Guideline for the Management of Pelvic Inflammatory Disease 2011. Available at: https://from www.bashh.org/documents/3572.pdf [Online].

British Committee for Standards in Haematology, 2014. BCSH guidelines for the use of anti-D immunoglobulin for the prevention of haemolytic disease of the fetus and newborn. *Transfus Med* **24**(1):8–20.

Faculty of Sexual and Reproductive Healthcare, updated 2012. Emergency Contraception clinical effectiveness unit 2011 Clinical Guidance. Available at: https://www.fsrh.org [Online].

National Institute for Health Care and Excellence, 2010. NICE clinical guideline107. Hypertension in pregnancy: diagnosis and management. Available at: https://from www.nice.org.uk/guidance/cg107 [Online].

National Institute for Health and Care Excellence, February 2015. NICE Clinical Knowledge Summaries. Contraception—emergency. Available at: https://from cks.nice.org.uk/contraception-emergency [Online].

National Institute for Health and Care Excellence, December 2012. NICE clinical guideline 154. Ectopic pregnancy and miscarriage: diagnosis and initial management. Available at: https://www.nice.org.uk/guidance/cg154 [Online].

Royal College of Obstetricians and Gynaecologists, 2009. Green-top Guideline 52. Prevention and management of postpartum haemorrhage. Available at: https://www.rcog.org.uk [Online].

Royal College of Obstetricians and Gynaecologists, 2010. Green-top Guideline 21. The Management of Tubal Pregnancy. Available at: https://www.rcog.org.uk [Online].

Cardiac emergencies

9.1 Acute coronary syndrome

9.1.1 Pathophysiology of acute coronary syndrome

Acute coronary syndrome (ACS) encompasses a range of conditions from unstable angina to ST-segment elevation myocardial infarction (STEMI), arising from thrombus formation on an atheromatous plaque.

The development of cholesterol-rich plaques within the walls of coronary arteries (atherosclerosis) is the pathological process that underlies coronary artery disease. However, the clinical manifestations of this generic condition are varied.

In stable angina the atherosclerotic process advances insidiously, gradually narrowing the lumen of the coronary artery. The blood supply to the myocardium is progressively compromised and the patient develops predictable, exertional chest discomfort. Stable angina is not an ACS.

At any stage in the development of atherosclerosis, an unstable plaque may develop. A tear develops in the intima of the plaque exposing the underlying cholesterol-rich atheroma, within the vessel wall, to the blood flowing in the lumen. This exposure stimulates platelet aggregation and thrombus formation. The lumen is further restricted by haemorrhage into the plaque and coronary vasospasm. The extent to which these events reduce blood flow to the myocardium determines the clinical nature of the ACS that ensues:

- STEMI—the thrombus completely occludes the lumen of the artery resulting in progressive necrosis of myocardium. The electrocardiogram (ECG) shows acute ST-segment elevation.
- Non-ST-segment elevation myocardial infarction (NSTEMI)—the volume of thrombus is insufficient to occlude the artery or does so only temporarily. There is some myocardial necrosis, evidenced by a rise in cardiac biomarkers (e.g. troponin), and often non-specific ECG abnormalities (e.g. ST-segment depression or T-wave inversion).
- Unstable angina—myocardial ischaemia is present, but without evidence of actual myocardial necrosis (normal serum troponin level).

There is now a universal definition of a myocardial infarction (MI). This is the detection of a rise and/or fall of cardiac biomarkers (preferably troponin), together with evidence of myocardial ischaemia with at least one of the following:

- Symptoms of ischaemia
- New or presumed new significant ST-T-wave changes or left bundle branch block on 12-lead) in the ECG
- Development of pathological Q waves in the ECG
- Imaging evidence of new or presumed new loss of viable myocardium or regional wall motion abnormality
- Intracoronary thrombus detected on angiography or autopsy

The clinical classification of MI includes:

Type 1: Spontaneous MI related to ischaemia due to a primary coronary event such as plaque erosion and/or rupture, fissuring, or dissection.

Type 2: MI secondary to ischaemia due to increased oxygen demand or decreased oxygen supply (e.g. coronary spasm, coronary embolism, anaemia, arrhythmias, hypertension, or hypotension).*

9.1.2 Causes of non-ischaemic chest pain and distinguishing features

The differential diagnosis of patients presenting with chest pain is extensive, ranging from relatively benign musculoskeletal aetiologies and gastro-oesophageal reflux, to life-threatening cardiac and pulmonary disorders. Chest pain is a very common ED presentation and knowledge of the different causes and features that help distinguish them, both for the exam and everyday clinical practice, is important (Table 9.1).

9.1.3 Clinical features of ischaemic chest pain

Features that may indicate ACS include:

- Pain—typically in the chest and/or other areas (e.g. the arms, back, or jaw) lasting longer than 15 minutes. The pain is classically described as a constricting discomfort/tightness.
- Associated autonomic symptoms—nausea, vomiting, sweating, breathlessness, or a combination of these.
- Chest pain associated with haemodynamic instability.
- New onset chest pain or abrupt deterioration in previously stable angina, with recurrent chest pain occurring frequently and with little or no exertion, and with episodes often lasting longer than 15 minutes.

9.1.4 Risk factors for acute coronary syndrome

Assessment for cardiovascular risk factors is an important part of determining if the pain is likely to be cardiac. Risk factors include:

- Hypertension
- Hyperlipidaemia (raised triglycerides, high LDL-cholesterol, low HDL-cholesterol)
- Smoking

* Reprinted from *Journal of the American College of Cardiology*, volume 60, issue 16, Kristian Thygesen, Joseph S. Alpert, Allan S. Jaffe, Maarten L. Simoons, Bernard R. Chaitman, Harvey D. White, Kristian Thygesen, Joseph S. Alpert, Harvey D. White, Allan S. Jaffe, Hugo A. Katus, Fred S. Apple, Bertil Lindahl, David A. Morrow *et al.*, Third Universal Definition of Myocardial Infarction, pp. 1581-1598, Copyright (2012), with permission from Elsevier.

Table 9.1 Causes of non-ischaemic chest pain and distinguishing features

Disease	Differentiating features
Reflux oesophagitis, oesophageal spasm	Heartburn.
	Worse in recumbent position.
	No ECG changes.
Pulmonary embolism	Tachypnoea, hypoxia, hypocarbia.
	Hyperventilation.
	May resemble inferior wall infarction on ECG: ST ↑ in II, III, and aVF.
	Other ECG changes include sinus tachycardia, right ventricular strain, RBBB, 'S1, Q3, T3' pattern.
	No pulmonary congestion on CXR.
	PaCO2 ↓, PaO2 ↓
Hyperventilation	Dyspnoea.
	Often a young patient.
	Tingling and numbness of limbs and lips; dizziness.
	PaCO2 ↓, PaO2 ↑ or normal.
	NB An organic disease may cause secondary hyperventilation (e.g. diabetic ketoacidosis).
Spontaneous pneumothorax	Dyspnoea; unilateral pleuritic chest pain.
	Often a young patient (typically a tall, slim, male) or older patient with underlying lung pathology (e.g. COPD).
	Auscultation of the chest may be normal or reveal decreased air entry on the affected side. The percussion note may be normal or hyper-resonant on the affected side.
	CXR confirms the diagnosis.
Aortic dissection	Severe pain with changing localization (as dissection extends).
	Pain described as tearing and inter-scapular.
	New aortic regurgitation murmur.
	Pulse deficit (asymmetry of pulses or difference of >20 mmHg between arms).
	In type A dissections, the coronary ostium may be obstructed resulting in signs of an inferior-posterior infarct on ECG.
	CXR may reveal a broad mediastinum.
Pericarditis	Change of posture and breathing influence pain.
	Pericardial friction rub may be heard.
	ST-elevation (saddle-shaped) but no reciprocal ST-depression.
Pleurisy	A jabbing pain when breathing.
	Cough is the most common symptom.
	CXR may reveal the underlying cause (e.g. pneumonia, lung malignancy, rib fractures, rheumatoid arthritis, snd so on).
Costochondritis	Palpation tenderness.
	Movements of the chest influence pain.
Early herpes zoster	No ECG changes.
	Dermatomal rash.
	Localized paraesthesia before rash.

(continued)

Table 9.1 Continued

Disease	Differentiating features
Peptic ulcer, cholecystitis, pancreatitis	Clinical examination of the abdomen reveals tenderness (inferior wall ischaemia can resemble an acute abdomen).
	Serum biochemistry (LFTs, amylase).
Depression	Continuous feeling of heaviness in the chest.
	No correlation to exercise.
	Normal ECG.

- Diabetes mellitus
- Obesity
- Male gender
- Advanced age
- Family history of coronary artery disease (coronary artery disease in a first-degree male relative diagnosed at 55 years of age or under, or in a first-degree female relative aged 65 years or under)
- Past medical history of coronary artery disease—previous MI, known coronary artery stenosis, previous coronary intervention (angioplasty, coronary stents, bypass grafts)

KEY POINTS

ACS encompasses a range of conditions from unstable angina to STEMI, arising from thrombus formation on an atheromatous plaque.

An MI is defined as the detection of a rise and/or fall of cardiac biomarkers together with evidence of myocardial ischaemia with at least one of the following:

- Symptoms of ischaemia
- ECG changes indicative of new ischaemia (new ST-T changes or new LBBB)
- Development of pathological Q waves in the ECG
- Imaging evidence of new loss of viable myocardium or new regional wall motion abnormality

Clinical features suggestive of ACS include:

- Pain, typically in the chest and/or other areas (e.g. the arms, back, or jaw) lasting >15 minutes. The pain is classically described as a constricting discomfort/tightness.
- Associated autonomic symptoms (e.g. nausea, vomiting, sweating, breathlessness).
- Chest pain associated with haemodynamic instability.
- New onset chest pain or abrupt deterioration in previously stable angina, with recurrent chest pain occurring frequently and with little or no exertion, and with episodes often lasting >15 minutes.

9.2 Investigations in acute coronary syndrome

9.2.1 Electrocardiogram

A 12-lead ECG should be performed as soon as possible, ideally within 10 minutes of arrival (College of Emergency Medicine clinical standard for MI). The initial ECG is predictive of early risk. If the initial ECG is normal or equivocal, serial ECGs should be performed. A normal resting 12-lead ECG is not sensitive enough to exclude ACS.

ECG changes suggestive of NSTEMI or unstable angina include:

• Regional ST-segment depression. ST-depression of 0.05 MV or greater in two or more contiguous leads is suggestive of NSTE-ACS in the appropriate clinical context.
• Deep T-wave inversion.

Other ECG findings (e.g. Q waves and T-wave changes) are less specific for ACS but may increase the suspicion of ACS in a patient with a significant history.

ECG changes suggestive of STEMI evolve over time, however reperfusion therapy may halt or reverse the changes:

• Hyperacute T-waves develop in the first 30 minutes.
• ST-segment elevation starts within minutes and evolves over one to two hours, eventually becoming 'tombstones'.
• Q waves start to develop after 1–2 hours and continue developing over the next 6–24 hours.
• ST-segments start returning to the isoelectric baseline over the next 24 hours.
• Terminal T-wave inversion, followed by full T-wave inversion, starts within 24 hours.
• Q waves persist but other changes usually resolve.

The ECG criteria for thrombolysis or referral for primary percutaneous coronary intervention (PCI) (in the presence of chest pain starting <12 hours ago) are:

• New onset LBBB
• 2 mm ST-segment elevation in two contiguous chest leads
• 1 mm ST-segment elevation in two contiguous limb leads

EXAM TIP

Identifying new LBBB can be difficult in the absence of an old ECG. If a patient presents with ischaemic-sounding cardiac chest pain and LBBB, it should be assumed to be new and the patient considered for reperfusion therapy.

The territory of the MI and likely coronary artery involved can be determined from the ECG (Table 9.2).

Additional ECG leads

Additional ECG leads are sometimes indicated, particularly in inferior MIs where there may be associated posterior and/or right ventricular involvement (Figures 9.1 and 9.2).

Posterior leads (V7–9) should be performed in patients with an inferior MI and those with anteroseptal ST-segment depression, which may be masking a true posterior MI. The leads are positioned in the same horizontal plane as V4–6. V7 is positioned at the left posterior axillary line, V8 at the left mid-scapular line, and V9 at the left spinal border. ST-segment elevation of 1 mm is considered indicative of a STEMI in leads V7–9.

Right ventricular MIs usually occur as a complication of an inferior MI. Right-sided leads (V1R–V6R) should be performed in patients with an inferior MI and patients who develop hypotension and have symptoms of a MI but a non-diagnostic 12-lead ECG. Patients may present with cardiogenic shock characterized by hypotension, an elevated JVP, and signs of right-sided heart failure (clear lung fields). Echocardiography, if available, will help confirm the diagnosis. The initial management is IV fluids to maintain right ventricular preload, often with CVP monitoring. Inotropes (e.g. dobutamine) may be required. Vasodilators, such as nitrates, opiates, and diuretics, should be avoided because they reduce preload and may precipitate cardiovascular collapse.

Table 9.2 Regional ECG changes and associated territory of myocardial infarction (MI)

MI territory (area involved)	ECG leads showing ST↑	ECG leads showing reciprocal changes	Artery involved
Septal	V1–2	None	Left anterior descending (LAD)
Anterior (left ventricle)	V3–4	None	LAD
Anteroseptal (septum and left ventricle)	V1–4	None	LAD
Anterolateral (left ventricle)	I, aVL, V3–6	II, II, aVF	LAD or circumflex
Inferior (left ventricle and apex)	II, III, and aVF	I, aVL	Right coronary artery
Posterior (posterior wall of left ventricle)	V7–9	Tall R waves and ST↓ V1–3	Right coronary artery or circumflex
Right ventricular	II, III, aVF, V1, V4R	I, aVL	Right coronary artery

Other causes of ST-elevation

MIs are not the only cause of ST-segment elevation. Other causes of ST-segment elevation include:

- Pericarditis—the ST-elevation is widespread (not territorial) and concave upwards 'saddle-shaped'. There may also be PR depression.
- Myocarditis—the ST-elevation is widespread and not territorial. The history is usually of fever, myalgia, and dyspnoea.
- Early repolarization—usually seen in young, athletic men. The T-wave begins early resulting in ST-segments that are minimally elevated (<2 mm) and concave upwards. The T-waves are of large amplitude. There may be associated J waves (notching in the terminal QRS complex).
- Left ventricular hypertrophy—the initial up-sloping of the ST-segment is usually concave as opposed to the flat/convex ST-elevation in ACS. The ECG should also meet the diagnostic criteria for LVH (S wave in V1 + R wave in V5 or V6 >35 mm).
- Left ventricular aneurysm.
- Brugada syndrome—ST-elevation is limited to leads V1–3, the elevation is concave upwards.
- Electrolyte disturbances—hyper- and hypokalaemia may cause ST-elevation.
- Hypothermia—J waves (a 'hump-like' deflection between the QRS complex and early part of the ST-segment).
- CNS pathologies—subarachnoid haemorrhage, ischaemic stroke, head trauma, acute meningitis, intracranial tumours.
- Prinzmetal's angina—coronary vasospasm resulting in transient chest pain and ST-segment elevation.
- Cocaine and amphetamines—can cause coronary vasospasm and ST-elevation in the absence of atherosclerosis.
- Cardiac trauma—blunt and penetrating can cause ST-segment changes.
- Electrical cardiac injury—either post-defibrillation or accidental.

(a)

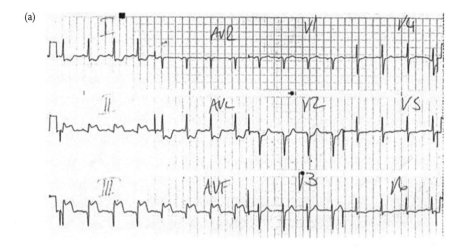

(b)

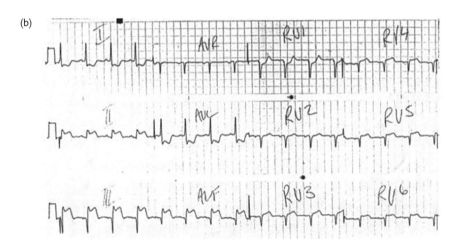

Figure 9.1 (a) Inferior ST-segment elevation myocardial infarction. (b) Inferior ST-segment elevation myocardial infarction with right ventricular involvement (note the right ventricular chest leads, with ST-segment elevation in lead RV4).

Reproduced from David A. Warrell, Timothy M. Cox, and John D. Firth, *Oxford Textbook of Medicine*, 2010, Figure 16.3.1.18, p. 2650, with permission from Oxford University Press.

9.2.2 Cardiac biomarkers

Cardiac biomarkers are proteins that are released into the cardiac interstitium due to the compromised integrity of myocyte cell membranes as a result of myocardial ischaemia.

Troponin I and T have the highest sensitivities and specificities for the diagnosis of acute MI compared to CK-MB, CK, and myoglobin. Troponin I and T peak 6 to 12 hours after the onset of an acute MI. The duration of detection of troponin I is 7–10 days and troponin T, 7–14 days. NICE recommend that blood samples for troponin I or T are taken on arrival at hospital and repeated 10–12 hours after the onset of symptoms. The use of high-sensitivity troponins has become useful in ruling out ACS protocol in low-risk patients. They involve baseline admission

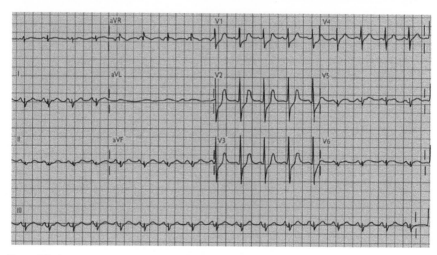

Figure 9.2 Acute posterior myocardial infarction: Note dominant R wave and ST-depression in V1-V3 (often seen with ST-elevation in V5/V6 reflecting posterolateral infarction).

Reproduced from Tim Raine, Katherine McGinn, James Dawson, Stephan Sanders, and Simon Eccles, *Oxford Handbook for the Foundation Programme*, 2011, Figure 17.9, p. 570, with permission from Oxford University Press.

high-sensitivity troponin and then a repeat level three hours later. The exact protocol depends on local guidelines, however a rise of less than 20% is not consistent with an ACS and greater than 20% confirms ACS.

NICE do not recommend the use of other biochemical markers in the assessment of patients with acute chest pain (e.g. natriuretic peptides, high-sensitivity C-reactive protein, or ischaemia-modified albumin).

Despite the high specificity for acute MI, troponin may rise in the absence of acute coronary disease. The following conditions may cause a troponin rise:

- Pulmonary embolism
- Aortic dissection
- Acute heart failure
- Peri/myocarditis
- Septic shock
- Post-angioplasty
- Post-electrical cardioversion
- Acute arrhythmias
- Renal failure
- Cardiac contusion

9.2.3 Other investigations in acute coronary syndrome

Further ED investigations should be directed at detecting risk factors for cardiovascular disease, possible triggers for ACS, and other diagnoses.

- Haemoglobin—anaemia may exacerbate stable angina.
- Creatinine—patients with impaired renal function may have a chronically raised troponin. Certain types of heparin are not recommended or require dose adjustment in renal impairment.
- Glucose—patients may be diabetic and require treatment of hyperglycaemia.

- Lipids—will aid secondary prevention of cardiovascular disease but will not alter ED management.
- CXR—may detect evidence of complications such as pulmonary oedema, or other diagnoses such as pneumonia or pneumothorax.
- Echocardiography—is useful if the diagnosis is equivocal looking for evidence of regional wall abnormalities.

KEY POINTS

The Royal College of Emergency Medicine clinical standards for MI include a 12-lead ECG performed within 10 min of a patient's arrival.

A normal ECG is not sensitive enough to exclude ACS.

The ECG criteria for thrombolysis or referral for primary PCI (in the presence of chest pain starting <12 h ago) are:

- New onset LBBB.
- 2 mm ST-segment elevation in two contiguous chest leads.
- 1 mm ST-segment elevation in two contiguous limb leads.

Additional ECG leads (posterior and/or right-sided) should be considered in patients with an inferior MI or patients who develop hypotension and have symptoms of a MI but a non-diagnostic 12-lead ECG.

Prior to diagnosing a STEMI always consider the history and other possible causes of ST-segment elevation.

Troponin is the most useful blood test in the investigation of patients with suspected ACS.

High-sensitivity troponins are useful in rule out pathways for low-risk individuals.

Troponin may rise in the absence of acute coronary disease. Always interpret the troponin result in the context of the clinical picture.

9.3 Management of acute coronary syndrome

The following is based on the guidance from NICE: Clinical Guideline 94—Unstable angina and NSTEMI; and Clinical Guideline 95—Chest pain of recent onset (see Further reading).

The management of STEMIs is discussed in section 9.4.

9.3.1 Generic management of suspected acute coronary syndrome

Patients presenting with acute chest pain suggestive of ACS should be assessed and treated in an ABCDE manner.

Oxygen should not be routinely administered but saturations should be checked. Supplemental oxygen should be administered to:

- patients with oxygen saturations <94% who are not at risk of hypercapnic respiratory failure, aiming for saturations of 94–98%;
- patients with COPD, who are at risk of hypercapnic respiratory failure, to achieve saturations of 88–92%, pending blood gas analysis.

Pain relief should be offered as soon as possible, using GTN (sublingual or buccal) and/or intravenous opiates.

A single loading dose of aspirin 300 mg should be given unless the patient is allergic to it.

9.3.2 Management of confirmed acute coronary syndrome

As soon as a diagnosis of unstable angina or NSTEMI (ECG changes and/or troponin rise) is made, the following treatment is recommended:

- Aspirin 300 mg unless contraindicated or already given (if aspirin is contraindicated due to hypersensitivity, clopidogrel can be given).
- Anti-thrombin therapy—the recommended low molecular weight heparin (LMWH), for patients without a high bleeding risk, is fondaparinux. If the patient has a high bleeding risk (advancing age, renal impairment—creatinine >265 mmol/L, known bleeding complication, low body weight), unfractionated heparin is an alternative. If patients are due to have angiography within 24 hours, then unfractionated heparin is recommended.

Patient should then be formally assessed for the risk of future adverse cardiovascular events using a risk scoring system that predicts six-month mortality.

9.3.3 Risk scoring in ACS

Risk scoring of patients with ACS is important to select the most appropriate treatment strategy. Antithrombotic and antiplatelet agents reduce the rate of adverse cardiovascular events but carry the risk of bleeding complications. The risk assessment is used to guide clinical management and balance the benefit of treatments against any possible adverse events.

The risk scoring system recommended by NICE is the Global Registry of Acute Cardiac Events (GRACE) which predicts six-month mortality.

The GRACE risk score was derived from the large GRACE registry of patients with ACS to predict death and death or MI, both in hospital and at six months. The GRACE scoring system uses eight variables to derive a score:

- Age.
- Killip class: (1) no evidence of heart failure; (2) mild to moderate heart failure (third heart sound, rales <1/3 up lung fields, raised JVP); (3) overt pulmonary oedema; (4) cardiogenic shock.
- Heart rate.
- Systolic blood pressure.
- Serum creatinine.
- ST-segment deviation.
- Cardiac arrest at admission.
- Elevated serum cardiac enzymes.*

In order to calculate the score (predicted six-month mortality), computer software or a nomogram is required (Table 9.3).

Other risk scores exist and NICE acknowledge that none is clearly superior. TIMI (thrombolysis in myocardial infarction) is a scoring system that is commonly used to risk stratify patients with ACS in the ED. However, the NICE guidance comments that GRACE discriminates better for mortality than TIMI.

The TIMI score has the advantage of being simpler to calculate because each variable carries the same prognostic weight and calculation of the score is a simple arithmetic sum. The TIMI score has appeared in previous SAQs.

* Reprinted from *American Heart Journal*, Volume 141, issue 2, The GRACE Investigators*, Rationale and design of the GRACE (Global Registry of Acute Coronary Events) Project: A multinational registry of patients hospitalized with acute coronary syndromes, pp.190-199, Copyright 2001, with permission from Elsevier.

Table 9.3 Risk of future adverse cardiovascular events based on predicated six-month mortality

Predicted 6-month mortality	Risk of future adverse cardiovascular events
≤1.5%	Lowest
>1.5 to 3%	Low
>3 to 6%	Intermediate
>6 to 9%	High
>9%	Highest

Date from Granger CB, Goldberg RJ, Dabbous O, et al. 'Predictors of hospital mortality in the Global Registry of Acute Coronary Events'. Arch Intern Med. 2003; 163(19):2345–2353.

Previous MRCEM question

EXAM TIP

Risk scoring is an important part of the management of ACS and has appeared in previous SAQs.

NICE recommends the GRACE risk score. GRACE comprises eight variables and requires computer software to calculate the score. It is better at discriminating for mortality at six months than the TIMI score.

TIMI has been widely used in UK EDs. It comprises seven equally weighted variables and is calculated as a simple arithmetic sum.

9.3.4 Ongoing management of acute coronary syndrome

The risk score is used to determine further antiplatelet and antithrombotic therapy, and the timing of coronary intervention.

Antiplatelets

Circulating blood platelets are involved early in the development of thrombus formation. They are stimulated by exposure to atheromatous material rich in lipid and collagen when the intimal lining of a plaque ruptures. The platelets aggregate, release vasoactive substances from their granules, and encourage the development of a blood clot rich in fibrin and red blood cells. Antiplatelet drugs can interfere with these pathways and therefore influence the pathophysiological mechanisms underlying ACS (Table 9.4).

Antithrombin therapy

Unfractionated heparin inhibits the conversion of fibrinogen to fibrin and therefore reduces the likelihood of thrombus formation. LMWH inhibit the coagulation system in a similar way and also binds Factor Xa.

The risk of bleeding with anticoagulants is higher in the following groups:

- Elderly
- Low body weight (<50 kg)
- Impaired renal function (creatinine >265 mmol/L)
- Known bleeding complications

Table 9.4 Antiplatelet agents used in the management of acute coronary syndrome (ACS)

Antiplatelet agent and mechanism of action	Indications	Long-term use
Aspirin Blocks cyclooxygenase, an enzyme involved in the pathway of prostaglandin and thromboxane synthesis, agents which are highly vasoactive and prothrombotic. Platelets do not synthesize new cyclooxygenase once exposed to aspirin and so effects persists for the life of each inhibited platelet.	Aspirin 300 mg should be offered to all patients with suspected ACS, unless there is clear evidence that they are allergic to it.	Aspirin should be continued indefinitely unless contraindicated by bleeding risk or hypersensitivity.
Clopidogrel Antiplatelet agent and part of the thienopyridine group that block platelets by inhibition of the adenosine diphosphate (ADP) pathway.	Patients with ACS and a predicted 6-month mortality >1.5% and no contraindications should be given 300 mg clopidogrel.	This should be continued for 12 months at a standard dose (e.g. 75 mg).
Ticagrelor Oral antagonist of P2Y12 ADP receptor, inhibiting platelet aggregation and thrombus formation.	Recommended by NICE for patients with STEMI or NSTEMI and high-risk features. Superior alternative to clopidogrel.	Used as dual therapy with aspirin. Loading dose of 180 mg followed by 90 mg BD for 12 months.
Glycoprotein IIb/IIIa inhibitors Glycoprotein IIb/IIIa antibodies and receptor antagonists inhibit the final common pathway of platelet aggregation. NB The potential reduction in a patient's ischaemic risk must be balanced with any increased risk of bleeding.	Consider eptifibatide or tirofiban for patients at intermediate or higher risk (>3%) if angiography is scheduled within 96 h of admission. Consider abciximab as an adjunct to PCI for patients at intermediate or higher risk (>3%) who are not already receiving a glycoprotein IIb/IIIa inhibitor.	Not used for long-term therapy.

NICE recommendations for heparin, in patients with confirmed ACS, are:

- Offer fondaparinux to all patients who do not have a high bleeding risk, unless coronary angiography is planned within 24 hours of admission.
- Offer unfractionated heparin as an alternative to fondaparinux to patients who are likely to undergo coronary angiography within 24 hours of admission.
- Consider unfractionated heparin, with dose adjustment guided by monitoring of clotting function, as an alternative to fondaparinux for patients with a significant bleeding risk.

Coronary intervention

Coronary angiography (with follow on PCI, if indicated) should be offered to patients with intermediate or higher risk (>3%) within 96 hours of admission.

Angiography should be performed as soon as possible for patients who are clinically unstable or at high ischaemic risk.

Other medical therapies

Nitrates provide symptomatic benefits to patients with ischaemic chest pain via systemic and coronary vasodilatation. In the United Kingdom they are usually given to patients who have ongoing ischaemic chest pain despite initial therapy.

α-blockers reduce myocardial oxygen demand by reducing cardiac contractility and rate. They are recommended in NSTEMI patients in the absence of contraindications (e.g. acute heart failure, hypotension, bradycardia, and so on). The most commonly used agents are atenolol or metoprolol, which may be given orally or intravenously.

KEY POINTS

All patients with confirmed ACS (unstable angina or NSTEMI) should be formally assessed for the risk of future adverse cardiovascular events using a risk scoring system that predicts six-month mortality (e.g. GRACE).

ED ACS management includes:

- Aspirin 300 mg to all patients unless contraindicated.
- LMWH (fondaparinux) to all patients unless the patient has a high bleeding risk or is undergoing PCI within 24 h (in which case use unfractionated heparin).
- Clopidogrel 300 mg to patients with a six-month mortality risk >1.5%.
- Ticagrelor 180 mg to patients with STEMI or NSTEMI.
- Consider glycoprotein IIb/IIIa inhibitors for patients with a six-month mortality risk >3% and undergoing PCI within 96 h.
- Intravenous opiates for pain.
- Sublingual or intravenous nitrates for ischaemic pain.
- α-blockers.
- Oxygen if indicated (use BTS Emergency Oxygen Guidelines see Chapter 10, section 10.7).

9.4 Management of STEMI/new LBBB

The following is based on guidance by the European Society of Cardiology (see Further reading). Generic management of STEMI/new LBBB:

- Analgesia—nitrates (sublingual or intravenous) and/or opiates.
- Oxygen—titrated to saturations (as per BTS Emergency Oxygen Guidance).
- Antiplatelets—aspirin 300 mg and clopidogrel 300 mg, or ticagrelor 180 mg.
- Antithrombin therapy—the agent recommended depends on the subsequent reperfusion therapy. If primary PCI is performed, bivalirudin or unfractionated heparin is recommended. If thrombolysis is used, enoxaparin or unfractionated heparin is recommended.

EXAM TIP

The Royal College of Emergency Medicine publish clinical standards for EDs, produced by the Clinical Effectiveness Committee. Myocardial infarction is included in those standards. The standards for reperfusion therapy are:

- Door to ECG 10 min (90%)
- Door to needle 30 min (75%)

- Call to needle 60 min (75%)
- Aspirin given 90% (if not contraindicated)

Knowledge of these standards could appear in a SAQ.

9.4.1 Reperfusion therapy

Early reperfusion of the occluded artery is the mainstay of treatment in STEMI/new LBBB. Reperfusion may be achieved by primary PCI or thrombolytic therapy.

Indications for reperfusion therapy:

- All patients with chest pain or discomfort of <12 hours duration and with persistent ST-segment elevation or (presumed) new LBBB.
- Consider in patients with clinical and/or ECG evidence of ongoing ischaemia even if symptoms started >12 hours before.

Primary percutaneous coronary intervention

Primary PCI with stenting, when performed by an experienced team within the recommended time, is the best reperfusion treatment to save lives.

Primary PCI should be performed within two hours of ECG diagnosis (first medical contact) in all patients. In patients presenting within two hours of pain onset and with a large infarct, the target is within 90 minutes.

If thrombolysis is contraindicated or the patient has cardiogenic shock primary PCI is indicated regardless of the time delay.

Thrombolytic therapy

If primary PCI cannot be performed within the recommended time (<2 hours from first medical contact), thrombolytic therapy should be started as soon as possible.

Thrombolytic agents currently used are tissue plasminogen activators (alteplase, reteplase, and tenecteplase) or streptokinase. They are given with heparin, either unfractionated or low molecular weight (enoxaparin), depending on local policy.

Prior to thrombolytic therapy, patients must be informed of the risks and benefits of treatment and give their consent. Approximately 30 early deaths are prevented per 1000 patients treated with thrombolysis. However, thrombolytic therapy is associated with a small but significant excess risk of stroke. The strokes are largely attributable to cerebral haemorrhage occurring in approximately 1% of patients. Major non-cerebral bleeds (bleeding which is life-threatening or requires transfusion) can occur in 4–13% of patients treated. The risk of complications is higher in the elderly, those with a low body weight, hypertension, prior cerebrovascular disease, and women.

There are relative and absolute contraindications to thrombolysis (Table 9.5). These have appeared in previous SAQ papers.

Previous MRCEM question

After successful thrombolysis, patients should be transferred to a hospital capable of PCI for coronary angiography (ideally 3–24 hours after thrombolytic therapy).

Rescue percutaneous coronary intervention

Rescue PCI is defined as PCI performed on a coronary artery which remains occluded despite thrombolytic therapy.

Identifying failed thrombolysis non-invasively is a challenge but <50% ST-segment resolution in the lead(s) with the highest ST-segment elevations 60–90 minutes after the start of thrombolytic therapy can be used as a surrogate.

Table 9.5 Contraindications to thrombolysis

Absolute contraindication	Relative contraindication
Haemorrhagic stroke or stroke of unknown origin at any time	Transient ischaemic attack in preceding six months
Ischaemic stroke in preceding 6 months	Oral anticoagulant therapy
CNS trauma or neoplasm	Pregnancy or within one week post-partum
Recent major trauma/surgery/head injury (within preceding three weeks)	Refractory hypertension (systolic BP >180 mmHg or diastolic BP>110 mmHg)
GI bleeding within last three months	Advanced liver disease
Known bleeding disorder	Infective endocarditis
Aortic dissection	Active peptic ulcer disease
Non-compressible puncture (e.g. liver biopsy, lumber puncture)	Refractory resuscitation

9.4.2 Complications of STEMI

Many of the early complications of STEMI can be treated or prevented by early reperfusion (Table 9.6).

KEY POINTS

Early reperfusion therapy is the mainstay of treatment in STEMI.

Primary PCI when performed within the recommended time is the best reperfusion therapy.

Primary PCI should be performed within 2 h after ECG diagnosis (and within 90 min in those presenting within 2 h of the onset of pain and with a large infarct).

If primary PCI cannot be performed within 2 h of diagnosis then thrombolysis should be started as soon as possible.

Thrombolysis is given with heparin (unfractionated or enoxaparin depending on local policy).

Irrespective of the reperfusion therapy used patients should receive aspirin, clopidogrel/ticagralor, oxygen (if required), opiates, nitrates, and β-blockers (once stable).

9.5 Atrial fibrillation

9.5.1 Introduction

Atrial fibrillation (AF) is an atrial tachycardia characterized by predominantly uncoordinated atrial activation with consequent deterioration of atrial mechanical function. On the ECG there are absent P waves, which are replaced by rapid fibrillatory waves that vary in size, shape, and timing. The ventricular response is usually irregular and depends on many things including: AV nodal properties; the level of vagal and sympathetic tone; and drugs that affect AV nodal conduction such as β-blockers, calcium-channel blockers, and digoxin.

AF is the commonest sustained cardiac arrhythmia. The prevalence of AF approximately doubles with each advancing decade of age, from 0.5% at age 50–59 years to almost 9% at age 80–89 years.

The adverse effects of AF are the result of haemodynamic changes related to the rapid and/or irregular heart rhythm, and the thromboembolic complications related to the prothrombotic state associated with the arrhythmia. Onset of AF can result in a reduction in cardiac output of

Table 9.6 Complications of STEMI

Complication	Management
Pulmonary oedema	Reperfusion therapy.
	Diuretics, nitrates, non-invasive ventilation.
Cardiogenic shock	Reperfusion therapy (primary PCI is superior to thrombolysis in this group).
	Inotropes and/or intra-aortic balloon pump.
Right ventricular failure	Reperfusion therapy.
	Maintenance of preload with IV fluids and avoidance of vasodilators (e.g. opiates, diuretics, and nitrates) which may cause cardiovascular collapse.
	Inotropes may be required.
Mitral regurgitation	Echocardiography to confirm the diagnosis.
(due to chordal rupture, papillary muscle rupture, or dilatation of the mitral valve)	Urgent surgery.
Ventricular septal rupture	Echocardiography to confirm the diagnosis.
	Urgent surgery.
Cardiac rupture and tamponade	Echocardiography to confirm the diagnosis
	Emergency pericardiocentesis may temporarily improve haemodynamic status.
	Urgent surgery.
Ventricular arrhythmias	VF/pulseless VT should be managed with defibrillation as per ALS guidance.
	Pulsed VT should be treated with electrical cardioversion if compromised and amiodarone if not.
	Accelerated idioventricular rhythm may occur during reperfusion and does not require treatment, resolving spontaneously.
Supraventricular arrhythmias	AF is the commonest supraventricular arrhythmia post-MI. It may self-terminate or require treatment as per the AF guidelines in this chapter (section 9.5).
Conduction defects	1st degree heart block requires no intervention.
	2nd degree heart block (Mobitz type 1 or Wenckebach) is usually self-limiting in inferior MIs but has a poorer prognosis in anterior MIs and may require pacing.
	2nd degree (Mobitz type 2) and 3rd degree heart block require pacing.

up to 10–20%, regardless of ventricular rate. The presence of fast ventricular rates can push an already compromised ventricle into heart failure. An uncontrolled AF rate may precipitate critical cardiac ischaemia. The prothrombotic state predisposes to stroke and thromboembolism, with an approximately fivefold greater risk than in people without AF.

NICE have produced guidance on the management of AF (see Further reading) and the recommendations here are based on that guideline.

9.5.2 Classification of atrial fibrillation

NICE classify AF based on the temporal pattern of the arrhythmia. This classification is used to guide the different treatment options:

- Initial event—first detected episode, which may or may not recur.
- Recurrent—when a patient experiences two or more episodes.
- Paroxysmal—episodes terminate spontaneously, defined by consensus as within seven days.
- Persistent—episodes require electrical or pharmacological cardioversion for termination.
- Permanent—episodes that are not successfully terminated by cardioversion, or when cardioversion is not pursued.

9.5.3 Causes and risk factors of atrial fibrillation

There are many risk factors for AF including:

- Increasing age
- Diabetes
- Hypertension
- Valvular heart disease

AF is often caused by co-existing medical conditions which can be cardiac or non-cardiac (Table 9.7).

9.5.4 Clinical features of atrial fibrillation

AF can present in a multitude of ways:

- Asymptomatically—incidental finding on a pulse check or ECG
- Non-specifically—breathlessness, dyspnoea, palpitations, syncope/dizziness, or chest discomfort
- With complications—stroke, thromboembolism, or heart failure

9.5.5 Investigations in atrial fibrillation

- ECG—should be performed in all patients (whether symptomatic or not) in whom AF is suspected.
- Echocardiography—is rarely performed in patients presenting acutely to the ED with AF. It is useful for ongoing management in certain patient groups: young patients requiring a baseline

Table 9.7 Causes of atrial fibrillation (AF)

Cardiac causes of AF	Non-cardiac causes of AF
Common: • Ischaemic heart disease • Rheumatic heart disease • Hypertension • Sick sinus syndrome • Pre-excited syndromes (e.g. WPW) Less common: • Cardiomyopathy • Pericardial disease • Atrial septal defect • Atrial myxoma	• Acute infections, especially pneumonia • Electrolyte abnormalities • Lung carcinoma • Other intrathoracic pathology (e.g. pleural effusion) • Pulmonary embolism • Thyrotoxicosis • Post-surgery (especially cardiac) • Excessive alcohol or caffeine

echocardiogram; patients having an elective rhythm control strategy; patients with suspected structural heart disease.

- Other investigations—should be directed according to the likely cause (e.g. thyroid function tests, electrolytes, CXR, septic screen, and so on).

9.5.6 Management of haemodynamically unstable atrial fibrillation

Most patients in AF present without haemodynamic compromise. However, a small group of patients are significantly compromised by the onset of AF. There are also those patients with permanent AF who have haemodynamic instability caused by a poorly controlled ventricular response rate.

NICE define non-life-threatening haemodynamic instability, caused by AF, as:

- Ventricular rate >150 bpm
- Ongoing chest pain
- Critical perfusion

In patients with non-life-threatening haemodynamic instability, due to AF, the treatment depends on whether the AF is thought to be permanent or not:

- AF not permanent—electrical cardioversion should be performed. Where there is a delay in organizing electrical cardioversion, intravenous amiodarone should be used.
- AF permanent—pharmacological rate control strategy should be used. Treatment should be with intravenous β-blockers or rate-limiting calcium antagonists. If these are contraindicated, amiodarone should be used.
- AF in WPW—flecainide may be used as an alternative for attempting pharmacological cardioversion. AV node-blocking agents (e.g. diltiazem, verapamil, or digoxin) should not be used.

Management of AF must include treatment of the underlying cause (e.g. electrolyte abnormalities, thyrotoxicosis), otherwise attempts at cardioversion are unlikely to be successful.

A very small proportion of patients may have a life-threatening deterioration in haemodynamic stability following the onset of AF. The recommended treatment for such patients is emergency electrical cardioversion, irrespective of the duration of the AF. (NB NICE do not define what a life-threatening deterioration in haemodynamic stability is.)

9.5.7 Treatment of persistent atrial fibrillation

The majority of patients attending the ED in AF do not have haemodynamic instability and for these patients there are two main treatment strategies:

- Rate control—use of chronotropic drugs to reduce the ventricular response rate.
- Rhythm control—use of electrical or pharmacological cardioversion to restore sinus rhythm.

NICE have given guidance on the most appropriate treatment strategy for certain groups of patients with persistent AF. NICE recommend that all patients should initially be rate controlled unless:

- AF is thought to be reversible
- Presence of heart failure thought to be caused by AF
- New onset AF
- Atrial flutter thought to benefit from ablation
- Rhythm strategy thought to be more suitable based on clinical judgement

Rate control

- The aims of rate control are to minimize symptoms associated with excessive heart rates and prevent tachycardia-associated cardiomyopathy. Rate control is used in those with permanent AF and those with persistent AF, where a rate control treatment strategy has been chosen.
- The recommended agents for rate control are β-blockers or rate-limiting calcium antagonists. Digoxin is only recommended in predominantly sedentary patients or in addition to β-blockers or calcium antagonists where monotherapy is inadequate.
- Amiodarone is not recommended for long-term rate control.

Rhythm control

Rhythm control may be achieved via electrical or pharmacological cardioversion. It should be considered in patients who remain symptomatic despite rate control, or where a rate control strategy has been unsuccessful. In patients without haemodynamic compromise, this can be performed electively. NICE recommend that a transthoracic echocardiogram is performed prior to elective cardioversion.

Where AF onset is within 48 hours, the patient should be anticoagulated with heparin (either unfractionated heparin or LMWH) and cardioverted electrically or pharmacologically. If pharmacological cardioversion is performed, IV amiodarone is the drug of choice in those with structural heart disease, and flecainide in those without structural heart disease. Intravenous magnesium or calcium is not recommended for pharmacological cardioversion.

Where AF onset is greater than 48 hours the treatment of choice is electrical cardioversion. To reduce the risk of stroke and thromboembolism, the patient should have a transoesophageal echocardiogram or therapeutic anticoagulation with warfarin for three weeks prior to the intervention.

Factors which make a patient unsuitable for cardioversion:

- Contraindication to anticoagulation
- Structural heart disease that precludes long-term maintenance of sinus rhythm
- Long duration of AF (>12 months)
- History of multiple failed attempts/relapses
- Ongoing reversible cause (e.g. thyrotoxicosis)

9.5.8 Treatment of paroxysmal AF

The three main aims of treatment for paroxysmal AF are:

- To suppress paroxysms of AF and maintain long-term sinus rhythm
- To control heart rate during paroxysms of AF if they occur
- To prevent complications associated with paroxysmal AF (e.g. stroke, tachycardia induced cardiomyopathy)

The long-term management of paroxysmal AF is usually directed by a cardiologist and therefore unlikely to appear in a FRCEM SAQ. The main treatment options are:

- A 'no-drug treatment' strategy
- A 'pill-in-the-pocket' strategy (e.g. flecainide, propafenone)
- Long-term prophylaxis (e.g. β-blocker)

9.5.9 Thromboprophylaxis in atrial fibrillation

All patients with AF should be risk stratified for stroke and thromboprophylaxis considered.

Stroke risk stratification in atrial fibrillation

NICE recommends using the CHA2DS2VASc stroke risk score (Table 9. 8) to assess the risk of stroke in the following individuals:

Table 9.8 CHA2DS2VASc Stroke risk score

Risk factor		Score
Age	<65 years	0
	66–74 years	1
	>75 years	2
Sex	Female	0
	Male	1
CCF History	Yes	1
Hypertension history	Yes	1
Diabetes	Yes	1
TIA/stroke/thromboembolism history	Yes	2
Vascular disease history	Yes	1

- Symptomatic or asymptomatic paroxysmal, persistent, or permanent atrial fibrillation
- Atrial flutter
- Continuing risk of arrhythmia in individuals in sinus rhythm post cardioversion
- Low risk—CHA2DS2VASc Score 0 (or 1 in women): anticoagulation not required
- Moderate risk—CHA2DS2VASc Score 1 in men: consider anticoagulation based on bleeding risk
- High risk—CHA2DS2VASc Score 2: recommends offering anticoagulation based on bleeding risk

Anticoagulation can be with either rivaroxaban; apixaban; dabigatran; or vitamin K antagonists such as warfarin.

Thromboprophylaxis and acute atrial fibrillation

In cases of acute AF, where the patient is haemodynamically unstable, any emergency intervention should be performed as soon as possible and the initiation of anticoagulation should not delay this.

In patients with acute AF, who are receiving no or subtherapeutic anticoagulation therapy, heparin (unfractionated or LMWH) should be started at the initial presentation. Heparin should be continued until a full assessment has been made and appropriate antithrombotic therapy has been started, based on the risk stratification.

Patients with AF of less than 48 hours duration, who are successfully cardioverted to sinus rhythm, do not require further anticoagulation.

Thromboprophylaxis and persistent atrial fibrillation

Patients undergoing elective cardioversion for persistent AF, longer than 48 hours, should be maintained on therapeutic anticoagulation with warfarin for a minimum of three weeks.

Following successful cardioversion, patients should remain on therapeutic anticoagulation with warfarin for a minimum of four weeks.

Anticoagulation should be continued long-term in patients with a high risk of AF recurrence or where it is recommended by the stroke risk stratification algorithm.

Factors leading to a high risk of AF recurrence include:

- History of AF >12 months
- Mitral valve disease
- LV dysfunction

Table **9.9** HAS-BLED major bleeding risk assessment

Risk Factor	Score
Hypertension (SBP > 160)	1
Renal disease (dialysis, transplant, creatinine >200 ummol)	1
Liver disease (cirrhosis, Bil.) > 2× normal, Alt/Ast/Alp >3× normal	1
Stroke	1
Prior major bleeding or predisposition to bleeding	1
Labile INR	1
Age >65 years	1
Medication predisposing bleeding (NSAIDs/antiplatelets)	1
Alcohol or drug use (>8 drinks/week)	1

- Enlarged left atrium
- History of AF recurrence

Thromboprophylaxis and permanent atrial fibrillation

Decisions about long-term anticoagulation therapy in permanent AF should be based on a risk-benefit assessment of prevention of stroke versus risk of bleeding.

NICE recommends the use of HAS-BLED score (estimation of risk of major bleeding in patients anticoagulated for atrial fibrillation) (Table 9.9) and offering modification and monitoring to individuals with the following risk factors:

- Concomitant use of antiplatelet drugs (e.g. aspirin or clopidogrel) or NSAIDs
- Uncontrolled hypertension
- Labile INR
- Heavy alcohol consumption

NB Risk of falls is not a sole indication for withholding anticoagulation.

Thromboprophylaxis and paroxysmal atrial fibrillation

The need for anticoagulation therapy in patients with paroxysmal AF should not be based on the frequency or duration of paroxysms but on appropriate risk stratification as for permanent AF.

KEY POINTS

AF is the commonest sustained cardiac arrhythmia.

NICE define non-life-threatening haemodynamic instability, caused by AF, as:

- Ventricular rate >150 bpm
- Ongoing chest pain
- Critical perfusion

A life-threatening deterioration in haemodynamic stability secondary to AF should be treated with emergency electrical cardioversion, irrespective of the duration of the AF.

In patients with haemodynamic instability, which is not life-threatening, the management of AF is determined by whether it is thought to be permanent or not:

- AF not permanent—electrical cardioversion
- AF permanent—pharmacological rate control strategy (β-blocker, calcium-channel antagonist, or amiodarone)

In haemodynamically stable patients with persistent AF, the decision between rate versus rhythm control is based on the following factors:

Rate control is achieved with β-blockers or rate-limiting calcium antagonists.

Rhythm control is achieved with elective cardioversion:

- Less than 48 h—electrically or pharmacologically, with heparin anticoagulation.
- More than 48 h—electrically after a TOE or three weeks therapeutic anticoagulation with warfarin.

All patients with AF should be risk stratified for stroke and thromboprophylaxis considered.

9.6 Arrhythmias

Arrhythmia management is a complex subject that lots of candidates find difficult. The most important arrhythmias to understand for the exam are the peri-arrest arrhythmias. Peri-arrest arrhythmia management is covered in Chapter 2, sections 2.5–2.7.

Arrhythmias that may cause sudden cardiac death are discussed in section 9.8.

This section focuses on the causes and types of arrhythmias.

9.6.1 Causes of arrhythmias

There are many causes of arrhythmias, which can be broadly grouped into the following categories:

- Cardiac disease (e.g. post-cardiac arrest, acute coronary disease, valvular heart disease, cardiomyopathy, accessory pathways, long QT syndrome)
- Drugs, for example antiarrhythmics (e.g. amiodarone, digoxin, β-blockers, and so on), tricyclic antidepressants, sympathomimetics (adrenaline, noradrenaline, dopamine), recreational drugs (e.g. cocaine, amphetamines)
- Metabolic, for example electrolyte abnormalities (hyper- or hypokalaemia, calcaemia or magnesaemia), hypoglycaemia
- Systemic illness (e.g. sepsis, anaemia, hypoxia, hypo- or hyperthyroidism, hypo- or hyperthermia)

9.6.2 Categories of arrhythmias

Arrhythmias can be categorized in various ways, including: stable or unstable; tachycardias or bradycardias; regular or irregular. Arrhythmias can also be categorized according to the site of origin. Tables 9.10 and 9.11 categorize arrhythmias according to their site of origin and the typical ECG features (see also Figures 9.3 and 9.4).

Tachyarrhythmias

Bradyarrhythmias

9.6.3 Arrhythmia management

It is not necessary to know all the different treatment options for the multitude of arrhythmias that may present to the ED. ED management should focus on peri-arrest arrhythmia identification and treatment (Chapter 2, sections 2.5–2.7); the identification of arrhythmias that require urgent inpatient management (e.g. haemodynamically unstable AF, Mobitz type II block, and so on); and those that may lead to serious complications (e.g. Brugada syndrome—section 9.8).

Table 9.10 Classification of tachyarrhythmias

Site of origin	Nature of arrhythmia	ECG findings
Atria	Premature atrial complexes	An early P wave is seen on the ECG, which is misshapen. The following QRST is normal.
	Multifocal atrial tachycardia	Three or more P waves of varying morphology and varying P–R intervals. The electrical impulse is generated at different focuses within the atria.
	Atrial flutter	'Saw-tooth' appearance. The ventricular rate depends upon the type of block (e.g. 2:1, 3:1, variable). It is due to a re-entry circuit within the atria.
	Atrial fibrillation	Absent P waves, with disorganized atrial activity in their place, and irregular R–R intervals.
AV node	AV nodal re-entry tachycardia (AVNRT)	Regular narrow complex tachycardia. Due to a re-entry circuit within or near the AV node (see Chapter 2, section 2.6).
	Junctional ectopic tachycardia	Rare tachycardia caused by increased automaticity of the AV node (often drug induced). The P waves have an abnormal morphology and may fall anywhere in relation to a regular, narrow QRS complex.
Atrio-ventricular	AV re-entry tachycardia (re-entry circuit crosses between the atria and ventricles other than at the AV node)	Wolff–Parkinson–White syndrome—short PR interval and delta wave (slurred upstroke in QRS complex; see Chapter 2, Figure 2.6). Lown–Ganong–Levine syndrome—short PR interval with a normal QRS complex (no delta wave).
Ventricular	Premature ventricular contractions (PVCs)	Ventricular bigeminy—PVC that occurs after every normal beat. Ventricular trigeminy—a PVC occurring after every two normal beats. Ventricular tachycardia—runs of three or more PVCs.
	Accelerated idioventricular rhythm	Similar morphology to VT but has a slower rate (<120 bpm). The depolarization rate of the ventricles exceeds that of the SA and AV nodes. Usually seen during reperfusion.
	Monomorphic VT	Each beat looks the same because they are generated from the same point in the ventricles. Usually due to an area of myocardial scarring. (see Chapter 2, Table 2.7)
	Polymorphic VT	Beat-to-beat variation in morphology. Usually due to an abnormality of ventricular repolarization.

KEY POINTS

Arrhythmia management is a complex subject. The most important arrhythmias to understand for the exam are the peri-arrest arrhythmias.

There are many causes of arrhythmias, which can be broadly grouped into the following categories: cardiac, drugs, metabolic, systemic illness.

Table 9.11 Classification of bradyarrhythmias

Site of origin	Nature of arrhythmia	ECG findings
SA node	Sick sinus syndrome	Due to ischaemia or fibrosis/degeneration of the SA node.
		Resulting in sinus pauses (>2 s) or sinus arrest. Junctional or other escape rhythms (e.g. AF) may emerge, often known as 'tachy-brady' syndrome. Patients ultimately need a pacemaker to manage the bradyarrhythmias and medical therapy (e.g. β-blockers) to manage the tachyarrhythmias.
AV node	1st degree heart block	Delayed conduction between the atria and ventricles resulting in a prolonged PR interval (>0.2 s).
	2nd degree heart block	Only a proportion of the P waves are conducted to the ventricles. There are two main types: • Mobitz type I (Wenkebach)—the PR interval gets progressively longer until a P wave fails to conduct. • Mobitz type II—constant PR but occasionally a P wave fails to conduct. This may be in a regular pattern (e.g. 2:1 or 3:1 block) or irregular.
	3rd degree heart block (complete heart block)	Atrial activity is not conducted to the ventricles. The atria and ventricles work independently of each other (P waves and QRS complexes are not related to each other).
		The rate and breadth of the QRS complexes depends upon the level of the block. With a proximal block (e.g. at the AV node) the escape rhythm will arise from the AV node or bundle of His resulting in a narrower QRS complex and a rate of approximately 50 bpm. With a more distal block, the escape rhythm will produce broader QRS complexes at a slower rate (approximately 30 bpm).
	Junctional rhythm	The AV node takes over as the pacemaker (due to SA or AV block). The rate is approximately 40–60 bpm. The atria may still contract prior to the ventricles due to retrograde conduction. The ECG usually shows an absent or inverted P wave which may appear before or after the QRS.

9.7 Transient loss of consciousness

9.7.1 Introduction

Transient loss of consciousness (TLoC) is a sudden, spontaneous, complete loss of consciousness with rapid recovery. TLoC is not a diagnosis but a symptom with a number of potential causes.

NICE clinical guideline 109—transient loss of consciousness was published in August 2010. The following section includes recommendations based on that guideline (see Further reading).

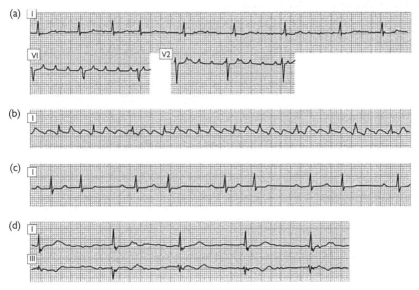

Figure 9.3 Atrial tachycardia (a), atrial flutter (b), and frequent atrial premature beats (c) that may mimic the irregular RR intervals typical for atrial fibrillation. Note first-degree atrioventricular block in (c). Atrial fibrillation may coexist with complete heart block, particularly, in elderly, and result in a regular slow rhythm (d).

Reproduced from A. John Camm, Thomas F. Lüscher, and Patrick W. Serruys, *The ESC Textbook of Cardiovascular Medicine*, 2009, Figure 28.15, p. 1037, with permission from Oxford University Press.

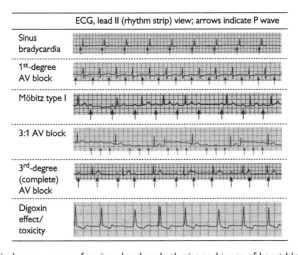

Figure 9.4 Typical appearances of various bradyarrhythmias and types of heart block.

Reproduced from Tim Raine, Katherine McGinn, James Dawson, Stephan Sanders, and Simon Eccles, *Oxford Handbook for the Foundation Programme*, 2011, Figure 7.7, p. 251, with permission from Oxford University Press.

9.7.2 Pathophysiology of transient loss of consciousness

The NICE guidance divides TLoC into three main causes:

- Syncope—due to dysfunction of the cardiovascular system (Table 9.12)
- Epilepsy—due to dysfunction of the nervous system (see Chapter 11, section 11.5)
- Psychogenic seizures—due to dysfunction of the psyche

The underlying pathophysiology of syncope is transient global cerebral hypoperfusion caused by hypotension secondary to low cardiac output or low peripheral vascular resistance.

9.7.3 Clinical features in transient loss of consciousness

Gaining an accurate history of events is vital in the assessment of a patient who has had a TLoC. Ideally a witness account should be sought.

An accurate description of events before, during, and after the TLoC may identify the likely cause (Table 9.13).

The following history should be established:

- Circumstances of the event
- Posture immediately before the loss of consciousness
- Prodromal symptoms (sweating, feeling hot)
- Appearance and colour of the patient during the event
- Presence or absence of movement during the event (e.g. limb-jerking)

Table 9.12 Types of syncope

Types of syncope	Mechanism	Examples
Neurally mediated (reflex syncope)	TLoC due to a reflex hypotensive response and/or reflex bradycardia	Vasovagal syncope—may be triggered by pain, prolonged standing, emotional stress, and so on.
		Carotid sinus syncope—pressure on the carotid artery causes syncope.
		Situational syncope—situations that increase intra-abdominal pressure (e.g. coughing, micturition, defecation).
Orthostatic hypotension	Changes in posture provoke a marked fall in BP	1° autonomic failure—Parkinson's disease, Lewy body dementia, multi-system atrophy, pure autonomic failure.
		2° autonomic failure—diabetes, amyloidosis, uraemia, spinal cord injury.
		Drugs (e.g. EtOH, diuretics, antihypertensives).
		Volume depletion (vomiting, diarrhoea, haemorrhage).
Cardiac	Arrhythmias	Bradyarrhythmias.
	Structural heart disease	Tachyarrhythmias.
		Valvular heart disease.
		Cardiomyopathy.
		Congenital heart disease.

Table 9.13 Features suggesting a specific diagnosis in transient loss of consciousness (TLoC)

Features suggesting vasovagal syncope	Features suggesting situational syncope	Features suggesting epilepsy
Posture—prolonged standing, or similar episodes that have been prevented by lying down. Provoking factors, (e.g. pain, medical procedure). Prodromal symptoms—sweating, feeling hot.	Syncope provoked by straining during micturition (usually while standing), coughing, or swallowing.	Bitten tongue. Head-turning to one side during TLoC. No memory of abnormal behaviour. Unusual posturing. Prolonged limb-jerking. Confusion after event. Prodromal *déjà vu* or *jamais vu*.

- Tongue-biting
- Any injuries occurrin
- Duration of event
- Presence or absence of confusion during the recovery
- Weakness down one side during the recovery period

9.7.4 Investigations for transient loss of consciousness

All patients with TLoC should have a 12-lead ECG.

The following ECG findings are considered red flags:

- Conduction abnormality (e.g. complete RBBB or LBBB or any degree of heart block)
- Evidence of a long (corrected QT >450 ms) or short (corrected QT <350 ms) QT interval
- Any ST-segment or T-wave abnormalities
- Inappropriate persistent bradycardia
- Any ventricular arrhythmia (including ventricular ectopic beats)
- Brugada syndrome
- Ventricular pre-excitation (part of WPW syndrome)
- Left or right ventricular hypertrophy
- Abnormal T-wave inversion
- Pathological Q waves
- Atrial arrhythmia (sustained)
- Paced rhythm

Other investigations should be directed by the suspected underlying cause:

- Blood glucose—if hypoglycaemia suspected
- Haemoglobin—if anaemia or bleeding suspected
- Urinary pregnancy test—in women of childbearing age
- Lying and standing blood pressures (with repeated measurements while standing for 3 minutes)—if orthostatic hypotension suspected

9.7.5 Risk scoring/red flags in transient loss of consciousness

There have been a number of different clinical decision rules developed for patients presenting with syncope. The NICE guidance has reviewed the available evidence and published a set of red flags. Patients presenting with red flags are at greater risk of adverse outcomes and should be referred for urgent specialist cardiovascular assessment within 24 hours.

Red flags:

- An ECG abnormality (as detailed in section 9.7.4)
- Heart failure (history or physical signs)
- TLoC during exertion
- Family history of sudden cardiac death in people aged younger than 40 years
- New or unexplained breathlessness
- A heart murmur
- 65 years or older without prodromal symptoms

9.7.6 Management of transient loss of consciousness

Vasovagal or situational syncope

If a diagnosis of vasovagal or situational syncope is made, the patient can be discharged from the ED. The patient should be advised to take a copy of their ECG and discharge summary to their GP.

Patients should be given the following information:

- An explanation of the mechanism causing their syncope.
- Advice on possible trigger events and strategies for avoiding them.
- If their trigger events are unclear, they should be advised to keep a record of their symptoms, when they occur and what they were doing at the time, in order to understand what causes their TLoC.
- Reassurance that their prognosis is good.
- Advice to consult their GP if they experience further TLoC, particularly if it differs from their recent episode.

Orthostatic hypotension

If orthostatic hypotension is diagnosed the likely cause should be considered (e.g. drug therapy) and managed appropriately. Patients may benefit from referral to a falls clinic.

Suspected epilepsy

Patients with suspected epilepsy should be referred for assessment by an epilepsy specialist and seen within two weeks. The management of epilepsy is discussed in Chapter 11, section 11.5.

Specialist cardiovascular assessment

Patients who do not have a diagnosis of vasovagal syncope, situational syncope, orthostatic hypotension, or suspected epilepsy should be referred on for specialist cardiovascular assessment. This should be within 24 hours in patients with red flags.

Further investigations will be guided by a specialist in TLoC; this may be a general physician, cardiologist, or neurologist, depending on local arrangements. The investigations will be directed according to the suspected underlying cause and may include ambulatory ECG, echocardiography, exercise testing, tilt testing, and carotid sinus massage.

9.7.7 Driving restrictions in TLoC

Patients diagnosed with simple faints have no driving restrictions.

Patients who require specialist cardiovascular assessment or those with suspected epilepsy must be advised not to drive while waiting for assessment. The patient is responsible for reporting the TLoC to DVLA. The driving licence restrictions will be determined by the underlying cause of the TLoC and risk of recurrence (see Chapter 21, section 21.5).

KEY POINTS

TLoC is a sudden, spontaneous, complete loss of consciousness with rapid recovery.

Causes of TLoC can be divided into three main categories:

- Syncope—due to dysfunction of the cardiovascular system.
- Epilepsy—due to dysfunction of the nervous system.
- Psychogenic seizures—due to dysfunction of the psyche.

Syncope is due to transient global cerebral hypoperfusion caused by hypotension secondary to low cardiac output or low peripheral vascular resistance. There are three main types of syncope:

- Neurally mediated—vasovagal, situational, carotid sinus syndrome.
- Orthostatic hypotension—autonomic failure, drugs, volume depletion.
- Cardiac—arrhythmias or structural heart disease.

9.8 Sudden cardiac death

9.8.1 Introduction

One of the main management priorities of patients presenting with transient loss of consciousness is to identify those at risk of sudden cardiac death (SCD). SCD is unexpected death due to a cardiac cause occurring in a short time period (<1 hour) after symptom onset. The patient may have known cardiac disease or SCD may be the first presentation of cardiac disease.

Most cases of SCD are related to cardiac arrhythmias, typically VF or VT. Interruption of the tachyarrhythmia with defibrillation or an implantable cardioverter defibrillator is the most effective treatment. Approximately 20–30% of patients with SCD have a bradyarrhythmia or PEA at the time of presentation, which may be the initial rhythm or the consequence of sustained VT.

9.8.2 Causes of sudden cardiac death

Most cases of SCD occur in patients with structural abnormalities of the heart. MI and post-MI remodelling of the heart are the most common structural abnormalities in patients with SCD. Hypertrophic cardiomyopathy, dilated cardiomyopathy, and valvular heart disease are associated with an increased risk of SCD. Acute illnesses, such as myocarditis, may provide both an initial and sustained risk of SCD due to inflammation and fibrosis of the myocardium.

Less commonly, SCD happens in patients who do not have structural heart disease usually due to inherited arrhythmia syndromes that predispose them to VT or VF.

Structural heart disease

Ischaemic heart disease—may lead to cardiac arrest due to ventricular arrhythmias. This can be due to the acute MI or post-MI remodelling of the heart where scar formation acts as a focus for re-entrant ventricular tachyarrhythmias.

Dilated cardiomyopathy—results in a dilated LV with poor systolic function. Causes include viral infection, autoimmune conditions, alcohol, thyrotoxicosis, peripartum, and idiopathic.

Hypertrophic cardiomyopathy—is a genetic disorder that is typically inherited in an autosomal-dominant fashion with variable penetrance and variable expressivity. It is characterized by myocardial hypertrophy in the absence of an identifiable cause (e.g. hypertension, aortic stenosis). Hypertrophic cardiomyopathy is the commonest cause of SCD in people younger than 30 years. The vast majority of young people who die are previously asymptomatic. The SCD event typically occurs after vigorous exertion. Common ECG findings include ST-T-wave abnormalities and LV hypertrophy. An echocardiogram is diagnostic.

Valvular heart disease—is a less common cause of SCD following the advent of valve replacement surgery. Aortic stenosis is the commonest valvular cause of SCD.

Congenital heart disease—is associated with SCD. Abnormalities associated with SCD include Tetralogy of Fallot, transposition of the great vessels, Fontan operation, aortic stenosis, Marfan syndrome, mitral valve prolapse, hypoplastic left heart syndrome, Eisenmenger syndrome, and Ebstein anomaly.

Arrhythmia syndromes

Patients may have no apparent structural heart disease but a primary electrophysiological abnormality that predisposes them to VT or VF. A history of syncopal episodes and a family history of SCD should raise suspicion of an underlying arrhythmia.

Long QT syndrome—results in a propensity to ventricular tachyarrhythmias, typically Torsades de Pointe (Table 9.14).

The QT interval should be measured from the beginning of the QRS complex to the end of the T-wave, which represents the duration of activation and recovery of the ventricular myocardium. QT intervals corrected for heart rate (QTc) longer than 0.44 seconds are generally considered abnormal, although a normal QTc can be more prolonged in females (up to 0.46 seconds).

EXAM TIP

Calculating the QTc has appeared in previous SAQ papers:

$$QTc = \frac{QT \text{ interval}}{\sqrt{R-R \text{ interval (in seconds)}}}$$

Normal QTc stands at <0.44 seconds in men and <0.46 seconds in women.

Short QT syndrome—is a recently discovered syndrome which can lead to lethal arrhythmias and SCD. It is due to mutations in the potassium channel. ECG shows a short QTc less than 0.33 seconds and tall, peaked T-waves.

Table 9.14 Causes of a long QT

Inherited long QT syndrome	Acquired long QT syndrome
Jervell–Lange–Nielsen syndrome Romano–Ward syndrome	Antiarrhythmics—class Ia (e.g. quinidine) and class III (e.g. sotalol, amiodarone)
	Other drugs (e.g. tricyclic antidepressants, erythromycin, phenothiazines, phenytoin, terfenadine)
	Electrolyte abnormalities (hypokalaemia, hypocalcaemia, hypomagnesaemia)
	Hypothyroidism
	Hypothermia
	Intracranial haemorrhage (especially subarachnoid haemorrhage)

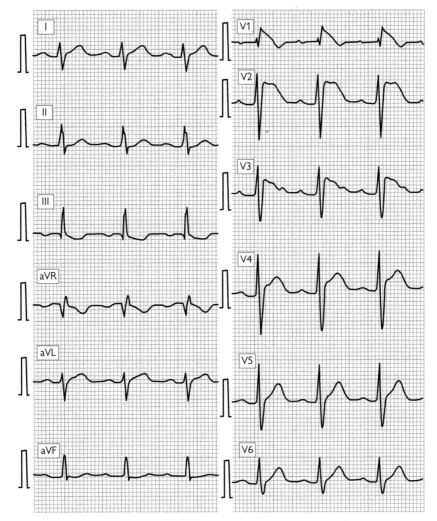

Figure 9.5 Typical Brugada syndrome ECG ('type 1'). Note 'r' and down sloping ST-elevation in V1–V3. PR interval is borderline prolonged (220 ms).

Reproduced from A. John Camm, Thomas F. Lüscher, and Patrick W. Serruys, *The ESC Textbook of Cardiovascular Medicine*, 2009, Figure 2.58, p. 69, with permission from Oxford University Press.

Brugada syndrome—is a genetic disorder resulting in a sodium channelopathy (Figure 9.5). Patients are at risk of polymorphic VT, VF, and SCD. ECG changes of coving ST-elevation in V1–V3 with downsloping ST-segments and inverted T-waves, and/or a RBBB appearance without terminal S-waves in the lateral leads is diagnostic for Brugada syndrome. Other ECG changes are recognized but are not diagnostic. The ECG changes may be transient and precipitated by drugs (class Ic antiarrhythmics, e.g. flecainide) or exercise.

WPW syndrome—is a recognized but rare cause of SCD. If a patient develops AF with a rapid ventricular response, conducted via the accessory pathway, VF can be induced.

> **EXAM TIP**
>
> Brugada syndrome has appeared in previous SAQs.
>
> If a SAQ involves a young male patient presenting with a syncopal episode, consider Brugada syndrome.
>
> If the ECG shows incomplete RBBB and ST elevations in the anterior precordial leads, consider Brugada syndrome.

9.8.3 Clinical features, investigations, and management of patients at risk of sudden cardiac death

Patients at risk of SCD may be asymptomatic prior to their arrhythmia. However, patients may have a prodrome of chest pain, fatigue, palpitations, syncope, and other non-specific complaints. The NICE TLoC red flags should be used to identify high-risk patients.

The ECG is the most important investigation. An echocardiogram may be diagnostic in structural heart disease. Further investigations should be directed by a cardiologist.

ED management is as per ALS guidance (Chapter 2) for patients presenting in cardiac arrest or in peri-arrest arrhythmias. If patients are stable, they should be referred for specialist cardiology review.

> **KEY POINTS**
>
> SCD is unexpected death due to a cardiac cause occurring in a short time period (<1 h) after symptom onset.
>
> Most cases of SCD occur in patients with structural abnormalities of the heart or inherited arrhythmia syndromes which predispose them to VT or VF.

9.9 Heart failure

9.9.1 Introduction

Heart failure is a clinical syndrome in which patients have the following features:

- Symptoms typical of heart failure—breathlessness at rest or on exertion, fatigue, tiredness, ankle swelling, orthopnoea, and paroxysmal nocturnal dyspnoea.
- Signs typical of heart failure—tachycardia, tachypnoea, pulmonary crackles, pleural effusion, raised jugular venous pressure, peripheral oedema, and/or hepatomegaly.
- Objective evidence of a structural or functional abnormality of the heart—cardiomegaly, third heart sound, cardiac murmurs, abnormality on echocardiogram, raised natriuretic peptide.

There are many words and phrases used to characterize patients with heart failure, which can cause confusion. Here chronic heart failure refers to patients with known, persistent heart failure. Acute heart failure refers to those with a rapid onset or change in signs and symptoms of heart failure, resulting in the need for urgent therapy.

Right and left heart failure are syndromes predominantly presenting with congestion of the systemic or pulmonary veins, leading to signs of fluid retention with ankle swelling or pulmonary oedema, respectively. The most common cause of right ventricular failure is a raised pulmonary artery pressure due to failure of the LV leading to poor perfusion of the kidney, retention of salt and water, and accumulation of fluid in the systemic circulation.

High and low output heart failure are other commonly used terms: low output refers to a low cardiac output due to heart pump failure; and high refers to medical conditions that increase the demands on the heart mimicking the signs and symptoms of heart failure. Causes of high output failure include anaemia, thyrotoxicosis, septicaemia, liver failure, arteriovenous shunts, and Paget's disease.

9.9.2 Causes of chronic heart failure

- Coronary artery disease
- Hypertension
- Cardiomyopathies—hypertrophic, dilated, restrictive, peripartum, acute myocarditis
- Valvular heart disease
- Arrhythmias (e.g. AF)
- Drugs—β-blockers, calcium antagonists, antiarrhythmics, cytotoxic agents
- Toxins—alcohol, cocaine, trace elements (mercury, cobalt)
- Endocrine—diabetes, hypo/hyperthyroidism, Cushing's syndrome, adrenal insufficiency, phaeochromocytoma
- Infiltrative—sarcoidosis, amyloidosis, haemochromatosis

9.9.3 Severity of heart failure

There are several classification systems for determining the severity of heart failure. The New York Heart Association (NYHA) functional classification is commonly used clinically and is employed in most randomized clinical trials. The Killip classification is used for the severity of heart failure in the context of acute MI (Table 9.15).

9.9.4 Investigations in heart failure

ECG—should be performed in every patient with suspected heart failure. Changes are common but non-specific and may demonstrate evidence of ischaemia, infarction, LVH, arrhythmias, and so on. If the ECG is completely normal, heart failure is unlikely (<10%).

CXR—is an essential component in the diagnostic work up. The CXR may show pulmonary congestion, pleural fluid accumulation, or demonstrate the presence of pulmonary disease or infection causing or contributing to the dyspnoea. CXR changes in pulmonary oedema include:

- Upper lobe diversion (distension of upper pulmonary veins)
- Cardiomegaly (LV and/or LA dilatation)
- Kerley B septal lines (increased lymphatic pressure)
- Fluid in interlobar fissures
- Peribronchial/perivascular cuffing and micronodules
- Pleural effusions
- Bat's wing hilar shadowing

Table 9.15 Classification of heart failure

Killip classification
Stage I—no heart failure
Stage II—heart failure; rales in lower 1/3 of lung fields, S3 gallop, raised JVP
Stage III—severe heart failure; frank pulmonary oedema with rales throughout the lung fields
Stage IV—cardiogenic shock; signs include hypotension (systolic BP <90 mmHg) and evidence of peripheral vasoconstriction (oliguria, sweating, cyanosis)

Table 9.16 Common blood test abnormalities in heart failure

Test	Possible abnormality	Cause(s)
Haemoglobin	Anaemia	Chronic heart failure (chronic disease), renal failure, iron loss, or poor utilization
Serum creatinine	Raised	Renal disease. Angiotensin converting enzyme inhibitors (ACEI), angiotensin receptor blockers (ARB), or aldosterone antagonist use
Serum sodium	Low	Chronic heart failure, diuretic use, haemodilution
	High	Dehydration
Serum potassium	Low	Diuretics, 2° hyperaldosteronism
	High	Renal failure, ACEI, ARB, or aldosterone antagonist use
Glucose	High	Diabetes, insulin resistance
Troponin	Raised	Mild elevation common in chronic heart failure ACS Myocarditis
Thyroid function	High or low TSH	Hypo/hyperthyroidism
INR	High	Anticoagulant overuse Liver congestion
CRP	High	Infection, inflammation

Blood tests—there are many that may be indicated in patients with heart failure. MRCEM questions often ask for the most useful test, which may depend on the clinical picture presented (see Table 9.16).

Natriuretic peptides—are useful biomarkers in heart failure, often used in the initial diagnosis and to manage chronic heart failure. They rise in response to myocardial wall stress. A normal level in an untreated patient makes heart failure unlikely.

Echocardiography—should be performed on all patients who have suspected heart failure. This is not usually performed in the ED unless it will alter the acute management (e.g. suspected prosthetic valve failure).

9.9.5 Acute heart failure

Acute heart failure may be new heart failure or worsening of pre-existing chronic heart failure.

Multiple cardiovascular and non-cardiovascular morbidities may precipitate acute heart failure. These causes can be subdivided according to components of the cardiac output or factors that increase demand on the heart. The cardiac output is determined by heart rate and stroke volume, which is determined by the preload, myocardial contractility, and afterload. Chapter 2, section 2.8 contains further details on the physiology of the cardiac output.

EXAM TIP

Cardiac Output = Heart rate × Stroke volume

Stroke volume is determined by the:

- Preload
- Myocardial contractility
- Afterload

Causes of acute heart failure include:

- Increased preload—due to volume overload or fluid retention
- Failure of myocardial contractility—due to ischaemia, infarction, cardiomyopathy, drugs, or toxins
- Increased afterload—due to systemic or pulmonary hypertension, or valvular dysfunction
- Abnormalities in cardiac rhythm—commonly AF
- Increased cardiac demands (high output states)—infection, anaemia, thyrotoxicosis, or drugs

Other conditions that may precipitate acute heart failure include non-adherence to medications, or the introduction of medications such as NSAIDs or cyclooxygenase inhibitors.

Clinical features of acute heart failure

Acute heart failure is usually characterized by pulmonary congestion, although in some patients, reduced cardiac output and tissue hypoperfusion may dominate the clinical presentation (Table 9.17). Patients will typically present in one of six clinical categories, although they may overlap. Pulmonary oedema may complicate all of these clinical presentations.

9.9.6 Emergency department management of acute heart failure

Multiple agents are used to manage acute heart failure (Table 9.18). There is a paucity of clinical trials data and their use is largely empirical. Most agents improve haemodynamic parameters but no agent has been shown to reduce mortality.

Table 9.17 Clinical presentations of acute heart failure

Clinical presentation	Features
Decompensated chronic heart failure	Usually a history of progressive worsening of symptoms.
	Systemic and pulmonary congestion.
Pulmonary oedema	Severe respiratory distress.
	Tachypnoea, orthopnoea.
	Wide spread crackles on chest auscultation.
	Oxygen saturations typically <90% on air.
Hypertensive heart failure	Signs and symptoms of heart failure accompanied by hypertension.
	There is evidence of increased sympathetic tone with tachycardia and vasoconstriction.
	The patient may be euvolaemic or only mildly hypervolaemic.
	Often there are signs of pulmonary congestion without signs of systemic congestion.
Cardiogenic shock	Evidence of tissue hypoperfusion induced by heart failure after adequate correction of preload and major arrhythmia.
	Pulmonary congestion and organ hypoperfusion develop rapidly.
Isolated right heart failure	Absence of pulmonary congestion.
	Raised JVP with or without hepatomegaly.
ACS and heart failure	Symptoms, ECG, and laboratory evidence of ACS.

Table 9.18 Treatment of acute heart failure

Treatment	Rationale
Morphine	Improves symptoms in those with chest pain, dyspnoea, anxiety, or restlessness.
	May improve co-operation with NIV.
Oxygen therapy	Restore saturations to 94–98% (88–92% in those at risk of hypercapnic respiratory failure).
Non-invasive ventilation (usually CPAP starting with a PEEP of 5 cmH$_2$0 and titrating up to 10 cmH$_2$0)	Should be considered early in patients with acute cardiogenic pulmonary oedema and hypertensive acute heart failure.
	Improves clinical parameters including respiratory distress.
	PEEP improves LV function by reducing afterload, improves oxygenation, and reduces the work of breathing.
	NIV should be used with caution in cardiogenic shock and RV failure.
Loop diuretics (furosemide 40 mg IV)	Reduces systemic and pulmonary congestion.
	Higher doses may be required in patients with volume overload. IV nitrates may reduce the need for high dose diuretics in such patients.
	Patients with hypotension, severe hyponatraemia, or acidosis are unlikely to respond to diuretic therapy.
Vasodilators (e.g. nitrates which may be sublingual or buccal initially followed by an IV infusion)	Recommended early in the treatment of acute heart failure.
	Relieves pulmonary congestion by reducing systemic vascular resistance and decreasing left and right heart filling pressures.
	Decreases systolic blood pressure and should not be used in patients with a systolic BP<90 mmHg (cautiously in those with a systolic BP 90–110 mmHg).
Fluid challenge	Patients with cardiogenic shock due to heart failure may be hypovolaemic and require restoration of preload.
	A fluid challenge of 250 ml every 10 min should be given and the response monitored. If systolic BP remains low despite restoration of preload inotropes will be required.
Inotropic agents (e.g. dopamine, dobutamine)	Should be considered in patients with low output states, in the presence of hypoperfusion or congestion despite the use of vasodilators, diuretics, and/or fluid challenges.
	Dobutamine has positive inotropic and chronotropic effects through stimulation of β_1 receptors. The β_2 actions cause peripheral vasodilatation.
	Dopamine at low doses stimulate dopaminergic receptors and at higher doses acts on α_1 and β_1 receptors, leading to vasoconstriction and increased CO due to improved myocardial contractility. The α stimulation at higher doses may increase systemic vascular resistance and worsen heart failure.

The main ED treatment goals in acute heart failure are:

- Improve symptoms
- Restore oxygenation
- Improve organ perfusion and haemodynamics
- Limit cardiac and renal damage
- Minimize ICU length of stay

In patients with isolated right-sided heart failure, the standard management for heart failure is inappropriate. Vasodilators such as nitrates, opiates, and diuretics should be avoided because they may precipitate cardiovascular collapse. The right ventricular preload must be maintained with IV fluids. Inotropes may be required. CVP monitoring may be necessary to guide treatment.

Monitoring in acute heart failure

Monitoring of patients with acute heart failure should be started as soon as possible and concurrently with assessment and treatment.

- Non-invasive monitoring—should be continual or very frequent for the basic observations (temperature, heart rate, BP, oxygen saturations, respiratory rate, and ECG).
- Arterial line—should be considered in patients requiring continually monitoring of the BP due to haemodynamic instability, or the requirement for frequent arterial blood samples.
- Central venous line—should be considered if monitoring of the central venous pressure and venous oxygen saturations are required. It also provides access to the central circulation if inotrope infusions are required.
- Urinary catheter—should be considered to accurately monitor urine output and assess treatment response.

KEY POINTS

Causes of acute heart failure include:
- Increased preload—due to volume overload or fluid retention
- Failure of myocardial contractility—due to ischaemia, infarction, cardiomyopathy, drugs, or toxins
- Increased afterload—due to systemic or pulmonary hypertension, or valvular dysfunction
- Abnormalities in cardiac rhythm—commonly AF
- Increased cardiac demands (high output states)—infection, anaemia, thyrotoxicosis, or drugs

The main ED treatment goals in acute heart failure are:
- Improve symptoms
- Restore oxygenation
- Improve organ perfusion and haemodynamics
- Limit cardiac and renal damage
- Minimize ICU length of stay

The mainstay of acute heart failure treatment is:
- Oxygen
- Opiates
- Loop diuretics
- Nitrates
- Non-invasive ventilation
- Fluid (as required)
- Inotropes

9.10 Hypertensive emergencies

9.10.1 Introduction and terminology

Hypertensive emergencies are severe forms of high blood pressure (diastolic BP usually >140 mmHg) associated with acute damage to end organs (heart, eyes, kidneys, and brain). This is different from hypertensive urgency, where there is marked elevation of blood pressure but no evidence of acute progressive end organ damage (although there may be pre-existing end organ involvement).

Hypertensive emergencies require immediate treatment to lower the blood pressure and minimize end organ damage. In contrast, hypertensive urgencies do not require immediate treatment and the elevated blood pressure may be a physiological response (e.g. acute ischaemic stroke). Rapid blood pressure reductions in such patients may cause harm due to cardiac, renal, or cerebral hypoperfusion.

Other terms that are commonly used are malignant hypertension and accelerated hypertension. Malignant hypertension is a syndrome of severe elevation of blood pressure with vascular damage that manifests as retinal haemorrhages, exudates, and/or papilloedema. The term accelerated hypertension is sometimes used to describe the syndrome when papilloedema is absent. Malignant and accelerated hypertension are both hypertensive emergencies, because they are associated with acute end organ damage.

Conditions that define hypertensive emergencies when associated with acute elevation of blood pressure include:

- Hypertensive encephalopathy
- Acute left ventricular failure
- Acute myocardial infarction or ischaemia
- Dissection of the aorta
- Intracranial haemorrhage
- Acute kidney injury
- Eclampsia

9.10.2 Causes of hypertension

Most hypertension is essential hypertension where no specific cause is found. Secondary hypertension accounts for approximately 10% of cases (Table 9.19).

9.10.3 Pathophysiology of hypertensive emergencies

Most hypertensive emergencies occur in patients with known hypertension and are the result of inadequate treatment or poor compliance.

The hypertensive emergency is thought to be triggered by an abrupt rise in systemic vascular resistance and failure of the normal autoregulatory mechanisms. The characteristic vascular lesion is fibrinoid necrosis of arterioles and small arteries, which causes the clinical manifestations of end organ damage. Red blood cells are damaged as they flow through vessels obstructed by fibrin deposits, resulting in microangiopathic haemolytic anaemia.

Loss of autoregulation results in endovascular damage. In the brain, this manifests as cerebral oedema and microhaemorrhage, which result in the clinical features of hypertensive encephalopathy. This can progress to macroscopic haemorrhage. In the eyes, flame haemorrhages and/or soft exudates may be seen. Endovascular damage in the kidneys results in acute kidney injury.

9.10.4 Clinical features of hypertensive emergencies

A hypertensive emergency may present in a number of different ways depending upon the end organ(s) involved (Table 9.20).

Table 9.19 Causes of hypertension

Cause	Examples
Essential hypertension	No specific cause.
	Associated risk factors: increasing age, obesity, salt intake, smoking, hyperlipidaemia, and family history.
Renal disease	Renal artery stenosis (excessive production of renin due to renal ischaemia).
	Parenchymal disease (e.g. glomerulonephritis).
	Polycystic kidneys.
Arterial disease	Coarctation of the aorta.
	Loss of elasticity of large arteries.
Endocrine disease	Phaeochromocytoma (excessive catecholamine release).
	Conn's syndrome (primary hyperaldosteronism).
	Cushing's syndrome (excessive glucocorticoid).
Drugs	Cocaine, amphetamines, oral contraceptive pill, steroids.

9.10.5 Investigations for hypertensive emergencies

Investigations should be directed at identifying end organ damage.

- ECG—looking for ischaemia, infarction, left ventricular hypertrophy, or strain.
- CXR—looking for evidence of pulmonary oedema, cardiomegaly, or a wide mediastinum suggestive of aortic dissection.
- Renal function—looking for evidence of acute kidney injury or electrolyte abnormalities.
- Urinalysis—looking for evidence of renal disease (haematuria, proteinuria, casts) and to check pregnancy status.
- Haemoglobin—looking for evidence of haemolytic anaemia.
- CT scan—of the head or aorta may be indicated if a cerebral haemorrhage or aortic dissection is suspected.

Table 9.20 Clinical features of hypertensive emergency

Clinical features	Cause
Chest pain	Myocardial ischaemia or infarction.
	Aortic dissection.
Dyspnoea	Pulmonary oedema due to left ventricular failure.
Headache	Cerebral oedema.
Visual disturbance	Cerebral oedema and/or haemorrhage.
Focal neurological abnormality	Cerebral haemorrhage.
Hypertensive encephalopathy	Symptom complex of severe hypertension, headache, vomiting, visual disturbance, reduced level of consciousness, seizure, and retinopathy with papilloedema.
Oliguria	Acute kidney injury.

9.10.6 Emergency department management of hypertensive emergencies

Hypertensive urgencies

Most patients with significantly elevated blood pressures in the ED will have hypertensive urgencies, not emergencies. These patients do not require aggressive blood pressure lowering and can usually be referred to the GP to monitor and treat their hypertension.

Hypertensive emergencies

Patients with true hypertensive emergencies (evidence of acute end organ damage) require urgent management of their blood pressure. Sudden large drops in blood pressure should be avoided because they may compromise blood flow to vital organs in which autoregulatory mechanisms are already damaged.

There is no universally agreed appropriate rate of reduction in blood pressure. The following advice is based on the Royal College of Emergency Medicine Guidelines on Hypertensive Emergencies, available at http://www.rcemlearning.co.uk/modules/hypertensive-emergencies/treatment-general-approach/, which recommends an initial reduction in the mean arterial pressure (MAP) of up to 25% in the first hour of treatment.

> **EXAM TIP**
>
> The MAP is calculated as follows:
>
> $$MAP = \frac{(2 \times \text{diastolic pressure}) + \text{systolic pressure}}{3}$$
>
> In order to achieve a controlled reduction in blood pressure, a titratable, intravenous, short-acting antihypertensive agent is recommended. The three most commonly used drugs to achieve this are:
>
> - Nitroprusside—this is the agent of choice for most hypertensive emergencies. It is a potent vasodilator reducing preload and afterload. It has a rapid onset and offset, and is titratable.
> - Labetalol—is a mixed α- and β-blockers and lowers blood pressure by vasodilatation and reducing cardiac contractility. It is not associated with reduced cerebral blood flow and is the agent of choice when used for hypertensive stroke syndromes.
> - Nitrates—cause vasodilatation of capacitance vessels, which reduces preload and is a coronary vasodilator. It is particularly useful when hypertension is associated with myocardial ischaemia/infarction or pulmonary oedema. The response of the blood pressure can be unpredictable.
>
> Patients being treated for hypertensive emergencies should be transferred to a high dependency area and should have continual ECG monitoring, invasive arterial blood pressure monitoring, and frequent assessment of neurological status and urine output.

> **KEY POINTS**
>
> Hypertensive emergencies are severe forms of high blood pressure (diastolic BP usually >140 mmHg) associated with acute progressive damage to end organs (heart, eyes, kidneys, and brain).
> The aim is an initial reduction in the MAP of up to 25% in the first hour of treatment.
> Nitroprusside, labetalol, and nitrates are the main agents used in a hypertensive emergency.
> Patients should have continual ECG and invasive blood pressure monitoring and be managed in a high dependency area.

9.11 Infective endocarditis

9.11.1 Introduction

Infective endocarditis is inflammation of the endocardium, particularly affecting the heart valves, caused mainly by bacteria but occasionally by other infectious agents. It is a rare condition, with an annual incidence of fewer than 10 per 100,000 cases in the normal population. Infective endocarditis is a life-threatening disease with a significant mortality (approximately 20%) and morbidity.

Predisposing factors:

- Prosthetic heart valves
- Intravenous drug use
- Degenerative valve sclerosis
- Invasive procedures at risk of bacteraemia
- Congenital heart disease
- Hypertrophic cardiomyopathy
- Nosocomial infection
- Rheumatic heart disease (less common now)
- Previous history of infective endocarditis

9.11.2 Causes of infective endocarditis

The commonest causes of infective endocarditis on blood culture are:

- *Streptococcus viridans*
- *Staphylococcus aureus*
- *Enterococci*
- *Streptococcus bovis*

Blood cultures may be negative and in such cases the cause is usually due to the HACEK group of Gram-negative bacilli:

- *Haemophilus* species
- *Actinobacillus*
- *Cardiobacterium hominis*
- *Eikenella corrodens*
- *Kingella kingae*

Other blood culture negative causes include:

- *Brucella*
- Fungi
- *Coxiella burnetii*
- *Bartonella*
- *Chlamydia*

9.11.3 Clinical features of infective endocarditis

Infective endocarditis can present in a multitude of ways depending on the presence or absence of pre-existing cardiac disease and the causative organism.

Clinical features include:

- Fever (up to 90% of patients present with fever)
- New regurgitant murmur
- Arthropathy
- Poor appetite and weight loss
- Immunological phenomenon—Osler nodes, Roth spots, glomerulonephritis

- Vascular phenomenon—Janeway lesions, splinter haemorrhages
- Emboli—stroke, splenomegaly, pulmonary embolism, digital ischaemia

9.11.4 Investigations for infective endocarditis

Blood cultures—are the cornerstone of diagnosis. Three sets should be taken from separate peripheral sites at 30-minute intervals. Bacteraemia is almost constant in infective endocarditis, so there is no rationale for delaying blood sampling to coincide with the peaks of fever.

Echocardiography—should be performed as soon as infectious endocarditis is suspected. A transthoracic echocardiogram is usually more readily available than a transoesophageal but a transoesophageal has a greater sensitivity.

Other investigations (e.g. white cell count, CRP, and so on) are supportive but not diagnostic for infective endocarditis.

9.11.5 Diagnostic criteria for infective endocarditis—Duke's criteria

The Duke's criteria based upon clinical, echocardiographic, and microbiological findings provide high sensitivity and specificity (~80% overall) for the diagnosis of infective endocarditis (Table 9.21).

Diagnosis of infective endocarditis is made in the presence of:

- 2 major criteria; or
- 1 major and 3 minor criteria; or
- 5 minor criteria.

Table 9.21 Duke's criteria for infective endocarditis

Major criteria	
Blood cultures positive for infective endocarditis	Typical microorganisms for infective endocarditis from two separate blood cultures (e.g. *Strep. viridans, Strep. bovis*, HACEK group, *Staph. aureus, Enterococci*)
Blood cultures persistently positive for atypical organism	At least two positive blood cultures drawn >12 h apart; or three of a majority of ≥4 separate cultures of blood
Evidence of endocardial involvement	Echocardiogram demonstrating vegetation, abscess, or dehiscence of prosthetic valve
	Or, new valvular regurgitation
Minor criteria	
Predisposition	Predisposing heart condition, IVDU
Fever	Temperature >38°C
Vascular phenomena	Major arterial emboli, septic pulmonary infarcts, mycotic aneurysm, intracranial haemorrhage, conjunctival haemorrhage, Janeway lesions
Immunologic phenomena	Glomerulonephritis, Osler's nodes, Roth's spots, rheumatoid factor
Microbiological evidence	Positive blood cultures but does not meet major criteria

Data from Li J, Sexton D, Mick N, et al (2000). 'Proposed Modifications to the Duke Criteria for the Diagnosis of Infective Endocarditis'. Clinical Infectious Diseases 30 (4): 633.

Table 9.22 Possible antibiotic regime for initial empirical treatment of infective endocarditis

Patient group	Antibiotic regime (empirical)
Native valve	Co-amoxiclav and gentamicin IV for 4–6 weeks
	If penicillin allergic:
	Vancomycin IV, gentamicin IV, and ciprofloxacin PO for 4–6 weeks
Prosthetic valve	Vancomycin IV, gentamicin IV, and rifampicin PO for 6 weeks

9.11.6 Emergency department management of infective endocarditis

Supportive management should be instituted as for any patient with sepsis.

Antibiotic therapy in the ED will be empirical and adjusted once blood cultures and sensitivities are known (Table 9.22). The appropriate empirical antibiotics depends on whether the patient has received prior antibiotic treatment or not, whether the infection is of a native or prosthetic valve, and local antibiotic resistance. Guidance should be taken from the local microbiology team.

KEY POINTS

The commonest cause of infective endocarditis is *Streptococcus viridans*.

The most useful investigations are blood cultures and echocardiography.

Diagnosis is made using Duke's criteria which are based on clinical, echocardiographic, and microbiological findings.

ED management should comprise of early antibiotics and supportive management.

9.12 Pericardial disease

9.12.1 Pericarditis

Pericarditis is inflammation of the pericardium.

Causes include:

- Viral infections (e.g. coxsackie B virus, HIV, cytomegalovirus)
- Bacterial infections (e.g. TB, pneumococcus)
- Post-myocardial infarction—early pericarditis or Dressler's syndrome. Early pericarditis occurs within 24–96 hours due to inflammation of the pericardial tissue overlying infarcted myocardium. Dressler's syndrome is an autoimmune pericarditis occurring 2–14 weeks later
- Uraemia
- Rheumatic fever
- Malignancy—as a paraneoplastic syndrome or due to a locally invasive tumour
- Collagen vascular disease (e.g. SLE, rheumatoid arthritis, polyarteritis nodosum)
- Post-cardiac surgery or radiotherapy
- Chest trauma—blunt or penetrating
- Drugs (e.g. isoniazid, ciclosporin, hydralazine, warfarin)
- Idiopathic

Clinical features of pericarditis

The classic triad for pericarditis is:

- Chest pain (pleuritic, retrosternal, exacerbated by inspiration, eased by sitting forwards)
- Pericardial friction rub
- ECG showing concordant ST-elevation

Other clinical features include:

- Low-grade fever
- Shortness of breath—either due to pain on inspiration or pericardial effusion
- Dry cough
- Dysphagia—due to compression of the oesophagus from the effusion
- Lethargy

Investigations for pericarditis

An ECG is the most useful initial investigation in suspected pericarditis (Figure 9.6). The ECG changes include:

- Widespread, saddle-shaped, ST-elevation (present in at least two limb leads and all the chest leads)
- PR depression (very specific for pericarditis)
- Tall, peaked T-waves
- Arrhythmias (typically sinus tachycardia but AF, atrial flutter, or atrial ectopics may occur)

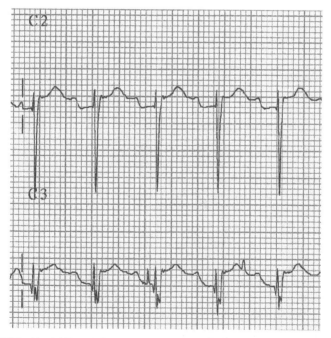

Figure 9.6 ECG of leads V1 and V2 showing PR segment depression and ST-elevation in pericarditis.

Reproduced from Saul G. Myerson, Robin P. Choudhury, and Andrew R. J. Mitchell, *Emergencies in Cardiology*, 2010, Figure 12.1, p. 207, with permission from Oxford University Press.

Other investigations include:

- CXR—usually unremarkable but may show a globular heart due to effusion or an associated pathology (e.g. TB, tumour)
- Troponin—may be raised in myopericarditis
- Inflammatory markers (ESR and CRP)
- FBC
- Renal function—looking for evidence of uraemia
- Blood cultures—if there is evidence of sepsis
- Echocardiography—may show a bright pericardium, a pericardial effusion, or impaired LV function

Management of pericarditis

- **Hospital admission**—is usually required for further investigation and monitoring of response to treatment. Some young patients with viral pericarditis and an echocardiogram which has excluded a large pericardial effusion may be managed as outpatients.
- **NSAIDs**—are the mainstay of treatment. Ibuprofen is the preferred NSAID and usually continued for two weeks.
- **Colchicine**—may be added to a NSAID if symptoms fail to respond or be used as monotherapy in patients who have contraindications to NSAIDs.
- **Steroids**—are not usually given in the ED and are reserved for patients who fail to respond to NSAIDs and colchicine, or have pericarditis secondary to connective tissue diseases, autoimmune conditions, or uraemia.

9.12.2 Pericardial effusion and cardiac tamponade

A pericardial effusion may occur with any type of pericarditis. Effusions that develop slowly may be fairly asymptomatic, while rapidly accumulating effusions (e.g. following myocardial rupture, aortic dissection, or post-cardiac surgery) can present with tamponade. Cardiac tamponade is the decompensated phase of cardiac compression caused by effusion accumulation and increased intrapericardial pressure (Table 9.23).

Table 9.23 Features of cardiac tamponade

Clinical features	Beck's triad (pathognomonic of tamponade): • Low arterial blood pressure. • Jugular venous distension that rises on inspiration (Kussmaul's sign). • Muffled heart sounds.
	Pulsus paradoxus (drop in systolic BP of >10 mmHg on inspiration)
	Tachycardia.
	Dyspnoea.
	Typically clear lungs.
ECG	May be normal or show non-specific ST-T-wave changes.
	QRS complexes may have reduced amplitude.
	Electrical alternans is rarely seen but is diagnostic of an effusion.
CXR	Globular cardiomegaly usually with clear lung fields.
Echocardiogram	Pericardial effusion.
	'Swinging heart'—the heart can move freely within the pericardial cavity.
	Diastolic collapse of the right heart (in severe cases the left heart may also collapse).

Pericardiocentesis

Emergency pericardiocentesis may be required in the ED for rapidly developing cardiac tamponade. Ideally, if time allows, pericardiocentesis should be guided by fluoroscopy in the cardiac catheterization laboratory.

If performed in the ED, pericardiocentesis should be guided by ultrasound but if this is not available and the patient is in peri-arrest, it may have to be performed blind.

Technique for 'blind' emergency pericardiocentesis:

- Long 18-G needle connected to a 20-ml syringe and 3-way tap;
- Puncture the skin 1–2 cm below the xiphisternum at 45° to the skin;
- Aspirate while advancing the needle cephalad, aiming towards the tip of the left scapula;
- Observe the ECG for evidence of cardiac irritation suggesting the needle has been advanced too far;
- Aspiration of a small amount of blood (e.g. 20–40 ml) may improve cardiac output temporarily.

KEY POINTS

Pericarditis is inflammation of the pericardium. The classic triad is:

- Chest pain
- Pericardial friction rub
- ECG showing concordant ST-elevation

ECG changes in pericarditis include:

- Widespread, saddle-shaped, ST-elevation
- PR depression
- Tall, peaked T-waves

Treatment of pericarditis is with NSAIDs. Colchicine may be used if NSAIDs are contraindicated or monotherapy fails.

A pericardial effusion may develop with any type of pericarditis.

Cardiac tamponade is the decompensated phase of cardiac compression caused by effusion accumulation and increased intrapericardial pressure.

Cardiac tamponade is a medical emergency and requires urgent pericardiocentesis.

9.13 SAQs

9.13.1 Hypertensive emergencies

A 65-year-old man presents with a headache and hypertension. The nurse comes to see you because she is worried about his blood pressure.

a) What is a hypertensive emergency? (1 mark)
b) List three classes of drugs to treat a hypertensive emergency? (3 marks)
c) Name four ED investigations you should do and a reason why for each? (4 marks)

After the initiation of treatment the patient has the following observations:

HR 90, BP 190/100, RR 20, saturations 97% on air.
d) What is this patient's mean arterial pressure? Show your calculation. (2 marks)

Suggested answer

a) What is a hypertensive emergency? (1 mark)
   A hypertensive emergency is severe high blood pressure (diastolic BP usually >140 mmHg) associated with acute damage to end organ(s) (heart, eyes, kidneys, and brain).
   (Definition must include end organ damage to gain mark)

b) List three classes of drugs to treat a hypertensive emergency? (3 marks)
   Vasodilator antihypertensive such as nitroprusside or hydralazine (used historically in eclampsia but has now been superseded by other agents).
   β-blocker, such as labetalol (has advantage of being a mixed α- and β-blocker).
   Nitrates (e.g. glyceryl trinitrate or isosorbide dinitrate)
   Calcium-channel blocker such as nicardipine (used in some countries as an alternative to nitroprusside but no parenteral form is available in the United Kingdom).
   NB Nifedipine or amlodipine may be started in 'hypertensive urgency' but are not recommended in an emergency.
   α-blocker such as phentolamine or phenoxybenzamine (used in hypertensive crisis secondary to excess catecholamine release, e.g. phaeochromocytoma or cocaine overdose).

c) Name four ED investigations you should do and a reason why for each? (4 marks)
   ECG—ischaemia, infarction, left ventricular hypertrophy, or strain
   CXR—pulmonary oedema, cardiomegaly, or a wide mediastinum suggestive of aortic dissection
   Renal function—acute kidney injury or electrolyte abnormalities
   Urinalysis—renal disease (haematuria, proteinuria, casts) and to check pregnancy status
   Haemoglobin—haemolytic anaemia
   CT scan—of the head (cerebral haemorrhage) or aorta (dissection)

d) What is this patient's mean arterial pressure? Show your calculation. (2 marks)

$$\text{Calculation MAP} = \frac{(2 \times 100) + 19)}{3} \quad \text{Answer} = 130$$

9.13.2 Atrial fibrillation

A 50-year-old man presents to the ED at 8 a.m. with a history of palpitations starting at 10 p.m. the previous night. He has no history of chest pain. He is normally fit and well. He is on no regular medications.
   His observations are: BP 140/80, HR 140, saturations 97% on air.
   His ECG shows atrial fibrillation.

a) (i)   What criteria do NICE use to define non-life-threatening haemodynamically unstable AF? (3 marks)

a) (ii)   You decide he does not have haemodynamically unstable AF and that a rhythm control strategy would be appropriate. (3 marks) Give three factors from a patient's history which favours a rhythm control strategy over rate control. (3 marks)

b)   He has a normal echocardiogram performed in the ED and has received a therapeutic dose of low molecular weight heparin. You decided to perform the cardioversion pharmacologically—what drug is the recommended first line agent in this patient? (1 mark)

c)   You decide to assess his risk for a future stroke or thromboembolic event. What factors do NICE consider 'high risk' for a future stroke? (3 marks)

Suggested answer

a) (i)   What criteria do NICE use to define non-life-threatening haemodynamically unstable AF? (3 marks)

Ventricular rate >150 bpm

Ongoing chest pain

Critical perfusion

a) (ii)   You decide he does not have haemodynamically unstable AF and that a rhythm control strategy would be appropriate. Give three factors in this patient's history which favour a rhythm control strategy? (3 marks)

New onset

Reversible cause

Presence of heart failure

b)   He has a normal echocardiogram performed in the ED and has received a therapeutic dose of low molecular weight heparin. You decided to perform the cardioversion pharmacologically—what drug is the recommended first line agent in this patient? (1 mark)

Flecanide (because the patient has no structural heart disease)

c)   You decide to assess his risk for a future stroke or thromboembolic event. What factors do NICE consider 'high risk' for a future stroke? (3 marks)

Previous stroke, TIA, or thromboembolic event

Age >75 years with hypertension, diabetes, or vascular disease

Structural heart disease (valvular heart disease, heart failure, or impaired LV function on echo)

Further reading

Dickstein K1, Cohen-Solal A, Filippatos G, et al. 2008. ESC Guidelines for the diagnosis and treatment of acute and chronic heart failure 2008: The Task Force for the Diagnosis and Treatment of Acute and Chronic Heart Failure 2008 of the European Society of Cardiology, 2008. Eur Heart J 29(19):2388–442.

National Institute for Health and Care Excellence, 2010. NICE clinical guideline 94. Unstable angina and NSTEMI. Available at: http://www.nice.org.uk/guidance/CG94 [Online].

National Institute for Health and Care Excellence, 2010. NICE clinical guideline 95. Chest pain of recent onset. Available at: www.nice.org.uk/guidance/CG95 [Online].

National Institute for Health and Care Excellence, 2010. NICE clinical guideline 109. Management of transient loss of consciousness in adults and young people. Available at: http://www.nice.org.uk/CG109 [Online].

National Institute for Health and Care Excellence, 2014. NICE clinical guideline 180. Atrial fibrillation: management. Available at: http://www.nice.org.uk/guidance/CG180 [Online].

RCEM Learning. *Hypertensive Emergencies*. Royal College of Emergency Medicine. Available at: http://www.rcemlearning.co.uk/modules/hypertensive-emergencies/treatment-general-approach/ [Online].

Sgarbossa EB, Pinski SL, Barbagelata A, *et al.* 1996. Electrocardiographic diagnosis of evolving myocardial infarction in the presence of left bundle branch block. *N Engl J Med* **334**(8):481–7.

Thygesen K, Alpert JS, Jaffe AS, *et al.* 2012. Third universal definition of myocardial infarction. *J Am Coll Cardiol* **60**(16):1581–98.

Van de Werf F, Bax J, Betriu A, *et al.* 2008. Management of acute myocardial infarction in patients presenting with persistent ST-segment elevation: The Task Force on the Management of ST-segment elevation acute myocardial infarction of the European Society of Cardiology. *Eur Heart J* **29**:2909–45.

Respiratory emergencies

CONTENTS

10.1 Asthma

10.1.1 Introduction

Asthma is a chronic, inflammatory disorder of the airways resulting in variable airflow obstruction. The national clinical guideline for asthma is summarized in the discussion that follows.

EXAM TIP

The British Thoracic Society (BTS) (https://www.brit-thoracic.org.uk) produces guidance on the management of many acute respiratory conditions. Knowledge of these guidelines is mentioned in the curriculum (e.g. asthma, COPD, pneumonia, pulmonary embolism, and pneumothorax) and has previously appeared in short-answer questions (SAQs).

It is worth looking at the BTS website prior to the exam for any new or updated guidance.

Throughout this chapter parts of the BTS guidelines, relevant to emergency department (ED) management, have been summarized.

10.1.2 Diagnosis of asthma

The diagnosis of asthma is based on the recognition of a characteristic pattern of symptoms and signs. Central to all diagnoses is one or more of the following symptoms: wheeze; breathlessness; chest tightness; and cough.

Clinical features that increase the probability of asthma are:

- Diurnal variation in symptom severity
- Symptoms in response to exercise, allergen exposure, and cold air
- Patient or family history of atopic disorders
- Low peak expiratory flow (PEF) rate
- Peripheral blood eosinophilia
- History of improvement with treatment

10.1.3 Severity markers for asthma

FREQUENT MRCEM QUESTION

Previous MRCEM SAQs have included the severity markers of asthma as defined by the BTS asthma guidelines (Table 10.1). All patients presenting with an asthma attack should have their level of severity assessed. The severity level determines the nature of the treatment required. Symptoms are a more sensitive measure of severity than peak expiratory flow rate (PEFR) at the onset of an exacerbation, as an increase in symptoms usually precedes deterioration in PEFR. Thereafter, PEFR is a more reliable indicator of severity than symptoms. The most clinically useful value is PEFR measured as a percentage of the person's best reading.

10.1.4 Investigations for asthma

- Peak expiratory flow rate—should be measured in all acute presentations. It should be expressed as a percentage of the patient's previous best value or predicted best.
- Arterial blood gas—is recommended by BTS if $SpO2$ <92% or other features of life-threatening asthma are present. Markers of severity include 'normal' or raised $PaCO2$ (> 4.6 kPa), severe hypoxia ($PaO2$ <8 kPa), and low pH.
- Chest radiographs—are not routinely recommended. They should be performed if a pneumothorax, pneumomediastinum, or consolidation is suspected; in life-threatening asthma; if there is failure to respond to treatment; or if mechanical ventilation is required.

10.1.5 Treatment of acute asthma

- Oxygen should be given immediately to hypoxic patients. Oxygen should be titrated to maintain SpO2 between 94–98%.

Table 10.1 Severity markers in asthma

Severity	Clinical features	Measurements
Moderate asthma	• No features of acute severe asthma • Increasing symptoms	• PEF >50–75% of best or predicted
Severe asthma	• Inability to complete sentences in one breath	• PEF 33–50% of best or predicted (use % predicted if recent best unknown) • Respiratory Rate ≥25 breaths per minute • Heart Rate ≥110 beats per minute
Life-threatening	• Silent chest • Cyanosis • Feeble respiratory effort • Arrhythmia, hypotension • Exhaustion, altered conscious level	• PEF <33% of best or predicted • $SpO2$ <92% • $PaO2$ < 8 kPa • Normal $PaCO_2$ (4.6–6.0)
Near fatal		• Respiratory acidosis (raised $PaCO_2$) and/or requiring positive pressure ventilation with raised inflation pressures

SpO2 Arterial oxygen saturation. PaO2 Arterial partial pressure of oxygen.

Adapted from the BTS/SIGN British Guideline on the Management of Asthma, 2014

- β_2 agonist (e.g. salbutamol or terbutaline) should be given as the first-line therapy to try and relive bronchospasm. In moderate and severe asthma this can be given as repeated doses via a metered-dose inhaler with a large spacer. Four puffs initially of salbutamol can be followed by two puffs, every two minutes according to response to a maximum of 10 puffs. In asthma with life-threatening features, the nebulized route (oxygen driven) is recommended (e.g. salbutamol 5 mg or terbutaline 10 mg). In patients with a poor response to initial β_2 agonist therapy, it can be nebulized continuously. Intravenous β_2 agonists should be reserved for those patients in whom inhaled therapy cannot be used reliably.
- Ipratropium bromide is an anticholinergic bronchodilator, which when combined with a β_2 agonist produces significantly greater bronchodilation than a β_2 agonist alone. Nebulized ipratropium bromide (500 mcg) should be added to β_2 agonist therapy in severe and life-threatening asthma or in those with a poor initial response to β_2 agonist. It can be repeated every four to six hours.
- Steroids reduce mortality, relapses, subsequent hospital admissions, and requirements for β_2 agonist therapy. Oral steroids are as effective as intravenous steroids, provided they can be swallowed and retained. The dose of oral prednisolone is 40–50 mg for at least five days or until recovery. The dose of intravenous hydrocortisone is 100 mg every six hours. Inhaled steroids should be started, or continued, as soon as possible to commence the chronic asthma management plan.
- Magnesium sulfate is a bronchodilator. It should be given in life-threatening and near fatal asthma, and in those with severe asthma who have had a poor response to inhaled therapy. Magnesium can be nebulized or given intravenously. Currently BTS recommend an intravenous dose 1.2–2 g over 20 minutes.
- Aminophylline is unlikely to result in any additional bronchodilation compared to standard care (nebulizers and steroids) and side effects, such as arrhythmias and vomiting, are increased. BTS recommend that aminophylline is used only after consultation with senior medical staff. Some patients with life-threatening or near fatal asthma and a poor initial response to therapy may gain some benefit. The dose is 5 mg/kg loading dose over 20 minutes (unless on oral maintenance therapy) followed by an infusion of 0.5 mg/kg/hour.
- Sedatives are contraindicated.

The management of acute severe asthma is summarized in Figure 10.1.

EXAM TIP

Learn the BTS asthma severity markers for adults and children (see Chapter 19, section 19.12).

10.1.6 Admission criteria for acute asthma
- Life-threatening or near fatal attack.
- Any features of a severe attack persisting after initial treatment.

10.1.7 Discharge criteria for acute asthma
Patients whose PEF is greater than 75% best or predicted one hour after initial treatment may be discharged from the ED. Patients should be discharged with:

- Oral prednisolone 40–50 mg for five days and inhaled steroids (e.g. beclometasone inhaler)
- Sufficient and in-date inhaled bronchodilator (e.g. salbutamol)
- PEF meter
- Written asthma action plan
- GP follow-up arranged for within two working days
- Consideration of referral to asthma liaison nurse or chest clinic

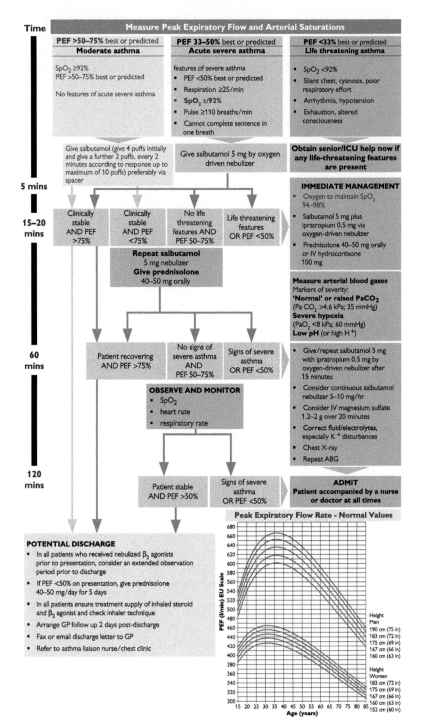

Figure 10.1 Management of severe acute asthma in adults in the emergency department

Reproduced from *Thorax*, British Thoracic Society Scottish Intercollegiate Guidelines Network, British guideline on the management of asthma, volume 69, suppl 1, p 93 & 149, copyright notice 2014, with permission from BMJ Publishing Group Ltd.

Adapted by permission from BMJ Publishing Group Limited. The BMJ, A. J. Nunn, I. Gregg, New regression equations for predicting peak expiratory flow in adults, vol 298, pp.1068-70, copyright 1989.

10.1.8 Intensive care referral

An intensive care referral is required for patients:

- requiring ventilatory support
- with severe or life-threatening asthma, failing to respond to therapy, evidenced by:
  - deteriorating PEF
  - persisting or worsening hypoxia
  - hypercapnea
  - arterial blood gas analysis showing ↓ pH
  - exhaustion, feeble respiration
  - drowsiness, confusion
  - reduced Glasgow coma scale (GCS) or respiratory arrest.

KEY POINTS

Asthma is a chronic, inflammatory disorder of the airways resulting in variable airflow obstruction.

The severity markers for asthma can be remembered by those which are clinical features (e.g. inability to complete sentences) and those which are measured (e.g. PEF).

The ED treatment of acute asthma includes:

- Oxygen
- β_2 agonist
- Ipatropium bromide
- Steroids
- Magnesium sulfate

Give written discharge advice to those patients able to be discharged from the ED. Ensure patients have a five-day course of prednisolone (40–50 mg) plus sufficient and in-date inhalers (steroid and β_2 agonist). Check the patient's inhaler technique before discharge and issue a peak flow meter. Arrange follow-up for 48 h.

10.2 Chronic obstructive pulmonary disease

10.2.1 Introduction

NICE have produced guidelines on the management of chronic obstructive pulmonary disease (COPD) patients endorsed by BTS. Section 10.2.2 is based on that guidance.

10.2.2 Diagnosis of chronic obstructive pulmonary disease

A diagnosis of COPD should be considered in patients over the age of 35 who have a risk factor (generally smoking) and who present with any of the following:

- Exertional breathlessness
- Chronic cough
- Regular sputum production
- Frequent winter 'bronchitis'
- Wheeze

The presence of airflow obstruction should be confirmed by performing spirometry. Although spirometry would not be performed in the ED, an understanding of the results could appear in a SAQ on COPD.

Spirometry

Spirometry measures functional lung volumes (Figure 10.2). Forced expiratory volume in 1 second (FEV_1) and forced vital capacity (FVC) are measured from a full, forced expiration into a spirometer. The FEV_1/FVC ratio gives a good estimate of severity of airflow obstruction.

Normal FEV_1/FVC ratio is 0.8. In obstructive disease (e.g. asthma, COPD), the FEV_1 is reduced more than the FVC and the FEV_1/FVC ratio is <0.7. In restrictive disease (e.g. lung fibrosis), FVC is reduced and the FEV1/FVC ratio is >0.8.

One of the diagnostic features that distinguish asthma from COPD is the degree of reversibility, with asthma being more responsive to treatment than COPD.

10.2.3 Exacerbations of chronic obstructive pulmonary disease

An exacerbation of COPD is a sustained worsening of the patient's symptoms from their usual stable state, which is beyond normal day-to-day variations, and is acute in onset.

There is no single defining symptom of an exacerbation but changes in breathlessness, cough, sputum production, and change in sputum colour are common.

Exacerbations of COPD can be associated with the following symptoms:

- Increased breathlessness
- Increased sputum purulence
- Increased sputum volume

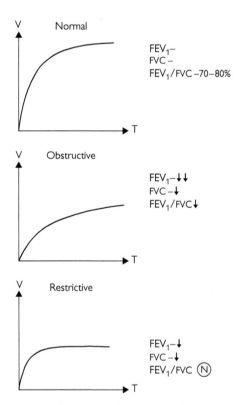

Figure 10.2 Spirograms showing obstructive and restrictive volume–time graphs

Reproduced from James Thomas and Tanya Monaghan, *Oxford Handbook of Clinical Examination and Practical Skills*, 2007, Figure 18.69, p. 725, with permission from Oxford University Press.

- Increased cough
- Upper airway symptoms (e.g. colds and sore throats)
- Increased wheeze
- Chest tightness
- Reduced exercise tolerance
- Fluid retention, with new or worsening peripheral oedema
- Increased fatigue
- Acute confusion, or impaired level of consciousness
- Marked reduction in activities of daily living

10.2.4 Causes of an exacerbation of chronic obstructive pulmonary disease

A number of factors are known to cause an exacerbation of COPD; however, the cause may be unidentifiable in up to 30% of cases.

Factors known to cause exacerbations include:

- Viral infections (e.g. rhinovirus, influenza, parainfluenza, adenovirus, and so on)
- Bacterial infections (e.g. *Haemophilus influenzae, Streptococcus pneumoniae, Moraxella catarrhalis, Staphylococcus aureus, Pseudomonas aeruginosa*)
- Environmental pollutants (e.g. nitrogen dioxide, particulates, sulphur dioxide)

10.2.5 Differential diagnosis of an exacerbation of chronic obstructive pulmonary disease

Other conditions may present with similar symptoms in patients with known COPD including:

- Pneumonia
- Pneumothorax
- Left ventricular failure/pulmonary oedema
- Pulmonary embolus
- Lung cancer
- Upper airway obstruction
- Pleural effusion
- Recurrent aspiration

The stem of the SAQ must be read carefully to ensure that the wrong conclusion is not made about the diagnosis. An exacerbation is not the only cause of breathlessness and cough in a COPD patient.

10.2.6 Assessing severity of an exacerbation of chronic obstructive pulmonary disease

COPD is not categorized into different grades of severity like asthma. However, the NICE guidance recommends that an exacerbation be considered severe if any of the following features are present:

- Marked dyspnoea
- Tachypnoea
- Pursed lip breathing
- Use of accessory muscles at rest
- Acute confusion
- New onset cyanosis
- New onset peripheral oedema
- Marked reduction in activities of daily living

10.2.7 Investigations for chronic obstructive pulmonary disease

The diagnosis of an exacerbation of COPD is made clinically and does not depend on the results of investigations; however, investigations assist in ensuring appropriate treatment is given.

The NICE guidance recommends the following investigations are performed in all patients presenting to hospital with an exacerbation of COPD:

- Chest radiograph
- Arterial blood gas with the inspired oxygen concentration recorded
- ECG (to exclude co-morbidities)
- FBC
- Urea and electrolytes
- Theophylline level in patients on theophylline therapy on admission
- Sputum culture
- Blood cultures if the patient is pyrexial

10.2.8 Assessment of need for hospital treatment

Not all patients presenting to the ED with an exacerbation of COPD require inpatient management. The NICE guidance has produced a list of factors to be considered when assessing the need for inpatient management.

10.2.9 ED management of an exacerbation of COPD

- Oxygen—therapy should be guided by the recommendation in the BTS emergency oxygen guidelines (see section 10.9.2). Oxygen saturations and an arterial blood gas should be performed to guide therapy. Initially, target saturations of 88–92% are appropriate.
- Bronchodilators—salbutamol and ipratropium bromide should be administered. These can be delivered by an inhaler or nebulizer, depending on the dose required and the severity of the exacerbation. If the patient is acidotic or hypercapnic, the nebulizer should be air-driven and oxygen, if required, delivered via nasal cannulae.
- Corticosteroids—should be administered to all patients admitted to hospital with an exacerbation of COPD. Prednisolone 30 mg should be given orally for 7–14 days.
- Antibiotics—should be used to treat exacerbations associated with a history of more purulent sputum, consolidation on chest X-ray (CXR), or clinical signs of pneumonia. Initial empirical treatment should be with an aminopenicillin, a macrolide, or a tetracycline (guided by local antibiotic policy).
- Theophylline—should only be used as adjunct to the management of an exacerbation if there is an inadequate response to nebulized bronchodilators.
- Non-invasive ventilation (NIV)—is the treatment of choice for persistent hypercapnic ventilatory failure despite optimal medical therapy. (Respiratory stimulants should only be used if NIV is not available.)
- Physiotherapy—should be considered to help patients clear sputum.
- Invasive ventilation and intensive care—should be considered for patients with exacerbations of COPD when this is thought to be necessary and appropriate.

KEY POINTS

An exacerbation of COPD is a sustained worsening of the patient's symptoms from their usual stable state, which is beyond normal day-to-day variations, and is acute in onset.

There is no single defining symptom of an exacerbation, but changes in breathlessness, cough, and sputum production are common.

ED management of an exacerbation of COPD includes:

- Oxygen—aiming for saturations 88–92%
- Inhaled bronchodilators—salbutamol and ipratropium bromide
- Steroids—prednisolone 30 mg for 7–14 days
- Antibiotics—if history of more purulent sputum, consolidation on CXR, or clinical signs of pneumonia
- Theophylline—if not responding to nebulized bronchodilators
- Non-invasive ventilation—for persistent hypercapnic ventilatory failure
- Physiotherapy—to aid sputum clearance
- ITU/ventilation—if failing to respond to medical therapy

10.3 Non-invasive ventilation

10.3.1 Introduction

Non-invasive ventilation is ventilatory support though a patient's upper airway using a mask. In the ED, NIV is often used to describe both continuous positive airways pressure (CPAP) and bi-level positive airways pressure (BiPAP); however, CPAP strictly speaking does not constitute ventilatory support.

10.3.2 Mechanism of action of non-invasive ventilation

CPAP

Continuous positive airways pressure (CPAP) provides a constant positive pressure throughout a patient's respiratory cycle. It is analogous to positive end expiratory pressure in a ventilated patient.

CPAP is provided by a tight-fitting face mask and a high gas flow (which must be greater than the patient's peak inspiratory flow rate to avoid rebreathing). A valve on the expiratory port ensures that pressure in the system, and the patient's airways, never falls below the set level.

The main effects of CPAP are to reduce the work of breathing and improve oxygenation. It achieves these effects via several mechanisms.

Increase in functional residual capacity

Functional residual capacity (FRC) is the volume of gas remaining in the lungs at the end of normal expiration. In a patient with a low FRC, the lungs collapse, and atelectasis occurs. This leads to a ventilation/perfusion (V/Q) mismatch and reduced pulmonary compliance with increased airway resistance. These effects result in hypoxia and an increase in the work of breathing.

Improved FRC has the following effects:

- Recruitment of alveoli—closed or underventilated alveoli are opened (recruited), which reduces intrapulmonary shunting (perfusion of unventilated alveoli) and improves oxygenation.
- Splinting of the airways—alveoli are splinted open, improving oxygenation and reducing airway resistance.
- Reduction in the work of breathing—CPAP reduces the work required to initiate inspiratory flow, which is why it is sometimes considered to provide ventilatory support, and may reduce the respiratory rate and $PaCO_2$. The increased FRC also allows the lungs to function on the more favourable part of the compliance curve, reducing the work of breathing further.

Reduction in left ventricular transmural pressure

This may be the main mechanism by which CPAP improves oxygenation in acute cardiogenic pulmonary oedema. CPAP also reduces preload and after-load, to which the failing heart is sensitive.

CPAP does not necessarily drive pulmonary oedema fluid back in to circulation, and total lung water may not change despite clinical improvement.

Delivery of high inspired oxygen concentrations

Certain CPAP systems are able to deliver 100% oxygen. The oxygen flow rate exceeds the patient's peak inspiratory flow rate, without rebreathing.

BiPAP

BiPAP is a combination of CPAP with pressure support (increased ventilatory support as the patient starts inspiration). The machine is set with two pressure settings: a higher inspiratory positive airway pressure (IPAP) and a lower expiratory positive airway pressure (EPAP). The difference between them generates a tidal volume which assists ventilation of the patient.

BiPAP improves oxygenation and reduces the work of breathing via the same mechanisms as CPAP. In addition, the tidal volume improves alveolar ventilation which helps clear CO_2 and reduces the respiratory rate.

When the patient is breathing spontaneously, the respiratory effort triggers both the inspiratory and expiratory phase of the respiratory cycle. If the patient becomes apnoeic, no respiratory assistance will occur; however, many BiPAP machines incorporate a back-up rate of 6–8 breaths per minute to prevent apnoea.

10.3.3 Indications for non-invasive ventilation

CPAP is generally used for patients with acute cardiogenic pulmonary oedema and BiPAP for those with acute hypercapnic respiratory failure in COPD. However, NIV may be used in other conditions, particularly if intubation and ventilation is not considered suitable for the patient.

Potential indications for CPAP:

- Cardiogenic pulmonary oedema refractory to medical therapy
- Acute hypoxaemic respiratory failure (if not suitable for immediate intubation)

Potential indications for BiPAP:

- Acute hypercapnic respiratory failure in COPD
- Acute hypercapnic respiratory failure in patients with chest wall deformity, neuromuscular disorder, or decompensated obstructive sleep apnoea
- Cardiogenic pulmonary oedema refractory to CPAP
- Patients where intubation may not be appropriate
- Type 1 respiratory failure resistant to oxygen therapy (only in HDU/ITU setting)
- Patients weaning from mechanical ventilation

COPD

BiPAP is a well-recognized treatment modality for patients with an acute exacerbation of COPD. It should be considered when patients fulfil the following criteria:

- pH 7.25–7.35 (below 7.25 patients respond poorly to NIV)
- $PaCO_2$ >6 kPa
- Despite maximal medical treatment (controlled oxygen to maintain saturations 88–92%; nebulized salbutamol 5 mg; nebulized ipratropium bromide 500 mcg; prednisolone 30 mg; antibiotics when indicated)

Cardiogenic pulmonary oedema

CPAP is widely used for the treatment of acute cardiogenic pulmonary oedema. There is not a set of blood gas criteria for cardiogenic pulmonary oedema as there is for COPD. The judgement to start CPAP is a clinical one.

CPAP has been shown to improve physiological parameters and reduce intubation rates, but has not been shown to reduce mortality in cardiogenic pulmonary oedema.

10.3.4 Contraindications for non-invasive ventilation

The most important contraindication for NIV is the need for immediate intubation and ventilation.

As experience with NIV has increased, many of the factors previously considered to be contraindications are now relative (Table 10.2). If NIV is the 'ceiling' of treatment for a patient, then many of the contraindications are negated. There is evidence to support the use of NIV in patients who are comatose secondary to COPD-induced hypercapnea, who may quickly become conscious as the $PaCO_2$ decreases.

10.3.5 Patient selection for non-invasive ventilation

Prior to commencing NIV, a plan should be made of the next management step if NIV is unsuccessful. Patients who may require NIV should be stratified into one of five groups, which should be clearly documented in the notes:

- Requires immediate intubation and ventilation (NIV contraindicated).
- Suitable for NIV and suitable for escalation to intensive care treatment/intubation and ventilation if required.
- Suitable for NIV but not suitable for escalation to intensive care treatment/intubation and ventilation.
- Not suitable for NIV but for full active medical management.
- Palliative care agreed as most appropriate management.

10.3.6 Settings for non-invasive ventilation

- CPAP—start at 5 cmH_2O and increase to a maximum of 15 cmH_2O as tolerated.
- BiPAP—start with an EPAP of 3–5 cmH_2O and an IPAP of 10 cmH_2O. Increase the IPAP by 2–5 cmH_2O increments to a target of 20 cmH_2O as tolerated. Increasing the inspired oxygen concentration will improve oxygenation and increasing the IPAP will improve respiratory acidosis. Target oxygen saturations are 88–92%, in patients with hypercapnic respiratory failure. Target pH $\geq$ 7.35.

Table 10.2 Inclusion and exclusion criteria for non-invasive ventilation (NIV)

Inclusion criteria	Exclusion criteria
<ul><li>*Able to protect airway</li><li>*Conscious and cooperative</li><li>Potential for recovery to quality of life acceptable to the patient</li><li>Patient's wishes considered</li><li>*Consider NIV if the patient is unconscious and endotracheal intubation deemed inappropriate or NIV is to be provided in a critical care setting</li></ul>	<ul><li>Life-threatening hypoxaemia</li><li>Severe co-morbidity</li><li>Confusion/agitation/severe cognitive impairment</li><li>Facial burns/trauma/recent facial or upper airway surgery</li><li>Vomiting</li><li>Fixed upper airway obstruction</li><li>Undrained pneumothorax</li><li>Upper gastrointestinal surgery</li><li>Inability to protect the airway</li><li>Copious respiratory secretions</li><li>Haemodynamically unstable requiring inotropes or vasopressors (unless in a critical care unit)</li><li>Patient moribund</li><li>Bowel obstruction</li></ul>

10.3.7 Monitoring for non-invasive ventilation

- The patient should be managed in the resuscitation room.
- Regular assessment of respiratory rate, effort of breathing, coordination of respiratory effort with the ventilator, GCS, and heart rate should be made. The patient should have continual oxygen saturation monitoring.
- The frequency of arterial blood gas analysis should be determined by the patient's condition but should be measured one hour after starting NIV and one hour after every subsequent change in settings.

10.3.8 Complications of non-invasive ventilation

- Hypotension—due to increased intrathoracic pressure, which reduces preload. The effects are exacerbated if the patient is hypovolaemic.
- Barotrauma—may occur due to gas trapping and overinflation. Pneumothorax is a rare complication.
- Gastric distension—may occur. However, not every patient requires a prophylactic nasogastric (NG) tube.
- Pulmonary aspiration—may occur if the patient vomits or regurgitates into a tight-fitting facemask.
- Pressure necrosis—of the bridge of the nose. This is less problematic with more modern masks.
- Discomfort—for the patient due to the tight-fitting mask.

KEY POINTS

Non-invasive ventilation is ventilatory support though a patient's upper airway using a mask.

CPAP provides a constant positive pressure throughout a patient's respiratory cycle.

BiPAP is a combination of CPAP with pressure support, which augments a patient's own respiratory effort and increases tidal volume.

CPAP works by improving oxygenation and reducing the work of breathing.

BiPAP provides the benefits of CPAP in addition to improving alveolar ventilation and reducing the respiratory rate.

CPAP should be considered for those with acute cardiogenic pulmonary oedema.

BiPAP should be considered for those with acute hypercapnic respiratory failure secondary to COPD.

The only absolute contraindication to NIV is an immediate indication for intubation and ventilation.

The 'ceiling' of treatment should be decided and documented before starting NIV.

10.4 Venous thromboembolism

10.4.1 Introduction

Venous thromboembolism (VTE) is the term used to describe the formation of a thrombus in a vein, which may dislodge from its site of origin and embolize. Venous thromboembolic disease represents a spectrum that includes deep venous thrombosis (DVT) and pulmonary embolism (PE).

VTE has a significant morbidity and mortality, with 25,000 people dying each year.

10.4.2 Deep vein thrombosis

Deep venous thrombosis commonly affects the veins of the legs (e.g. popliteal or femoral) or the deep veins of the pelvis. Occasionally a DVT may form in an upper limb.

The main risk from a DVT is that it may embolize, causing a fatal PE. There is also the potential of developing post-thrombotic syndrome, which causes chronic leg swelling and ulceration.

Clinical features of deep vein thrombosis

The classic presentation of a DVT is:

- Leg pain
- Swelling
- Warmth
- Tenderness
- Dilated superficial veins

However, a DVT may be completely asymptomatic. History and clinical examination alone cannot reliably exclude a DVT and, if it is suspected, further investigation is required.

Risk stratification in suspected DVT

There are multiple risk factors for DVT and risk stratification scores have been developed to guide investigations. The most commonly used risk stratification tool is the modified (two-level) Wells' criteria. This dichotomous scoring system replaced the original Wells' score.

Investigations for deep vein thrombosis

- D-dimer is a marker of endogenous fibrinolysis. It is a sensitive but non-specific marker of DVT. Patients who score <2 on the modified Wells' criteria are suitable for D-dimer testing. If the D-dimer is negative a DVT can be excluded. Patients with a score ≥2 require further investigation and therefore a D-dimer is not indicated.
- Compression ultrasound of proximal leg veins—ultrasound imaging is required in those patients who score ≥2 on the modified Wells' criteria or have a positive D-dimer. The ultrasound scan should be carried out within four hours of being requested, or within 24 hours of being requested after provision of an interim 24 hour dose of parenteral anticoagulant. The proximal leg vein ultrasound scan should be repeated in six to eight days for all patients with a positive D-dimer test and a negative proximal leg vein ultrasound scan.
- Alternative diagnoses must be considered in patients with an unlikely Wells score (1 point or less) and either a negative D-dimer test, or a positive D-dimer test and a negative proximal leg vein ultrasound scan.

Treatment of deep vein thrombosis

- Low molecular weight heparin (LMWH) should be commenced once a DVT is suspected until the diagnosis if confirmed or excluded.
- Warfarin is indicated if a DVT is confirmed. Treatment is usually for three months but may be longer in patients with persisting risk factors.

10.4.3 Pulmonary embolism

Pulmonary embolism is a common, life-threatening condition that can be notoriously difficult to diagnose.

Clinical features of pulmonary embolism

Most patients with PE are breathless and/or tachypnoeic (respiratory rate >20 breaths per minute) but the absence of these features is not sensitive enough to reliable exclude the diagnosis. The classic clinical features are:

- Pleuritic chest pain
- Haemoptysis
- Dyspnoea
- Tachycardia
- Tachypnoea
- Mild fever
- Cyanosis
- Elevated JVP

Risk factors for pulmonary embolism

There are many predisposing factors for a PE. All patients with a possible PE should have their clinical probability assessed and documented. The two most commonly used risk stratification tools are the BTS guidance and the Wells' criteria.

The BTS guidelines recommend that the clinical probability of a PE be assessed by asking two questions:

1. Is another diagnosis unlikely?
2. Is there a major risk factor? (see list below)

The patient is considered low probability if the answer to both these questions is no; intermediate probability if one answer is positive; and high if both are positive.

Major risk factors for VTE (BTS guidance):

- Recent immobility
- Major surgery
- Lower limb trauma or surgery
- Pregnancy/post partum
- Major medical illness
- Previous proven VTE

The Wells' criteria for pre-test probability of PE are shown in Table 10.3.

Confusion can sometimes arise about the cut-off values for the Wells' score. Some of this confusion is due to the multitude of publications about the subject, some of which suggest alternative cut-off values. The cut-off can also depend on the D-dimer assay used in certain hospitals. Therefore, there is local variation and some hospitals place the cut-off at 4 points dividing patients into two categories: high risk (>4) or low risk (≤4). The values in Table 10.3 are based on the publication by Wells et al. in 2001.

EXAM TIP

The most commonly used risk-assessment tools for PE are the BTS guidance and the Wells' criteria for PE. It is not necessary to know both scoring systems for the exam—one will suffice. Both have been included here for completeness.

It is probably easiest to remember the tool used in your local hospital because you can revise it each time you assess a patient with a possible PE.

Table 10.3 Wells' score for pre-test probability of pulmonary embolism (PE)

Feature	Score
Clinical signs or symptoms of DVT (objectively measured leg swelling and pain with palpation in the deep vein region)	3
Alternative diagnosis less likely than PE	3
Heart rate >100 bpm	1.5
Immobilization or surgery in the previous four weeks	1.5
History of DVT or PE	1.5
Haemoptysis	1
Malignancy (active treatment, treatment in the last six months, or palliative)	1

Total score

Score <2 = low pre-test probability of PE (1.6% chance of PE)
Score 2-6 = moderate pre-test probability of PE (16.2% chance of PE)
Score >6 = high pre-test probability of PE (37.5% chance of PE)

Data from Wells P, Anderson D, Rodger M, et al. Excluding Pulmonary Embolism at the Bedside without Diagnostic Imaging: Management of Patients with Suspected Pulmonary Embolism Presenting to the Emergency Department by Using a Simple Clinical Model and D-Dimer. Ann Intern Med July 17, 2001 135:98–107.

Investigations for pulmonary embolism

- D-dimer:
  - It should not be used as a routine screening test for PE and should only be considered after the assessment of clinical probability.
  - It should not be performed in those with a high clinical probability of PE.
  - It is indicated in patients with low clinical probability (unlikely Wells score of 4 points or less); a negative D-dimer can reliably exclude a PE in this group.
  - The use of D-dimer in patients with intermediate clinical probability depends on the assay used. ELISA (Vidas) and latex (MDA) tests are considered sensitive enough to exclude PE in patients with intermediate clinical probability. Agglutination (SimpliRED) tests are only suitable for patients with a low pre-test clinical probability of PE.
- ECG—may be useful for excluding other causes. The commonest abnormality in a PE is sinus tachycardia. Other abnormalities include AF, RBBB, RAD, right ventricular strain. The 'S_1, Q_3, T_3' pattern is rarely seen.
- CXR—may show pulmonary oligaemia, an elevated hemidiaphragm, a small pleural effusion, or linear opacities (the result of previous PEs). It may also reveal an alternative diagnosis such as a pneumonia, pneumothorax, or lobar collapse.
- CT pulmonary angiogram (CTPA)—is the recommended initial lung imaging modality for patients with a suspected pulmonary embolism and a likely Wells score (more than 4 points). CTPA should be performed immediately or preceded by immediate interim parenteral anticoagulant therapy, if not immediately available. A proximal leg vein ultrasound scan should be considered if the CTPA is negative and DVT is suspected.
- For patients with contrast media allergy, renal impairment, or at high risk from radiation, ventilation/perfusion single photon emission computed tomography (V/Q SPECT) scan or a V/Q planar scan should be considered.

- Bedside echocardiography is useful in unstable patients with suspected massive PE, as right ventricular dilatation, right ventricular hypokinesia/dysfunction, free-floating thrombus, or pulmonary arterial hypertension can be detected.
- Thrombophilia screening is recommended in patients with unprovoked DVT or PE or who have a first-degree relative who has had DVT or PE, if it is planned to stop anticoagulant therapy. It should not be measured acutely, because the thrombus can distort the results.
- Arterial blood gases—are useful if there are concerns about the patient's ventilatory status. However, they do not have a role in diagnosing a PE due to a lack of sensitivity and specificity. Normal arterial blood gases do not exclude PE.
- Consider alternative diagnoses in patients with a likely Wells score and both negative CTPA and no suspected DVT, and in patients with an unlikely Wells score and either a negative D-dimer test or a positive D-dimer test and a negative CTPA.
- Patients with unprovoked pulmonary embolism should be investigated for the possibility of undiagnosed cancer, including a full history and physical examination, CXR, blood tests (including full blood count, serum calcium and liver function tests) and urinalysis, with the consideration of abdominopelvic Computed tomography (CT) scanning and mammography in all patients over 40.

Treatment of pulmonary embolism

- Supplemental oxygen should be given if the patient is hypoxic.
- LMWH should be started once a PE is suspected and until it is confirmed or excluded. Heparins are of animal origin and this may be of concern to patients with certain religious or other beliefs.
- Unfractionated heparin may be considered in the following circumstances: as an initial first dose due to its quicker onset; if rapid reversal may be needed; or in a massive PE.
- Warfarin is indicated once a PE is confirmed. The length of anticoagulation depends on the risk factors present.
- Novel oral anticoagulant agents such as dabigatran and rivaroxaban are increasingly being used.

10.4.4 Massive pulmonary embolism

Massive PE is likely in patients with collapse, hypotension, unexplained hypoxia, engorged neck veins, and right ventricular gallop.

Thrombolysis is the first-line treatment in massive PE and it may be instituted on clinical grounds alone if cardiac arrest is imminent.

CTPA or echocardiography will reliably diagnose clinically massive PE if the patient's condition permits.

Alteplase is the thrombolysis agent recommended by BTS:

- The dose is 100 mg in stable patients with a confirmed diagnosis.
- The dose is 50 mg in unstable patients.
- Thrombolysis is followed by unfractionated heparin after three hours.

Other invasive options available in some units are clot fragmentation via a pulmonary artery catheter or embolectomy.

10.4.5 Venous thromboembolism in pregnancy

VTE remains the main direct cause of maternal death in the United Kingdom and sequential reports of Confidential Enquiries into Maternal Deaths have highlighted failures in obtaining objective diagnoses and employing adequate treatment.

VTE is up to 10 times more common in pregnant women than in non-pregnant women of the same age, and can occur at any stage of pregnancy but the puerperium is the time of highest risk.

The following section, 'D-dimer in preganancy' is based on the guidance in the Royal College of Obstetricians and Gynaecologists (RCOG) Green-top guideline 'Thrombosis and embolism during pregnancy and the puerperium, reducing the risk' (see Further reading).

D-dimer in pregnancy

The recommendation from the RCOG is that a D-dimer should not be performed to diagnose acute VTE in pregnancy.

In pregnancy, D-dimer can be elevated because of the physiological changes in the coagulation system and levels become 'abnormal' at term and in the postnatal period in most healthy women. D-dimer levels are also elevated by conditions such as pre-eclampsia. Therefore, a positive D-dimer is not necessarily consistent with VTE and objective testing is required.

A low level of D-dimer is likely, as in the non-pregnant woman, to suggest that there is no VTE. However, pregnancy increases the pre-test probability of a PE and, therefore, even if the D-dimer is negative a proportion of women will still have a VTE (how many depends on the sensitivity of the D-dimer assay). Therefore, the RCOG do not recommend testing D-dimer in pregnant women.

The BTS guidance does allow for the use of D-dimer in pregnancy provided another diagnosis is more likely than a PE (i.e. the patient is intermediate risk), and the D-dimer assay is sufficiently sensitive.

Therefore, careful consideration needs to be given to the patient's clinical probability of a VTE before performing a D-dimer.

Suspected deep venous thrombosis in pregnancy

- LMWH should be started once a DVT is suspected and continued until a diagnosis is achieved.
- D-dimer testing is not recommended by the RCOG.
- Compression duplex ultrasound is the investigation of choice for patients with a suspected DVT.
- If a DVT is confirmed, the patient should continue LMWH. LMWH does not cross the placenta. Warfarin is teratogenic and should not be prescribed in pregnancy, but is safe for use in breast feeding.

Suspected pulmonary embolism in pregnancy

- If a PE is clinically suspected, a CXR should be performed. The CXR may identify other pulmonary disease such as pneumonia, pneumothorax, or lobar collapse. The radiation dose to a foetus at any stage of pregnancy is negligible.
- If there is clinical suspicion of a DVT, Doppler ultrasound leg studies should be performed. The diagnosis of DVT may indirectly confirm a diagnosis of PE. The anticoagulant treatment for DVT and PE is the same and therefore further investigation may not be necessary, limiting the radiation dose given to the mother and foetus.
- In the case of a normal Doppler ultrasound (USS) or the absence of signs of a DVT and ongoing clinical suspicion of acute PE, then a V/Q scan or CTPA should be performed.
- V/Q scan is recommended over CTPA scan in the presence of a normal CXR.
- Women should be advised that a V/Q scan carries a slightly increased risk of childhood cancer compared with CTPA (1/280,000 versus less than 1/1,000,000) but carries a lower risk of maternal breast cancer (lifetime risk increased by up to 13.6% with CTPA, background risk of 1/200 for study population).
- Women should be involved in the decision to undergo CTPA or V/Q scanning and, ideally, informed consent should be obtained before these tests are undertaken.
- Treatment with LMWH should be commenced and continued until VTE has been excluded.
- LMWH dose should be based on pre-pregnancy or early pregnancy weight. There is no convincing evidence of dosing regimens (e.g. once daily or split dosing).

- In the case of massive PE, treatment should involve a multidisciplinary team. Intravenous heparin is preferred over thrombolysis.

KEY POINTS

Venous thromboembolic disease represents a spectrum that includes DVT and PE.

All patients with a possible VTE should have their clinical probability assessed and documented.

The most commonly used risk stratification tool for DVT is the modified Wells' criteria. It is composed of 10 variables with a potential score of –2 to + 8. Score ≥2 indicates that the probability of a DVT is likely. Score <2 indicates that the probability of a DVT is unlikely.

The two most commonly used risk stratification tools for PE are the BTS guidance and the Wells' criteria. The scores categorize patients as low, intermediate, or high risk.

D-dimer is a marker of endogenous fibrinolysis. It is a sensitive but non-specific marker of VTE. A D-dimer should only be considered after assessment of clinical probability. It should not be used as a screening test.

Patients with a suspected VTE should be started on LMWH until a diagnosis is made.

Massive PE is likely in patients with collapse, hypotension, unexplained hypoxia, engorged neck veins, and right ventricular gallop.

Thrombolysis (alteplase) is the first-line treatment in massive PE and it may be instituted on clinical grounds alone if cardiac arrest is imminent.

10.5 Pneumonia

10.5.1 Introduction

Pneumonia is a common ED presentation. The BTS have published guidance on the management of adults and children who have a community-acquired pneumonia. The main points for adults are detailed in this section. The management of pneumonia in children is covered in Chapter 19, section 19.13.

10.5.2 Definition of community-acquired pneumonia

The BTS guidance defines community-acquired pneumonia (CAP) in patients admitted to hospital as:

- symptom and signs consistent with an acute lower respiratory tract infection (e.g. cough, dyspnoea, tachypnoea, pleural pain, fever, new focal signs on chest examination, and so on), and;
- new radiographic shadowing for which there is no other explanation (e.g. not pulmonary oedema or infarction).

10.5.3 Causes of community-acquired pneumonia

The commonest causes of CAP are:

- Bacterial—*Strep. pneumoniae* (commonest), *H. influenza*, *Legionella*, *Staph. aureus*.
- Viral—influenza A and B, respiratory syncytial virus.

The atypical pathogens that may cause CAP are:

- *Mycoplasma pneumoniae*.
- *Chlamydia pneumoniae*.

- *Chlamydia psittaci.*
- *Coxiella burnetii.*

Atypical pathogens are characterized by being difficult to diagnose early in the illness and being sensitive to antibiotics other than β lactams, such as macrolides, tetracyclines, or fluoroquinolones.

10.5.4 Severity assessment of community-acquired pneumonia

Previous MRCEM question

CURB-65 is a well-established tool for assessing the severity of pneumonia in adults and has appeared in previous SAQs; 1 point is gained for each feature present (Table 10.4).

10.5.5 Investigations in community-acquired pneumonia

The following investigations are recommended on patients requiring hospital admission for CAP.

- CXR—should be performed on all admitted patients with suspected CAP as soon as possible to confirm or refute the diagnosis.
- Blood tests—FBC, urea and electrolytes (to inform severity), LFTs, and CRP (to aid diagnosis and as a baseline measure) are recommended by BTS.
- Oxygen saturations and, if necessary, arterial blood gases in accordance with the BTS guideline for emergency oxygen use (section 10.7).
- Microbiological testing—guided by the severity of the CAP. Patients with moderate (CURB-65 = 2) or high severity (CURB-65 = 3–5) CAP should have the following performed:
  - blood cultures
  - sputum culture
  - pneumococcal and legionella urine antigen testing.
- Sputum testing for *Mycobacterium tuberculosis* should be considered in patients with a persistent productive cough, especially if they have malaise, night sweats, weight loss, or risk factors for TB (e.g. social deprivation, ethnic origin, elderly).
- Patients with mild pneumonia do not routinely require a full range of microbiological tests and these should be guided by clinical factors, epidemiological factors, and prior antibiotic therapy.

Table 10.4 CURB-65 score

Feature	Parameter
Confusion	Abbreviated mental test score ≤8
Urea	>7 mmol/L
Respiratory rate	≥30/min
Blood pressure	Systolic <90 mmHg or diastolic ≤60 mmHg
Age	≥65

Score 0 or 1: Low risk (<3% mortality risk)
Score 2: Intermediate risk (3–15% mortality risk)
Score 3 to 5: High risk of death and hospital treatment urgently required (mortality risk >15%). Early review by critical care should be considered.

Data from Lim WS, van der Eerden MM, Laing R, et al. 'Defining community acquired pneumonia severity on presentation to hospital: an international derivation and validation study'. Thorax 2003;58:377–82.

10.5.6 Emergency department treatment of community-acquired pneumonia

- Oxygen therapy—should be given, if required, to maintain saturations between 94 and 98%. If the patient is at risk of hypercapnic respiratory failure, target saturations between 88% and 92% initially and then guide oxygen therapy as based on arterial blood gas measurements.
- Intravenous fluids—should be given if there is evidence of volume depletion.
- Antibiotic therapy—guided by local microbiology policy (see Table 10.7 for possible regimes).
- A five-day course of a single antibiotic should be offered to patients with low-severity community-acquired pneumonia; amoxicillin should be considered in preference to a macrolide or a tetracycline in the absence of penicillin allergy. A fluoroquinolone or dual antibiotic therapy should not be routinely offered. A 7–10 day course of dual antibiotic therapy with amoxicillin and a macrolide should be considered for patients with moderate-severity community-acquired pneumonia.
- Prophylaxis of VTE with LMWH should be considered in patients who are not fully mobile.
- Critical care involvement should be considered for patients with high severity CAP.

KEY POINTS

The definition of community-acquired pneumonia in patients admitted to hospital is symptoms and signs consistent with an acute lower respiratory tract infection and new radiographic shadowing, for which there is no other explanation.

Strep. pneumoniae is the commonest cause of community-acquired pneumonia.

A CXR should be performed on all admitted patients with suspected CAP as soon as possible to confirm or refute the diagnosis.

CURB-65 is a well-established tool for assessing the severity of pneumonia in adults.

- Confusion—abbreviated mental test score ≤8
- Urea—>7 mmol/L
- Respiratory rate—≥30/min
- Blood pressure—systolic <90 mmHg or diastolic ≤60 mmHg
- Age ≥65

Table 10.5 Possible antibiotic therapies for community-acquired pneumonia

Pneumonia severity	Antibiotic guidance	
	Preferred treatment	Alternative treatment
Low (CURB-65 = 0–1)	Amoxicillin 500 mg tds orally	Doxycycline 200 mg loading dose then 100 mg orally or clarithromycin 500 mg bd orally
Moderate (CURB-65 = 2)	Amoxicillin 500 mg–1.0 g tds orally plus clarithromycin 500 mg bd orally	Doxycycline 200 mg loading dose then 100 mg orally or levofloxacin 500 mg od orally or moxifloxacin 400 mg od orally
High (CURB-65 ≥3)	Co-amoxiclav 1.2 g tds IV plus clarithromycin 500 mg bd IV	Benzylpenicillin 1.2 g qds IV plus either levofloxacin 500 mg bd IV or ciprofloxacin 400 mg bd IV, or
		cefuroxime 1.5 g tds IV or cefotaxime 1 g tds IV, or ceftriaxone 2 g od IV, plus clarithromycin 500 mg bd IV

10.6 Spontaneous pneumothorax

10.6.1 Introduction

A pneumothorax is air in the pleural space.

- Primary pneumothoraces arise in patients with no previous lung disease.
- Secondary pneumothoraces arise in patients with underlying lung pathology (most commonly COPD).

10.6.2 Clinical features of pneumothorax

The size of the pneumothorax cannot reliable be determined from the history and in smaller pneumothoraces clinical examination may be entirely normal.

Characteristic features include:

- Chest pain
- Dyspnoea
- Reduced air entry on affected side
- Hyperresonance on affected side
- Reduced expansion on the affected side

If a patient has severe symptoms accompanied by signs of cardiorespiratory distress, a tension pneumothorax should be considered.

10.6.3 Investigations for pneumothorax

- CXR is the recommended initial investigation for suspected pneumothorax. The BTS guidance on the management of a spontaneous pneumothorax is based on the size, degree of clinical compromise, and history of pre-existing lung disease.
  - Small—<2 cm rim of air on CXR, between the lung margin and chest wall (at the level of the hilum).
  - Large—≥2 cm rim of air on CXR (this approximates to a ≥50% pneumothorax).
- On bedside ultrasound scanning, if a pneumothorax is present, there is lack of dynamic pleural sliding with respiration (sliding sign) and loss of vertical comet-tail artefacts at the pleural interface. Horizontal hyperechoic lines (A-lines) secondary to reverberation, found at twice the distance from the skin to pleura, provide further confirmation. Bedside USS cannot, however, be used to comment on the size of the pneumothorax.
- CT scanning is recommended if the diagnosis is uncertain or for complex cases.
- Arterial blood gas analysis is not required if the oxygen saturations are adequate (>92%) on breathing room air.

10.6.4 Management strategies for spontaneous pneumothoraces

Patients with pre-existing lung disease tolerate a pneumothorax less well, and the distinction between primary and secondary pneumothorax should be made at the time of diagnosis to guide appropriate management.

Breathlessness indicates the need for active intervention regardless of the size, as well as supportive treatment (including oxygen).

The size of the pneumothorax determines the rate of resolution and is a relative indication for active intervention.

Figure 10.3 shows a flowchart for the management of spontaneous pneumothorax based on the BTS guidance.

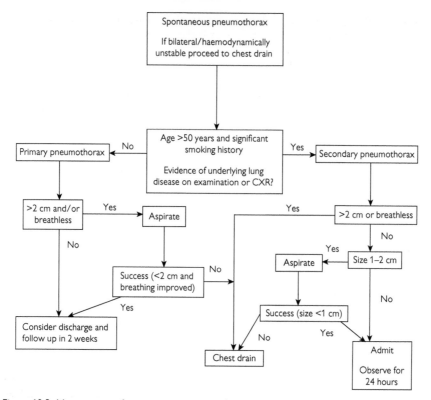

Figure 10.3 Management of spontaneous pneumothorax

Reproduced from *Thorax*, Andrew MacDuff, Anthony Arnold, John Harvey, on behalf of the BTS Pleural Disease Guideline Group, Management of spontaneous pneumothorax: British Thoracic Society pleural disease guideline 2010, volumn 65, suppl 2 pp.ii18-ii31, copyright 2010 with permission from BMJ Publishing Group Ltd.

10.6.5 Emergency department treatment for a spontaneous pneumothorax

- The size of the pneumothorax is less important than the degree of clinical compromise. Accurate pneumothorax size calculations require CT scanning.
- Active intervention is needed for patients with primary or secondary spontaneous pneumothorax and significant breathlessness, irrespective of size.
- Patients with a small primary spontaneous pneumothorax (PSP), without significant breathlessness, and selected asymptomatic patients with a large PSP may be managed by observation alone.
- Supplemental oxygen should be given to patients with secondary spontaneous pneumothoraces who are breathless and hypoxaemic. Oxygen should be titrated as per BTS emergency oxygen guidelines.
- Needle aspiration with a 14–16-G cannula should be performed in eligible patients (as per Figure 10.3). Infiltrate just above the third rib with 10 ml 1% lidocaine. Insert 16 gauge or 18 gauge intravenous cannula in second intercostal space in the mid-clavicular line and remove the inner needle. Aspirate with 20 ml syringe to confirm release of air. Remove syringe and replace with a three-way tap and 50 ml syringe. The third port should have a cut piece of IV tubing

attached, running into a jug of sterile water. Aspirate air into the 50 ml syringe and expel into the water jug. Continue until resistance is felt or more than 2.5 litres of air have been aspirated, because further expansion is unlikely since the patient is likely to have a persistent air leak. Stop aspiration if the patient coughs excessively. Needle aspiration should not be repeated unless there were technical difficulties.

- If indicated (Figure 10.3), an intercostal drain should be inserted in the fifth intercostal space just anterior to mid-axillary line. A small bore (8–14 F) Seldinger drain is recommended.
- Analgesia should be prescribed, as necessary.

10.6.6 Discharge advice following a spontaneous pneumothorax

Patients with primary pneumothorax who are managed conservatively or have a successful aspiration can be discharged from the ED. Follow-up should be arranged with a respiratory physician.

Patients should be given the following discharge advice:

- Repeat CXR at two to four weeks.
- Air travel is not possible until a CXR has confirmed resolution (airlines have previously arbitrarily stated a six-week interval between having a pneumothorax and flying but this has since been amended to one week after full resolution).
- Diving should be permanently avoided.
- Advice to stop smoking (cessation reduces the risk of recurrence).
- Resume work and normal activities once all symptoms have resolved.
- Return immediately to the ED if symptoms recur.

KEY POINTS

Primary pneumothoraces arise in patients with no previous lung disease.

Secondary pneumothoraces arise in patients with underlying lung pathology.

The management of spontaneous pneumothorax depends on whether it is primary or secondary; symptomatic or asymptomatic; large or small.

The main treatment options are:

- 1°, asymptomatic, small pneumothorax—observe as an outpatient (repeat CXR after two to four weeks).
- 1°, symptomatic (breathlessness) or large pneumothorax—aspirate and discharge if successful. If unsuccessful, then insert a small intercostal drain.
- 2° pneumothorax, which is small (1–2 cm) and with minimal symptoms—aspirate and admit for 24 h observation. If following aspiration the pneumothorax is still >1 cm, then insert an intercostal drain.
- 2° pneumothorax which is very small (<1 cm) and with minimal symptoms—manage conservatively and admit the patient for 24 h observation.
- 2° pneumothorax which is symptomatic or large—insert an intercostal drain.

10.7 Haemoptysis

Haemoptysis is the act of coughing up blood or blood stained mucous which can originate from anywhere along the respiratory tract (larynx/trachea/bronchi/lungs). In addition to the pulmonary causes of haemoptysis, there are also extrapulmonary causes (see Table 10.6).

Table 10.6 Causes of haemoptysis

Pulmonary	Cardiac	Vasculitis
Tracheobronchitis	Pulmonary embolism	Systemic lupus erythematosus
Chronic bronchitis	Left ventricular failure	Wegener's granulomatosis
Bronchiectasis	Mitral stenosis	Goodpasture's syndrome
Pneumonia	Pulmonary hypertension	
Pulmonary infarction	Aortobronchial fistula	
Tuberculosis		
Pulmonary mycetoma		
Pulmonary sequestration		
Arteriovenous malformations		
Bronchogenic carcinoma		
Lung abscess		
Aspergilloma		
Trauma		
Iatrogenic		

10.7.1 Causes of haemoptysis

10.7.2 Massive haemoptysis

Massive haemoptysis is classified as:

● >400 ml over 3 hours
● > 600 ml over 24 hours

Massive haemoptysis is usually from systemic bronchial arteries rather than the low pressure pulmonary arterial system. The amount of bleeding has no relationship to the gravity of the underlying pulmonary lesion. The primary goals of intervention are to lateralize the source of bleeding and to directly protect the contralateral lung from drowning.

   Management of massive haemoptysis includes:

● High-flow inspired oxygen.
● Place bleeding lung dependent.
● Bronchoscopy to clear the airway, localize the site of bleeding, and institute local control measures. This is best achieved by a combination of rigid and fibre-optic flexible bronchoscopy under general anaesthesia.
● In patients not suitable for lung (lobe) resection but who continue to bleed (especially from cavities in the lung, which are almost always fed by bronchial arteries), embolization of the bronchial artery under radiographic control is an alternative.
● Radiation treatment may be helpful if the bleeding is due to cavitating cancer.

10.8 Respiratory failure and oxygen therapy

10.8.1 Respiratory failure

Respiratory failure occurs when gas exchange is inadequate leading to hypoxia. It is defined as a PaO_2 below 8 kPa. There are two types of respiratory failure:

- Type 1 failure (oxygenation failure): hypoxaemia (PaO_2 < 8 kPa) with a normal or low $PaCO_2$. It is usually due to a ventilation/perfusion mismatch. Causes include pneumonia, asthma, pulmonary oedema, PE, and ARDS.
- Type 2 failure (ventilatory failure): hypoxaemia with hypercapnea ($PaCO_2$ > 6.5 kPa). Due to hypoventilation, most commonly caused by COPD but also obstructive sleep apnoea, chest wall deformities, neuromuscular disease, and reduced respiratory drive (e.g. sedatives, head trauma).

10.8.2 Hypoxaemia

The causes of hypoxaemia are multifactorial but there are several distinct mechanisms:

- Alveolar hypoventilation
- Ventilation–perfusion mismatch
- Pulmonary diffusion defects
- Reduced inspired oxygen concentration

In nearly all patients hypoxaemia can initially be improved by increasing the inspired oxygen concentration.

Alveolar hypoventilation

This results in insufficient oxygen entering the alveoli to replace that taken up by the blood. It may be caused by airway obstruction (e.g. blood, vomit, tongue, bronchospasm); respiratory depression (e.g. head injury, stroke, drugs, alcohol); or impaired ventilation (e.g. pneumothorax, haemothorax, pulmonary oedema, diaphragmatic splinting).

Hypoventilation causes the alveolar partial pressure of oxygen (P_AO_2) and the arterial pressure of oxygen (PaO_2) to decrease, and the arterial partial pressure of carbon dioxide ($PaCO_2$) to increase.

In most patients, increasing the inspired oxygen concentration will restore alveolar and arterial PO_2. However, if a patients tidal volume decreases below approximately 150 ml, there is no ventilation of the alveoli, only the 'dead space' (the volume of the airways that plays no part in gas exchange). Therefore, no oxygen reaches the alveoli, irrespective of the inspired concentration. Ventilatory support is required in addition to oxygenation to improve the patient's condition.

Ventilation–perfusion (V/Q) mismatch

This results in an imbalance between the ventilated alveoli and perfused areas of the lung. It may be caused by impaired perfusion (e.g. PE or hypovolaemia) or impaired ventilation (e.g. pulmonary oedema, pneumonia, asthma).

If ventilation exceeds perfusion (V/Q>1), then this can be considered wasted ventilation because oxygen is not taken up from the non-perfused areas. If a large area of the lung is not perfused (e.g. massive PE), then the patient may become profoundly hypoxic.

If perfusion exceeds ventilation (V/Q<1), then blood leaving areas of poor or no ventilation remains 'venous' and is often referred to as shunted blood. This blood mixes with oxygenated blood leaving ventilated areas of lung. The final oxygen content depends on the relative proportions of these two regions.

The effect of small regions of V/Q mismatch can be corrected by increasing the inspired oxygen concentration; however, once more than 30% of the pulmonary blood flow passes through regions where V/Q <1 hypoxaemia is inevitable, even when breathing 100% oxygen. This is because the oxygen content of pulmonary blood flowing through regions ventilated with 100% oxygen can increase by only a small, finite amount, and this is insufficient to offset regions of low V/Q.

Pulmonary diffusion defects

This result from conditions which thicken the alveolar membrane (e.g. fibrosing alveolitis). This thickening impairs oxygen transfer into the blood. In the ED, this is managed by giving supplemental oxygen to increase the P_AO2.

Reduced oxygen concentration

This will result in a reduced amount of oxygen in the alveoli. In the ED it should not be possible to give a hypoxic mix (<21% oxygen); however, some anaesthetic machines may be able to deliver less than 21% oxygen.

10.8.3 Chronic CO_2 retention

Chronic CO_2 retention is a significant concern for the management of acutely short-of-breath patients in the ED. Inappropriate oxygen therapy in this group can result in a worsening of the patient's condition. There are several theories as to why patients with chronic CO_2 retention become increasingly hypercapnic with oxygen therapy.

Hypoxic drive theory

This is the most commonly cited reason in COPD patients but is increasingly disputed. The theory is that, due to the chronically high CO_2 levels, patients' chemoreceptors desensitize and rely on hypoxia to stimulate respiration. When high concentrations of oxygen are applied, this drive is lost and the respiratory rate decreases.

Release of pulmonary vasculature vasoconstriction

Poorly ventilated alveoli have low oxygen tensions, which causes reflex pulmonary vasoconstriction. This reflex avoids areas of lung being perfused that are hypoxic (avoiding a ventilation/perfusion mismatch). When high concentrations of oxygen are given, the alveoli are less hypoxic and the vasoconstriction is released. However, these alveoli are still poorly ventilated and have high CO_2 levels, resulting in worsening hypercapnoea.

Haldane effect

Unsaturated haemoglobin carries CO_2; however, when haemoglobin is saturated with oxygen, the CO_2 is displaced into the plasma resulting in an increase $PaCO_2$ level. In patients with normal lungs, increased ventilation can remove the extra CO_2 but in patients with diseased lungs and chronic hypoventilation, this is not possible.

10.8.4 Emergency oxygen guidelines

BTS published guidelines for the emergency use of oxygen in 2008 (see Further reading). The essence of the guidelines is that oxygen should be prescribed to achieve a target saturation range and patients receiving oxygen should be regularly monitored to keep within that range. The guidelines suggests aiming to achieve normal or near-normal oxygen saturations for all acutely ill patients, apart from those at risk of hypercapnic respiratory failure.

The main points relevant to ED management are summarized here:

- Oxygen is a treatment for hypoxaemia, not breathlessness.
- High-concentration oxygen should be administered to all critically ill patients.
- Oxygen saturations should be checked in all breathless and acutely ill patients (supplemented by arterial blood gases when necessary).
- Inspired oxygen concentration should be documented.
- Oxygen should be prescribed to achieve a target saturation of 94–98% for most acutely ill patients.
- Patients at risk of hypercapnic respiratory failure should have a target saturation of 88–92%.
- Oxygen delivery devices and flow rates should be adjusted to keep the oxygen saturations in the target range.
- Patients at risk of hypercapnic respiratory failure should have oxygen commenced at 28% via a Venturi mask with an initial target saturation of 88–92% pending blood gas analysis. Patients with a previous history of respiratory failure should start at 24%.

- If patients have an oxygen alert card, saturations should be aimed at the pre-specified range.
- Patients at risk of hypercapnic respiratory failure should have nebulizers driven by compressed air and supplemental oxygen given via nasal cannulae.

10.8.5 Pulse oximetry

Key points in the use of pulse oximeters in emergency medicine:

- Pulse oximeters are calibrated for adult haemoglobin.
- Do not indicate the adequacy of ventilation, especially if supplementary oxygen is being given.
- Must not be used with patients suspected of having inhaled carbon monoxide or other abnormal haemoglobins.
- There is a non-linear relationship between SpO_2 and oxygen partial pressure, which depends on the oxyhaemoglobin dissociation curve.

Potential sources of error with pulse oximetry

- Poorly adherent probe
- Dark skin
- Excessive motion: motion artefact
- Low signal-noise ratio with impaired peripheral perfusion—shock, cardiac arrest
- False nails—or blue, black, or green nail varnish
- Lipaemia—hyperlipidaemia, propofol infusion
- Bright ambient light
- Abnormal haemoglobins—carboxyhaemoglobin, methaemoglobin
- Intravenous dyes—methylene blues
- SpO_2 <80%
- Venous pulsations—obstructed venous return, severe right heart failure, dependent limb, tourniquet constriction

---

KEY POINTS

Respiratory failure occurs when gas exchange is inadequate leading to hypoxia. There are two types of respiratory failure:

- Type 1 failure (oxygenation failure): hypoxaemia (PaO_2 < 8 kPa) with a normal or low $PaCO_2$
- Type 2 failure (ventilatory failure): hypoxaemia with hypercapnea ($PaCO_2$ > 6.5 kPa)

The causes of hypoxaemia are multifactorial but there are several distinct mechanisms:

- Alveolar hypoventilation
- Ventilation–perfusion mismatch
- Pulmonary diffusion defects
- Reduced inspired oxygen concentration

There are several theories as to why patients with chronic CO_2 retention become increasingly hypercapnic with oxygen therapy:

- Hypoxic drive theory
- Release of pulmonary vasculature vasoconstriction
- Haldane effect

The essence of the BTS emergency oxygen guideline is that oxygen should be prescribed to achieve a target saturation range and patients receiving oxygen should be regularly monitored to keep within that range.

10.9 Arterial blood gas analysis

10.9.1 Introduction

Arterial blood gases (ABGs) are a very useful ED investigation when performed appropriately. They provide information about the acid-base balance, oxygenation, and ventilation of a patient.

10.9.2 Indications for arterial blood gases

The BTS emergency oxygen guidelines provide indications for when ABGs should be performed. These are:

- All critically ill patients.
- Unexpected or inappropriate hypoxaemia (oxygen saturations <94%) or any patient requiring oxygen to achieve this target range.
- Deteriorating oxygen saturations or increasing breathlessness in a patient with previously stable hypoxaemia (e.g. severe COPD).
- Any previously stable patient who deteriorates and requires significantly increased inspired oxygen concentration to maintain constant oxygen saturations.
- Any patient with risk factors for hypercapnic respiratory failure who develops acute breathlessness, deteriorating oxygen saturations, drowsiness, or other symptoms of CO_2 retention.
- Breathless patients who are thought to be at risk of metabolic conditions (e.g. diabetic ketoacidosis, acute renal failure).
- Acutely breathless or critically ill patients with poor peripheral circulation in whom a reliable oximetry signal cannot be obtained.
- Any other evidence from the patient's medical condition that would indicate that blood gas results would be useful in the clinical management (e.g. unexpected change in patient's clinical status).*

10.9.3 Normal values for an arterial blood gas

When performing an arterial blood gas, the concentration of inspired oxygen (FiO_2) must be known and documented. If the inspired oxygen concentration has recently changed, and if the patient's condition allows, the blood gas should be postponed for 15 minutes to give a truer reflection of the FiO2.

The 'normal' arterial blood gas values are:

- pH 7.35–7.45
- PaO_2 10.5–13.5 kPa (breathing room air)
- $PaCO_2$ 4.5–6.5 kPa
- HCO_3^- 22–28 mmol/L

10.9.4 Interpreting an arterial blood gas

Interpreting arterial blood gases can initially seem complicated and often worries candidates. One of the easiest ways to start interpreting an ABG is to ask five questions about the blood gas result:

1. Is the patient hypoxic?
   - Normal PaO_2 10.5–13.5 kPa (breathing room air).
   - Hypoxia can be present with a PaO_2 > 10.5 kPa if the patient is breathing supplemental oxygen and therefore the FiO_2 must always be recorded.

---

* Reproduced from *Thorax*, B R O'Driscoll, L S Howard, A G Davison, BTS guideline for emergency oxygen use in adult patients, vol 63, suppl 6, vi1-vi68, copyright 2008, with permission from BMJ Publishing Group Ltd.

2. Is the patient acidotic or alkalotic?
   - pH <7.35 is acidaemia.
   - pH >7.45 is alkalaemia.
3. What is the respiratory component? If the CO_2 is abnormal is it in keeping with the pH?
   - Normal $PaCO_2$ 4.5–6.5 KPa.
   - CO_2 is an acidic gas.
   - If there is an acidosis and the CO_2 is raised there is a primary respiratory acidosis.
   - It there is an acidosis and the CO_2 is low there is respiratory compensation (e.g. hyperventilation in diabetic ketoacidosis) or a mixed disorder (e.g. salicylate overdose).
   - If there is an alkalosis and the CO_2 is low there is a primary respiratory alkalosis.
   - If there is an alkalosis and the CO_2 is high there is respiratory compensation or a mixed disorder.
4. What is the metabolic component? If the HCO_3^- is abnormal is it in keeping with the pH?
   - Normal HCO_3^- 22–28 mmol/L.
   - HCO_3^- is alkaline.
   - If there is an alkalosis and the HCO_3^- is raised, there is a primary metabolic alkalosis.
   - If there is an alkalosis and the HCO_3^- is low, there is metabolic compensation or a mixed disorder.
   - If there is an acidosis and the HCO_3^- is raised, there is metabolic compensation (e.g. chronic type 2 respiratory failure) or a mixed disorder (e.g. recurrent vomiting).
   - If there is an acidosis and the HCO_3^- is low, there is a primary metabolic acidosis.
5. Combine the information in questions 2, 3, and 4 to determine the primary disturbance and if there is any compensation or a mixed picture.
   Once the primary disturbance has been assessed on a blood gas, it is necessary to determine if any compensation is occurring or if there is a mixed picture. Often the history given in the question stem enables the candidate to work out if there is compensation or a mixed picture.

10.9.5 Causes of acid-base disturbance

Metabolic acidosis ($\downarrow pH$, $\downarrow HCO3-$)

Metabolic acidosis may result from increased acid production, exogenous acid absorption, loss of HCO_3^-, or decreased acid elimination.

Mechanisms of increased acid production/absorption include:

- Tissue hypoxia due to cardiorespiratory depression, recurrent seizures, or impaired oxygen carrying capacity (e.g. carbon monoxide poisoning or methaemoglobinaemia).
- Poisoning by substances that are acids (e.g. salicylates).
- Poisoning by substances that have acid metabolites (e.g. toxic alcohols—methanol, ethylene glycol).
- Poisons that affect adenosine triphosphate consumption or production in mitochondria (e.g. paracetamol, sodium valproate, metformin, carbon monoxide, cyanide) by uncoupling oxidative phosphorylation or inhibiting cytochromes of the electron transport chain. This results in a lactic acidosis.
- Production of ketones (e.g. DKA, alcoholic ketoacidosis, or poisoning with ethanol or isoniazid).

Mechanism of HCO_3^- loss:

- Loss from the gastrointestinal tract (e.g. diarrhoea, pancreatic fistula).
- Loss from the renal tract (e.g. renal tubular acidosis).

Mechanisms of impaired acid elimination:

- Acute kidney injury.
- Toxic metabolites causing renal impairment (e.g. ethylene glycol).
- Poisons causing renal tubular acidosis (e.g. toluene).

Table 10.7 Causes of a metabolic acidosis

Metabolic acidosis with a raised anion gap	Metabolic acidosis with a normal anion gap
Methanol **U**raemia **D**iabetic ketoacidosis **P**araldehyde **I**ron/Isoniazid **L**actic acid **E**thanol/Ethylene glycol **S**alicylates Other causes include: Paracetamol toxicity Amphetamines Carbon monoxide Cocaine Metformin Rhabdomyolysis Alcoholic ketoacidosis	Gastrointestinal tract losses for HCO_3^- (e.g. diarrhoea, pancreatic fistula, small bowel fistula) Renal loss of HCO_3^- (e.g. renal tubular acidosis; type 2) Renal dysfunction and/or failure Hypoaldosteronism (e.g. type 4 renal tubular acidosis) Carbonic anhydrase inhibitor (acetazolamide) Extra chloride (e.g. ingestion of ammonium chloride, magnesium chloride)

The causes of metabolic acidosis can be divided into those with a raised or normal anion gap (Table 10.7). Calculation of the anion gap can help identify the most likely cause of metabolic acidosis.

The anion gap is equal to the difference between the plasma concentrations of the measured cations (Na^+ and K^+) and the measured anions (HCO_3- and $Cl-$). The anion gap estimates the unmeasured anions (e.g. phosphate, ketones, lactate, and so on).

The anion gap is calculated by the following formula:

$$(Na^+ + K^+) - (HCO_3 - C1).$$

An anion gap <18 mmol/L is considered to be normal. A high anion gap (>18) metabolic acidosis is associated with the addition of endogenous or exogenous acids, which is paired with an unmeasured anion. It can be remembered by the mnemonic 'MUDPILES'.

A normal anion gap metabolic acidosis occurs when there is gain of both H^+ and $Cl-$ ions, or a loss of HCO_3- and retention of $Cl-$. The anion gap is normal because HCO_3- and $Cl-$ are measured anions.

Osmolar gap

Osmolality is the number of osmoles per kg of solvent.

The serum osmolality can be measured in the laboratory and calculated. The difference between the two values is the osmolar gap and suggests the presence of another low molecular weight substance in the serum.

$$The calculated osmolality = 2(Na + K) + urea + glucose.$$

$$Osmolar gap = Measured - Calculated.$$

$$Normal < 10 mosmol/kg.$$

Causes of an increased osmolar gap include:

- Ethanol
- Ethylene glycol
- Methanol
- Mannitol
- Lactic acid
- Acetone
- Formaldehyde
- End-stage renal failure
- Paraldehyde

Metabolic alkalosis ($\uparrow$pH, $\uparrow$ HCO$_3^-$)

Metabolic alkalosis results from the loss of acid, the gain of alkali, or the contraction of the extra-cellular fluid compartment with a consequent change in bicarbonate concentration.

Causes of metabolic alkalosis include:

- Loss of acid—which may be via the gastrointestinal tract (e.g. vomiting or NG suction) or via the kidney (e.g. due to excess aldosterone—Conn's syndrome—increasing sodium–hydrogen exchange in the kidney).
- Shift of hydrogen ions into the intracellular space—mainly seen in hypokalaemia, where hydrogen ions move into the intracellular space to maintain neutrality.
- Alkali administration (e.g. bicarbonate infusion, excessive antacid consumption). Massive blood transfusion can also cause an alkalosis because citrate in the transfused blood is converted to bicarbonate.
- Contraction alkalosis—results from loss of bicarbonate-poor, chloride-rich extracellular fluid. This is mainly due to thiazide and loop-diuretics, which leads to contraction of the extracellular fluid volume and a relative increase in bicarbonate concentration.

Respiratory compensation occurs via hypoventilation. Treatment is directed at the underlying cause.

Respiratory acidosis ($\downarrow$pH, $\uparrow$CO$_2$)

Any cause of type two respiratory failure results in a primary respiratory acidosis. For example:

- Central nervous system (CNS) depression
- Neuromuscular disease
- Impaired lung ventilation (e.g. COPD)
- Acute airway obstruction

Respiratory alkalosis ($\uparrow$pH, $\downarrow$CO$_2$)

Any cause of hyperventilation can result in respiratory alkalosis:

- Increased CNS drive (e.g. stroke, SAH, meningitis)
- Anxiety
- Altitude
- Fever
- Pregnancy
- Medications (e.g. salicylates, aminophylline)
- Sepsis

- Carbon monoxide poisoning
- Hyperthyroidism
- Liver failure

10.9.6 Alveolar–arterial gradient (A–a gradient)

The A–a gradient is useful at determining whether hypoxia is due to a ventilation/perfusion mismatch. SAQs on PE may require an A–a gradient to be calculated.

The formula to calculate the A–a gradient is:

$$P_AO_2(\text{alveolar}) - PaO_2 \text{ arterial}$$

The P_AO_2 is calculated by the alveolar gas equation:

$$P_AO_2 - FiO2 \times (P_B - P_{SVP}) - (PaCO_2/RQ)$$

- P_B = The atmospheric pressure (101.3 kPa) at sea level
- P_{SVP} = The saturated vapour pressure of water (6.3 kPa)
- RQ = Respiratory quotient (0.8)

This formula can be abbreviated to:

$$FiO2 \times 95 - (PaCO_2/0.8).$$

The normal A–a result varies depending on age but an A–a gradient <2 kPa is normal in young adults up to 5 kPa in the elderly.

EXAM TIP

Interpretation of blood gases frequently appears in SAQs.

Here is an example blood gas interpretation.

A 19-year-old patient presents with suspected diabetic ketoacidosis and the following ABG result:

- pH 7.15
- $PaCO2$ 3.0 kPa
- $PaO2$ 14.5 kPa (on air)
- HCO_3^- 12 mmol/L
- Na^+ 144 mmol/L
- K^+ 3.2 mmol/L
- Cl^- 107 mmol/L
- Glucose 24 mmol/L
- Lactate 1.0 mmol/L

Interpretation of ABG result:

- Patient has an acidosis (pH 7.15)
- Primary metabolic acidosis (HCO_3^- 12 mmol/L) with respiratory compensation ($PaCO_2$ 3.0 kPa)
- Anion gap = (144 + 3.2)–(12 + 107) = 28.2 (raised due to ketoacidosis)
- A–a gradient = [(0.21 × 95)–(3.0/0.8)]–14.5 = 1.7 kPa (normal)

You are not allowed a calculator in the exam so ensure you show your workings out to gain marks even if the maths is incorrect.

KEY POINTS

ABGs can be interpreted using a five-step approach.

1. Is the patient hypoxic?
2. Is the patient acidaemic or alkalaemic?
3. What is the respiratory component? If the CO_2 is abnormal is it in keeping with the pH?
4. What is the metabolic component? If the HCO_3^- is abnormal is it in keeping with the pH?
5. Combine the information in questions 2, 3, and 4 to determine the primary disturbance and if there is any compensation or a mixed picture.

- The anion gap is calculated by the following formula:

$$(Na^+ + K^+) - (HCO_3^- + Cl^-)$$

An anion gap <18 mmol/L is considered to be normal.

Causes of a raised anion gap can be remembered by the mnemonic 'MUDPILES'.

- Osmolar gap = Measured–Calculated osmolality

$$\text{The calculated osmolality} = 2\,(Na + K) + urea + glu$$

Nor006Dal osmolar gap <12 mosmol/kg.

- The A–a gradient is calculated by:

$$P_AO_2\,(alveolar) - P_aO_2\,(arterial).$$

The P_AO_2 is calculated by:

$$FiO_2 \times 95 - (PaCo_2/0.8)$$

The normal A–a result varies depending on age but an A–a gradient <2 kPa is normal in young adults up to 5 kPa in the elderly.

10.10 SAQs

10.10.1 Asthma

You are asked to assess a 35-year-old gentleman in the resuscitation room. He is having an exacerbation of his asthma. The following observations have been recorded:

RR 40/min; SpO2 90% on 15 L O_2; P 144/min; BP 95/60; PEF 145 (best 450).

a) (i) Give four features of life-threatening asthma. (2 marks, ½ mark per answer)

a) (ii) List three severity markers found on the arterial blood gas. (3 marks)

b) You identify that he has life-threatening asthma. What is your immediate first-line management? Give dose and mechanism of action of any drugs. (4 marks)

c) Give two indications for calling intensive care. (1 mark)

Suggested answer

a) (i) Give four features of life-threatening asthma. (2 marks, ½ mark per answer)

PEF <33% best or predicted

Silent chest

SpO2 <92%

Cyanosis

PaO_2 <8 kPa

Feeble respiratory effort

Normal $PaCO_2$ (4.6–6.0 kPa)

Bradycardia, arrhythmia, hypotension

Exhaustion, confusion, coma

a) (ii) List three severity markers found on the arterial blood gas. (3 marks)

PaO_2 <8 KPa

$PaCO_2$ normal or high

Acidosis

b) You identify that he has life-threatening asthma. What is your immediate first-line management? Give dose and mechanism of action of any drugs. (4 marks)

Salbutamol 5 mg nebulizer—ß2 agonist or bronchodilator

Ipratropium bromide 500 mcg nebulizer—antimuscarinic action, blocks bronchoconstriction

Prednisolone 40–50 mg orally or hydrocortisone 100 mg IV—reduces inflammatory component of airway constriction

Magnesium sulfate 1.2–2g IV over 20 minutes—bronchodilator

Not oxygen—patient already receiving high flow

c) Give two indications for calling intensive care. (1 mark)

Patient requiring ventilatory support

Patient with acute severe or life-threatening asthma, failing to respond to therapy

10.10.2 Pulmonary embolism

A 30-year-old lady attends your emergency department. She is complaining of pleuritic right-sided chest pain that started earlier that day. She feels breathless on minimal exertion. She has no past medical history of note and is on no medications. Observations: RR 30, SpO_2 97% on air, HR 100 bpm, BP 110/60 mmHg.

a) (i) The most important differential diagnosis in this lady is a PE. What is the most useful initial investigation in this patient and why? (2 marks)

a) (ii) Describe four features you may see on her ECG. (2 marks)

> She has a CTPA confirming a saddle embolus. On return to the ED she becomes increasingly short of breath. Repeat observations are: HR 160, RR 30, BP 60 mmHg systolic, SpO_2 unrecordable.

b) (i) What emergency treatment does this patient require and what agent would you use? (2 marks)

b) (ii) If this treatment is contraindicated, what other treatment could be tried? (1 mark)

c) (i) Her blood gas shows pH 7.38, $PaCO_2$ 3.0 kPa, PaO_2 10.0 kPa, HCO_3^- 28 mmol/L. She is breathing 60% oxygen via a Venturi mask. What is her A–a gradient? (1 mark calculation, 1 mark answer).

c) (ii) What would you expect a normal A–a gradient to be in this patient? (1 mark)

Suggested answer

a) (i) The most important differential diagnosis in this lady is a PE. What is the most useful initial investigation in this patient and why? (2 marks)

> D-dimer
>
> Low-probability patient (using Wells or BTS)

a) (ii) Describe four features you may see on her ECG. (2 marks)

> Sinus tachycardia
>
> S1 Q3 T3 pattern
>
> Right bundle branch block
>
> Right ventricular strain
>
> AF
>
> RAD
>
> (½ mark per answer)

b) (i) What emergency treatment does this patient require and what agent would you use? (2 marks)

> Thrombolysis—Alteplase

b) (ii) If this treatment is contraindicated, what other treatment could be tried? (1 mark)

> Unfractionated heparin
>
> Thrombolectomy
>
> Clot fragmentation

c) (i) Her blood gas shows pH 7.38, $PaCO_2$ 3.0 kPa, PaO_2 10.0 kPa, HCO_3^- 28 mmol/L. She is breathing 60% oxygen via a Venturi mask. What is her A–a gradient? (1 mark calculation, 1 mark answer).

> $PaO_2 = 10.0$
>
> $PAO_2 = (0.6 \times 95)-(3.0/0.8) = 53.25$.
>
> A–a gradient $= 53.25-10 = 43.25$ kPa.

c) (ii) What would you expect a normal A–a gradient to be in this patient? (1 mark)

> Normal A–a gradient in young healthy person <2 kPa

Further reading

British Thoracic Society, 2003. BTS guidelines for the management of suspected acute pulmonary embolism. Available at: https://www.brit-thoracic.org.uk [Online].

British Thoracic Society, 2008. BTS guidelines for emergency use of oxygen in adult patients. Available at: https://www.brit-thoracic.org.uk [Online].

British Thoracic Society, 2009 (Updated). BTS guidelines for the management of community acquired pneumonia in adults. Available at: https://www.brit-thoracic.org.uk [Online].

British Thoracic Society, 2010. BTS Pleural disease Guidelines 2010: Management of spontaneous pneumothorax. Available at: https://www.brit-thoracic.org.uk [Online].

National Institute for Health and Care Excellence, January 2010. NICE Clinical Guideline 92. Venous thromboembolism: reducing the risk of venous thromboembolism (deep vein thrombosis and pulmonary embolism) in patients admitted to hospital. Available at: https://www.nice.org.uk/guidance/CG92 [Online].

National Institute for Health and Care Excellence, June 2010. NICE clinical guideline CG101. Chronic obstructive pulmonary disease in over 16s: diagnosis and management. Available at: https://www.nice.org.uk/Guidance/cg144 [Online].

National Institute for Health and Care Excellence, June 2012. NICE clinical guideline 144. Venous thromboembolic diseases: diagnosis, management and thrombophilia testing. Available at: https://www.nice.org.uk/Guidance/cg144 [Online].

National Institute for Health and Care Excellence, Dec 2014. NICE clinical guideline 191. Guideline for diagnosis and management of community and hospital-acquired pneumonia in adults. Available at: https://www.nice.org.uk/guidance/cg191 [Online].

Royal College of Obstetricians and Gynaecologists, 2015. Green-top guideline 37a. Thrombosis and embolism during pregnancy and the puerperium, reducing the risk. Available at: https://www.rcog.org.uk/en/guidelines-research-services/guidelines/gtg37a/ [Online].

Royal College of Obstetricians and Gynaecologists, 2015. Green-top guideline 37b. Thromboembolic disease in pregnancy and the puerperium: Acute management. Available at: https://www.rcog.org.uk/globalassets/documents/guidelines/gtg-37b.pdf [Online].

Royal College of Physicians, British Thoracic Society, Intensive Care Society, 2008. Chronic obstructive pulmonary disease: non-invasive ventilation with bi-phasic positive airways pressure in the management of patients with acute type 2 respiratory failure. Concise Guidance to Good Practice series, No 11. London: RCP. Available at: https://www.rcplondon.ac.uk/guidelines-policy/non-invasive-ventilation-chronic-obstructive-pulmonary-disease [Online].

Scottish Intercollegiate Guideline Network, October 2014. SIGN guideline 141. British guideline on the management of asthma. Available at: https://www.sign.ac.uk/guidelines/fulltext/141 [Online].

Wells PS, Anderson DR, Rodger M, et al. 2001. Excluding pulmonary embolism at the bedside without diagnostic imaging: management of patients with suspected pulmonary embolism presenting to the emergency department by using a simple clinical model and D-dimer. Ann Intern Med **135**(2):98–107.

Wells PS, Anderson DR, Rodger M, et al. 2003. Evaluation of D-dimer in the diagnosis of suspected deep-vein thrombosis. N Engl J Med **349**:1227–35.

Neurological emergencies

CONTENTS

11.1 The unconscious patient

11.1.1 Introduction

Patients who are unconscious are a common emergency department (ED) presentation. There are many different causes of a reduced level of consciousness and the ED physician must have a structured approach to produce a differential diagnosis, establish safe monitoring, investigate appropriately, and formulate an initial management plan.

A patient may be unconscious due to serious illness and/or serious injury. Patients can have different levels of unconsciousness and unresponsiveness, depending on how much or how little of the brain is functioning, and the intensity of the stimulus. The ED physician must be able to initiate treatment and investigations based on a limited history, and therefore a good understanding of the conditions that can cause unconsciousness is required.

Management of the unconscious patient is one of the major presentations included in the ACCS curriculum and therefore a likely topic in the FRCEM examination.

11.1.2 Pathophysiology of unconsciousness

Consciousness requires two key components of the central nervous system to be functioning: the ascending reticular activating system in the pons and midbrain, and at least one cerebral hemisphere.

Causes of failure of the reticular activating system include:

- Brainstem stroke (ischaemic or haemorrhagic)
- Raised intracranial pressure resulting in herniation of the brain and compression of the brainstem

Failure of both cerebral hemispheres may occur due to:

- Inadequate blood supply
- Inadequate substrate for normal metabolism (e.g. oxygen or glucose)
- Direct or indirect trauma to the cerebrum
- Exposure of the brain to a toxic insult (e.g. infection, toxic metabolites, or exogenous poisons)

A stroke affecting one cerebral hemisphere does not result in coma, because the other hemisphere and the reticular activating system are still functioning. A brainstem stroke may lead to coma due to failure of the reticular activating system.

11.1.3 Causes of unconsciousness

There are multiple causes of unconsciousness, which should be assessed for in a systematic manner. Causes include:

Supratentorial lesions:

- Intracranial haemorrhage: extradural haematoma, subdural haematoma, intracerebral haemorrhage, subarachnoid haemorrhage
- Tumour
- Infarction
- Abscess
- Venous sinus thrombosis
- Head injury (intracranial haemorrhage, cerebral oedema, diffuse axonal injury, hydrocephalus)

Infratentorial lesions:

- Infarction
- Haemorrhage
- Tumour
- Inflammatory lesion

Diffuse lesions

- Metabolic causes: hypoglycaemia, hyperglycaemia, hyponatraemia, hypernatraemia, hypercalcaemia, hypocalcaemia, hypoxia, and/or hypercarbia, acidosis (including diabetic ketoacidosis), liver failure, hypothyroidism, Wernicke's encephalopathy
- Hypoxic-ischaemic injury: hypoxia and/or hypercarbia (respiratory failure), hypovolaemia (shock); near drowning, strangulation
- Drugs and toxins: opiates, alcohol, carbon monoxide, tricyclic antidepressants, barbiturates, organophosphates, and so on
  - Epilepsy: non-convulsive status epilepticus
  - Hypothermia
  - Infections: meningitis, encephalitis, cerebral malaria, systemic sepsis

11.1.4 Clinical assessment and management of an unconscious patient

Patients should be assessed with the standard ABCDE approach (Table 11.1). Assessment and treatment should occur simultaneously. It is essential to ensure the patient is not hypoxic, hypercarbic, or hypotensive, because these can all cause unconsciousness, and will worsen the outcome in other causes.

Once the initial ABCDE assessment has been performed attention can be directed at a detailed neurological examination.

11.1.5 Investigations for the unconscious patient

Investigations should be directed by the most likely cause of the reduced level of consciousness. Careful clinical examination is the key to efficiently and effectively identifying the most probable cause of the coma. There is no merit to simply scanning all unconscious patients.

Table 11.1 ABCDE approach to assessing the unconscious patient

Airway and breathing	• Unless the cause of unconsciousness is associated with a brief or easily reversible aetiology (e.g. post-ictal, hypoglycaemia, opiate overdose, and so on), intubation and ventilation should be considered early. This will enable protection of the patient's airway and optimize ventilatory function. • Patients should receive high-flow oxygen until an arterial blood gas determines the concentration of oxygen required.
Circulation	• Hypotension may be the cause of a reduced conscious level and will exacerbate other aetiologies. Patients should be managed with intravenous fluids and inotropic support if required. Any cause for hypotension should be sought and corrected (e.g. haemorrhage, sepsis, cardiac failure, and so on). • Intra-arterial pressure monitoring and serum lactate are useful to guide therapy.
Disability	• The patient's GCS and pupillary reaction should be assessed regularly. Any abnormal ocular movements or limb posturing should be noted. • Hypoglycaemia should always be considered and bedside blood glucose checked. If hypoglycaemia is present the patient should receive intravenous glucose (50-ml boluses of 50% glucose). • Patients who may have taken an opiate overdose (history suggestive, needle track marks, pin-point pupils, and so on) should be given naloxone (0.4-mg boluses IV). • Flumazenil should only be administered to those with a clear history of a benzodiazepine overdose and when there is no suspicion of a mixed overdose including tricyclic antidepressants, due to the risk of precipitating intractable seizures. • Patients who are malnourished or suspected of being alcoholics are at risk of Wernicke's encephalopathy due to thiamine deficiency. Indiscriminate glucose infusions can precipitate further acute neurological damage. Therefore, such patients should receive thiamine IV prior to the administration of glucose.
Exposure	The patient should be examined, looking for evidence of a potential cause for the reduced conscious level. The clinical examination should particularly look for evidence of: • Head injury (e.g. scalp lacerations, haematomas, signs of base of skull fracture, injuries to suggest a seizure—bitten tongue, posterior dislocation of the shoulder, and so on). • Organ failure (e.g. hypoxia, hypercapnea, tachycardia, hypotension, and so on). • Infection (e.g. fever, rash, neck stiffness, and so on). • Toxins (e.g. needlestick marks, dry skin (suggests tricyclic overdose), cherry red skin (suggests carbon monoxide poisoning), profuse sweating (suggests hypoglycaemia or organophosphate poisoning), and so on).

• Blood glucose—is the most useful bedside test for the unconscious patient and may reveal a rapidly reversible cause.
• Computed tomography (CT) scanning—is the most useful investigation for the unconscious patient. However, it is not always required urgently and sometimes not at all in those patients in whom the diagnosis is clear (e.g. hypothyroidism, diabetic ketoacidosis, some post-ictal patients, and so on) or those who, following emergency treatment, regain consciousness

(e.g. opiate overdose, hypoglycaemia). CT may reveal intracranial haemorrhage, skull fractures, intracranial air, hydrocephalus, diffuse cerebral oedema, and so on.

- Arterial blood gas analysis—should be performed to identify hypoxia, hypercarbia, and acidosis. A raised anion gap may suggest a toxic or metabolic cause.

Other investigations should be guided by the clinical picture (e.g. full blood count (FBC), renal function, blood cultures, chest X-ray, and so on).

11.1.6 Emergency department management of the unconscious patient

Management of the unconscious patient should start concurrently with assessment (see Table 11.1). Hypoxia and hypotension must be identified and treated in all patients. Failure to do so increases morbidity and mortality.

Further management depends on the likely cause and the details of such management are included in other sections of this book.

- Head injury—the priority in patients who have sustained a head injury is to maintain adequate cerebral perfusion pressure and oxygenation. Head injury management is covered in Chapter 4, section 4.5.
- Acute cerebrovascular event—most patients who have a stroke do not present in coma but those with a brainstem event might. The management of stroke is discussed in this chapter (section 11.7). Patients suffering from seizures will have a reduced level of consciousness both during the seizure and in the post-ictal phase. The management of seizures and epilepsy is covered in sections 11.5 and 11.6.
- Cerebral infection—the priority is to commence appropriate antibiotic therapy. The management of central nervous system (CNS) infections is covered in Chapter 15, sections 15.3 and 15.4.
- Metabolic and endocrine causes—the management of patients with hypothyroidism, diabetic ketoacidosis, and other endocrine pathologies is covered in Chapter 14. The management of alcoholic liver disease and acute withdrawal is covered in Chapter 13, sections 13.7 and 13.8.
- Toxins—the management of poisoning is covered in Chapter 17.

KEY POINTS

Unconsciousness may be due to failure of the reticular activating system and/or both cerebral hemispheres.

Patients should be managed with an ABCDE approach. Hypoxia and hypotension must be identified and treated in all patients with a reduced level of consciousness.

Hypoglycaemia is a reversible cause of reduced conscious level. It must be recognized and treated promptly.

Patients who are malnourished or suspected of being alcoholics should receive intravenous thiamine prior to any glucose-containing fluids to avoid precipitating Wernicke's encephalopathy.

Patients suspected of having an opiate overdose should receive naloxone.

Patients should only be given flumazenil if there is a clear history of a benzodiazepine overdose and when there is no suspicion of a mixed overdose including tricyclic antidepressants.

A raised anion gap on an arterial blood gas may suggest a toxic or metabolic cause.

Patients with a reduced level of consciousness and pyrexia should be given broad spectrum antibiotics to cover for meningitis.

11.2 Headache

11.2.1 Introduction

Headache affects nearly everyone at least occasionally and is a common ED presentation. The majority of patients presenting to the ED with a headache have a benign cause; however, the challenge is identifying the small percentage with a potentially life-threatening cause.

Section 11.2.2 is based on the guidance from the British Association for the Study of Headache (BASH) and the SIGN guidance on the diagnosis and management of headache in adults.

11.2.2 Headache classification

The International Classification of Headache Disorders (ICHD) is the recognized standard for categorizing headaches. It classifies headache disorders into two broad groups: primary headaches and secondary headaches (Table 11.2).

• Primary headaches are those with no organic or structural aetiology.
• Secondary headaches are those due to an underlying structural or organic disease.

11.2.3 Clinical features of acute headache

Most patients presenting to the ED with a headache have a benign primary headache. The history is of prime importance in the evaluation of headache and could well be examined in an OSCE station. Knowledge of clinical features that suggest a particular cause of headache and 'red flag' features that suggest a potential secondary cause could appear in a SAQ (Table 11.3).

Table 11.2 The International Classification of Headache Disorders

Primary headaches	• Migraine • Tension-type headache • Cluster headache • Miscellaneous (benign cough headache, benign exertional headache, headache associated with sexual activity)
Secondary headaches	• Head injury (including post-traumatic headache) • Vascular disorders (e.g. subarachnoid haemorrhage (SAH), stroke, intracranial haematoma, cavernous sinus thrombosis, hypertension, unruptured arteriovenous malformation, temporal arteritis) • Non-vascular disorders (e.g. idiopathic intracranial hypertension, intracranial tumour, post-lumbar puncture) • Headaches associated with substances or their withdrawal (including analgesia, caffeine, nitrates, alcohol, and carbon monoxide) • Infections (e.g. encephalitis, meningitis, sinusitis) • Metabolic (e.g. hypoxia, hypercapnea, hypoglycaemia) • Craniofacial disorders (e.g. pathology of skull, neck, eyes, nose, ears, sinuses, mouth, and temporomandibular joints causing pain; this includes headache secondary to glaucoma) • Headache attributed to psychiatric disorders • Cranial neuralgias (e.g. trigeminal neuralgia)

Data from 'International Headache Society Classification Subcommittee. The International Classification of Headache Disorders'. 2nd edition. Cephalalgia 2004; 24 (Suppl 1): 1–160.

Table 11.3 Clinical features of different types of headache

Type of headache	Clinical features
Primary	
Migraine	Pulsating, unilateral headache
	Builds up over minutes to hours
	Variable duration but may last up to 72 h
	May be preceded by an aura (15–33% of patients)
	Moderate to severe in intensity; often disabling
	Associated with nausea and vomiting
	Exacerbated by light (photophobia), sound (phonophobia), and physical activity
	Episodic (patient may have a history of previous migraines)
	Sensitivity to light between attacks
	Positive family history of migraine
	See section 11.3
Tension-type headache	Pain is typically bilateral
	Pressing or tightening ('band-like') in quality
	Mild to moderate intensity
	No nausea or vomiting
	Not aggravated by physical activity
	May have pericranial tenderness
	May have sensitivity to light or noise
Cluster headache	Severe unilateral pain in a trigeminal distribution
	Associated with ipsilateral cranial autonomic features (e.g. watering of the eye, injection of conjunctiva)
	Recurrent lasting 30–120 min. Occurs in clusters that can last several weeks
	No aura or vomiting
Headache associated with sexual activity (coital cephalgia)	Explosive headache indistinguishable from a SAH
	Related to sexual activity usually at or near orgasm
	Classically the headache is severe and throbbing
	The first time a patient experiences coital cephalgia a subarachnoid haemorrhage should be actively excluded
Secondary	
Subarachnoid haemorrhage (SAH)	Sudden onset, 'worst-ever' headache
	Maximum intensity usually reached in less than one min
	Usually occipital and may be described like a blow to the back of the head
	May be associated with vomiting, neck pain, and photophobia
	The patient may present with a transient loss of consciousness or fits
	The patient may be drowsy and/or confused
	May have a history of a 'warning headache' days to weeks earlier
	Fundoscopy may show subhyaloid retinal haemorrhage (haemorrhage near the optic nerve head)
	May have focal neurological deficits depending on the location of the aneurysm (e.g. IIIrd nerve palsy with posterior communicating artery aneurysms)
	See section 11.4

Table 11.3 Continued

Type of headache	Clinical features
Meningitis	Generalized headache in an unwell/drowsy patient
	May have neck stiffness and photophobia
	May be pyrexial
	May have a rash (meningococcal)
	See Chapter 15, section 15.4
Space-occupying lesion (raised intracranial pressure—ICP)	Headache exacerbated by lying down and valsalva manoeuvres (e.g. coughing, straining, laughing, bending forwards)
	Headache may wake the patient from sleep
	Visual obscurations (transient changes in vision) with change in posture or valsalva suggest raised intracranial pressure
	Seizures
	Cognitive change or focal neurological signs
	Papilloedema
Temporal arteritis	Diffuse, throbbing headache
	Patient age >50 years
	Scalp tenderness, jaw claudication, and tender temporal artery with reduced pulsation
	Visual disturbance
	(A normal ESR makes the diagnosis unlikely). For further details on temporal arteritis see Chapter 7, section 7.17
Acute angle closure glaucoma	Unilateral headache
	Eye pain
	Mid-dilated, red eye
	Halos around lights
	Reduced visual acuity
	For further details on acute angle closure glaucoma see Chapter 7, section 7.13
Carbon monoxide poisoning	Headache that improves on leaving the environment
	Nausea and vomiting
	Dizziness
	Muscle weakness
	Blurred vision
	For further details on carbon monoxide poisoning see Chapter 17, section 17.7

Red flag features

A secondary headache should be considered in patients presenting with new onset headache, or a headache that differs from their usual pattern. If a patient has any of the following 'red flags', it suggests a potential secondary headache and the need for further investigation.

- New onset or change in headache in patients who are aged over 50.
- Thunderclap headache: rapid time to peak headache intensity (seconds to 5 minutes).
- Focal neurological symptoms (e.g. limb weakness, aura <5 minutes or >1 hour).

- Non-focal neurological symptoms (e.g. cognitive disturbance).
- Change in headache frequency, characteristics, or associated symptoms.
- Abnormal neurological examination.
- Headache that changes with posture.
- Headache that wakes the patient up. (NB Migraine is the most frequent cause of morning headache.)
- Headache precipitated by physical exertion or valsalva manoeuvre (e.g. coughing, laughing, straining).
- Patients with risk factors for cerebral venous sinus thrombosis (e.g. coagulopathies, such as thrombophilia, polycythaemia; dehydration; nephrotic syndrome; chronic inflammatory diseases, such as inflammatory bowel disease, lupus, Behcet's disease; pregnancy; oestrogen-containing oral contraceptives; infections, such as meningitis, sinusitis, or mastoiditis; head trauma).
- Jaw claudication or visual disturbance.
- Neck stiffness.
- Fever.
- New onset headache in a patient with a history of HIV infection.
- New onset headache in a patient with a history of cancer.

Examination of a patient with headache

Patients presenting to the ED with headache for the first time or with headache that differs from their usual symptoms should have the following examination:

- Fundoscopy
- Cranial nerve assessment, especially pupils, visual fields, eye movements, facial power and sensation, and bulbar function (soft palate and tongue movement)
- Assessment of tone, power, reflexes, and coordination in all four limbs
- Plantar responses
- Assessment of gait, including heel-toe walking

Further examination should be directed by the patient's history. The patient must have their blood pressure recorded.

11.2.4 Investigations for acute headache

A detailed history and examination is the mainstay of assessing a patient with headache. Further investigations are determined by the most likely cause. The vast majority of primary headaches do not require neuroimaging.

Neuroimaging

SIGN recommend that neuroimaging is not indicated in patients with a clear history of migraine, no red flag features for potential secondary headache, and a normal neurological examination.

CT scanning is the most commonly requested neuroimaging from the ED. Potential indications for requesting an urgent CT in a patient with headache include:

- Suspected subarachnoid haemorrhage (SAH) (CT should be performed as soon as possible to maximize sensitivity)
- Suspected stroke
- Unexplained abnormal neurological signs
- Reduced level of consciousness
- Signs and symptoms suggestive of raised intracranial pressure

MRI is more sensitive than CT for many secondary causes of headache. It is less readily available than CT in most UK EDs and is often requested on the advice of a neurologist or after discussion with a radiologist. MRI is particularly useful for the early detection of ischaemic brain lesions, posterior fossa lesions, white matter disease, and tumours.

Lumbar puncture

Lumbar puncture with cerebrospinal fluid (CSF) analysis is appropriate for patients with thunderclap headache and normal neuroimaging to exclude a diagnosis of subarachnoid haemorrhage.

Lumbar puncture should be delayed 12 hours from the onset of the thunderclap headache because xanthochromia (bilirubin and oxyhaemoglobin) can only be reliably detected in the CSF after 12 hours. In delayed presentations lumbar puncture can be performed up to two weeks after the onset of symptoms.

The opening pressure should be measured routinely in all lumbar punctures.

Features of a lumbar puncture and CSF analysis that suggest an SAH include:

- Raised opening pressure
- Xanthochromia (spectrophotometry is the recommended method of analysis)
- Increased number of red blood cells (RBC >50 mm^{-3})
- Normal gram stain
- Elevated protein
- White cells may occasionally be slightly elevated
- Normal glucose

Inflammatory markers

Erythrocyte sedimentation rate (ESR) and C-reactive protein (CRP) have been shown to be useful in the diagnosis of temporal arteritis in patients with suggestive symptoms. The SIGN guideline recommends measuring both the ESR and CRP because the sensitivity and specificity for temporal arteritis is increased.

KEY POINTS

Headache disorders can be broadly classified into two groups:

- Primary headaches—those with no organic or structural aetiology
- Secondary headaches—those due to an underlying structural or organic disease

Patients should be assessed for clinical features that suggest a particular cause of headache and 'red flag' features. 'Red flag' features include:

- New onset or change in headache in patients who are aged over 50
- Thunderclap headache
- Abnormal neurological examination (focal and non-focal signs)
- Headache that changes with posture
- Headache that wakes the patient up
- Headache precipitated by physical exertion or valsalva manoeuvre
- Patients with risk factors for cerebral venous sinus thrombosis
- Jaw claudication or visual disturbance
- Neck stiffness
- Fever
- New onset headache in a patient with a history of cancer or HIV

The following patients should have an urgent CT arranged in the ED:

- Suspected SAH
- Suspected stroke
- Unexplained abnormal neurological signs
- Reduced level of consciousness
- Signs and symptoms suggestive of raised intracranial pressure

Lumbar puncture with CSF analysis is appropriate for patients with thunderclap headache and normal neuroimaging to exclude a diagnosis of subarachnoid haemorrhage.

ESR and CRP should be performed in patients with symptoms suggestive of temporal arteritis.

11.3 Migraine

11.3.1 Introduction

Migraine occurs in 15% of the UK adult population, in women more than men in a 3:1 ratio.

Patients with migraine typically describe recurrent episodic, moderate, or severe headaches (which may be unilateral and/or pulsating) lasting part of the day up to three days. The headache may be associated with gastrointestinal symptoms, photophobia, and phonophobia.

Patients with recurrent migraine rarely attend the ED unless symptoms are different from their usual pattern; therefore, caution is required to avoid missing a more serious condition.

11.3.2 Pathophysiology of migraine

The pathophysiology of migraine is not entirely clear, but there are two main schools of thought. The first is the vascular theory, which proposes that initial intracranial vasoconstriction is responsible for the aura of migraine and subsequent rebound vasodilatation results in the headache. The other theory is that of neurovascular dysfunction, in which a complex series of neural and vascular events initiate migraine.

11.3.3 Types of migraine

There are two main types of migraine as classified by the ICHD:

- Migraine without aura
- Migraine with aura (~1/3 of patients with migraine)

The aura

A typical aura involves premonitory visual symptoms that occur 5–60 minutes before the headache. These symptoms include flashes of light, wavy linear patterns on the visual fields (fortification spectra), scintillating scotomata (an area of decreased or absent vision surrounded by moving zigzag lines), or blurred vision. Other reversible focal neurological disturbances may occur, including unilateral paraesthesia, dysphasia, ataxia, and mild unilateral weakness.

Rare forms of migraine

These include:

- Hemiplegic migraine—profound hemiplegia precedes the development of the headache by 30–60 minutes.
- Basilar migraine—brainstem disturbance results in impaired consciousness, vertigo, dysarthria, diplopia, and limb weakness.
- Acephalgic migraine—very occasionally, neurological defects may be present without headache.

11.3.4 Triggers for migraine

Migraine may be precipitated by:

- Fatigue
- Alcohol
- Menstruation
- Oral contraceptive pill
- Stress
- Strenuous unaccustomed exercise
- Certain foods (e.g. chocolate, cheese)

11.3.5 ED treatment of acute migraine

The treatment of acute migraine attacks should proceed in a stepped approach, commencing with simple analgesics and anti-emetics, and, if required, escalating to 5HT receptor agonists (e.g. triptans).

- Step 1—simple analgesics (e.g. aspirin (600–900 mg) or ibuprofen (400–600 mg)) ± an anti-emetic (e.g. prochlorperazine, domperidone, or metoclopramide). Domperidone and metoclopramide act as a prokinetic to promote gastric emptying, in addition to their anti-emetic properties.
- Step 2—rectal analgesics (e.g. diclofenac 100 mg PR) ± an anti-emetic.
- Step 3—specific anti-migraine drugs. Triptans (e.g. sumatriptan orally or subcutaneously) are useful in the acute treatment of migraine in patients who have had previous attacks not controlled by simple analgesics. Triptans should be taken at the start of the headache phase due to evidence of greater efficacy, and appear to be ineffective if taken during the aura. Patients should be warned about the potential for a rebound headache and may require a further dose. Triptans are contraindicated in patients with ischaemic heart disease, previous myocardial infarction, coronary vasospasm, uncontrolled or severe hypertension, hemiplegic migraine, or following recent ergotamine use (<12 hours).
- Step 4—combination therapy. Patients presenting to the ED with uncontrolled symptoms may require a combination of a non-steroidal anti-inflammatory (NSAID), anti-emetic, and triptans. Patients may also benefit from intravenous fluids.

NB Opiates—are not recommended routinely in acute migraine due to the risk of developing medication-overuse headache. Ergotamine—is not recommended by SIGN for the treatment of acute migraine.

KEY POINTS

Clinical features of a migraine include:

Pulsating, unilateral headache.

Build-up over minutes to hours.

Variable duration (may last up to 72 h).

Preceding aura in 15–33% of patients.

Moderate to severe in intensity. Often disabling.

Associated nausea and vomiting.

Exacerbated by light, sound, and physical activity.

Episodic (patient may have a history of previous migraines).

Patients with recurrent migraine rarely attend the ED unless symptoms are different from their usual pattern; therefore, caution is required to avoid missing a more serious condition.

The treatment of acute migraine attacks should proceed in a stepped approach, commencing with simple analgesics and anti-emetics, and, if required, escalating to 5HT-receptor agonists (e.g. triptans).

11.4 Subarachnoid haemorrhage

11.4.1 Introduction

Atraumatic SAH can occur at any age and is an important cause of sudden collapse and death. The typical clinical features of an SAH are described in Table 11.3.

SAH has a significant morbidity and mortality, with up to 40% of patients dying in the first week and more than one-third of survivors having significant neurological deficit.

11.4.2 Causes of subarachnoid haemorrhage

- Saccular ('berry') aneurysms in the circle of Willis (commonest cause ~85% cases)
- Arteriovenous malformations
- Mycotic aneurysmal rupture (secondary to an infective process)
- Angioma
- Neoplasm
- Trauma

11.4.3 Risk factors for subarachnoid haemorrhage

- Past medical history of SAH
- Family history
- Polycystic kidney disease
- Marfan syndrome
- Ehlers–Danlos syndrome
- Coarctation of the aorta
- Hypertension
- Smoking
- Atherosclerosis

11.4.4 Differential diagnosis of thunderclap headache

Thunderclap headache is defined as a headache that reaches its maximum intensity rapidly (seconds to five minutes) mimicking a SAH. Other causes of a thunderclap headache include:

- Intracerebral haemorrhage
- Cerebral venous sinus thrombosis
- Arterial dissection
- Pituitary apoplexy
- Coital cephalgia

There are no reliable features to differentiate between benign (e.g. coital cephalgia) and sinister (e.g. SAH) causes of a thunderclap headache. Therefore, when a patient presents for the first time with a sudden severe headache, they should be investigated further. A negative CT and LP, with CSF fluid analysis, within two weeks of onset of a thunderclap headache, are considered sufficient to exclude a diagnosis of SAH, based on the SIGN guidance.

11.4.5 Grading of subarachnoid haemorrhage

The two most commonly used clinical scales to grade the severity of SAH are the Hunt and Hess and the World Federation of Neurological Surgeons (WFNS) grading systems. They are used as predictors of prognosis, with higher grades correlating to lower survival rates.

The Hunt and Hess grading system is as follows:

- Grade 1—asymptomatic or mild headache (~70% survival rate).
- Grade 2—moderate-to-severe headache, nuchal rigidity, and no neurological deficit other than possible cranial nerve palsy (~60% survival rate).

- Grade 3—mild alteration in mental status (confusion, lethargy), mild focal neurological deficit (~50% survival rate).
- Grade 4—stupor and/or hemiparesis (~40% survival rate).
- Grade 5—comatose and/or decerebrate rigidity (~10% survival rate).*

The WFNS scale is as follows:

- Grade 1—Glasgow coma score (GCS) of 15, motor deficit absent.
- Grade 2—GCS of 13–14, motor deficit absent.
- Grade 3—GCS of 13–14, motor deficit present.
- Grade 4—GCS of 7–12, motor deficit absent or present.
- Grade 5—GCS of 3–6, motor deficit absent or present.**

11.4.6 Clinical features of increasing intracranial pressure

An SAH may lead to increased intracranial pressure (ICP). The clinical features to suggest an acutely raised ICP include:

- Vomiting, headache, irritability
- Seizures
- Reducing GCS
- Cushing's triad—hypertension, bradycardia, irregular respirations
- Focal neurology
- Papilloedema
- Abnormal posturing: decorticate or decerebrate
- Dilated or unequal pupils

11.4.7 Investigations for subarachnoid haemorrhage

The two most important investigations in a suspected SAH are a CT and lumbar puncture. The CT should be performed as soon as possible to maximize its sensitivity. A lumbar puncture is indicated if the CT is negative. It should be delayed 12 hours after the onset of headache to enable detection of xanthochromia (see section 11.2).

Other investigations that may be abnormal and/or useful in a SAH are:

- Blood glucose—as a potentially reversible cause of reduced conscious level or seizures.
- Clotting—is useful if the patient is anticoagulated because reversal may be required.
- FBC and Group and Save—because an intraoperative blood transfusion may be required.
- Urea and electrolytes—due to the subsequent risk of syndrome of inappropriate antidiuretic hormone.
- Electrocardiogram (ECG)—because the increased circulation of catecholamines may lead to ischaemic or non-specific ST/T wave changes.

11.4.8 Emergency department management of subarachnoid haemorrhage

The most important element of ED management is prompt diagnosis of a patient with a SAH.

The ED treatment required will depend on the grade of the SAH. Those with grade I and II SAH require rapid diagnosis, supportive management, and urgent transfer to the neurosurgical team. Those with higher grade SAHs will require more extensive care.

Supportive management of a patient with a subarachnoid haemorrhage

Table 11.4 details the supportive management of a patient with a SAH.

* Reproduced from Hunt WE and Hess RM, 'Surgical risk as related to time of intervention in the repair of intracranial aneurysms', *Journal of Neurosurgery*, 28, 1, pp. 14–20, Copyright 1968, with permission from the American Association of Neurological Surgeons.

** Reproduced with permission of the World Federation of Neurological Surgeons.

Table 11.4 Supportive management of a patient with a SAH

A and B	Ensure adequate oxygenation (aim for oxygen saturations >94%)
	Aim for $PaCO_2$ in normal range
	Intubate and ventilate as required to achieve these aims and protect the airway
	Tape the endotracheal tube in place rather than tie it to avoid increases in ICP
	Avoid excessive intrathoracic pressures to prevent rises in ICP
C	Maintain end organ perfusion (aim for MAP≥80 mmHg)
	Use urine output as indicator of adequate renal perfusion
D	Maintain normoglycaemia
	Treat seizures (benzodiazepines, prophylactic phenytoin)
	Position—30° head-up tilt to help reduce ICP
	Avoid cervical collars/compression if possible to avoid increased ICP
	Monitor for signs of neurological deterioration
E	Pain management to avoid increases in ICP (if the patient has severe pain titrate morphine IV in 1-mg increments)
	Temperature control (aim for normothermia)

Specific management for subarachnoid haemorrhage

On the advice of the neurosurgical team, the following treatments may be recommended:

- Nimodipine (60 mg orally or via nasogastric tube (NG) tube)—used to prevent and treat ischaemic neurological deficits secondary to cerebral vasospasm.
- Mannitol (e.g. 200 ml of 10% IV)—an osmotic diuretic may be given if there is evidence of raised intracranial pressure.

11.4.9 Complications of SAH

- Re-bleeding (peak incidence the day after the initial SAH).
- Hydrocephalus.
- Cerebral vasospasm.
- Neurological deficits from cerebral ischaemia.
- Syndrome of inappropriate antidiuretic hormone, resulting in hyponatraemia.
- Neurogenic pulmonary oedema.
- Aspiration pneumonia.
- Myocardial ischaemia or infarction due to excessive catecholamine release.
- Left ventricular dysfunction due to excessive catecholamine release.
- Death.

KEY POINTS

Causes of SAH include:
- Saccular ('berry') aneurysms in the circle of Willis
- Arteriovenous malformations
- Mycotic aneurysmal rupture (secondary to an infective process)
- Angioma
- Neoplasm
- Trauma

Typical clinical features of a SAH include:

- Sudden onset, 'worst-ever' headache.
- Maximum intensity reached in less than one min.
- Usually occipital and may be described like a blow to the back of the head.
- May be associated with vomiting, neck pain, and photophobia.
- The patient may present with a transient loss of consciousness or fits.
- The patient may be drowsy and/or confused.
- May have a history of a 'warning headache' days to weeks earlier.
- Fundoscopy may show subhyaloid retinal haemorrhage.
- May have focal neurological deficits depending on the location of the aneurysm.

The two most important investigations in a suspected SAH are a CT and lumbar puncture. The CT should be performed as soon as possible to maximize its sensitivity. A lumbar puncture is indicated if the CT is negative and should be delayed 12 h after the onset of headache.

ED management should focus on prompt diagnosis, supportive management, and urgent transfer to the neurosurgical team.

Specific treatments that may be required on advice of a neurosurgeon include nimodipine (to reduce cerebral vasospasm) and mannitol (an osmotic diuretic to reduce ICP).

11.5 Epilepsy

11.5.1 Introduction

Epilepsy is the most common neurological condition in the United Kingdom, affecting 1 in every 131 people. Epilepsy is more common in children and people over 65, but can develop in anyone of any age.

Epilepsy is a neurological condition characterized by recurrent epileptic seizures unprovoked by any immediately identifiable cause. An epileptic seizure is the clinical manifestation of an abnormal and excessive discharge of neurons in the brain. This is thought to arise from an imbalance between excitatory and inhibitory neurotransmitters, most commonly between glutamate and gamma-aminobutyric acid (GABA), leading to a failure of inhibitory processes.

Seizures

Many people will have a one-off seizure at some point in their lives, but not all seizures are due to epilepsy. There are different types of seizures, which may happen for many reasons. Seizures not due to epilepsy are called non-epileptic seizures. Non-epileptic seizures are different from epileptic seizures because they are not caused by disrupted electrical activity in the brain.

Causes of non-epileptic seizures include:

- Hypoglycaemia
- Arrhythmias
- Structural heart disease
- Syncope
- Febrile convulsions
- Psychogenic seizures
- Panic attacks

11.5.2 Causes of epilepsy

Epilepsy can have a number of causes. The three main categories of epilepsy are:

- Symptomatic epilepsy—due to a known cause (e.g. head injury).
- Idiopathic epilepsy—where there is no apparent cause.

- Cryptogenic epilepsy—where there is no apparent cause but there is evidence that it may be the result of brain damage due to other associated conditions (e.g. learning difficulties).

Symptomatic epilepsy

Causes of symptomatic epilepsy include:

- Conditions that affect the structure of the brain (e.g. cerebral palsy)
- Drug and alcohol misuse
- Birth defects
- Hypoxia at birth
- CNS infections (e.g. meningitis)
- Head injuries
- Strokes
- Brain tumours

Idiopathic epilepsy

No apparent cause for epilepsy can be found. However, it has been suggested that small genetic changes in the brain could be the cause of the epilepsy.

Cryptogenic epilepsy

The term cryptogenic epilepsy is used when no definite cause for epilepsy can be found but there is strong evidence that the symptoms are due to damage or disruption of the brain.

Evidence supportive of cryptogenic epilepsy includes:

- Learning difficulties
- Developmental condition (e.g. autistic spectrum disorder)
- Unusual electroencephalogram (EEG) readings

11.5.3 Types of epilepsy

There are about 40 different types of epileptic seizure. People with epilepsy can experience any of the varieties of seizures, although most people follow a consistent pattern of symptoms. This pattern is known as an epilepsy syndrome.

Seizures are divided into two main types: partial seizures and generalized seizures.

Partial seizures

Partial seizures originate from a specific area of the cortex; they are sometimes called 'focal' seizures because the seizure affects just one area or 'focus'. There are two types of partial seizure:

- Simple partial seizures—involve only one area of the brain and consciousness is maintained.
- Complex partial seizures—arise from a single region of the brain and are associated with a degree of consciousness impairment.

The clinical features of a simple partial seizure depend on the region of the brain affected (see Table 11.5).

Complex partial seizures affect a larger part of one hemisphere than a simple partial seizure. The patient's conscious level is reduced and they may be confused and have no memory of the seizure. Patients may be able to hear during a seizure but will often not fully understand what is being said.

Complex partial seizures often happen in the temporal lobes ('temporal lobe epilepsy') but can affect other areas of the brain.

Clinical features of complex partial seizures in the temporal lobe include:

- Picking up objects for no reason or fiddling with clothing
- Mumbling or making chewing or lip-smacking movements

Table 11.5 Clinical features of a simple partial seizure

Frontal lobe	Temporal lobe	Parietal lobe	Occipital lobe
A strange feeling like a 'wave' going through the head Regular rhythmic contractions of a single limb or muscle group	_Déjà vu_ An unusual smell or taste Sudden intense emotion, such as fear or joy	Tingling/'pins and needles' in the limbs A sensation that an arm or leg feels bigger or smaller than they actually are	Visual disturbance (e.g. coloured or flashing lights) Hallucinations

- Incomprehensible speech
- Wandering around in a confused way

Clinical features of complex partial seizures in the frontal lobe include:

- Making a loud cry or scream
- Making a strange posture or movements such as cycling or kicking

Complex partial seizures in the parietal or occipital lobes are less common but like simple partial seizures can affect vision or senses.

Secondary generalization

Partial seizures sometimes spread from one hemisphere to both hemispheres. This is called a secondary generalized seizure because it starts as a partial seizure and then becomes generalized. When this happens, the patient loses consciousness and will usually have a tonic–clonic seizure. Sometimes the partial seizure is so brief that it is not noticed.

Generalized seizures

Generalized seizures affect both sides of the brain at once and can happen without warning. The patient is unconscious (except in myoclonic seizures). Following the seizure, the patient has no recollection of what happened during the attack.

There are six main types of generalized seizure:

- Absences (sometimes called _petit mal_)—are more common in children, and are typically very short-lived (i.e. a few seconds). During an absence the patient becomes unconscious for a short time. Patients may stare vacantly and not respond to what is happening around them.
- Myoclonic seizures—are characterized by brief muscle jerks. They can happen in clusters and often occur shortly after waking. They are not always due to epilepsy and some people experience them as they fall asleep. Conscious is maintained during myoclonic seizures but they are classified as generalized seizures because they do not usually happen on their own but alongside other seizure types.
- Tonic seizures—result in all of a patient's muscles contracting. If the patient is standing they often fall, usually backwards, and may sustain a head injury. Tonic seizures are usually very brief and happen without warning.
- Atonic seizures (or 'drop attacks')—results in all of a patient's muscles relaxing. If the patient is standing, they often fall, usually forwards, and may sustain an injury. Like tonic seizures, atonic seizures are usually brief and happen without warning.
- Clonic seizures—cause the same sort of twitching as myoclonic jerks but the symptoms last longer, normally up to two minutes.
- Tonic–clonic seizures (sometimes called _grand mal_)—are the seizure most people think of as epilepsy. They are the commonest type of seizures, accounting for 60% of seizures

experienced by patients with epilepsy. It begins with a sudden powerful contraction of the muscles (tonic phase), often associated with a fall to the floor, followed by regular rhythmic contraction and relaxation (clonic phase) of the musculature of all limbs. The patient may bite their tongue or experience urinary incontinence during the seizure. Following the seizure the patient is usually tired, confused, and may have a headache ('post-ictal' phase).

11.5.4 Triggers for epileptic seizures

Certain triggers are recognized for epileptic seizures, and may contribute to the development of seizure clusters. These triggers include:

- Stress.
- Sleep deprivation.
- Alcohol, particularly binge drinking and during a hangover.
- Substance abuse, such as cocaine, amphetamines, ecstasy, and any opiate-based drugs, such as heroin, methadone, or codeine.
- Concurrent infections that cause a fever.
- Flashing lights (this is an uncommon trigger that affects only 5% of people with epilepsy, and is also known as photosensitive epilepsy).
- Menstruation.

11.5.5 First-fit management

Patients frequently present to the ED following a first seizure. Patients should not be labelled with the diagnosis of epilepsy in the ED. The main role of the ED is to screen patients for potential reversible causes and refer on for specialist assessment.

Clinical features of a 'first fit'

A detailed history is crucial for the diagnosis and this should be obtained from the patient and any available witnesses.

No one feature enables the diagnosis of an epileptic seizure but certain clinical features may suggest a particular diagnosis (Table 11.6).

Patients should have a cardiovascular, respiratory, and neurological examination as part of their assessment in the ED.

Table 11.6 Clinical features suggesting a particular cause of a seizure

Epileptic seizure	Non-epileptic seizure	Vasovagal episode	Cardiac disorders
Bitten tongue	Poorly controlled thrashing	Posture—prolonged standing precipitates an attack or similar episodes have been prevented by lying down	Short-lived, irregular myoclonic jerking
Head-turning to one side	Back arching		Palpitations
No memory of abnormal behaviour	Eyes held shut		Chest pain
	Head rolling	Provoking factors (e.g. pain, medical procedure)	Shortness of breath
Unusual posturing	Pelvic thrusting		May occur during exercise
Prolonged limb-jerking		Prodromal symptoms (e.g. sweating, feeling hot)	
Confusion after event			Reduced exercise tolerance or fatigue
Prodromal *déjà vu* or *jamais vu*		May have short-lived, irregular myoclonic jerking	
Incontinence		Full, rapid recovery	

Examination findings that may suggest an underlying precipitant include:

- Fever: suggestive of an infective process such as meningitis.
- Purpuric rash: suggestive of meningococcal disease.
- External signs of head trauma, which may be indicative of intracranial bleeding (e.g. subdural haematoma).
- Retinal haemorrhages: in keeping with a diagnosis of subarachnoid haemorrhage.
- Jaundice, spider naevi, or other signs suggestive of chronic alcohol abuse.
- Focal limb or facial weakness: supportive of a diagnosis of thromboembolic stroke.

Investigations following a first fit

The following investigations should be performed on patients presenting with a first fit:

- 12 lead ECG—to screen for an underlying arrhythmia (e.g. abnormal QT interval).
- Blood glucose—to exclude hypoglycaemia as a cause.
- FBC—to screen for a potential underlying infective cause.
- U&E, magnesium, and calcium—to screen for potential metabolic causes.

If the patient is pyrexial, then further investigation may be appropriate to identify the infective cause:

- Urinalysis
- Chest X-ray (CXR)
- Blood cultures

A CT head scan is not routinely required in patients following a first fit but should be performed in those where an underlying focal cause is likely, for example focal neurological signs, head injury, suspected intracranial infection, bleeding disorder (including anticoagulants), or where full consciousness is not regained.

Follow-up and discharge advice

The NICE guidance on the management of epilepsy recommends that all patients having a first fit should be seen as soon as possible (within two weeks) by a specialist in the management of epilepsy.

Upon discharge from the ED, the patient and relatives should be given the following advice (verbally and written):

- How to recognize a seizure.
- First-aid advice on how to manage a subsequent seizure.
- Safety advice (e.g. not locking bathroom doors, swimming unsupervised, operation of heavy machinery, and so on).
- Driving advice—the patient must be informed they cannot drive and they must inform the DVLA. They must refrain from driving for six months from the date of the seizure. A subsequent diagnosis of epilepsy extends this to one year.
- Appointment with an epilepsy specialist and contact details for the service.

KEY POINTS

Epilepsy is a neurological condition characterized by recurrent epileptic seizures unprovoked by any immediately identifiable cause.

- An epileptic seizure is the clinical manifestation of an abnormal and excessive discharge of neurons in the brain.
- Seizures are divided into two main types: partial seizures and generalized seizures.

Partial seizures originate from a specific area of the cortex. There are two types of partial seizure:

Simple partial seizure—involve only one area of the brain and consciousness is maintained.

Complex partial seizures—arise from a single region of the brain and are associated with a
    degree of consciousness impairment.

Partial seizures sometimes spread from one hemisphere to both hemispheres. This is called a
secondary generalized seizure. When this happens, the patient loses consciousness, and will
usually have a tonic–clonic seizure.

Generalized seizures affect both sides of the brain at once and can happen without warning.
The patient is unconscious. Following the seizure, the patient has no recollection of what
happened during the attack. The commonest type of generalized seizure is tonic–clonic.

Patients attending the ED following a first seizure should be screened for potential reversible
causes. Those who are fit for discharge should be referred on for specialist assessment and
seen within two weeks.

All patients who have had a seizure should have a blood glucose check and an ECG.

Patients should be given verbal and written advice upon discharge from the ED. They should
be advised not to drive and that it is their responsibility to inform the DVLA.

11.6 Status epilepticus

11.6.1 Introduction

Status epilepticus is a state of prolonged, uncontrolled seizures. It is a common ED presentation
that is potentially life-threatening. Untreated, the mortality approaches 30%.

Status epilepticus shows a bimodal distribution with highest incidences in the first year of life and
after the age of 60 years.

Rapid diagnosis and emergency treatment is essential to terminate the seizure and to minimize
the risk of any long-term neurological damage. Various treatment strategies are available but the
mainstay of treatment is benzodiazepines.

11.6.2 Definition of status epilepticus

Traditional definitions of status epilepticus refer to either:

- a single seizure persisting for more than 30 minutes; or
- multiple seizures of shorter duration without full neurological recovery in between seizures.

More recently, the term 'impending status epilepticus' has been advocated to describe continuous
or intermittent seizures that last longer than five minutes.

The reason for the term 'impending status epilepticus' relates to evidence that:

- A significant proportion of seizures that continue for five minutes will persist for longer than
  30 minutes.
- The average seizure duration in adults is less than one minute, therefore seizures that persist
  beyond five minutes represent a significant deviation from the norm.
- There is evidence that neuronal injury can result after just five minutes of seizure activity.

Refractory status epilepticus refers to persistent convulsions despite adequate doses of two intravenous antiepileptic agents.

11.6.3 Causes of status epilepticus

In one-third of patients presenting with status epilepticus, there will be a previous diagnosis of epilepsy. In two-thirds of patients with status epilepticus, there will be no previous history of epilepsy;
however, half of these patients will subsequently go on to be diagnosed with epilepsy.

Table 11.7 Causes of status epilepticus

Previous history of epilepsy	No history of epilepsy
Most common causes for status epilepticus: • Drug non-compliance • Drug withdrawal • Drug therapy alteration Other causes include: • Inter-current illness • Metabolic abnormalities • Co-ingestion of drugs that lower the seizure threshold	• Drug withdrawal syndromes (e.g. alcohol, barbiturates, benzodiazepines) • Acute structural brain injury (e.g. stroke, SAH, trauma, and cerebral hypoxia) • CNS infection (e.g. meningitis, encephalitis, and abscess)

The most likely cause of status epilepticus depends on whether there is a previous diagnosis of epilepsy or not (Table 11.7).

11.6.4 Clinical presentation of status epilepticus

Status epilepticus refers to a prolonged seizure of any type. Presentations may vary from clinically obvious tonic–clonic convulsions, to subtle focal seizures, to seemingly bizarre sensory alterations associated with partial seizures.

Numerous systemic and metabolic changes occur in association with prolonged seizures, including:

• Tachycardia
• Hypertension
• Hyperglycaemia
• Lactic acidosis

Most of these changes are thought to result from a surge in catecholamine release that accompanies the seizure and resolve with seizure resolution.

Beyond 30 minutes of seizure duration, cerebral autoregulation may become impaired and cerebral perfusion will fall as hypotension occurs, with potential for ischaemic injury and cerebral oedema.

11.6.5 Investigations for status epilepticus

All ED patients presenting with status epilepticus should have the following investigations:

• Blood glucose.
• Urea and electrolytes.
• Magnesium.
• Calcium.
• Full blood count.
• Arterial blood gas—an acidosis is commonly seen in status epilepticus, typically with metabolic (lactic acidosis) and respiratory (hypoventilation) components. The induced acidosis does not correlate with any degree of neuronal injury and is thought to act as anticonvulsant contributing to the termination of seizures. Typically the acidosis resolves on termination of the seizure.

Further investigations will be determined by the specific circumstances of individual cases. These may include:

• CT brain scan
• Blood cultures

- Serum antiepileptic drug levels
- Lumbar puncture for CSF evaluation
- Toxicology screen

An EEG is rarely required in the acute setting. However, it may be of value in patients with suspected non-convulsive status, or in those patients who are paralysed and sedated in order to monitor seizure activity.

11.6.6 Emergency department management of status epilepticus

Status epilepticus is a medical emergency that requires urgent aggressive therapy in order to limit any long-term damage. The outcome for a patient worsens with increasing duration of status epilepticus and there is progressive loss of responsiveness to benzodiazepines. Therefore, early initiation of antiepileptic drug therapy is the key to successful treatment.

The management for status epilepticus in adults and children is similar but not identical. Table 11.8 details the stepwise management of status epilepticus for adults and Table 11.9 for children.

11.6.7 Drug therapy in status epilepticus

Benzodiazepines

Benzodiazepines are first-line agents for treating status epilepticus. They prevent propagation of the seizure rather than affecting the original focus. They enhance the effect of the neurotransmitter GABA, which decreases neuronal activity. All benzodiazepines carry the risk of respiratory depression and hypotension.

All have a rapid onset of action due to their lipid solubility and consequent ability to cross the blood–brain barrier.

Table 11.8 The management of status epilepticus in adults

Time	Management	No IV access
0 minutes	Manage ABC	
	Administer high-flow oxygen	
	Measure the blood glucose and administer IV glucose if hypoglycaemia is found	
	Intravenous Pabrinex® or thiamine should be given in patients with known, or suspected, alcohol abuse, or poor nutritional status	
5 minutes	If the seizure persists beyond five minutes treat as status epilepticus	Diazepam 10 mg PR or midazolam 10 mg buccal
	Lorazepam 4 mg IV	
15 minutes	Lorazepam 4 mg IV	Diazepam 10 mg PR or midazolam 10 mg buccal
25 minutes	Request senior help if not already present	Consider intraosseous access or cutdown if IV access has not been achieved
	Phenytoin 15–18 mg/kg IV and/or phenobarbital 10–15 mg/kg IV	
40 minutes	Rapid sequence induction with one of propofol, midazolam, or thiopental	
	Transfer to intensive care unit	

Table 11.9 The management of status epilepticus in children

Time	Management	No IV access
0 minutes	Manage ABC Administer high-flow oxygen Measure the blood glucose and administer IV glucose if hypoglycaemia is found	
5 minutes	If the seizure persists beyond 5 minutes treat as status epilepticus Lorazepam 0.1 mg/kg IV	Diazepam 0.5 mg/kg PR or midazolam buccal (age 1–6 months 300 mcg/kg; age 6 months to 1 year, 2.5 mg; age 1–5 years, 5 mg; age 5–10 years, 7.5 mg; age >10 years, 10 mg)
15 minutes	Lorazepam 0.1 mg/kg IV	Paraldehyde 0.4 ml/kg (in same volume of olive oil) PR
25 minutes	Request senior help if not already present. Phenytoin 18 mg/kg IV. If already on phenytoin, give phenobarbital 20 mg/kg IV AND paraldehyde 0.4 ml/kg PR if not already given	Consider intraosseous access or cutdown if IV access has not been achieved
40 minutes	Rapid sequence induction using thiopental 4 mg/kg IV Transfer to intensive care unit	

The agents used most frequently are:

- Diazepam (lipid-soluble).
- Lorazepam (lipid-soluble).
- Midazolam (water-soluble at pH less than 4, lipid-soluble at physiological pH).

Diazepam is available as both intravenous and rectal preparations. Rectal diazepam will terminate seizures in 70% of patients; intravenous diazepam will terminate seizures in 60–80% of patients in status epilepticus.

Lorazepam is less lipophilic, has a smaller volume of distribution, and a longer intracerebral half-life (12 hours) than diazepam. It may therefore provide more prolonged suppression of seizures. Intravenous lorazepam will terminate seizures in 60–90% of patients in status epilepticus.

Midazolam is water-soluble at pH<4 making it available for buccal or intranasal use. At physiological pH (7.4) it is lipid-soluble enabling it to cross the blood–brain barrier.

Phenytoin

Phenytoin is a long-acting drug whose advantage is the prevention of seizure recurrence over an extended period of time. Its delayed onset (10 to 30 minutes) necessitates use in combination with a rapidly acting agent, typically a benzodiazepine.

Phenytoin is not water-soluble and is formulated with propylene glycol, which has the potential to cause significant side effects including:

- Local infusion site reactions.
- Arrhythmias mandating cardiac monitoring during infusion.
- Hypotension.

Phenytoin is associated with the 'purple glove syndrome' characterized by local oedema, skin discoloration, and pain distal to the infusion site. Skin necrosis and limb ischaemia have been reported.

Complications are reduced by keeping infusion rates below 50 mg per minute and by avoiding co-infusion with glucose-containing fluids, which can lead to the formation of precipitates.

Fosphenytoin is the inactive prodrug of phenytoin, which is broken down into the active drug by serum phosphatases. It has the advantage that it is water-soluble and hence is associated with fewer of the local side effects. It may also be infused at a faster rate. However, the time taken for the active metabolite to be formed means it has a similar time to onset as phenytoin.

Paraldehyde

Paraldehyde is recommended in paediatric treatment algorithms as a second-line agent to be used after benzodiazepines in the absence of intravenous access. It is given via the rectal route, mixed with an equal volume of olive oil. While there is little published evidence to support its use, there is a large body of anecdotal evidence.

Barbiturates

Barbiturates have a similar mode of action to benzodiazepines by modification of the actions of GABA. These agents are not standard first-line drugs but may be used for patients with refractory status epilepticus.

Side effects include respiratory depression and sedation, particularly if used after benzodiazepines. Agents used include:

- Phenobarbital.
- Thiopental.
- Pentobarbital, a short-acting agent with a rapid onset of action that is very effective at terminating seizures.

KEY POINTS

Status epilepticus refers to a single seizure lasting >30 min or multiple shorter seizures without full neurological recovery in between.

Impending status epilepticus refers to multiple or continuous seizures lasting >5 min without full neurological recovery in between.

Two-thirds of patients with status epilepticus will have no prior history of epilepsy or convulsions. Causes in these patients include drug withdrawal syndromes, acute structural brain injury, and CNS infections.

In patients with epilepsy, status epilepticus most commonly results from reduced intake of normal antiepileptic medication.

After 30 min of seizure activity, there may be failure of cerebral autoregulation with potential for ischaemia and oedema.

Intravenous benzodiazepines will terminate seizures in over 80% of patients in a matter of minutes and hence should be used as first-line agents. As seizure duration increases, responsiveness to benzodiazepines reduces.

Lorazepam is more effective at terminating seizures than diazepam and is more effective at preventing seizure recurrence.

Ten minutes should be left between doses of antiepileptic agents to allow time for the drug to work and avoid compounding any adverse effects.

11.7 Acute stroke

11.7.1 Introduction

The World Health Organization defines stroke as the sudden onset of focal neurological signs, of presumed vascular origin, lasting longer than 24 hours or causing death.

Stroke accounts for 11% of all deaths and is a significant cause of morbidity.

NICE produced guidance on the diagnosis and management of acute stroke and transient ischaemic attack (TIA) in 2008. The following section is based on that guidance.

11.7.2 Causes of stroke

Stroke can be classified as ischaemic, due to an interruption of blood supply, or haemorrhagic, due to rupture of a cerebral artery. Approximately 85% of strokes are caused by ischaemia and the remainder by haemorrhage.

An ischaemic stroke can be due to:

- Thrombosis—atherosclerotic disease typically affects the extracranial internal carotid artery but may also affect the vertebral and basilar arteries.
- Embolism—common sources of cardiac emboli are atrial fibrillation, mural thrombus, and valvular heart disease. Typically, emboli involve the territory of large intracerebral arteries, particularly the middle cerebral.
- Small vessel disease (e.g. striate arteries).
- Systemic hypoperfusion (e.g. due to shock).
- Venous thrombosis—rare cause of stroke due to thrombosis of the dural venous sinuses (e.g. hypercoaguable states, sickle cell disease).
- Carotid artery dissection—rare but should be suspected in patients younger than 50 years old. There is usually a history of ipsilateral head, face, or neck pain.

Haemorrhagic stroke generally occurs in small arteries or arterioles and is commonly due to hypertension, vascular malformations (e.g. berry aneurysms, AVMs, cavernous angiomas), cerebral amyloid angiopathy, or infarcts into which secondary haemorrhage has occurred.

11.7.3 Clinical features of stroke

The clinical features of stroke reflect the vascular territory involved (see Table 11.10).

The anterior circulation is served by the internal carotid arteries, the main branches of which are the middle cerebral artery and anterior cerebral artery. The anterior circulation supplies blood to the anterior three-fifths of the cerebrum. The posterior circulation is served by the vertebral and basilar arteries. The vertebra-basilar arteries supply the posterior two-fifths of the cerebrum, part of the cerebellum, and the brainstem. The basilar artery gives off the posterior cerebral arteries.

The anterior and posterior circulations are linked via posterior communicating arteries, forming the circle of Willis (Figure 11.1).

The Oxford clinical classification is often used to categorize stroke (Table 11.11). It describes four subtypes of stroke:

- Total anterior circulation stroke (TACS)
- Partial anterior circulation stroke (PACS)
- Lacunar stroke (LACS)
- Posterior circulation stroke (POCS)

11.7.4 Recognition of stroke

Distinguishing acute stroke from 'stroke mimics' is vitally important in the ED to ensure prompt and appropriate treatment. Stroke mimics include:

Table 11.10 Clinical features of stroke according to arterial territory

Arterial territory	Clinical features
Middle cerebral artery	• Contralateral motor deficit (weakness of the face and arm is greater than the leg) • Contralateral sensory deficit • Gaze deviated towards side of lesion • If dominant hemisphere involved—receptive/expressive dysphasia • If non-dominant hemisphere involved—neglect/inattention
Anterior cerebral artery	• Disinhibition • Speech preservation • Altered mental status • Contralateral motor deficit (weakness in leg greater than arm) • Contralateral cortical sensory deficit (e.g. gait apraxia)
Posterior cerebral artery	• Visual disturbance • Contralateral homonymous hemianopia • Impaired memory
Vertebrobasilar artery	• Cerebellar signs (intention tremor, dysdiadochokinesia, nystagmus, and ataxia) • Vertigo • Dysarthria • Visual field defects, diplopia • Syncope • Ipsilateral cranial nerve deficits • Contralateral motor deficit

• Seizures (e.g. with Todd's paresis)
• Space-occupying lesions (primary or secondary cerebral tumours)
• Hypoglycaemia
• Subdural haemorrhage
• Cerebral abscess
• Encephalitis
• Cerebral vasculitis (e.g. temporal arteritis)
• Migraine
• Spinal cord lesions

Table 11.11 Oxford clinical classification of stroke

Total anterior circulation stroke	Partial anterior circulation stroke	Lacunar stroke	Posterior circulation stroke
All three of: • Contralateral motor or sensory deficit • Homonymous hemianopia • Higher cortical dysfunction	Two of: • Contralateral motor or sensory deficit • Homonymous hemianopia • Higher cortical dysfunction	Any one of: • Pure motor deficit • Pure sensory deficit • Sensorimotor deficit	Any one of: • Isolated homonymous hemianopia • Brainstem signs • Cerebellar ataxia

Data from Bamford J, Sandercock P, Dennis M, et al (June 1991). 'Classification and natural history of clinically identifiable subtypes of cerebral infarction'. Lancet 337 (8756): 1521–6.

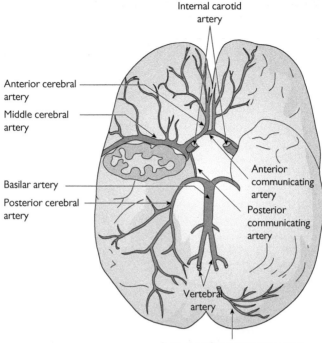

Figure 11.1 The arterial circle of Willis, at the base of the brain

Reproduced from David A. Warrell, Timothy M. Cox, and John D. Firth, Oxford Textbook of Medicine, 2010, Figure 24.10.1.2, p. 4935, with permission from Oxford University Press

- Sepsis (may exacerbate old neurological signs)
- Delirium
- Vestibular pathology
- Mononeuropathies
- Functional disorders
- Dementia

Two formal assessment tools for the recognition of stroke are commonly used in pre-hospital medicine and the ED; these are the face arm speech test (FAST) and the Recognition of Stroke in the Emergency Room (ROSIER) scale.

The face arm speech test

The FAST scale is predominantly used by the ambulance service to identify patients suffering from an acute stroke. It is also suitable for use by the general public.

The face arm speech test is composed of three equally weighted clinical signs:

- Facial asymmetry: 1 point
- Arm (or leg) weakness: 1 point
- Speech disturbance: 1 point

A stroke should be suspected if any of these signs are present (score >0). The sensitivity for stroke is 82% and specificity 83%.

Table 11.12 ROSIER scale

Negative predictive symptoms	Positive predictive symptoms
• Loss of consciousness or syncope? Yes: −1 point Seizure activity? Yes: −1 point.	New acute onset: • Asymmetric facial weakness? Yes: + 1 point • Asymmetric arm weakness? Yes: +1 point • Asymmetric leg weakness? Yes: + 1 point • Speech disturbance? Yes: + 1 point • Visual field defect? Yes: +1 point

The total score range is −2 to + 5.
Stroke is likely if the score ≥1, in the absence of hypoglycaemia. The sensitivity for stroke diagnosis is 93% and specificity 83%.

Data from Nor AM, Davis J, Sen B et al. The Recognition of Stroke in the Emergency Room (ROSIER) scale: development and validation of a stroke recognition instrument. Lancet Neurology 2005;4(11):727–734.

ROSIER

The ROSIER scale is designed for ED use. It comprises two negative predictive symptoms, to help screen for stroke mimics, and five positive predictive symptoms (Table 11.12).

11.7.5 Assessing the severity of stroke

National Institute for Health Stroke Score (NIHSS)

The NIHSS is a systematic assessment tool that provides a quantitative measure of stroke-related neurological deficit. It was initially designed as a research tool but is now widely used to evaluate the severity of a stroke, determine appropriate treatment, and provide prognostic information. Patients with an acute stroke who may be eligible for thrombolysis should have a NIHSS calculated.

The score involves a neurological examination to evaluate the effects of an acute cerebral infarction.

The components of the NIHSS are:

- Level of consciousness
- Language
- Neglect
- Visual field loss
- Extraocular movements
- Motor strength
- Ataxia
- Dysarthria
- Sensory loss

The total possible score is 42. A higher score indicates a more severe stroke and a worse prognosis.

11.7.6 Investigations for acute stroke

Brain imaging

Brain imaging should be performed immediately (i.e. the next available slot and definitely within one hour) for patients with acute stroke, if any of the following apply:

- Indications for thrombolysis or early anticoagulation treatment
- On anticoagulant treatment
- A known bleeding tendency
- A depressed level of consciousness

- Unexplained or fluctuating symptoms
- Papilloedema, neck stiffness, or fever
- Severe headache at onset of stroke symptoms

For patients without an immediate indication, brain imaging should be performed as soon as possible (i.e. within 24 hours).

Typically in the ED, a non-contrast CT scan is the most commonly used brain imaging technique. This can help exclude an intracerebral haemorrhage or important mimics, such as brain metastases. However, the sensitivity for detection of ischaemia is low in the very early stages of stroke. Some hospitals may offer MRI scanning, which has a greater sensitivity for early ischaemia.

Other investigations in acute stroke

- Blood glucose—is paramount and the most useful bedside test to exclude an easily reversible stroke mimic. Blood glucose should be maintained between 4 and 11 mmol/L.
- Clotting—should be checked if the patient is on anticoagulants. Urgent reversal will be required if imaging reveals an intracranial bleed.
- ECG—may suggest a cardiac origin for thrombus (e.g. atrial fibrillation).
- ESR—may suggest a vasculitic cause.
- Other investigations, such as FBC, U&E, lipids, and CXR, should be requested but are unlikely to alter the acute ED management and therefore should not be the first answers given in an SAQ.

11.7.7 Emergency department management of acute stroke

Acute treatments with proven benefits in acute ischaemic stroke include admission to a dedicated stroke unit; administration of intravenous tissue plasminogen activator; antiplatelet agents; and surgical decompression of massive cerebral oedema.

Thrombolysis in acute ischaemic stroke

Alteplase is licensed for the thrombolysis of acute stroke. The indications for thrombolysis in acute stroke are detailed in Table 11.13.

The dose is 0.9 mg/kg (maximum 90 mg) infused over 60 minutes, with 10% of the total dose given as an initial bolus.

The European licence for alteplase permits administration within three hours of symptom onset but many centres now administer up to 4.5 hours, based on research evidence.

The benefit of alteplase is reducing long-term disability. The earlier alteplase is given the greater benefit. Alteplase does not improve overall survival or immediately improve neurological function.

The main concern of administering alteplase is the potential for iatrogenic intracerebral haemorrhage. The highest risk of intracerebral haemorrhage is in those with a high NIHSS score, a large area of ischaemia on CT, or hypertension. Therefore, patient selection guidance is designed to minimize the risk.

Table 11.13 Indications for thrombolysis in acute stroke

Indications for thrombolysis in acute stroke	CT appearance consistent with an ischaemic stroke
	Onset <3 h (<4.5 h in some centres)
	Clinical diagnosis of stroke (plus NIHSS calculated)
	Risk and benefits explained to patient and/or relative
	No contraindications to thrombolysis

Table **11.14** Contraindications to thrombolysis in stroke

Rationale	Contraindications
Timing	• Onset of symptoms >4.5 h • Unclear time of onset
Age	• Age <18 or >80 years old (patients older than 80 years old were excluded from most clinical trials, however many centres will give thrombolysis to selected older patients)
Stroke severity	• Mild stroke (NIHSS <5) or rapid improvement • Severe stroke (NIHSS >25 or extensive stroke on imaging)
Possible stroke mimic	• Evidence of intracranial haemorrhage • Seizure at onset of stroke • Symptoms indicating a subarachnoid haemorrhage (even if CT normal)
General increased bleeding risk	• Oral anticoagulant use (INR >1.4) • Platelet count <100 × 10⁶/L • Heparin within the last 48 h with raised APTT • Known bleeding diathesis • Active internal bleeding • Recent (<3 months) major surgery or trauma
Increased risk of intracerebral bleeding	• Previous stroke within past three months • Previous stroke and concomitant diabetes • Previous intracranial haemorrhage • Intracranial neoplasm, AVM, or aneurysm • Systolic BP >185 mmHg or diastolic BP >110 mmHg

Increasingly ED physicians are administering alteplase for the treatment of acute ischaemic stroke as part of a well-organized stroke service. ED physicians should be appropriately trained and experienced in acute stroke management and be supported by neuroradiological and stroke physicians.

Contraindications to thrombolysis in acute stroke continue to evolve as experience with the technique develops. Table 11.14 details contraindications to thrombolysis.

Aspirin

- NICE guidelines recommend that patients with acute ischaemic stroke receive 300 mg aspirin daily for two weeks, followed by a long-term secondary preventative antiplatelet strategy.
- Aspirin should be withheld for 24 hours after thrombolysis.
- If a patient's swallowing is impaired, rectal aspirin should be given.
- If the patient is allergic or intolerant of aspirin, then an alternative antiplatelet agent should be used (e.g. clopidogrel or dipyridamole).

Supportive management in stroke

Failure of homeostatic mechanisms during the acute phase of stroke is common and supportive care delivered through a specialist stroke unit is crucial.

In the ED, management should focus on maintaining hydration, normoxia, normothermia, and blood glucose at 4–11 mmol/L.

The role of blood pressure control in the immediate phase after stroke is unclear. UK and international guidelines do not recommend routine lowering of blood pressure in acute stroke.

Treatment may be appropriate if there is a hypertensive emergency with one or more of the following:

- Hypertensive encephalopathy
- Hypertensive nephropathy
- Hypertensive cardiac failure/myocardial infarction
- Aortic dissection
- Pre-eclampsia/eclampsia
- Intracerebral haemorrhage with systolic BP >200 mmHg

Blood pressure reduction to 185/110 mmHg or lower should also be considered in patients who are eligible for thrombolysis.

KEY POINTS

A stroke is the sudden onset of focal neurological signs, of presumed vascular origin, lasting longer than 24 h or causing death.

Stroke can be classified as ischaemic, due to an interruption of blood supply, or haemorrhagic, due to rupture of a cerebral artery.

The clinical features reflect the vascular territory involved.

The face arm speech test (FAST) and ROSIER scales are formal assessment tools which are commonly used for the recognition of stroke.

Brain imaging should be performed (within one hour) if any of the following apply:

- Indications for thrombolysis or early anticoagulation treatment
- On anticoagulant treatment
- A known bleeding tendency
- A depressed level of consciousness
- Unexplained or fluctuating symptoms
- Papilloedema, neck stiffness, or fever
- Severe headache at onset of stroke symptoms

For patients without an immediate indication, brain imaging should be performed within 24 h.

Proven treatments for acute ischaemic stroke include admission to a dedicated stroke unit; thrombolysis; antiplatelet agents; and surgical decompression of massive cerebral oedema.

11.8 Transient ischaemic attack

11.8.1 Introduction

A transient ischaemic attack is defined as stroke symptoms and signs that resolve within 24 hours. TIA is part of the pathophysiological continuum of cerebrovascular disease. An acute TIA is the clinical consequence of an interruption of the blood supply to a focal part of the brain with consequent disruption of function.

11.8.2 ABCD^2 score

Previous MRCEM question

A substantial risk of stroke exists in the early period after TIA. The most commonly used risk stratification tool is the ABCD^2 score, which is recommended by NICE (Tables 11.15 and 11.16). The ABCD^2 score has appeared in previous SAQ papers.

Table 11.16 Risk of future stroke based on ABCD^2 score

ABCD^2 score	Risk of stroke		
	2 days	7 days	90 days
0–3 (low risk)	1%	1.2%	3.1%
4–5 (moderate risk)	4.1%	5.9%	9.8%
6–7 (high risk)	8.1%	11.7%	18%

Data from Johnston SC, Rothwell PM, Nguyen-Huynh MN et al. Validation and refinement of scores to predict very early stroke risk after transient ischaemic attack. Lancet 2007;369(9558):283–292.

11.8.3 Emergency department management of transient ischaemic attacks

The following section is based on the NICE guidance:

- All patients with TIA should be immediately started on aspirin 300 mg daily.
- The risk of subsequent stroke should be assessed using the ABCD^2 score.
- Patients with an ABCD^2 score of 4 or greater should have specialist assessment within 24 hours of symptom onset.
- Patients with crescendo TIA (two or more TIAs in a week) should have specialist assessment within 24 hours of symptom onset.
- Patients with an ABCD^2 score of 3 or below should have specialist assessment within one week of symptom onset.
- Patients presenting more than one week after symptoms have resolved should have specialist assessment within one week of presentation.
- Measures for secondary prevention should be introduced as soon as the diagnosis is confirmed (e.g. lipid lowering therapy, antihypertensives, treatment of diabetes, management of AF, and lifestyle advice).
- Patients who are discharged from the ED should be advised that they cannot drive for at least one month. They may resume driving after this period if clinical recovery is satisfactory. They

Table 11.15 ABCD^2 score

Characteristics		ABCD^2 score
Age	≥60 years	1 point
Blood pressure	≥140/90 mmHg	1 point
Clinical features	Focal weakness	2 points
	Speech disturbance without weakness	1 point
Duration	≥60 minutes	2 points
	10–59 minutes	1 point
Diabetes		1 point

Reprinted from *The Lancet*, volume 369, issue 9558, S Claiborne Johnston, Peter M Rothwell, Mai N Nguyen Huynh, Matthew F Giles, Jacob S Elkins, Allan L Bernstein, Stephen Sidney, Validation and refinement of scores to predict very early stroke risk after transient ischaemic attack, pp. 283–292, Copyright 2007, with permission from Elsevier

do not need to notify the DVLA unless there is a residual neurological deficit (see Chapter 20, section 20.5).

11.8.4 Imaging for transient ischaemic attacks

- Not all patients suffering a TIA require brain imaging. Patients should have specialist assessment before a decision on imaging is made.
- Patients who have a suspected TIA, in whom the vascular territory or pathology is uncertain, should undergo brain imaging (preferably a diffusion-weighted MRI).
- Patients at a high risk of stroke (e.g. $ABCD^2 \geq 4$ or crescendo TIA), who require imaging, should have this done within 24 hours of symptom onset. Patients at lower risk of stroke ($ABCD^2 \leq 3$), who require imaging, should have this done within one week of symptom onset.
- Brain imaging may also be helpful for patients being considered for carotid endarterectomy where it is uncertain if the stroke is in the anterior or posterior circulation.
- Carotid imaging is required to determine the presence and severity of carotid stenosis in those patients who may be appropriate for carotid endarterectomy (i.e. those with a TIA involving the anterior circulation who are fit and willing for surgery. NICE recommend that carotid imaging is performed within one week of symptom onset).

KEY POINTS

A transient ischaemic attack (TIA) is a brief episode of neurological dysfunction caused by focal brain or retinal ischaemia.

A substantial risk of stroke exists in the early period after TIA.

$ABCD^2$ score is the recommended risk stratification tool for TIA.

The $ABCD^2$ score can be used to determine the urgency of specialist assessment and further investigation.

Early specialist assessment and modification of risk factors (diabetes, AF, hypertension, hypercholesterolemia, and smoking) reduces the risk of subsequent stroke.

Aspirin should be started immediately unless there are contraindications.

Patients who have a TIA affecting the anterior circulation, and who are potentially fit for surgery, should have carotid imaging.

11.9 Motor weakness

11.9.1 Anatomy of motor system

The curriculum includes a broad understanding of the neuroanatomy of the motor system and the diseases that can affect the various components of this system.

The primary motor cortex is located in the precentral gyrus of the cerebrum. It is organized according to the body region it controls (motor homunculus). It contains neurons (upper motor neurons), which send long axons down the spinal cord to synapse with lower motor neurons.

As the motor axons travel down through the cerebral white matter, they move closer together, and form part of the posterior limb of the internal capsule. They continue down into the brainstem where the majority decussate in the medulla oblongata (pyramidal decussation). After crossing, the upper motor neurons travel down the spinal cord in the lateral corticospinal tracts. Fibres that do not decussate in the brainstem travel down the anterior corticospinal tract and cross over to the contralateral side in the spinal cord, shortly before reaching the lower motor neurons.

Upper motor neurons synapse with lower motor neurons in the anterior horn of the spinal column. Upper motor neurons secrete the chemical neurotransmitter glutamate.

Lower motor neurons travel in peripheral nerves to innervate muscles of the cervical, thoracic, and lumbosacral segments. Lower motor neurons secrete the chemical neurotransmitter acetylcholine at neuromuscular junctions to stimulate voluntary muscle contraction.

11.9.2 Clinical features of lesions in the motor system

Certain clinical features help identify the location of the lesion within the motor system (Table 11.17).

Table 11.17 Clinical features and sites of lesions within the motor system

Site of lesion	Clinical features	Examples
Upper motor neuron (above the level of the anterior horn cell, e.g. cerebral cortex, internal capsule, corticospinal tracts)	• Spasticity • Hyperreflexia • Plantars upgoing • Clonus • Hoffman's reflex may be positive (flicking a finger causes neighbouring digits to flex) • Minimal muscle wasting • Weakness affects muscle groups not individual muscles (leg flexors and arms extensors most affected) • Loss of skilled fine-movement is greater than expected for overall grade of weakness	• Stroke • Tumour • Abscess • Intracerebral bleed • Spinal cord injury (e.g. trauma, compression, infarction, bleed, syringomyelia, subacute combined degeneration of the cord)
Lower motor neuron (below or at the level of the anterior horn cell)	• Flaccidity • Hypotonia • Fasiculations (if lesion at or near the anterior horn cell) • Hyporeflexia • Plantars are absent or normal • Muscle wasting • Weakness equally affects extensors and flexors • Weakness in muscles supplied specifically by the nerve root or nerve affected	• Mononeuropathy • Polyneuropathy • Guillain–Barré syndrome • Subacute combined degeneration of the cord • Spinal cord compression (in the early stages of acute cord damage there are LMN signs; as the condition progresses LMN signs persist at the site of the compression and UMN signs develop below it)
Neuromuscular junction	• Muscle fatigability • Commonly affects extraocular, bulbar, face, and neck muscles • Reflexes may be normal or brisk • Ptosis is usually present • No sensory symptoms	• Myasthenia gravis
Muscle	• Muscle weakness (predominantly proximal) • Myotonia (delayed muscular relaxation after contraction) • Variable muscle wasting or hypertrophy • Usually symmetrical • No sensory symptoms • Reflexes are lost at a later stage than with neuropathies	• Myopathies (e.g. dystrophia myotonica, Duchenne's muscular dystrophy, polymyositis)

11.9.3 Upper motor neuron motor weakness

- Monoplegia—is weakness of one limb and is usually due to a motor cortex lesion (e.g. stroke or tumour) or very rarely a partial internal capsule, brainstem, or cord lesion (e.g. multiple sclerosis).
- Hemiplegia—is weakness of the arm and leg on the same side. Weakness of the leg, arm, and lower face on one side may be due to a lesion in the contralateral motor cortex or internal capsule, most commonly due to a stroke but also trauma, tumour, abscess, or multiple sclerosis. Crossed paralyses (e.g. ipsilateral facial and contralateral arm and leg weakness) are typical of brainstem lesions.
- Paraplegia—is weakness of both legs and is usually due to spinal cord injury (e.g. trauma, compression, infarction, bleed). Spinal cord injury may also result from subacute combined degeneration of the cord secondary to B12 deficiency or syringomyelia.
- Quadriplegia—is weakness of all four limbs and may result from similar causes as paraplegia, plus cervical cord injury, and repeated strokes.

Subacute combined degeneration of the spinal cord

Subacute combined degeneration of the spinal cord may be seen in any cause of low vitamin B12 (e.g. pernicious anaemia, low dietary intake seen in vegan diets, malabsorption syndromes, small bowel resection, and so on). It may be precipitated if a patient who has combined vitamin B12 and folic acid deficiency is treated with folic acid before the vitamin B12 deficiency is corrected.

It affects both upper motor neurones (UMNs) and lower motor neurones (LMNs). UMN signs result from damage of the posterior and lateral columns of the spinal cord. LMN signs result from peripheral neuropathy. Onset is usually insidious with joint position and vibration sense affected first (dorsal columns) followed by distal paraesthesia (neuropathy). Left untreated stiffness and weakness ensure. The classic triad is:

- Extensor plantars
- Brisk knee jerks
- Absent ankle jerks

Treatment is with vitamin B12 injections.

Syringomyelia

Syringomyelia is a generic term for disorders in which a cyst or cavity (syrinx) forms within the spinal cord. It may be a congenital abnormality or acquired as a complication of trauma, meningitis, tumour, or haemorrhage.

Symptoms result from destruction of the spinal cord. The damage may result in pain, paralysis, weakness, and stiffness in the back, shoulders, and extremities. Loss of temperature sensation may occur, particularly in the hands. The condition usually leads to a cape-like loss of pain and temperature sensation along the back and arms. Classically the dorsal columns are spared, leaving vibration and proprioception intact. Diagnosis is with MRI. Patients require referral to a neurosurgeon.

Spinal cord compression

The spinal cord runs from the foramen magnum down to the conus medullaris at approximately the level of second lumbar vertebrae. From here the spinal nerves for a band-like structure, the cauda equina that terminates at the filum terminale.

Spinal cord compression can occur at any point along its route. The spinal cord can be compressed by any external force such as from a fracture of vertebrae following trauma, abscess, haematoma, or a prolapsed intervertebral disc. Acute cord compression is syndrome of spastic paraparesis and is a medical emergency requiring urgent assessment and intervention to prevent long-term neurological damage.

Presentation of cord compression can vary between individuals. Clinical symptoms may include:

- Back pain
- Sensory level (an area of hyperaesthesia may be present at the level of an injury with sensory loss below)
- Paralysis below the level of the lesion
- Urinary/faecal incontinence
- Urinary retention
- Hyperreflexia

Management is dependent on the cause, however all patients presenting with signs and symptoms of acute cord compression should be investigated with an urgent MRI and discussion with regard to neurosurgery. Access to MRI scans in the ED, particularly out of hours, can vary widely and thus local guidelines will exist.

The difficulty in diagnosis includes the differentiation between progressive chronic cord compression and acute compression. For example, a slowly growing meningioma may slowly compress the cord causing symptoms of sensory loss and pain with preserved motor function, whereas injury following trauma may present with an acute paraplegia.

In the case of malignant cord compression, emergency radiotherapy may be indicated, and management should engage in discussion with the oncology/medical team. Many hospitals have their own local guidelines on malignant cord compression.

There are numerous different specific spinal cord syndromes, see Chapter 4, section 4.6—Spinal trauma.

Cauda equina syndrome

Cauda equina syndrome (CES) is a separate entity to spinal cord compression as it involves compression of the lumbar nerve roots after the termination of the spinal cord in the cauda equine. In comparison to cord compression, CES is a lower motor neurone lesion.

Symptoms include:

- Back pain
- Saddle anaesthesia
- Bladder/bowel disturbance
- Weakness
- Hyporeflexia

Management and assessment is similar to that of acute cord compression.

11.9.4 Lower motor neuron motor weakness

Mononeuropathy

A mononeuropathy is a single peripheral nerve lesion. Commonly mononeuropathies are caused by compressible lesions or have a vascular aetiology (Table 11.18). Two of the commonest mononeuropathies are carpal tunnel syndrome (see Chapter 5, section 5.19) and common peroneal nerve palsy.

Polyneuropathy

Polyneuropathies are generalized disorders of peripheral nerves that have a heterogeneous set of causes. Typically peripheral nerves are affected in a diffuse symmetrical fashion with symptoms and signs most prominent in the extremities. Different aetiologies may be associated with mainly motor, mainly sensory, or mainly autonomic fibres (Table 11.19).

Motor neuropathies cause partial denervation of muscle, of which fasiculations is a sign, particularly if the disorder is at or near the anterior horn cells. Patients may report weakness or clumsiness

Table 11.18 Common mononeuropathies

Nerve	Causes	Clinical features
Median nerve	Entrapment in the carpal tunnel at the wrist	Numbness and dysaesthesia in the radial 3½ fingers
	Associated with pregnancy, obesity, hypothyroidism, acromegaly, amyloidosis, rheumatoid arthritis	Weakness of the thenar eminence and lateral two lumbricals
Common peroneal nerve	Compression at the fibula neck (e.g. below knee plaster)	Weakness of tibialis anterior—dorsiflexion of the foot (foot drop) and inversion of the foot
	Fracture of the fibula neck	
	Diabetes mellitus	Weakness of peroneus—eversion of the foot
	Polyarteritis nodosa	
	Collagen-vascular disease	Loss of sensation over the dorsum of the foot
Ulnar nerve	Trauma at the elbow	Weakness/wasting of the hypothenar eminence
		Weakness of the interossei and ulnar 2 lumbricals—finger abduction
		Loss of sensation to the ulnar 1½ fingers and ulnar side of the hand
Radial nerve	Compression against the humerus (e.g. 'Saturday night' palsy)	Weakness of wrist and finger extension.
		Loss of sensation is variable but consistently absent on the dorsal aspect of the base of the thumb (first web space)

of the hands, difficulty walking with falls and stumbles, and respiratory difficulties. Signs are those of a LMN lesion: wasting and weakness most marked in the distal muscles of hands and feet; and reflexes which are reduced or absent.

Sensory neuropathies result in numbness, tingling or burning sensations often affecting the extremities first ('glove and stocking' distribution).

Autonomic neuropathies result in postural hypotension, impotence, reduced sweating, urinary retention, diarrhoea, or constipation.

Table 11.19 Causes of polyneuropathies

Mainly motor neuropathy	Mainly sensory neuropathy	Autonomic neuropathy
Guillain–Barré syndrome	Diabetes mellitus	Diabetes mellitus
Porphyria	Uraemia	Guillain–Barré syndrome
Lead poisoning	Vitamin B12 deficiency	Vascular or cord lesions
Diphtheria	Chronic alcohol abuse	Amyloidosis
Charcot-Marie-Tooth syndrome	Leprosy	Uraemia
	Amyloidosis	Chronic hepatic failure
		Secondary to drugs (e.g. tricyclics, levodopa)

Guillain–Barré syndrome

Guillain–Barré syndrome is a rare acute infective polyneuropathy. It is associated with demyelination of peripheral nerves.

The most common presentation is a post-infection disorder in an otherwise healthy patient. Approximately two-thirds of patients report symptoms of an infection (gastrointestinal or upper respiratory) in the preceding three weeks. Organisms implicated include *Campylobacter jejuni, Haemophilus influenzae, Mycoplasma pneumoniae, Cytomegalovirus,* and *Epstein–Barr virus.*

Guillain–Barré syndrome is characterized by rapidly progressive, bilateral weakness, accompanied by reduced or absent tendon reflexes. The symptoms and signs typically, but not always, move proximally.

Diagnostic features include:

- Progressive weakness in both arms and legs, often starting with legs
- Reduced, or absent, tendon reflexes
- Relative symmetry of symptoms
- Progression of symptoms up to four weeks
- Recovery
- Absence of fever at presentation
- Mild sensory symptoms or signs
- Facial weakness or other cranial nerve involvement
- Pain

Miller–Fisher syndrome is a variant of Guillain–Barré syndrome that has the cardinal feature of ophthalmoplegia, which is often part of a triad including ataxia and areflexia. Patients may also have ptosis, or facial or bulbar palsy, along with mild limb weakness.

Guillain–Barré syndrome is largely a clinical diagnosis, however raised CSF protein (>0.4 g/L) with a normal white cell count is the typical CSF finding.

Other useful initial investigations include:

- Stool culture (for *C. jejuni* and others).
- ECG—due to the risk of autonomic failure and cardiac arrhythmias.
- Lung function tests—if the patient has any respiratory compromise or is unable to walk.
- Creatine kinase—if raised suggests an alternative diagnosis such as myositis.
- Hypokalaemia and hypoglycaemia—may mimic Guillain–Barré symptoms, and should be excluded.

Poor prognostic features include:

- Rapid onset of symptoms
- Increasing age
- Prior infection with *C. Jejuni*
- Severe weakness

ED management should focus on identification of possible cases and ensuring hospital admission. Patients with seemingly mild symptoms can rapidly progress to respiratory compromise.

Serial lung function tests are important and patients with a FVC <20 ml/kg are candidates for prophylactic intubation and ventilation.

Initial treatment is supportive. Plasma exchange or intravenous immunoglobulins are indicated in severe cases (e.g. patients who are unable to walk). Corticosteroids are of no proven benefit.

Motor neuron disease

Motor neuron disease is a degenerative disorder affecting both LMN and UMN, supplying limb and bulbar muscles.

The cause of motor neuron disease is unknown. There are three principal types:

- Progressive muscular atrophy—lesion of the anterior horn cells typically presenting with LMN signs.
- Amyotrophic lateral sclerosis—combined LMN wasting and UMN hyperreflexia contribute to weakness.
- Progressive bulbar palsy—bulbar musculature is affected.

Clinical features include UMN signs (weakness, spasticity, brisk reflexes, upgoing plantars), and LMN signs (weakness, wasting, and fasiculations).

There is no sensory involvement, which helps distinguish motor neuron disease from multiple sclerosis and polyneuropathies. It never affects the extraocular muscles which distinguishes it from myasthenia gravis.

11.9.5 Disorders of the neuromuscular junction

Neuromuscular transmission is dependent on cholinergic transmission between the terminals of the motor nerves and the motor end plate.

The most commonly recognized condition at the neuromuscular junction is myasthenia gravis; however, it is also implicated in botulism and organophosphate poisoning.

Myasthenia gravis

Myasthenia gravis is an antibody-mediated, autoimmune disease affecting the neuromuscular junction. Antibodies are produced to the acetylcholine receptors, which prevent their functioning, leading to muscle weakness.

The typical presentation is muscle fatigability, which may progress to permanent weakness. Most patients have ptosis. Muscle groups commonly affected include extraocular, bulbar, face, and neck. Reflexes are usually normal but may be brisk. The patient does not have any sensory symptoms.

Diagnostic tests include a Tensilon® test (injection of edrophonium); anti-acetylcholine receptor antibodies (present in 85–90%); electrophysiology studies; and CT of the mediastinum (looking for evidence of a thyoma).

Symptomatic treatment is with anticholinesterase (e.g. pyridostigmine).

Botulism

Botulinum toxin prevents release of acetylcholine at the neuromuscular junction. It results in muscle weakness, diplopia, ataxia, bulbar palsy, and sudden cardiorespiratory failure. Patients require supportive treatment, ventilation, and botulinum antitoxin.

Organophosphate poisoning

Organophosphates inhibit acetylcholinesterase, which is the enzyme that degrades the neurotransmitter acetylcholine. Acetylcholine accumulates throughout the nervous system resulting in over-stimulation of muscarinic and nicotinic receptors. Clinical effects are manifested via activation of the autonomic and central nervous systems and at nicotinic receptors on skeletal muscle.

Organophosphate poisoning is discussed in more detail in Chapter 17, section 17.3.

11.9.6 Muscle disorders

Disorders of the muscle are known as myopathies. The most important feature is muscle weakness, variably accompanied by wasting, hypertrophy, and myotonia (delayed muscular relaxation after contraction). Signs are usually symmetrical. Myopathies are not usually painful, with the exception of inflammatory causes.

If fasiculations are seen, this is a sign of muscle denervation and indicates a disorder of the motor nerves or neuromuscular junction.

Causes of myopathies include:

- Inflammatory—polymyositis (idiopathic inflammatory disorder of skeletal muscle)
- Inherited—Duchenne's muscular dystrophy, dystrophia myotonica
- Drug-induced—alcohol, statins, steroids, chloroquine, colchicine, and so on
- Secondary to endocrine disease—hyperthyroidism, hypothyroidism

---

KEY POINTS

Diseases of the motor system can be classified according to their location, which can help explain the clinical features and causes.

Upper motor neuron lesions result in spasticity, hyperreflexia, clonus, upgoing plantars, and muscle weakness which predominantly affect leg flexors and arm extensors.

Lower motor neuron lesions result in flaccidity, hypotonia, fasiculations (if lesion at or near the anterior horn cell), hyporeflexia, muscle wasting, and muscle weakness which equally affects extensors and flexors.

Lesions at the neuromuscular junction (e.g. myasthenia gravis) result in muscle fatigability and the absence of sensory symptoms.

Myopathies result in predominantly proximal muscle weakness, myotonia, and the absence of sensory symptoms.

Subacute combined degeneration of the cord results from low vitamin B12 levels, most commonly secondary to pernicious anaemia. The posterior and lateral columns of the spinal cord are specifically damaged, but the clinical picture is complicated by the early development of coexistent peripheral nerve damage.

Guillain–Barré syndrome is rare acute infective polyneuropathy. It typically presents with progressive ascending bilateral weakness, with reduced or absent reflexes.

Myasthenia gravis is an antibody-mediated, autoimmune disease affecting the neuromuscular junction. Antibodies are produced to the acetylcholine receptors. The typical presentation is muscle fatigability which may progress to permanent weakness. Most patients have ptosis.

11.10 Falls in older people

11.10.1 Introduction

Falls are a major cause of disability and the leading cause of mortality, resulting from injury, in people aged over 75 in the United Kingdom. The Royal Society for the Prevention of Accidents estimates that one in three people aged 65 and over experience a fall at least once per year, rising to one in two among those older than 80.

Five per cent (5%) of falls result in a fracture and 95% of hip fractures are the result of a fall. This has significant consequences for individuals losing independence and quality of life, in addition to the financial cost to the NHS.

The College curriculum includes falls as one of the acute presentations assessed in ACCS. Therefore, the management of a patient who has fallen could appear as part of the FRCEM examination.

11.10.2 Risk factors for falling

Falls have a multifactorial aetiology. The major risk factors for falling are:

- A history of previous falls
- Gait deficit

- Balance deficit
- Mobility impairment
- Fear
- Visual impairment
- Cognitive impairment
- Urinary incontinence
- Home hazards
- Multiple medications

11.10.3 Identification of people who have fallen

The recommendation from the NICE guidance on the assessment and prevention of falls in older people is that all older people in contact with healthcare professionals should be routinely asked whether they have fallen in the past year and asked about the frequency, context, and characteristics of the fall. Therefore, all older patients (aged 65 or older) presenting to the ED for any condition should be asked about falls.

Older people who present to the ED following a fall or considered at risk of falling should be offered a multifactorial risk assessment (e.g. referred to a specialist falls service).

11.10.4 ED assessment of people who have fallen

Patients presenting to the ED following a fall frequently do so due to an associated injury or illness.

In addition to assessment of any injury, patients should have a thorough history and examination conducted to establish if the cause was a fall, collapse, or loss of consciousness. Chapter 9 includes guidance on the management of patients with transient loss of consciousness (section 9.7), which should always be considered in the differential of a patient who presents following a 'fall'. For any patients presenting to the ED with a fall, assessment should focus on identifying the cause of the fall and thus aim to prevent further falls.

History and examination

The history should ideally be obtained from the patient and, if available, a witness account of events should be sought. A detailed history is key in assessment of any patient with a fall. Pertinent points in the history include:

- Circumstances of events—is there a clear history of a simple trip or slip, or is there history suggestive of a preceding illness (e.g. chest pain, palpitations, limb weakness, dizziness, and so on)?
- Loss of consciousness—is there any reported loss of consciousness or amnesia pre or post fall?
- Does the patient have a history of falling or collapsing?
- Does the patient feel dizzy on sudden changes in posture?
- Vision—does the patient require glasses? When was their last eyesight test? Do they have cataracts?
- Recent illnesses—has the patient had any recent illnesses that could have precipitated the 'fall' (e.g. urinary tract infection)?
- What is the patient's past medical history—cardiac, respiratory, neurological, and metabolic?
- Have they previously sustained a fragility fracture?
- Drug history—are there medications that could have caused orthostatic hypotension or resulted in dizziness or poor balance (e.g. antihypertensives, antidepressants, antipsychotics, anticholinergics, opiates)? Are there any recent medication changes?
- Social history—what is the patient's social support? Do they have home hazards that are contributing to falls (e.g. loose fitting rugs, poor lighting, stairs, upstairs bathroom, and so on)?
- Alcohol history—is there a history of alcohol excess?

In addition to the examination of any injuries, the patient should have a focused assessment to screen for evidence of any underlying cause for the fall.

This includes specifically:

- Neurological examination for proximal muscle weakness; cerebellar signs; joint position sense; foot drop; spatial neglect; signs of Parkinsonism.
- Locomotor system examination for reduced range of movement, pain/ tenderness and deformity of lower limb joints. This includes a review of the feet and footwear, including pattern of wear of the soles.
- Cardiovascular system examination for heart rate and rhythm; cardiac murmurs (especially aortic stenosis); supine/standing blood pressure and pulse rate. In falls, clinics testing for carotid sinus hypersensitivity may be indicated.
- Gait, balance, and mobility assessment.
- Vision assessment, including visual acuity and visual fields.
- Medication review, as polypharmacy is a risk factor for recurrent falls.

11.10.5 Investigations for patients who have fallen

Investigations should be guided by the particular presentation of the patient and any injuries sustained. In addition, the following investigations should be considered:

- Blood glucose.
- 12 lead ECG.
- Postural blood pressures.
- Urinalysis.
- Creatine kinase and renal function should be checked if the patient has had a prolonged period of immobility, to screen for rhabdomyolysis.

When a detailed history of the fall is not possible, full investigation may be required to exclude possible reversible causes.

11.10.6 Emergency department management of a patient who has fallen

ED management should focus on treating the consequences of a fall and identifying any potential underlying causes, which may prevent future falls.

Patients who have fallen should be offered referral on to a specialist falls service for a multifactorial assessment. Prior to discharge, the patient and/or carers should be given written information about the assessment they are going to receive and how to prevent further falls. Many EDs also have access to physiotherapists and occupational therapists that can assess mobility and enable safe discharge. Follow-up assessment in a falls clinic may also be required.

11.10.7 Consequences of falls

Although most falls do not result in serious injury, the consequences for an individual of falling or of not being able to get up after a fall can include:

- Psychological problems (e.g. a fear of falling and loss of confidence in being able to move about safely)
- Loss of mobility, leading to social isolation and depression
- Increase in dependence and disability
- Hypothermia
- Pressure-related injuries
- Infection, including hypostatic pneumonia
- Dehydration
- Rhabdomyolysis

> **KEY POINTS**
>
> Falls are a major cause of disability and the leading cause of mortality, resulting from injury, in people aged over 75 in the UK.
>
> Falls have a multifactorial aetiology.
>
> All older patients (aged 65 or older) presenting to the ED, for any condition, should be asked about falls.
>
> Older people who present to the ED following a fall or considered at risk of falling should be offered a multifactorial risk assessment (e.g. referred to a specialist falls service).
>
> Patients presenting to the ED following a fall frequently do so due to an associated injury or illness. In addition to assessment of any injury, patients should have a thorough history and examination conducted to establish if the cause was a fall, collapse, or loss of consciousness. Investigations should be guided by the patient's presentation. The majority of patients should have blood glucose, ECG, postural blood pressures, and urinalysis checked.

11.11 Hydrocephalus

11.11.1 Introduction

Hydrocephalus is from the Greek, meaning 'water on the head' and is an abnormal accumulation of CSF in the brain resulting in increased intracranial pressure. Hydrocephalus can either be congenital or acquired and can be subclassified as either communicating or non-communicating.

CSF is produced in the lateral ventricles where it travels through the ventricular system into the subarachnoid space where it is reabsorbed. The brain makes approximately 500 ml of CSF a day and is constantly reabsorbed. It is produced by the choroid plexus in the lateral ventricles, travels through the intraventricular foramina into the third ventricle, and then into the fourth ventricle via the cerebral aqueduct. From the fourth ventricle, CSF travels into the subarachnoid space where it is reabsorbed by arachnoid granulations. Any condition that affects the flow of CSF or its reabsorption can result in build-up of CSF and thus hydrocephalus.

11.11.2 Communicating hydrocephalus

Communicating hydrocephalus is a problem with the reabsorption of CSF, resulting in its accumulation. In a normal individual the total volume of CSF is reabsorbed approximately three times a day.

Two types of communicating hydrocephalus are:

- Normal pressure hydrocephalus: enlarged ventricles with normal pressure (triad of gait instability, dementia, and urinary incontinence)
- Hydrocephalus ex vacuo: compensatory ventricular enlargement in response to parenchymal loss

11.11.3 Non-communicating (obstructive) hydrocephalus

Non-communicating hydrocephalus is due to an obstruction to CSF flow and can occur at any point along its route.

Individuals with known hydrocephalus will usually be under the care of a specialist neurosurgical team. Many individuals will have a shunt *in situ* to drain CSF and thus prevent the development of hydrocephalus. There are many different types of shunt, the two most common are ventricular peritoneal and lumbar peritoneal, excess CSF being drained into the peritoneal cavity from the ventricles and lumbar subarachnoid space respectively. Shunts typically consist of a proximal ventricular or lumbar catheter, a unidirectional valve, and a distal drainage catheter, which may be lumbar, peritoneal, or in the right atrium

Patients will typically present to the ED when they have developed a problem with their shunt such as blockage or infection. If shunt blockage is suspected, patients should be investigated with CT brain and shunt series imaging, followed by discussion with a neurosurgeon.

11.11.4 Shunt complications

Clinical features of shunt malfunction include:

- Headache
- Vomiting
- Drowsiness
- Papilloedema with/without failing vision
- Occasional temporal gaze failure
- Neck stiffness
- Thoracic back pain in patients with spina bifida
- Abdominal pain

Shunt assessment includes the following options, guided by early neurosurgical advice

- Blood tests, including blood counts and inflammatory markers.
- CT scan to assess ventricular size.
- Shunt series: plain X-rays of the whole of the shunt to look for breakages, disconnections, or migration of the shunt from its usual location. This usually involves a lateral skull X-ray, and anteroposterior (AP) views of the chest and abdomen.
- Shunt palpation: if the pumping chamber can be emptied, but does not refill readily, it suggests the ventricular catheter is blocked; if the pumping chamber is not compressible and cannot be easily emptied, the distal catheter is blocked.
- Shunt tap: a 23 or 25 gauge butterfly needle is inserted into the subcutaneous reservoir (not the valve pumping chamber) to measure CSF pressure using a manometer, and sample CSF for microbiology.

11.12 SAQs

1.12.1 Stroke and transient ischaemic attack

A 70-year-old lady presents to the ED following a 20-minute episode of right arm and leg weakness. Her symptoms are now fully resolved. She has a past medical history of hypertension for which she takes bendroflumethazide. She has no other past history of note and is not on any other medication. She has no known drug allergies.

Her observations at triage are: temperature 36.5°C, HR 70, BP 165/85, RR 16, oxygen saturations 98%, GCS 15, blood glucose 5.4.

a) (i)   You think this lady has had a TIA. What are the components and cut off values of the ABCD^2 score? (5 marks—½ for component, ½ for value)

a) (ii) What is this patient's ABCD^2 score? (1 mark)

b) (i)   You arrange urgent follow-up in the TIA clinic. What medication (including dose) should the patient be discharged with? (1 mark)

b) (ii) The patient asks if she can continue driving. What is your advice? (1 mark)

c) She returns to the ED one month later with a dense right hemiparesis that started one hour earlier. List two indications for stroke thrombolysis. (2 marks)

Suggested answer

a) (i)   You think this lady has had a TIA. What are the components and cut off values of the ABCD^2 score? (5 marks—½ for component, ½ for value) See Table 11.20

a) (ii) What is this patient's ABCD^2 score? (1 mark)

5

b) (i)   You arrange urgent follow-up in the TIA clinic. What medication (including dose) should the patient be discharged with? (1 mark)

Aspirin 300 mg OD

b) (ii) The patient asks if she can continue driving. What is your advice? (1 mark)

No driving for one month

Table 11.20 The ABCD^2 score

			Patient's score
Age	≥60 years	1 point	1
Blood pressure	≥140/90 mmHg	1 point	1
Clinical features	Focal weakness	2 points	2
	Speech disturbance without weakness	1 point	
Duration	≥60 min	2 points	
	10–59 minutes	1 point	1
Diabetes		1 point	
			Total 5

Reprinted from The Lancet, volume 369, issue 9558, S Claiborne Johnston, Peter M Rothwell, Mai N Nguyen Huynh, Matthew F Giles, Jacob S Elkins, Allan L Bernstein, Stephen Sidney, Validation and refinement of scores to predict very early stroke risk after transient ischaemic attack, pp. 283–292, Copyright 2007, with permission from Elsevier

c) She returns to the ED one month later with a dense right hemiparesis that started one hour earlier. List two indications for stroke thrombolysis. **(2 marks)**

Onset <3 hours

Clinical diagnosis of stroke

CT appearances consistent with an ischaemic stroke

No contraindications to thrombolysis

Risks and benefits explained to patient and/or relative

11.12.2 Subarachnoid haemorrhage and status epilepticus

A 35-year-old man presents to the ED with a sudden onset occipital headache, associated with nausea and neck stiffness. He is GCS 15 and apyrexial. You are concerned he may have a subarachnoid haemorrhage.

a) (i) List four risk factors for subarachnoid haemorrhage. **(2 marks)**

a) (ii) Give two other differential diagnoses for a thunderclap headache. **(2 marks)**

   A CT scan confirms a subarachnoid haemorrhage and the neurosurgical team request that the patient be transferred to them. The neurosurgical registrar asks you to give nimodipine 60 mg orally.

b) What is the reason for giving nimodipine? **(1 mark)**

   A 25-year-old patient with known epilepsy presents having a tonic–clonic seizure that has persisted for 35 minutes. He has been given 10 mg rectal diazepam by the paramedics but continues to fit.

   His blood glucose is 7 mmol/L. He has intravenous access. There is no suggestion of alcohol abuse. He weighs approximately 70 kg.

c) (i) List the next two drugs (and doses) you would give if he continues to fit? **(2 marks)**

c) (ii) In a patient with known epilepsy, what are the two commonest causes of status epilepticus. **(2 marks)**

d) What is the difference between a partial seizure and generalized seizure? **(1 mark)**

Suggested answer

a) (i) List four risk factors for subarachnoid haemorrhage. **(2 marks)**

   Past medical history of SAH

   Family history

   Polycystic kidney disease

   Marfan's syndrome

   Ehlers–Danlos syndrome

   Coarctation of the aorta

   Hypertension

   Smoking

   Atherosclerosis

a) (ii) Give two other differential diagnoses for a thunderclap headache. **(2 marks)**

   Intracerebral haemorrhage

   Cerebral venous sinus thrombosis

   Arterial dissection

   Pituitary apoplexy

   Coital cephalgia

b) What is the reason for giving nimodipine? (1 mark)

Prevent and treat ischaemic neurological deficits secondary to cerebral vasospasm

c) (i) List the next two drugs (and doses) you would give if he continues to fit? (2 marks)

Lorazepam 4 mg IV

Phenytoin 15–18 mg/kg IV (dose range 1050 mg–1260 mg)

(c) (ii) In a patient with known epilepsy, what are the two commonest causes of status epilepticus? (2 marks)

Any two of:

Drug non-compliance

Drug withdrawal

Drug therapy alteration

d) What is the difference between a partial seizure and generalized seizure? (1 mark)

Partial seizures originate from a specific area of the cortex and consciousness is not fully lost. Generalized seizures affect both sides of the brain at once and the patient is unconscious.

Further reading

British Association for the Study of Headache. Available at: https://www.bash.org.uk [Online].

International Headache Society Classification Subcommittee, 2004. The International Classification of Headache Disorders, 2nd edition. *Cephalalgia*. 24 (Suppl 1): 1–160. Available at: https://www.ihs-classification.org/en/ [Online].

National Institute for Health and Care Excellence, July 2008. NICE Clinical guideline 68. Diagnosis and initial management of acute stroke and transient ischaemic attack. Available at: https://www.nice.org.uk/CG68 [Online].

National Institute for Health and Care Excellence, November 2008. NICE Clinical guideline 75. Mestatstic spinal cord compression in adults: diagnosis and management. Available at: https://www.nice.org.uk/Guidance/CG75 [Online].

National Institute for Health and Care Excellence, January 2012. NICE Clinical guideline 137. Epilepsies: diagnosis and management. Available at: https://www.nice.org.uk/Guidance/CG137 [Online].

National Institute for Health and Care Excellence, June 2013. NICE Clinical guideline 161. Falls in older people: assessing risk and prevention. Available at: https://www.nice.org.uk/guidance/cg161 [Online].

Scottish Intercollegiate Guideline Network, 2008. SIGN guideline 107. Diagnosis and management of headache in adults. Available at: https://www.sign.ac.uk/pdf/sign107.pdf [Online].

CHAPTER 12

Renal emergencies

CONTENTS

12.1 Introduction

The curriculum includes knowledge of the differential diagnosis, investigation, and initial management of patients presenting to the emergency department (ED) with oliguria.

Acute kidney injury (AKI) has replaced the term 'acute renal failure'.

12.2 Acute kidney injury

12.2.1 Definition of acute kidney injury

The UK Renal Association has proposed a universal definition and staging system to allow the earlier detection and management of AKI.

Acute kidney injury is diagnosed when one of the following criteria is met:

- serum creatinine rises by ≥ 26 µmol/L from the baseline value within 48 hours; or
- serum creatinine rises ≥1.5-fold from the baseline value that is known, or presumed to have occurred, within one week; or
- urine output is <0.5 ml/kg/hour for >6 consecutive hours.*

If the patient does not have a baseline serum creatinine value within one week of their admission or presentation, it is acceptable to use a reference serum creatinine value within three months (acceptable up to one year).

12.2.2 Staging of acute kidney injury

Acute kidney injury staging can be performed using serum creatinine or urine output criteria (Table 12.1). Patients should be staged according to whichever criterion gives them the highest stage.

*Reproduced from Acute Kidney Injury (AKI), Guidelines AKI 1.1-3. http://www.renal.org/guidelines/modules/acute-kidney-injury#sthash.5QGpoQeb.dpbs.

Table 12.1 Staging system for acute kidney injury (AKI)

Stage	Serum creatinine (SCr) criteria	Urine output criteria
1	SCr increase ≥ 26 µmol/L or SCr increase ≥ 1.5 to 2-fold from baseline	<0.5 ml/kg/h for >6 consecutive hours
2	SCr increase ≥ 2 to 3-fold from baseline	<0.5mL/kg/h for >12 h
3	SCr increase ≥ 3-fold from baseline or SCr increase ≥ 354 µmol/L or commenced on renal replacement therapy irrespective of stage	<0.3mL/kg/h for >24 h or anuria for 12 h

Data from Acute kidney injury (March 2011). UK Renal Association. www.renal.org/Clinical/GuidelinesSection/AcuteKidneyInjury

12.2.3 Pathophysiology of acute kidney injury

The driving force for glomerular filtration is the pressure gradient across the glomerulus to Bowman's space of the proximal tubule. Glomerular capillary pressure depends on renal blood flow, which is maintained by cardiac output and autoregulated by the combined resistance of the renal afferent and efferent arterioles.

The causes of AKI can be classified as:

- Pre-renal—due to reduced renal blood flow
- Intrinsic renal—due to disease of the glomerulus, interstitium, or tubule
- Post-renal—due to obstruction impairing drainage of the kidneys

Pre-renal failure

Pre-renal failure is the commonest aetiology of patients presenting to the ED with AKI. Reduced renal blood flow can be due to:

- Volume loss (e.g. haemorrhage, vomiting, diarrhoea, dehydration, diuretics, and so on)
- Decreased cardiac output (e.g. MI, PE, valvular heart disease, tamponade, sepsis, and so on)
- Renal artery disease (e.g. renal artery stenosis, sickle cell disease, atheroembolism, pre-eclampsia, hypertension, vasculitis, and so on)

Intrinsic renal failure

Intrinsic renal failure results from damage to the glomerulus, tubule, interstitium, and/or vasculature (see Table 12.2).

Glomerulonephritis

Glomerulonephritis (see Table 12.2) is characterized by inflammation of the glomeruli. It can be divided into two broad categories based on the pathological pattern: non-proliferative and proliferative. The causes can be classified as primary (disease intrinsic to the kidney) or secondary due to infection, drugs, or systemic disorders (e.g. diabetes, systemic lupus erythematosus (SLE), vasculitis).

Non-proliferative glomerulonephritis

- Minimal change disease—this is the cause of nephrotic syndrome in the majority of children.
- Focal segmental glomerulosclerosis—may be primary or secondary to reflux nephropathy, Alport's syndrome, heroin, or HIV.
- Membranous glomerulonephritis—usually idiopathic and can present with a mixed nephrotic and nephritic picture.

Table 12.2 Causes of intrinsic renal failure

Tubular disease	• Ischaemic acute tubular necrosis • Nephrotoxic drugs (e.g. aminoglycosides, radio-contrast, NSAIDs) • Rhabdomyolysis
Interstitial disease	• Acute interstitial nephritis (usually due to a drug induced allergic reaction, e.g. penicillins, NSAIDs) • Infiltrative disease: sarcoidosis, lymphoma • Autoimmune disease: SLE
Glomerular disease	• Glomerulonephritis
Vascular disease	• Malignant hypertension • Haemolytic uraemic syndrome • Renal vein thrombosis • Thrombotic thrombocytopenic purpura

Proliferative glomerulonephritis

- IgA nephropathy—is the most common glomerulonephritis in adults. It may be primary or secondary, most commonly presenting in young men following an upper respiratory tract or gastrointestinal infection.
- Post-infectious—classically presents 10–14 days after a pharyngeal *Streptococcus pyogenes* infection.
- Membranoproliferative—may be primary or secondary to SLE or viral hepatitis.
- Rapidly progressive glomerulonephritis—any glomerulonephritis can progress to this. Goodpasture's syndrome (antibodies directed against basal membrane antigens) and Wegner's granulomatosis present solely as this.

Typically non-proliferative glomerulonephritis presents as nephrotic syndrome and proliferative glomerulonephritis presents with nephritic syndrome.

- Nephrotic syndrome—characterized by proteinuria (>3.5 g/day), hypoalbuminaemia, hyperlipidaemia, and oedema.
- Nephritic syndrome—characterized by haematuria (with red cell casts on microscopy), proteinuria (mild <3.5 g/day), hypertension, oedema, elevated serum creatinine, and oliguria.

Post-renal failure

Post-renal or obstructive renal failure accounts for approximately 10% of cases of AKI, becoming more common in the elderly. Table 12.3 details causes of obstruction which may lead to AKI.

> **EXAM TIP**
>
> It is easy to become overwhelmed when learning the causes and pathophysiology of AKI. The main points to remember are the broad categories of pre-renal, intrinsic, and post-renal failure. The finer details on tubular, interstitial, and glomerular disease are provided for clarity and completeness but are unlikely to be necessary for the exam. Please do not` waste revision time worrying about the minutiae. A question on the detailed pathophysiology of the kidney is highly unlikely and if it did appear would only be worth 1 or 2 marks of a question.

12.2.4 Clinical features of acute kidney injury

The development of AKI can be insidious and the clinical features can be non-specific. AKI is most frequently caused by ischaemia, sepsis, or nephrotoxins. The patient's history should be

Table 12.3 Level and causes of obstruction

Urethra and bladder	• Benign prostatic hypertrophy • Cancer of the bladder, prostate, cervix, or colon • Uretheral stricture • Neurogenic bladder (diabetes, spinal cord disease, multiple sclerosis, anticholinergic drugs)
Ureter	• Calculi • Cancer of the ureter, uterus, or colon • Vesicoureteric reflux • Aortic aneurysm • Pregnant uterus • Inflammatory bowel disease • Retroperitoneal fibrosis • Trauma • Papillary necrosis (sickle cell disease, diabetes, pyelonephritis)
Intra-renal	• Crystals: uric acid, aciclovir, sulphonamides • Protein casts: multiple myeloma, amyloidosis

carefully considered to identify risk factors, potential causes, and systemic symptoms suggestive of AKI.

Risk factors for AKI include:

- Age 65 years or over
- Deteriorating early warning scores
- Chronic kidney disease (adults with an estimated glomerular filtration rate <60 ml/min/ 1.73 m^2)
- Heart failure
- Sepsis
- History of acute kidney injury
- Peripheral vascular disease
- Hypertension
- Liver disease
- Diabetes mellitus
- Nephrotoxic medications within the past week, such as NSAIDs, aminoglycosides, ACE inhibitors, angiotensin II receptor antagonists, diuretics, especially if hypovolaemic
- Use of iodinated contrast agents within the past week
- Symptoms or history of urological obstruction

Potential causes of AKI:

- Reduced fluid intake
- Increased fluid losses
- Urinary tract symptoms
- Recent drug ingestion
- Sepsis

Systemic clinical features (suggestive of autoimmune vasculitis, acute interstitial nephritis, infection, and so on):

- Fever
- Rash
- Arthralgia
- Iritis

12.2.5 Investigation of acute kidney injury

Investigations should be aimed at determining the severity of AKI and the likely cause.

- Urea, creatinine, and electrolytes—to determine the stage of AKI and identify any associated electrolyte abnormalities.
- FBC—to diagnose any associated anaemia or elevated white cell count (WCC) suggesting infection.
- Arterial blood gas—to identify any acidosis.
- Electrocardiogram (ECG)—to identify any abnormalities secondary to electrolyte derangement.
- Urinalysis and microscopy—to identify any proteinuria, haematuria, or red cell casts.
- Urine culture—if infection is suspected.
- Blood culture—if infection is suspected.
- Renal ultrasound—if obstruction suspected.

Urinalysis

Urinalysis can provide important clinical information on patients with AKI.

- Positive protein values of 3 + on reagent strip testing of urine suggest intrinsic glomerular disease.
- A reagent strip positive for blood may indicate lower urinary tract obstruction (calculi, tumours), infection, severe renal ischaemia due to arterial or venous thrombosis, or glomerular disease. Glomerular disease is supported by finding red cell casts on microscopy. Haematuria in the presence of proteinuria suggests a glomerular cause for acute kidney injury. Myoglobinuria will cause a positive reagent strip reaction for blood without evidence of red cells on urine microscopy.
- Increased numbers of white cells are non-specific may suggest infection or acute interstitial nephritis.

Urinary biochemistry

Various measures are used to assist in the diagnosis of AKI including urine osmolality, urinary sodium, serum urea:creatinine ratio, creatinine clearance, and so on. All have limitations and their specificity and sensitivity in clinical practice often means a single measurement is inconclusive. If the patient has received diuretics the measures become difficult to interpret. Their usefulness as ED investigations are therefore limited and are probably best directed by a renal specialist.

These measurements would not be the priority when answering a question on the investigation of AKI. However, the curriculum includes knowledge of the methods used to assess renal function, so the following is a brief overview of some of the tests available.

- Urine and plasma osmolality—can be used to differentiate pre-renal from acute tubular necrosis (ATN). In pre-renal AKI, the kidney is functioning maximally to retain sodium and water, to improve the plasma volume. The urine is maximally concentrated with a high osmolality (600–900 mmol/L). In ATN, the renal tubules are not functioning normally and are unable to concentrate the urine and the urinary osmolality falls. Eventually the urinary osmolality approaches that of plasma (280 mmol/L).
- Urinary sodium—can be used to differentiate pre-renal from ATN. In pre-renal AKI, the urinary sodium is low (<10 mmol/L) due to the kidneys maximally reabsorbing sodium to try and restore plasma volume. In ATN the kidneys are unable to reabsorb sodium and the urinary sodium rises (>30 mmol/L).
- Serum urea:creatinine ratio—in pre-renal AKI there is increased urinary urea reabsorption. The urea is increased proportionally more than creatinine resulting in an increased serum urea:creatinine ratio.

- Fractional excretion of urea—is low in pre-renal AKI due to increased urinary urea reabsorption.
- Creatinine clearance—can be used to estimate the glomerular filtration rate (GFR) by calculating the creatinine content of a 24-hour urine collection. This is performed less commonly now due to the difficulties in ensuring an accurate 24-hour urine collection. GFR is usually estimated from the serum creatinine.

Criteria for detecting acute kidney injury

- A rise in serum creatinine of 26 micromol/L or greater within 48 hours
- A 50% or greater rise in serum creatinine known or presumed to have occurred within the past seven days
- A fall in urine output to less than 0.5 ml/kg/hour for more than six hours in adults and more than eight hours in children and young people
- A 25% or greater fall in eGFR in children and young people with or at risk of acute kidney injury

12.2.6 Emeregncy department management of acute kidney injury

In many cases AKI can be effectively treated and resolved by adequate volume replacement, treatment of the underlying medical condition (e.g. sepsis, haemorrhage), relief of any renal tract obstruction (e.g. urinary catheterization), and avoidance of nephrotoxic medications.

Recommendations from *Adding Insult to Injury*, a review of the care of patients who died in hospital with a primary diagnosis of acute kidney injury (acute renal failure), National Confidential Enquiry into Patient Outcomes and Death (NCEPOD) report (2009), and NICE guideline CG169 include:

- Initial clerking of all emergency patients should include a risk assessment for acute kidney injury.
- All patients admitted as an emergency, regardless of specialty, should have their electrolytes checked routinely on admission and appropriately thereafter.
- Predictable and avoidable AKI should never occur.
- Reagent strip urinalysis should be performed on all emergency admissions.
- All acute admitting hospitals should have access to either onsite nephrologists or a dedicated nephrology service within reasonable distance of the admitting hospital.
- All acute admitting hospitals should have access to a renal ultrasound scanning service 24 hours a day including the weekends and the ability to provide emergency relief of renal obstruction.
- All patients with upper tract urological obstruction should be referred to a urologist.
- A nephrologist should be consulted if there is a possible diagnosis that may require specialist treatment (vasculitis, glomerulonephritis, tubule-interstitial nephritis or myeloma), acute kidney injury with no clear cause, stage 3 acute kidney injury, a renal transplant, or chronic kidney disease stage 4 or 5.

Fluid management

Fluid management in patients with AKI presents a significant challenge. An assessment should be made of the patient's volume status (i.e. hypovolaemic, euvolaemic, hypervolaemic). Hypovolaemia potentiates and exacerbates all forms of AKI. In the acutely ill patient, fluid replacement is best achieved through the rapid infusion of repeated small volumes (250 ml of crystalloid or colloid) and close monitoring using a central venous pressure (CVP) line and urinary catheter. Lactate and base excess measurements may also be helpful in conjunction with clinical judgement in assessing response to volume loading. There is no evidence base to favour the use of colloid over crystalloid to protect kidney function. The fluid choice should take into consideration the nature of the fluid lost.

Urinary catheterization

Urinary obstruction is an easily reversible cause of AKI. A bladder scanner can quickly identify a large, distended bladder. Placement of a urinary catheter allows diagnosis and treatment of an uretheral or bladder outlet obstruction and accurate measurement of urine output. The routine use of urinary catheters should be balanced against the risk of introducing infection.

Prevention of further injury

Nephrotoxic drugs (e.g. NSAIDs, aminoglycosides, and radio-contrast) should be stopped or avoided in patients with AKI. Inappropriate drug dosing of patients with AKI is an important cause of adverse drug events. Drug doses need to be adjusted appropriately with the correct assessment of kidney function to reduce toxicity.

Patients may require imaging that necessitates radiological contrast, however alternative imaging techniques should be considered (e.g. ultrasound, MRI). If the only option is to use radio-contrast, the patient should receive appropriate volume expansion prior to the procedure with 0.9% sodium chloride. Using carbon dioxide to reduce the amount of contrast needed should be considered or a low osmolar agent can be used which is associated with a decreased risk of nephrotoxicity. Acetylcysteine has a protective effect against acute kidney injury.

Loop diuretics and dopamine

There is currently no evidence to support the use of a specific pharmacological therapy in the treatment of AKI (e.g. furosemide or dopamine).

The rationale behind the use of loop diuretics was based on their putative ability to reduce the energy requirements of the cells of the ascending loop of Henle and therefore ameliorate the resultant ischaemic damage. Loop diuretics have also been used to convert patients with oliguric AKI to non-oliguric AKI (recognized to have a better prognosis), to facilitate the management of fluid and electrolyte disturbances, and reduce the requirement for renal replacement therapy (RRT). The use of loop diuretics has been associated with an increased risk of failure to recover renal function and mortality, perhaps related to the resultant delay in commencing RRT appropriately.

Dopamine at low doses induces an increase in renal blood flow, natriuresis, and diuresis in healthy humans. It has been proposed that dopamine may potentially reduce ischaemic cell injury in patients with AKI by improving renal blood flow and reducing oxygen consumption through inhibition of sodium transport. A meta-analysis of studies investigating the use of dopamine in the prevention and treatment of AKI has found no good evidence to support any important clinical benefits to patients with or at risk of AKI.

12.2.7 Complications of acute kidney injury

Complications of AKI include:

- Biochemical—metabolic acidosis, hyperkalaemia, and other electrolyte disturbances (sodium, phosphate, and calcium)
- Cardiovascular—pulmonary oedema, hypertension, myocardial depression, arrhythmias, pericarditis
- Gastrointestinal—gastrointestinal (GI) bleeding, gastric stasis, ileus, anorexia, vomiting
- Haematological—anaemia, impaired haemostasis, platelet dysfunction
- Neurological—lethargy, memory impairment, encephalopathy, peripheral neuropathy

KEY POINTS

The commonest cause of AKI in the ED is pre-renal (reduced renal blood flow).

Acute tubular necrosis is the commonest intrinsic cause of AKI usually secondary to ischaemia or nephrotoxins (e.g. aminoglycosides, radio-contrast, and myoglobin).

Post-renal AKI accounts for approximately 10% of AKI. Post-renal AKI is more common in elderly men due to prostatic disease.

The main treatment modalities for AKI are:

- Fluid resuscitation and monitoring of volume status
- Prevention of further injury by stopping nephrotoxic drugs
- Urinary catheterization to relieve any urethral or bladder obstruction
- Treatment of complications (e.g. hyperkalaemia, pulmonary oedema)
- Treatment of the precipitant (e.g. sepsis, hypovolaemia)

12.3 Renal replacement therapy

The main methods of renal replacement therapy are:

- Intermittent haemodialysis (IHD)
- Peritoneal dialysis (PD)
- Continuous renal replacement therapy (CRRT)

Patients requiring long-term renal replacement therapy usually undergo IHD two or three times per week or alternatively PD. These modes are not commonly used in critically ill patients. IHD is associated with significant haemodynamic instability in critically ill patients and PD is not capable of removing large volumes of fluid or solute.

CRRT allows more gradual correction of biochemical abnormalities and removal of fluid, allowing better control of uraemia and clearance of solutes, and avoiding hypotension. CRRT is usually provided in intensive care.

Types of CRRT include:

- Continuous venovenous haemodialysis (CVVHD)—dialysis fluid is passed over a filter membrane in a counter-current manner to the patient's blood. Fluids, electrolytes, and small molecules can move in both directions across the filter, depending on hydrostatic pressure, ionic binding, and osmotic gradients. Fluid can be effectively removed by allowing more dialysate fluid to pass out of the filter than passes in.
- Continuous venovenous haemofiltration (CVVHF)—blood from the patient passes through a filter. Plasma water, electrolytes, and low molecular weight molecules pass through the filter down a pressure gradient. The filtrate is discarded and replaced by a balanced electrolyte solution. A negative fluid balance can be achieved by replacing less fluid than is removed.
- Continuous venovenous haemodiafiltration (CVVHDF)—dialysis fluid is passed across a filter to remove solute by osmosis and at the same time ultrafiltrate is removed and replaced, combining the techniques of haemodialysis and haemofiltration.

Indications for and timing of RRT in AKI is widely debated. The UK Renal Association advice for starting RRT in patients with AKI is that it should be a clinical decision based on the fluid, electrolyte, and metabolic status of the patient. However, Table 12.4 details the main indications for starting RRT.

Table 12.4 Indications to start renal replacement therapy in AKI

Biochemical indications	• Refractory hyperkalaemia >6.5 mmol/L • Serum urea >27 mmol/L • Refractory metabolic acidosis pH <7.15 • Refractory electrolyte abnormalities: hyponatraemia (<115 mmol/L), hypernatraemia (>165 mmol/L), hypercalcaemia • Tumour lysis syndrome with hyperuricaemia and hyperphosphataemia
Clinical indications	• Urine output <0.3 ml/kg for 24 h or absolute anuria for 12 h • AKI with multiorgan failure • Refractory volume overload • End organ involvement: pericarditis, encephalopathy, neuropathy, myopathy, uraemic bleeding • Severe poisoning or drug overdose (e.g. methanol, ethylene glycol, aspirin, theophylline, lithium) • Severe hypothermia or hyperthermia • Creation of intravascular space for plasma and other blood product infusions and nutrition

---

KEY POINTS

The main ED indications for initiation of RRT are:

• Resistant hyperkalaemia (K^+ >6.5)

• Pulmonary oedema

• Refractory metabolic acidosis (pH <7.15)

• Severe poisoning (e.g. methanol, ethylene glycol, aspirin, theophylline, lithium)

• Complications of uraemia (e.g. pericarditis)

12.4 Hyperkalaemia

Previous MRCEM question

12.4.1 Introduction

The management of hyperkalaemia has appeared in previous MRCEM SAQs.

Hyperkalaemia can be classified as:

• Mild (5.5–6.0 mmol/L)

• Moderate (6.1–6.9 mmol/L)

• Severe (>7.0 mmol/L)

12.4.2 Causes of hyperkalaemia

There are many causes of hyperkalaemia as detailed in Table 12.5.

12.4.3 Clinical features of hyperkalaemia

Clinical manifestations of hyperkalaemia result predominantly from the derangement of membrane polarization. Features include muscle weakness, paraesthesia, hypotonia, areflexia, ascending

Table 12.5 Causes of hyperkalaemia

Pseudo-hyperkalaemia	• Sample haemolysis • Tourniquet use • Sample taken from limb with IV fluids containing K^+
Intra- to extracellular shift	• Acidosis (e.g. DKA) • Heavy exercise • Insulin deficiency • Drugs (e.g. β-blockers, suxamethonium, digoxin toxicity)
Potassium load	• Potassium supplements (orally or IV) • Crush injury/rhabdomyolysis • Burns • Tumour cell necrosis • Massive or incompatible blood transfusion • GI bleed
Decreased potassium excretion	• Acute kidney injury • Chronic renal failure patients subjected to a K^+ load • Pre-dialysis • Drugs, for example NSAIDs, ACEI, K^+ sparing diuretics (amiloride, spironolactone), β-blockers • Aldosterone deficiency (e.g. Addison's disease)

paralysis, nausea, vomiting, and diarrhoea. Cardiac manifestations are the most serious consequence leading to arrhythmias and eventually cardiac arrest.

ECG changes in hyperkalaemia include:

- Tall peaked T waves
- Short QT
- Prolonged PR
- Widened QRS
- Flattened P waves
- Sinusoidal QRST
- AV dissociation
- VT/VF
- Asystole

In patients who slowly develop hyperkalaemia higher levels of serum potassium can be tolerated before ECG changes occur.

12.4.4 Management of hyperkalaemia

Provided there are no ECG abnormalities the serum potassium level should be confirmed to exclude a spurious result. This may be done via a blood gas analyser depending on the urgency of the situation.

Potassium levels greater than 6.5 mmol/L or with ECG changes require urgent treatment (see Table 12.6). Treatment can be divided into three categories:

- Cardiac protection (e.g. antagonizing the toxic effects of hyperkalaemia at the myocardial cell membrane)
- Shifting K^+ into the intracellular space
- Increasing excretion of K^+

Table 12.6 Methods of treating hyperkalaemia

Cardiac protection	• Calcium chloride or gluconate 10 ml of 10% IV
Shifting K⁺ into the intracellular space	• Salbutamol nebulizer 5 mg • Insulin and glucose (10 units of short-acting insulin with 50 ml of 50% glucose IV over 15–30 min) • Sodium bicarbonate (1.26% infusion or 8.4% 50 ml aliquots) • 0.9% normal saline to correct any volume deficits and therefore improve acidosis
Excretion of K⁺	• Potassium exchange resin (e.g. calcium resonium PO or PR) to enhance gastrointestinal excretion • Renal replacement therapy • (Hydrocortisone if secondary to Addison's disease)

KEY POINTS

Causes of hyperkalaemia include:
- Renal failure
- Drugs (e.g. NSAIDs, ACEIs, β-blockers, and so on)
- Rhabdomyolysis
- Burns
- Metabolic acidosis
- Addison's disease

ECG changes are progressive and include:
- First degree heart block
- Flattened P waves
- Tall, peaked T waves
- ST-segment depression
- Sine wave pattern (S and T waves merge)
- Widened QRS
- Bradycardia
- VT (pulsed)
- Cardiac arrest (PEA, VT/VF, asystole)

Urgent treatment is indicated for K⁺ >6.5 mmol/L or in the presence of ECG changes. The main treatment aims are:
- Cardiac protection—calcium chloride or gluconate
- Shift K⁺ into the intracellular space—salbutamol nebulizer, insulin/glucose infusion, sodium bicarbonate
- Increase excretion of K⁺—calcium resonium, RRT

12.5 Rhabdomyolysis

Rhabdomyolysis results from skeletal muscle injury and cell lysis with the release of myoglobin and other potentially toxic muscle breakdown products into the systemic circulation. Myoglobin is freely filtered by the kidneys and is directly toxic to the tubule epithelial cells. This toxicity is compounded by associated hypovolaemia and acidosis.

12.5.1 Causes of rhabdomyolysis

- Trauma
- Burns
- Electrical injuries
- Compartment syndrome
- Drugs (e.g. ecstasy, cocaine, alcohol, statins)
- Excessive exercise or prolonged seizures
- Prolonged immobilization
- Myositis
- Metabolic disorders—$\downarrow K^+$, $\downarrow PO_3{}^{4-}$, diabetic emergencies
- Neuroleptic malignant syndrome
- Malignant hyperthermia

12.5.2 Clinical features of rhabdomyolysis

There may be minimal or no symptoms initially and a high index of suspicion is required. The classical triad consists of myalgia, generalized weakness, and dark urine.

Clinical sequelae include:

- Hypovolaemia—sequestration of plasma water within injured myocytes
- Hyperkalaemia—release of cellular potassium into the systemic circulation
- Metabolic acidosis—release of phosphate and sulphate
- AKI—due to hypovolaemia, nephrotoxic effects of myoglobin, and obstruction of renal tubules by urate crystals
- Disseminated intravascular coagulation (DIC)

12.5.3 Investigation of rhabdomyolysis

- Urinalysis—myoglobin tests positive for blood on a reagent strip but no red blood cells are visible on microscopy.
- Creatine kinase (CK)—is released from damaged muscle and is a very sensitive but non-specific marker for rhabdomyolysis. Serial CK measurements should be checked to determine the peak level.
- Renal function—patients may have developed or be at high risk of developing AKI.
- Electrolytes—patients are at risk of life-threatening hyperkalaemia. They may also develop hyperphosphataemia and/or hypocalcaemia.
- Clotting and platelets—patients are at risk of DIC.
- ECG—to monitor for changes suggestive of hyperkalaemia.

12.5.4 Management of rhabdomyolysis

Management of rhabdomyolysis involves volume assessment and close monitoring (e.g. CVP line), with aggressive fluid resuscitation and alkalinization of the urine. If there is a reversible underlying cause this should be treated (e.g. fasciotomy for compartment syndrome). Complications such as hyperkalaemia should be monitored for and treated (see section 12.4).

- Fluids resuscitation—0.9% sodium chloride is recommended by the UK Renal Association at a rate of 10–15 ml/kg/h to achieve high urinary flow rates (>100 ml/h).
- Sodium bicarbonate (1.26%)—should be used cautiously to maintain a urinary pH>7.5.
- Mannitol—is an osmotic diuretic and free radical scavenger which is sometimes used. The evidence for this is limited and inappropriate use can precipitate pulmonary oedema especially if renal impairment is already present.
- Renal replacement therapy—may be required if AKI develops.

KEY POINTS

Rhabdomyolysis results from skeletal muscle injury and cell lysis, which releases myoglobin.
A useful screening test for myoglobinuria is a urinary dipstick. Myoglobin tests positive for haemoglobin on reagent strip testing.

- Creatine kinase should be checked serially to determine the peak level.
- ED management includes:
  - Identification and treatment of the cause (e.g. fasciotomy for compartment syndrome).
  - Fluid resuscitation.
  - Urinary alkalinization (sodium bicarbonate).
  - Treatment of any associated hyperkalaemia.
  - Identification of the need for renal replacement therapy (e.g. AKI).

12.6 SAQs

12.6.1 Rhabdomyolysis

An 85-year-old lady is brought to the ED via ambulance. Paramedics were called when her neighbours had not seen her for three days. The paramedics found her on the floor of her bedroom. She is confused and looks unwell. She is on high flow O_2, has IV access, and her initial bloods results are:

Na 134 mmol/L, K 6.9 mmol/L, urea 35 mmol/L, creatinine 350 μmol/L, pH 7.20 kPa, pO_2 12.1 kPa, pCO_2 6.9 kPa, HCO_3^- 8 mmol/L, BE −15.0.

a) (i) List four ECG abnormalities found in hyperkalaemia. (2 marks)

a) (ii) Interpret the arterial blood gas. (1 mark)

b) What are the three main treatment aims in managing hyperkalaemia in the ED and give examples of the drugs you would use to achieve this. (3 marks)

c) (i) What bedside test would support the diagnosis of rhabdomyolysis? (1 mark)

c) (ii) What blood test would confirm the diagnosis of rhabdomyolysis? (1 mark)

d) What would be your first two treatments in managing this patient's rhabdomyolysis? (2 marks)

Suggested answer

a) (i) List four ECG abnormalities found in hyperkalaemia. (2 marks)

    Tall peaked T waves

    Short QT

    Prolonged PR

    Widened QRS

    Flattened P waves

    Sinusoidal QRST

    AV dissociation

    VT/VF

    Asystole

a) (ii) Interpret the arterial blood gas. (1 mark)

    Mixed metabolic and respiratory acidosis (½ mark for each component)

b) What are the three main treatment aims in managing hyperkalaemia in the ED and give examples of the drugs you would use to achieve this. (3 marks)

    Cardiac protection—calcium chloride or gluconate 10 ml of 10% IV

    Shift K^+ into the intracellular space—salbutamol nebulizer 5mg; or insulin and glucose infusion (10 units of short-acting insulin with 50 ml of 50% glucose IV); or sodium bicarbonate (1.26% infusion or 8.4% 50 ml aliquots)

    Excretion of K^+—calcium resonium PO or PR to enhance GI excretion

    (½ mark for method, ½ mark for drug)

c) (i) What bedside test would support the diagnosis of rhabdomyolysis? (1 mark)

    Urinary dipstick positive for blood

c) (ii) What blood test would confirm the diagnosis of rhabdomyolysis? (1 mark)

    Creatine kinase

d) What would be your first two treatments in managing this patient's rhabdomyolysis? (2 marks)

Aggressive fluid resuscitation—0.9% sodium chloride to achieve high urinary flow rates (>100 ml/h)

Sodium bicarbonate (1.26%)—to maintain a urinary pH>7.5

12.6.2 Acute kidney injury

A 70-year-old man presents to the ED for a repeat blood test. His GP performed a routine check of his renal function and on receiving the result advised the patient to attend the hospital urgently. His blood results are:

Na 134 mmol/L, K 6.9 mmol/L, urea 35 mmol/L, creatinine 450 µmol/l.

a) List two likely pre-renal causes of acute kidney injury in this patient. (2 marks)

b) (i) The patient has a history of hypertension and is on some antihypertensive medications but he cannot remember their names. Name two classes of antihypertensive medications which may cause renal impairment. (2 mark)

b) (ii) What other conditions in this patient's past medical history may put him at risk of acute kidney injury? (2 marks)

c) Apart from rechecking his renal function, what is the most important investigation to perform in the ED on this patient? (1 mark)

Repeat renal function is performed. The results are: Na 134 mmol/L, K 7.1 mmol/L, urea 40 mmol/L, creatinine 550 µ mol/l.

d) What are the three main treatment aims in managing this patient? (3 marks)

Suggested answer

a) List two likely pre-renal causes of acute kidney injury in this patient. (2 marks)

Volume loss—vomiting, diarrhoea, dehydration, diuretics
Decreased cardiac output—valvular heart disease, heart failure
Renal artery disease—atheroemboli, hypertension

b) (i) The patient has a history of hypertension and is on some antihypertensive medications but he cannot remember their names. Name two classes of antihypertensive medications which may cause renal impairment. (2 mark)

ACE inhibitor
Angiotensin II receptor antagonist
Loop diuretic
Thiazide

b) (ii) What other conditions in this patient's past medical history may put him at risk of acute kidney injury? (2 marks)

Chronic kidney disease
Cardiac failure
Peripheral vascular disease
Liver disease
Diabetes mellitus

c) Apart from rechecking his renal function, what is the most important investigation to perform
    in the ED on this patient? (1 mark)
    ECG (due to the hyperkalaemia on the initial result)
d) What are the three main treatment aims in managing this patient? (3 marks)
    Treat the hyperkalaemia
    Fluid resuscitation
    Relieve any urinary tract obstruction
    Stop any nephrotoxic drugs

Further reading

National Institute for Health and Care Excellence, August 2013. NICE clinical guideline 169. Acute
    Kidney Injury: prevention, detection and management. Available at: https://www.nice.org.uk/
    Guidance/CG169 [Online].
UK National Confidential Enquiry into Patient Outcomes and Death (NCEPOD) Acute Kidney
    Injury: Adding Insult to Injury Report. Available at: http://www.ncepod.org.uk [Online].

CHAPTER 13

Gastrointestinal emergencies

CONTENTS

13.1 Acute gastrointestinal bleeding

Acute gastrointestinal (GI) bleeding is a common major medical emergency and one of the acute presentations included in the ACCS curriculum. The management discussed in this chapter is based on SIGN and NICE guidelines.

Upper GI bleeding is that arising proximal to the ligament of Treitz at the duodenojejunal flexure (i.e. oesophagus, stomach, and duodenum). Lower GI bleeding is that arising from the small bowel and colon.

Haematemesis is the vomiting of blood from the upper GI tract or occasionally after swallowing blood from a source in the nasopharynx. Bright red haematemesis usually implies active haemorrhage from the oesophagus, stomach, or duodenum. Patients presenting with haematemesis have a higher mortality than those presenting with melaena alone.

Coffee-ground vomit refers to the vomiting of black material, which is assumed to be partially digested blood. Its presence implies that bleeding has ceased or has been relatively modest.

Melaena is the passage of black tarry stools, usually due to acute upper GI bleeding but occasionally from bleeding within the small bowel or right side of the colon.

Haematochezia is the passage of fresh or altered blood per rectum usually due to colonic bleeding. Occasionally profuse upper GI or small bowel bleeding can be responsible.

13.2 Acute upper gastrointestinal bleeding

Previous MRCEM question

Upper GI bleeding is a significant cause of morbidity and mortality. Upper GI bleeding is about four times more common than lower GI bleeding.

The risk stratification and management of patients with upper GI bleeding has appeared in previous MRCEM examinations.

13.2.1 Causes of upper gastrointestinal bleeding

Causes of upper GI bleeding include:

- Peptic ulcer disease
- Oesophagitis
- Gastritis/erosions
- Duodenitis
- Oesophageal varices
- Malignancy (e.g. gastric carcinoma)
- Mallory–Weiss tear
- Coagulation disorders (e.g. thrombocytopenia, warfarin)
- Aortoenteric fistulas (rare, consider if the patient has had aortic surgery)
- Benign tumours (e.g. leiomyomas, angiomas)
- Congenital (e.g. Ehlers–Danlos syndrome)

Peptic ulcer disease

Peptic ulcer disease is the commonest cause of upper GI bleeding (35–50%), which may be the consequence of *Helicobacter pylori* infection and/or NSAID use.

There is a strong association between *Helicobacter pylori* infection and peptic ulcer disease. *Helicobacter pylori* disrupt the mucosal barrier and cause inflammation of the gastric and duodenal mucosa. Eradication therapy reduces the risk of recurrent ulcers and further upper GI bleeding.

NSAIDs are the second most important aetiological factor in the development of peptic ulcer disease. They exert an effect on cyclooxygenase-1, leading to impaired resistance of the mucosa to acid.

Varices

Variceal haemorrhage occurs from dilated veins (varices) at the junction between the portal and systemic venous systems. These collaterals are found in the oesophagus, stomach, rectum, small and large bowel. Portal hypertension due to chronic liver disease results in increased blood flow through the collaterals and resulting dilatation.

Bleeding from varices is characteristically severe and may be life-threatening. The size of varices and their propensity to bleed is directly related to the portal pressure, which, in the majority of cases, is related to the severity of the underlying liver disease. The severity of liver disease can be graded using the Child–Pugh score (Table 13.1).

Table 13.1 Child–Pugh grading of chronic liver disease

Score	1	2	3
Encephalopathy	None	Mild (grade 1–2)	Severe (grade 3–4)
Ascites	Absent	Mild	Severe
Bilirubin (mmol/l)	<34	34–51	>51
Albumin (g/l)	>35	28–35	<28
INR	<1.3	1.3–1.5	>1.5

Data from Pugh RN, Murray-Lyon IM, Dawson JL, et al. 'Transection of the oesophagus for bleeding oesophageal varices'. Br J Surg. 1973 Aug;60(8):646–9.

13.2.2 Risk factors for upper gastrointestinal bleeding

Certain factors are associated with a poorer outcome in patients with an acute upper GI bleed. Poor outcome is defined in terms of severity of bleed, uncontrolled bleeding, rebleeding, need for intervention, and mortality.

Risk factors include:

- Increasing age—mortality due to an upper GI bleed increases with age.
- Co-morbidity—patients without co-morbidities have the lowest mortality (~4%). If the patient has one co-morbidity, the mortality doubles. Patients with cardiac failure or malignancy have a significantly worse prognosis.
- Liver disease—cirrhosis is associated with a doubling of mortality. Patients presenting with varices have an overall mortality of 14%.
- Inpatients—have an approximately 3-fold increased risk of death compared to patients newly admitted with GI bleeding. This is due to the presence of co-morbidities in established inpatients rather than an increased severity of bleeding.
- Shock—patients with hypotension and tachycardia have an increased mortality and need for intervention.
- Continued bleeding—after admission is associated with up to a 50-fold increase in mortality.
- Haematemesis—on presentation doubles the mortality.
- Haematochezia—doubles the rebleeding, mortality, and surgery rates.
- Elevated blood urea—is associated with a need for intervention.

NSAIDs and anticoagulants are risk factors for developing an upper GI bleed but do not adversely affect the clinical outcomes of patients presenting with an upper GI bleed.

13.2.3 Clinical assessment of a patient with an upper gastrointestinal bleed

Resuscitation takes priority when assessing a patient with an upper GI bleed and an ABCDE approach should be followed if the patient is unstable.

If the patient is stable, a detailed history and examination can be performed. Important points in the history include:

- Nature of blood vomited—fresh blood suggests active bleeding and/or variceal bleeding. Coffee-ground vomit suggests that bleeding has ceased and is more likely to be caused by a peptic ulcer.
- Passage of melaena—supports the diagnosis of an upper GI bleed. The passage of haematochezia suggests either a lower GI bleed or a very brisk upper GI bleed.
- Abdominal pain—a duodenal ulcer is more likely to present with severe epigastric pain and features of peritonism. Variceal bleeding may be painless.
- Recent vomiting or retching—suggests a possible Mallory–Weiss tear.
- Associated symptoms to suggest hypovolaemia and/or anaemia (e.g. shortness of breath, lethargy, weakness, fainting, and so on).
- Symptoms that may suggest an underlying malignancy (e.g. weight loss, dysphagia, abdominal pain, anorexia, and so on).
- Past medical history (e.g. liver disease or alcoholism) predisposing to variceal bleeding; or a history of peptic ulcer disease or gastro-oesophageal reflux that may suggest a bleeding ulcer. Significant co-morbidities that increase the mortality from upper GI bleeding should be noted (e.g. heart failure, malignancy).
- Medication history (e.g. warfarin, NSAIDs, and corticosteroids) that can predispose the patient to an upper GI bleed.
- Social history—an alcohol history should be taken to determine the likelihood of alcoholic liver disease.

Examination should initially proceed in an ABCDE manner looking for signs of hypovolaemic shock (e.g. tachycardia, hypotension, prolonged capillary refill, tachypnoea, and reduced GCS).

The abdomen should be examined for evidence of masses, tenderness, peritonism, and previous surgical scars (e.g. previous aortic surgery). A rectal examination provides useful information about the presence of melaena or haematochezia. Any vomit should be inspected for evidence of blood or 'coffee-grounds'.

A variceal haemorrhage should be suspected in patients with stigmata of chronic liver disease, which include:

- Jaundice
- Ascites
- Splenomegaly
- Spider naevi
- Caput medusae
- Encephalopathy
- Gynaecomastia
- Palmar erythema

Signs of malignancy include:

- Nodularity and enlargement of the liver
- Ascites
- Lymphadenopathy

13.2.4 Risk stratification of upper gastrointestinal bleeding

Risk assessment for all patients with acute upper gastrointestinal bleeding includes a Blatchford score (table 13.2) at first assessment and a Rockall score after endoscopy.

In the validation group, scores of 6 or more were associated with a greater than 50% risk of needing an intervention.

The Rockall scoring system is one of the most widely used methods for risk assessment in upper GI bleeding and it has been validated in several studies. It was principally designed to predict death based on a combination of both clinical and endoscopic findings. The pre-endoscopy Rockall score is now widely used in emergency departments to risk stratify patients with upper GI bleeds and is included in the SIGN guidance (Table 13.3). The Rockall score has appeared in previous exam questions.

Only patients with a pre-endoscopy Rockall score or a Blatchford score of 0 can be safely managed as an outpatient. Patients with a score greater than 0 have a significant risk of mortality: a score of 1 has a predicted mortality of 2.4%; score 2 predicted mortality is 5.6%; score 7 predicted mortality is 50%.

Once the patient has had an endoscopy, a full Rockall score can be calculated (Table 13.4).

Based on the Rockall scoring system and expert opinion, SIGN have developed an initial assessment protocol for patients presenting with an acute upper GI bleed (Boxes 13.1 and 13.2).

13.2.5 Investigation of upper gastrointestinal bleeding

Bloods should be sent for:

- FBC—to determine the degree of anaemia. The full extent may not be apparent until the patient is fluid resuscitated. Platelets may be low if there is a consumptive coagulopathy.
- Clotting—patients are at risk of coagulopathy.
- Cross match—the number of units should be determined by the clinical picture.
- Liver function tests (LFTs)—to determine the presence and degree of any liver failure.
- Urea and electrolytes—urea may rise due to degradation of red blood cells in the GI tract.

Table 13.2 Blachford score

Admission risk factor	Score component value
Blood urea (mmol/L)	
6.5–8.0	2
8.0–10	3
10.0–25	4
>25	6
Haemoglobin (g/L) for men	
12.0–12.9	1
10.0–12.0	3
<10.0	6
Haemoglobin (g/L) for women	
10.0–11.9	1
<10	6
Systolic blood pressure (mmHg)	
100–109	1
90–99	2
<90	3
Other markers	
Pulse ≥100/per min	1
Presentation with malaena	1
Presentation with syncope	2
Hepatic disease	2
Cardiac failure	2

Table 13.3 Rockall score (pre-endoscopy)

Score	0	1	2	3
Age	<60	60–79	≥80	
Shock	'No shock' HR<100 Sys BP>100	'Tachycardia' HR>100 Sys BP>100	'Hypotension' HR>100 Sys BP<100	
Co-morbidity	No major co-morbidity		Cardiac failure, ischaemic heart disease, any major co-morbidity	Renal failure, liver failure, disseminated malignancy

Data from Rockall TA, Logan RF, Devlin HB, et al (1996). 'Risk assessment after acute upper gastrointestinal haemorrhage'. Gut 38 (3): 316–21.

Table 13.4 Rockall score (endoscopy criteria for full score)

Score	0	1	2	3
Diagnosis	Mallory–Weiss tear, no lesion identified	All other diagnoses	Malignancy of upper GI tract	
Major stigmata of recent haemorrhage	No evidence of recent haemorrhage		Blood in upper GI tract, visible or spurting vessel	

Data from Rockall TA, Logan RF, Devlin HB, et al (1996). 'Risk assessment after acute upper gastrointestinal haemorrhage'. Gut 38 (3): 316–21.

An erect chest X-ray (CXR) should be performed to detect any subdiaphragmatic air indicating a perforation (see Chapter 6, section 6.6).

The definitive investigation and treatment is endoscopy.

13.2.6 Emergency department management of upper gastrointestinal bleeding

Initial resuscitation

Initial resuscitation should proceed in an ABCDE manner:

- A and B—high-flow oxygen should be administered. Hypovolaemia may lead to a reduced level of consciousness, which carries the risk of airway compromise and hypoventilation. Recurrent vomiting and diminished airway reflexes may lead to aspiration. Intubation and ventilation are required if the patient becomes obtunded and is unable to maintain their airway, especially if they require an emergency endoscopy.
- C—patients who are shocked have a greater risk of death from an upper GI bleed than those who are not shocked. Shock needs to be recognized early and treated aggressively with IV fluid resuscitation. Crystalloid or colloid can be used as the initial resuscitation fluid to restore circulating volume. Once 30% of the circulating volume is lost, red cell transfusion should be used to restore volume. The haematology laboratory should be informed if the patient is having a major upper GI bleed so that they can initiate their major haemorrhage protocol. Patients with major bleeds may require additional blood products. Platelet transfusion is indicated for active bleeding in the presence of a platelet count $<50 \times 10^9$ /L. Prothrombin complex concentrate should be given to patients on warfarin with active bleeding. Fresh frozen plasma should be offered if the prothrombin time (INR) or activated partial thromboplastin time is greater than 1.5 times normal. If the fibrinogen level remains under 1.5 g/L despite fresh frozen plasma, cryoprecipitate administration should be considered. Recombinant factor VIIa should only be given when all other methods have failed.

Box 13.1 Initial assessment protocol for acute upper GI bleeding (patients that may be discharged)

Consider for discharge, or non-admission with outpatient follow up, if:

- age <60 years; and
- no evidence of haemodynamic disturbance; and
- no significant co-morbidity; and
- not a current inpatient or transfer; and
- no witnessed haematemesis or haematochezia.

Box 13.2 Initial assessment protocol for acute upper GI bleeding (patients that require admission)

Consider for admission and early endoscopy (and calculation of full Rockall score) if:

- age>60 years; or
- witnessed haematemesis or haematochezia; or
- haemodynamic disturbance; or
- liver disease or known varices.

- Balloon tamponade—should be considered as a temporary salvage procedure in uncontrolled variceal haemorrhage. This usually involves placement of a Sengstaken-Blakemore tube, which has oesophageal and gastric balloons and a gastric aspiration port, often after tracheal intubation to protect the airway.

Endoscopy

Endoscopy is usually the definitive treatment for acute upper GI bleeding, with a small percentage of patients requiring arterial embolization or surgery if endoscopy fails to control bleeding. For patients with uncontrolled variceal haemorrhage following endoscopy, the treatment of choice is transjugular intrahepatic portosystemic shunting (TIPS).

The timing of endoscopy depends upon the pre-endoscopy Rockall score and local facilities. If the patient is unstable, has ongoing active bleeding, or a suspected variceal bleed then endoscopy should be performed once appropriate resuscitation has taken place. For those without an immediate indication for endoscopy, the aim should be to perform the procedure within 24 hours of admission.

Endoscopic techniques to stop bleeding depend upon the cause but may include injection of sclerosants, thermal coagulation, clipping, and/or band ligation.

Pharmacological therapies

A variety of pharmacological therapies are available for treating patients with acute upper non-variceal GI bleeds. Certain therapies are recommended following endoscopy (e.g. proton pump inhibitors and *Helicobacter pylori* eradication therapy) and therefore are not usually administered in the ED.

- Proton pump inhibitors (PPIs) and H2-receptor antagonists are not recommended prior to an endoscopic diagnosis, due to a lack of evidence to support their use. Intravenous PPIs are indicated in patients with major peptic ulcer bleeding following endoscopic haemostatic therapy.
- Aspirin, NSAIDs, and anticoagulants—should be stopped when a patient presents with an upper GI bleed. Patients on warfarin may require reversal with prothrombin complex concentrate (e.g. Beriplex® or Octaplex®) or fresh frozen plasma.
- *Helicobacter pylori* eradication therapy—patients with peptic ulcer bleeding should be tested for *Helicobacter pylori*. Those who test positive should be treated with a one week course of eradication therapy (e.g. amoxicillin, clarithromycin, and a proton pump inhibitor), followed by three weeks of ulcer healing treatment. The eradication of *H. Pylori* reduces the incidence of rebleeding.

Patients with variceal bleeds, or a history strongly suggestive of variceal bleeding, may require other therapies.

- Vasoactive drugs—terlipressin is the only vasoactive drug shown to reduce mortality when given pre-endoscopy. SIGN recommends terlipressin should be given to patients with suspected variceal bleeding prior to endoscopy. It acts by causing generalized arteriolar and venous constriction. The resulting splanchnic vasoconstriction reduces portal pressure and the degree of variceal bleeding. Important side effects may occur due to vasoconstriction including myocardial ischaemia or infarction, and peripheral ischaemia. Therefore it should not be used in patients with vascular disease, especially those with coronary disease.

- Antibiotic therapy (e.g. ciprofloxacin or ceftriaxone)—should be commenced in all patients with an upper GI bleed and chronic liver disease. Antibiotics have been shown to reduce mortality from variceal bleeding by up to 27%.

Ongoing management

- Aspirin, NSAIDs, and COX-2 inhibitors should only be prescribed to patients following an upper GI bleed if there is a clear indication. If such treatments are required, proton pump inhibitors should be given concurrently.
- Selective serotonin reuptake inhibitors (SSRIs) should be used cautiously in patients who have had or are at risk of an upper GI bleed, especially those already taking NSAIDs or aspirin. In such cases, a non-SSRI antidepressant should be considered.
- Oral anticoagulants and corticosteroids should be used cautiously in patients who have had or are at risk of an upper GI bleed.
- β-blockers are recommended for secondary prevention of variceal bleeding.

KEY POINTS

Upper GI bleeding is a significant cause of morbidity and mortality.

Peptic ulcer disease is the commonest cause of upper GI bleeding.

Variceal haemorrhage occurs from dilated veins at the junction between the portal and systemic venous systems. The size of varices and their propensity to bleed is directly related to the portal pressure, which is related to the severity of the underlying liver disease.

Blatchford and Rockall scoring are used to risk stratify patients with upper GI bleeding. It has pre- and post-endoscopy components. The pre-endoscopy score is calculated from age, haemodynamic compromise, and co-morbidity.

Only patients with a pre-endoscopy Rockall score or Blatchford score of 0 can be safely managed as an outpatient.

Endoscopy is usually the definitive treatment for acute upper GI bleeding.

ED management should follow an ABCDE approach with prompt fluid resuscitation to correct any hypovolaemic shock.

There is a lack of evidence for the use of proton pump inhibitors prior to endoscopy.

Patients with variceal bleeding should be given terlipressin, if there are no contraindications, and broad-spectrum antibiotics.

13.3 Acute lower gastrointestinal bleeding

13.3.1 Introduction

Approximately 25% of GI haemorrhage originates from the lower GI tract. The majority (~80%) will stop spontaneously. Although lower GI haemorrhage originates from distal to the ligament of Treitz, approximately 15% of patients with haematochezia will have an upper GI source due to rapid transit through the GI tract. All patients with evidence of GI bleeding should have a rectal examination.

13.3.2 Causes of lower gastrointestinal bleeding

Causes include:

- Diverticular disease (commonest cause)
- Angiodysplasia
- Ischaemic colitis
- Haemorrhoids
- Inflammatory bowel disease
- Neoplasia
- Radiation enteropathy

13.3.3 Risk factors for lower gastrointestinal bleeding

There is limited evidence on the risk factors for a poor outcome in lower GI bleeding. Factors that have been shown to be associated with poorer outcome (e.g. uncontrolled bleeding and/or death) are:

- Increasing age—acute lower GI bleeding occurs most commonly in the elderly.
- Shock and gross rectal bleeding—predict subsequent severe bleeding.
- Co-morbidity—the presence of two or more co-morbid conditions double the chance of a severe bleed.
- Aspirin and NSAIDs—increase the risk of a severe lower GI bleed.
- Inpatients—who are hospitalized for another condition and have a lower GI bleed have a higher mortality than those presenting acutely with a lower GI bleed.

13.3.4 Clinical assessment of a patient with a lower gastrointestinal bleed

As with an upper GI bleed, resuscitation takes priority when assessing a patient with a lower GI bleed and an ABCDE approach should be employed if the patient is unstable.

If the patient is stable, a detailed history and examination can be performed.

Pertinent points in the history include:

- Nature of the stool—dark red blood in the stool suggests more proximal colonic bleeding or brisk upper GI bleeding. Bright red, fresh blood suggests a lower GI cause. Blood mixed in with the stool suggests a colonic cause. Blood on the outside of the stool or on the toilet paper suggests a local rectal cause (e.g. haemorrhoid or anal fissure). Mucus may suggest inflammatory bowel disease.
- Abdominal pain—left iliac fossa pain may suggest diverticulitis. Pain is a late sign in GI malignancies.
- Associated symptoms (e.g. fever and/or vomiting) support an infective cause. Dizziness, breathlessness, and/or fainting suggest anaemia.
- Altered bowel habit—may suggest an underlying GI malignancy.
- Weight loss—suggests an underlying GI malignancy.
- Past medical history (e.g. inflammatory bowel disease, diverticulitis, haemorrhoids, and so on).
- Family history—of bowel disorders, particularly malignancy.
- Medications (e.g. anticoagulants, NSAIDs, aspirin).

A thorough abdominal examination should be performed, including a rectal examination to detect bleeding haemorrhoids, anal fissures, or a rectal mass.

13.3.5 Investigation of lower gastrointestinal bleeding

Investigations should be performed as for an upper GI bleed. In addition, blood and stool cultures should be sent if an infective cause is suspected.

Plain abdominal X-rays should not be routinely requested unless bowel obstruction or toxic megacolon is suspected.

Box 13.3 Initial assessment protocol for acute lower GI bleeding (patients that may be discharged)

Consider for discharge or non-admission with outpatient follow up if:

- age <60 years; and
- no evidence of haemodynamic disturbance; and
- no evidence of gross rectal bleeding; and
- an obvious anorectal source of bleeding on rectal examination/sigmoidoscopy.

Colonoscopy or flexible sigmoidoscopy is the investigation of choice, but is rarely indicated in the ED.

Further imaging may include abdominal CT, double-contrast barium enema, or mesenteric angiography.

13.3.6 Risk stratification of a lower gastrointestinal bleed

There are no commonly used predictive models or scoring systems for lower GI haemorrhage. SIGN have produced guidance on whether a patient requires admission or not (Boxes 13.3 and 13.4).

13.3.7 Emergency department management of lower gastrointestinal bleeding

The majority of lower GI bleeding will stop spontaneously and supportive therapy is all that is required, with appropriate referral on for further investigation.

- ABC—should be assessed and managed appropriately as for upper GI bleeding.
- Fluid resuscitation—should be guided by the patient's haemodynamic status as for an upper GI bleed.
- Colonoscopy—is an effective way of controlling massive lower GI bleeding. Early colonoscopy should be used to determine the site of bleeding and to achieve haemostasis.
- Arterial embolization—may be considered if colonoscopy fails to control the bleeding.
- Surgical resection—is reserved for cases where other techniques fail to control the bleeding.

KEY POINTS

The majority of lower GI bleeding will stop spontaneously.

There is no commonly used risk assessment tool for lower GI bleeding.

ED management of lower GI bleeding is supportive. A small proportion of patients will require an urgent colonoscopy to control bleeding. If colonoscopy fails to control bleeding, arterial embolization or surgery may be required.

Box 13.4 Initial assessment protocol for acute lower GI bleeding (patients that require admission)

Consider for admission if:

- age>60 years, or;
- haemodynamic disturbance; or
- evidence of gross rectal bleeding; or
- taking aspirin or an NSAID; or
- significant co-morbidity.

13.4 Vomiting

13.4.1 Introduction

Vomiting is the forceful discharge of gastric contents. Regurgitation is the return of undigested food back up the oesophagus into the mouth, without the force of vomiting.

Persistent vomiting can lead to dehydration, severe alkalosis, bleeding, and rarely oesophageal perforation.

The curriculum includes knowledge of the differential diagnosis, investigation, and management of a patient with vomiting.

13.4.2 Pathophysiology of vomiting

The vomiting reflex is coordinated by the postrema area of the brain, which lies on the floor of the fourth ventricle. Adjacent to the postrema is the chemoreceptor trigger zone (CTZ), which contains chemoreceptors that sample both blood and cerebrospinal fluid.

The vomiting centre receives inputs from various sources:

- The CTZ contains dopamine, serotonin, 5-HT_3, opioid, and acetylcholine receptors, which sample blood and cerebrospinal fluid. Stimulation of these receptors can trigger pathways which result in emesis.
- The vestibular system sends information to the vomiting centre via the vestibulocochlear nerve (CN VIII). The vestibular system plays a major role in motion sickness and is rich in muscarinic and histamine H_1 receptors.
- The vagus nerve (CN X) is activated when the pharynx is irritated, leading to a gag reflex.
- The abdominal splanchnic and vagal nerves transmit information regarding the state of the gastrointestinal system. Irritation of the GI mucosa by chemotherapy, radiation, distension, or acute infection activates the 5-HT_3 receptors of these inputs.
- The cerebral cortex mediates vomiting that arises from emotion, stress, and psychiatric disorders.

Once the vomiting centre is stimulated, it initiates three types of output (motor, parasympathetic, and sympathetic) that lead to the act of vomiting. The events involved in vomiting are:

- Increased salivation (parasympathetic).
- Retro-peristalsis—starts from the middle of the small intestine and progresses up the digestive tract.
- Lowering of intrathoracic pressure (by inspiration against a closed glottis) coupled with increased intra-abdominal pressure (as abdominal muscles contract), which propels stomach contents into the oesophagus as the lower oesophageal sphincter relaxes. The stomach and oesophagus do not contract in the process of vomiting.
- Sweating and tachycardia (sympathetic).

13.4.3 Causes of vomiting

There are many of causes of vomiting. Table 13.5 lists potential causes.

13.4.4 Clinical assessment of a patient who is vomiting

A detailed history and examination will usually determine the most likely causes of vomiting. Table 13.6 details clinical findings that are suggestive of particular causes of vomiting.

The curriculum includes specific knowledge of 'red flags' that may suggest an upper GI malignancy in a patient who presents with vomiting, these include:

- Unexplained weight loss
- Chronic gastrointestinal bleeding
- Early satiety

Table 13.5 Causes of vomiting

Gastrointestinal tract	Gastroenteritis (e.g. viral or bacterial infection)
	Gastro-oesophageal reflux disease
	Acute abdomen (e.g. appendicitis, pancreatitis, cholecystitis)
	Bowel obstruction
	Ileus
	Food intolerance
Nervous system	Motion sickness
	Vertigo (e.g. due to benign paroxysmal positional vertigo, Ménière's disease, vestibular neuronitis, acute labyrinthitis)
	Intracranial haemorrhage
	Cerebral tumours
	Migraine
	Raised intracranial pressure
Endocrine system	Hyper or hypoglycaemia
	Hypercalcaemia
	Uraemia
	Adrenal insufficiency
Pregnancy	'Morning sickness'
	Hyperemesis gravidarum
Drugs	Alcohol
	Opiates
	Selective serotonin reuptake inhibitors
	NSAIDs
	Metronidazole
	Chemotherapy agents
	Many drugs can cause nausea and vomiting, a temporal relationship between starting the drug or altering dose is suggestive.
Other	Psychogenic (e.g. bulimia)
	Carbon monoxide poisoning
	Myocardial ischaemia or infarction

- Dysphagia
- Persistent vomiting
- Jaundice
- Family history of gastric cancer
- Palpable epigastric mass
- Lymphadenopathy (e.g. supraclavicular, periumbilical)
- Hepatomegaly
- Iron deficiency anaemia
- Rectal bleeding or melena

13.4.5 Complications of vomiting

Vomiting can result in a variety of complications which may present to the ED.

Table 13.6 Clinical features suggestive of particular causes of vomiting

Cause of vomiting	Suggestive clinical findings
Gastroenteritis	Vomiting and diarrhoea. Unremarkable abdominal examination.
Bowel obstruction	Absolute constipation, abdominal distension, tympanic percussion note, bilious vomiting, hyperactive bowel sounds, previous abdominal surgery (see Chapter 6, section 6.5).
Gastroparesis or ileus	Vomiting partially digested food a few hours after eating.
Acute abdomen	Significant abdominal pain, peritonism (see Chapter 6, section 6.1).
Intracranial haemorrhage	Evidence of external head injury, headache, focal neurological signs, reduced level of consciousness (see Chapter 4, section 4.5).
CNS infection	Gradual onset of headache, fever, neck stiffness, focal neurological signs, rash (see Chapter 15, section 15.3).
Acute labyrinthitis	Vertigo, nystagmus, hearing loss, recent URTI (see Chapter 7, section 7.8).
Benign paroxysmal positional vertigo	Symptoms exacerbated by head movement. Previous attacks (see Chapter 7, section 7.8).
Migraine	Pulsating, unilateral headache, visual symptoms, preceding aura, history of previous attacks (see Chapter 11, section 11.3).
Motion sickness	History of recent travel.
Diabetic ketoacidosis	Polyuria, polydipsia, dehydration, raised blood glucose, tachypnoea (see Chapter 14, section 14.1).
Pregnancy	Positive pregnancy test or known pregnancy (see Chapter 8, section 8.8).

Complications include:

- Dehydration and electrolyte imbalance
- Upper GI bleeding (e.g. Mallory–Weiss tear)
- Aspiration
- Oesophageal rupture (Boerhaave syndrome)

Boerhaave syndrome

Boerhaave syndrome is a surgical emergency which is caused by spontaneous rupture of the oesophagus secondary to vomiting. If left untreated the condition is fatal.

Symptoms of Boerhaave syndrome are non-specific and a high-index of suspicions is required to make a timely diagnosis. Symptoms include chest pain, abdominal pain, vomiting, and dyspnoea. Patients may have surgical emphysema on examination of the chest and neck. They may be profoundly shocked.

A CXR may show subcutaneous emphysema, pneumothorax, pneumomediastinum, pleural effusion, and/or free mediastinal air. However, up to one-third of patients have a normal CXR. If the diagnosis is suspected an oesophagogram or thoracic CT is required.

Patients should be urgently referred to a cardiothoracic surgeon and resuscitated with IV fluids, analgesia, and broad-spectrum antibiotics.

13.4.6 Emergency department management of vomiting

The ED management of vomiting depends on the suspected underlying cause and whether the patient has any complications.

Table 13.7 Indications, mode of action, and side effects of commonly used anti-emetics

Anti-emetic	Indications	Mode of action	Side effects
Phenothiazines (e.g. prochlorperazine)	Nausea and vomiting	Block dopamine receptors at the CTZ	Hypotension Extra-pyramidal side effects (e.g. dyskinesia, dystonia) Neuroleptic malignant syndrome
Prokinetics (e.g. metoclopramide, domperidone)	Gastric paresis Gastro-oesophageal reflux disease Nausea and vomiting	Enhance GI motility + Dopamine receptor antagonist at CTZ	Metoclopramide may cause extra-pyramidal side effects (NB Domperidone does not cross the blood-brain barrier and therefore does not cause the same extra-pyramidal effects)
Antihistamines (e.g. cyclizine)	Motion sickness Vertigo Raised intracranial pressure Mechanical bowel obstruction	Acts on the vestibular system and the CTZ. Plus exerts a central anticholinergic action	Drowsiness Dry mouth
5-HT$_3$ receptor antagonists (e.g. ondansetron)	Postoperative nausea Chemotherapy (Not effective for motion sickness)	Antagonize 5-HT$_3$ receptors peripherally (prokinetic) and centrally (CTZ)	Constipation Headache Transient rise in LFTs

The curriculum specifically includes knowledge of the use and adverse effects of commonly used anti-emetics (Table 13.7).

Anti-emetics may need to be given in combination when nausea and vomiting persist. It is recommended that metoclopramide and cyclizine are not given together because they counteract each other. Metoclopramide is a dopamine receptor antagonist, which enhances gastric emptying. The final common pathway of gastric emptying is via acetylcholine, which is blocked by the anticholinergic effects of cyclizine. Therefore, combination therapy blocks the prokinetic effect of metoclopramide and diminishes the anti-emetic benefits.

If metoclopramide or cyclizine have failed to control symptoms, then ondansetron is an appropriate next therapy.

KEY POINTS

Vomiting is the forceful discharge of gastric contents.

Persistent vomiting can lead to dehydration, severe alkalosis, bleeding, and rarely oesophageal perforation (Boerhaave syndrome).

'Red flags' for upper GI malignancy include:
- Unexplained weight loss
- Chronic gastrointestinal bleeding

- Early satiety
- Dysphagia
- Persistent vomiting
- Jaundice
- Family history of gastric cancer
- Palpable epigastric mass
- Lymphadenopathy (e.g. supraclavicular, periumbilical)
- Hepatomegaly
- Iron deficiency anaemia
- Rectal bleeding or melena

13.5 Diarrhoea

13.5.1 Introduction

The British Society of Gastroenterology defines diarrhoea as the abnormal passage of loose or liquid stools more than three times per day and/or a volume of stool greater than 200 g/day. Diarrhoea lasting less than four weeks is considered acute and longer than four weeks chronic.

13.5.2 Pathophysiology of diarrhoea

Diarrhoea can be the result of several different mechanisms including:

- Increased osmotic load in the gut lumen—soluble compounds (e.g. osmotic laxatives; magnesium-based antacids; foods containing mannitol, sorbitol, or xylitol), which cannot be absorbed by the small intestine draw fluid into the intestinal lumen resulting in osmotic diarrhoea.
- Increased secretion into the gut lumen—secretory diarrhoea results from active chloride secretion into the bowel lumen. Water follows the chloride ions, leading to a net loss of fluid. Infections (e.g. *Vibrio cholerae*), drugs (e.g. laxatives, diuretics, theophylline, caffeine, and ethanol), and gut allergies can cause secretory diarrhoea.
- Inflammation of the intestinal lining.
- Increased intestinal mobility.

13.5.3 Causes of diarrhoea

Diarrhoea is a symptom with many different causes, the commonest of which is infection (see Table 13.8).

13.5.4 Clinical assessment of a patient presenting with diarrhoea

Diarrhoea is one of the most common symptoms for which people seek medical attention. An accurate history and detailed clinical examination will often be sufficient to determine the cause of the diarrhoea.

Pertinent points in the history include:

- Time-scale of symptoms—most people with acute diarrhoea due to an infective cause will improve within two to four days. A history of chronic diarrhoea (>4 weeks) makes infection less likely and suggests other aetiologies.
- Quantity and character of stools (e.g. fatty, suggestive of chronic pancreatitis), bloody (see Table 13.9), watery, or mucus (as seen in inflammatory bowel disease).
- Associated symptoms suggesting infection (e.g. fever, recent travel, contact with a person with diarrhoea, recent antibiotics, and so on).

Table 13.8 Causes of diarrhoea

Causes of diarrhoea	Examples
Viral infection (commonest cause in the community)	Rotavirus, norovirus.
Bacterial infection	*Salmonella, Campylobacter jejuni, Shigella, Escherichia coli*
	Clostridium difficile (common in elderly patients who have recently taken antibiotics).
Drugs	Antibiotics, NSAIDs, metformin, proton pump inhibitors, selective serotonin reuptake inhibitors, statins, theophylline, thyroxine, allopurinol, angiotensin-II receptor blockers, digoxin, colchicine, H_2-receptor antagonists, laxatives, and so on.
	The list is extensive and most drugs will list diarrhoea as a potential adverse effect.
Gastrointestinal infections	Appendicitis, pancreatitis, diverticulitis.
Irritable bowel syndrome	
Inflammatory bowel disease	Ulcerative colitis, Crohn's disease.
Malabsorption syndromes	Coeliac disease, chronic pancreatitis, lactose intolerance, lymphoma, cystic fibrosis, gastrectomy, small bowel resection.
Colorectal cancer	
Other	Anxiety, food allergy, hyperthyroidism, diabetes, alcohol excess, factious diarrhoea.

- Recent medication changes.
- Assessing complications of diarrhoea (e.g. dehydration).

'Red flag' symptoms in patients with diarrhoea include:

- Blood in the stool (see Table 13.9).
- Recent hospital treatment or antibiotic use—suggests possible *Clostridium difficile*.
- Persistent vomiting—suggests possible GI tract obstruction with overflow diarrhoea, plus increases the risk of dehydration.
- Weight loss—suggests possible GI malignancy.
- Painless, watery, high-volume diarrhoea—increased risk of dehydration.

Table 13.9 Causes of bloody diarrhoea

Causes of bloody diarrhoea	Examples
Bacterial infection	*Campylobacter jejuni, Salmonella, Escherichia coli* 0157:H7, *Vibrio parahaemolyticus, Shigella, Yersinia, Clostridium difficile*
Viral infection	Cytomegalovirus
Parasitic infection	*Entamoeba histolytica*, Schistosomiasis
Malignancy	Colorectal cancer, anal cancer
Inflammatory bowel disease	Ulcerative colitis, Crohn's disease
Diverticular disease	
Ischaemic colitis	

- Nocturnal symptoms disturbing sleep—suggests an organic cause.
- Diarrhoea persisting >6 weeks in a patient older than 60.
- Diarrhoea persisting in a patient with a family history of bowel or ovarian cancer.
- Abdominal mass.
- Rectal mass.
- Unexplained anaemia.
- Raised inflammatory markers.

Examination of a patient presenting with diarrhoea should include: assessment for signs of dehydration; an abdominal examination; and a rectal examination in patients with an unclear aetiology and especially those aged older than 50 years.

13.5.5 Investigations for diarrhoea

Investigations are not always necessary for adults presenting with acute diarrhoea.
  Indications for stool culture and sensitivity include:

- Patient systemically unwell.
- Blood or pus in the stool.
- Patient immunocompromized.
- Recent foreign travel, to areas other than Western Europe, North America, Australia, or New Zealand.
- Recent antibiotic use or hospital admission.
- Persistent diarrhoea (>1 week).

A stool sample will routinely be tested for *Campylobacter, Cryptosporidium, E. coli* 0157:H7, *Salmonella,* and *Shigella*. If a parasitic infection is suspected, three specimens should be sent two to three days apart, to test for ova, cysts, and parasites of amoeba and *Giardia*.
  Blood tests should be directed by the clinical picture, for example renal function, FBC, LFTs, calcium, iron status, vitamin B12, folate, thyroid function tests, ESR, CRP, and antibody testing for coeliac disease.

13.5.6 Emergency department management of diarrhoea

Acute diarrhoea is usually self-limiting and will resolve without complications. Dehydration is the main concern in a patient presenting to the ED with diarrhoea, especially in children and the elderly.
  The need for fluid resuscitation should be based on the clinical picture, degree of dehydration, and supporting blood results (e.g. impaired renal function). In milder cases of dehydration, fluids can be given orally. Oral rehydration therapy formulations (e.g. Dioralyte®) contain glucose, sodium, potassium, chloride, and bicarbonate. They should be given as frequent small sips. If the patient is severely dehydrated, or unable to tolerate oral fluids, then IV fluids are required.
  Antibiotics are rarely required in the treatment of diarrhoea because it is usually the result of a viral infection. Patients with *Clostridium difficile* diarrhoea will require antibiotic treatment with oral metronidazole or vancomycin. Patients with amoebiasis, giardiasis, *Campylobacter*, or *Shigella* infections may need antibiotics. Antibiotic use in such cases is best guided by a consultant microbiologist.
  Anti-diarrhoeal agents (e.g. loperamide, codeine phosphate) are not recommended in children and rarely required in adults. They may aggravate nausea and vomiting and occasionally cause an ileus.
  Admission is required if:

- The patient is vomiting and unable to retain oral fluids.
- The patient has features of severe dehydration or shock.

Admission may also be necessary for the following patient groups:

- Elderly
- Poor level of home support
- Fever
- Bloody diarrhoea
- Abdominal pain and tenderness
- Co-existent medical problems (e.g. diabetes, immunodeficiency, renal impairment, inflammatory bowel disease, heart disease, and so on)

Patients with red flags, who are fit for discharge from the ED, should be referred urgently to gastro-enterology or the colorectal team for assessment of a potential serious underlying cause.

KEY POINTS

Diarrhoea is the abnormal passage of loose or liquid stools more than three times per day and/or a volume of stool greater than 200 g/day.

Causes of diarrhoea include:
- Infection—viral, bacterial, and parasitic
- Drugs
- Appendicitis, pancreatitis, diverticulitis
- Inflammatory bowel disease
- Irritable bowel disease
- Malabsorption syndromes
- Colorectal cancer
- Ischaemic colitis

'Red flag' symptoms in patients with diarrhoea include:
- Blood in the stool
- Recent hospital treatment or antibiotic use
- Persistent vomiting
- Weight loss
- Painless, watery, high-volume diarrhoea
- Nocturnal symptoms disturbing sleep
- Diarrhoea persisting >6 weeks in a patient older than 60
- Diarrhoea persisting in a patient with a family history of bowel or ovarian cancer
- Abdominal mass
- Rectal mass
- Unexplained anaemia
- Raised inflammatory markers

13.6 Inflammatory bowel disease

13.6.1 Introduction

The term inflammatory bowel disease (IBD) encompasses a group of conditions that cause inflammation of the gastrointestinal lining.

- Ulcerative colitis is characterized by diffuse mucosal inflammation limited to the colon.
- Crohn's disease is characterized by patchy, transmural inflammation, which may affect any part of the gastrointestinal tract.

- Indeterminate colitis is the term used when it is not possible to tell the difference between ulcerative colitis and Crohn's disease.
- Microscopic colitis is a rarer type of IBD, which includes collagenous colitis and lymphocytic colitis.

IBD is usually diagnosed in young adults (late teens or early twenties) but it can appear at any age.

Over time, inflammation damages the lining of the gastrointestinal tract causing ulcers, which may then bleed and produce mucus. In Crohn's disease the inflammation can make the gut narrower resulting in strictures or lead to the development of fistulas.

13.6.2 Clinical features of inflammatory bowel disease

The cardinal symptom of ulcerative colitis is bloody diarrhoea, associated with colicky abdominal pain, urgency, and tenesmus.

The symptoms in Crohn's disease are more heterogeneous, but typically include abdominal pain, diarrhoea, and weight loss. Systemic symptoms of malaise, anorexia, and fever are more common with Crohn's than ulcerative colitis.

Extraintestinal signs of IBD include:

- Clubbing
- Erythema nodosum
- Pyoderma gangrenosum
- Scleritis
- Acute iritis
- Arthritis
- Ankylosing spondylitis
- Fatty liver
- Primary sclerosing cholangitis
- Cholangiocarcinoma
- Osteomalacia
- Apthous ulcers (in ulcerative colitis)

13.6.3 Severity of inflammatory bowel disease

Severe ulcerative colitis correlates with more than six bloody stools per day and systemic signs of toxicity (fever-temperature greater than 37.8°C, pulse rate >90/minute, anaemia, raised ESR >30 mm/hour).

The severity of Crohn's is more difficult to assess than ulcerative colitis but evidence of systemic illness (fever, tachycardia, and raised inflammatory markers) warrants admission.

13.6.4 Complications of inflammatory bowel disease

Ulcerative colitis

- Bowel perforation
- Toxic megacolon—consider if bowel loops are >5.5 cm on abdominal X-ray
- Colonic cancer
- Colonic bleeding

Crohn's disease

- Toxic megacolon
- Small bowel obstruction due to strictures
- Abscess formation
- Fistulae (colovesical, colovaginal, perianal)
- Bowel perforation

- Rectal haemorrhage
- Colonic cancer

13.6.5 Emergency department management of inflammatory bowel disease

Patients with flares of their IBD or complications require hospital admission. Patients should be referred jointly to gastroenterology and surgery.

ED management is supportive with IV fluid resuscitation and analgesia.

Steroids (intravenous and per rectum) should be given on the advice of the gastroenterology team.

KEY POINTS

Inflammatory bowel disease encompasses a group of conditions that cause inflammation of the gastrointestinal lining; the commonest types are ulcerative colitis and Crohn's disease.

Ulcerative colitis is characterized by diffuse mucosal inflammation limited to the colon.

Crohn's disease is characterized by patchy, transmural inflammation, which may affect any part of the gastrointestinal tract.

ED management of IBD flares is supportive and early referral to gastroenterology.

13.7 Liver failure

13.7.1 Introduction

Liver failure is the inability of the liver to perform its normal synthetic and metabolic functions. It can broadly be divided into two forms, acute and chronic.

- Acute liver failure—coagulopathy and encephalopathy develop within 26 weeks of first symptoms and in the absence of pre-existing liver disease. This definition encompasses fulminant liver failure, where coagulopathy and encephalopathy develop within eight weeks, and subfulminant, where this occurs between 8 and 26 weeks.
- Chronic liver failure—progressive destruction and regeneration of the liver parenchyma leads to fibrosis and cirrhosis.

13.7.2 Investigating liver failure

Previous MRCEM question

Liver function tests

Interpretation of LFTs has appeared in previous short-answer questions (SAQs). Knowing how to differentiate between hepatocellular and cholestatic patterns of LFTs is important for the exam (Table 13.10).

- Transaminases (ALT, AST)—liver transaminases are involved in the metabolism of amino acids. Elevation suggests hepatocellular injury.
- Alkaline phosphatase (ALP)—elevation suggests cholestasis.
- Gamma glutamyltransferase (γGT)—is elevated in cholestasis and useful in verifying that a raised ALP is due to biliary disease and not another cause (e.g. bone metastases, Paget's, and so on). γGT is also elevated by large quantities of alcohol ingestion, often disproportionate to other liver enzymes.
- Albumin and prothrombin time (PT)—are markers of the liver's synthetic function and deranged in hepatocellular disease.

Table 13.10 Pattern of liver function tests

Hepatocellular pattern	Cholestatic pattern
Raised transaminases (ALT, AST)	Raised ALP
Reduced albumin	Raised γGT
Raised PT	Raised bilirubin
Raised bilirubin	

- Bilirubin—is elevated in pre-hepatic failure, hepatocellular damage, and post-hepatic obstruction. Excess bilirubin results in jaundice (see Box 13.5).

Further investigation of liver failure depends on the initial pattern of LFTs. A hepatocellular pattern of LFTs requires the following investigations:

- Viral serology
- Autoantibodies (e.g. anti-nuclear antibody, anti-smooth muscle antibody)
- Alpha-1 anti-trypsin
- Copper/caeruloplasmin (low in Wilson's disease)
- Ferritin and iron studies (useful in haemachromatosis)
- Liver biopsy may be required

Box 13.5 Production and excretion of bilirubin

Bilirubin metabolism

- Pre-hepatic

Bilirubin is produced from the breakdown of haem. Haem is oxidized to biliverdin, which is then reduced to bilirubin. At this stage, the bilirubin is unconjugated and water-insoluble. Any disease that causes haemolysis can cause pre-hepatic jaundice (e.g. malaria, sickle cell anaemia, spherocytosis, Glucose 6-PD deficiency, transfusion reaction). Due to the insoluble nature of unconjugated bilirubin, it does not appear in the urine.

- Hepatic

Unconjugated bilirubin travels to the liver bound to albumin where it is conjugated with glucuronic acid to from conjugated bilirubin. Any disease that impairs hepatic metabolic function can cause hepatic jaundice.

- Post-hepatic

Conjugated bilirubin is excreted into the biliary and cystic ducts as part of bile. It is converted to urobilinogen in the small intestine. Urobilinogen may be reabsorbed from the gastrointestinal tract and excreted in the urine, or converted to stercobilin and excreted in the faeces. Any disease that causes post-hepatic obstruction can cause obstructive jaundice (e.g. gallstones, malignancy—pancreatic or cholangiocarcinoma, primary sclerosing cholangitis, biliary atresia, bile duct strictures, pancreatitis). Due to the soluble nature of conjugated bilirubin, it appears in the urine but the stools are pale due to a lack of stercobilin.

A cholestatic pattern of LFTs requires:

- Liver ultrasound.
- ERCP/MRCP.
- Antimitochondrial antibody—if the biliary tree is normal on imaging, then this should be measured and if positive suggests primary biliary cirrhosis.

13.7.3 Acute liver failure

Acute liver failure is an uncommon condition in which the rapid deterioration of liver function results in coagulopathy and alteration in the mental status of a previously healthy individual. Acute liver failure often affects young people and carries a very high mortality.

Acute liver failure due to paracetamol toxicity is the most common type of liver failure to present to the ED.

Acute liver failure is potentially reversible and treatment is supportive to allow time for regeneration to occur or pending a transplant.

Causes of acute liver failure

- Paracetamol toxicity.
- Idiosyncratic drug reactions (e.g. isoniazid, halothane, NSAIDs, amitriptyline).
- Illicit drugs (e.g. cocaine, ecstasy).
- Viral infections (e.g. hepatitis A, B, especially if co-infection with hepatitis D), and E (seen in pregnant women in endemic areas). Hepatitis C rarely causes acute liver failure.
- HELLP syndrome.
- Metabolic—acute fatty liver of pregnancy, alpha-1 anti-trypsin deficiency.
- Toxins—amanita phalloides mushrooms.
- Vascular—hepatic or portal vein thrombosis, veno-occlusive disease.
- Malignancy—primary hepatocellular carcinoma or hepatic metastases.
- Autoimmune hepatitis.

Clinical features of acute liver failure

- Hepatic encephalopathy:
  - Grade I—Drowsy, but coherent, mood change
  - Grade II—Drowsy, confused at times, inappropriate behaviour
  - Grade III—Very drowsy and stuporose, confusion, gross disorientation
  - Grade IV—Coma*

- Jaundice
- Fetor hepaticus
- Asterixis
- Constructional apraxia
- Right upper quadrant tenderness
- Ascites (e.g. with Budd–Chiari syndrome)

Imaging in acute liver failure

- Liver ultrasound—useful if the cause of liver failure is unclear, to determine hepatic and portal vein blood flow, and look for evidence of malignancy.
- CT abdomen—may be required for further definition of intrahepatic anatomy.
- CT head—should be considered to exclude other causes of an altered mental status.

* Reproduced from *Gastroenterology*, Vol 72, issue 4 (pt1), Conn HO, Leevy CM, Vlahcevic ZR, et al., Comparison of lactulose and neomycin in the treatment of chronic portal-systemic encephalopathy. A double blind controlled trial, pp.573-583, Copyright Elsevier 1977.

Complications of acute liver failure

- Cerebral oedema is the main cause of morbidity and mortality. The exact mechanism of cerebral oedema is not fully understood but high ammonia levels and a failure of cerebral autoregulation are thought to be involved.
- Renal failure—due to dehydration, hepatorenal syndrome, or acute tubular necrosis.
- Hypoglycaemia—severe hypoglycaemia occurs in approximately 40% of patients with fulminant liver failure.
- Multiorgan failure—patients may develop SIRS leading to multiorgan failure (see Chapter 15, section 15.1).
- Coagulopathy—due to failure of the synthetic function of the liver.

Emergency department management of acute liver failure

The most important aspect of treatment in acute liver failure is good supportive care. The expertise of a liver specialist should be sought early.

- A and B—patients with grade 3–4 encephalopathy are at risk of airway compromise and require intubation and ventilation. A nasogastric tube should be placed in such patients to decompress the stomach and reduce the risk of aspiration.
- C—most patients with acute liver failure have some degree of circulatory dysfunction. Careful monitoring of haemodynamic status is required, often with a central venous pressure (CVP) and arterial line. Fluid resuscitation with crystalloid or colloid is appropriate in the initial phase of resuscitation. Vasopressors and inotropes may be required for patients who do not respond to adequate filling. If the patient is coagulopathic treatment with vitamin K, fresh frozen plasma, platelets, or recombinant factor VII may be required.
- D—the level of consciousness and grade of encephalopathy should be regularly assessed. Patients should be nursed 30° head up to reduce intracranial pressure. Patients with signs of raised intracranial pressure (typically grade 3–4 encephalopathy) require mannitol to reduce the degree of cerebral oedema.
- E—blood glucose levels should be regularly monitored and treated if low with IV boluses of 10% glucose. Patients should be examined for any evidence of concurrent infection (e.g. cellulitis, pneumonia, UTI, and so on) and, if present, treated with broad-spectrum antibiotics. Prophylactic antibiotics are not recommended routinely, especially in patients with mild hepatic encephalopathy.

Further management includes:

- Avoiding sedatives or drugs with hepatic metabolism metabolism (e.g. benzodiazepines, opiates) diuretics which produce hypokalaemia, and drugs which cause constipation. Such drugs can further impair cerebral function and may precipitate or exacerbate hepatic encephalopathy.
- Emptying the bowels with lactulose and phosphate enemas to reduce ammonia levels.
- Haemofiltration or haemodialysis if renal failure develops.
- Acetylcysteine for those with paracetamol overdose (see Chapter 17, section 17.4).
- Proton pump inhibitors to protect against gastric ulcers.

A liver transplant is the definitive treatment. Criteria for liver transplantation have been produced by King's College Hospital (Table 13.11).

13.7.4 Liver cirrhosis

Cirrhosis is the consequence of chronic liver disease and implies irreversible liver damage. Histologically there is loss of normal hepatic architecture with fibrosis and nodular regeneration. The commonest causes are alcohol, and hepatitis B and C.

Table 13.11 King's College Hospital Criteria for liver transplantation

Paracetamol induced acute liver failure	Non-paracetamol acute liver failure
• Arterial pH <7.3 or all of the following: • PT>100 s • Creatinine>300 µmol/L • Grade III/IV encephalopathy	• PT>100 s or three out of the following five: • Drug induced liver failure • Age <10 or >40 years • >7 days between onset of jaundice and encephalopathy • PT>50 s • Bilirubin>300 µmol/L

Data from J. O'Grady et al. Early indicators of prognosis in fulminant hepatic failure, *Gastroenterology*, 97(2), pp. 439–445.

Clinical features of liver cirrhosis include:

• Clubbing
• Leuconychia
• Palmar erythema
• Dupuytren's contracture
• Spider naevi
• Splenomegaly
• Gynaecomastia
• Testicular atrophy
• Parotid enlargement

Patients may present to the ED with chronic liver failure as an incidental finding or with a complication of chronic liver failure.

Complications of chronic liver failure include:

• Portal hypertension
• Variceal haemorrhage
• Ascites
• Spontaneous bacterial peritonitis
• Hepatic encephalopathy
• Hepatorenal syndrome
• Hepatocellular carcinoma.

KEY POINTS

The commonest cause of acute liver failure in the ED is a delayed presentation paracetamol overdose.

The commonest causes of chronic liver failure are alcohol, and hepatitis B and C.

Elevated transaminases (ALT, AST) suggest hepatocellular injury. Raised ALP suggests cholestasis.

Bilirubin can be raised due to pre-hepatic (e.g. malaria, sickle cell anaemia, spherocytosis), hepatic (e.g. hepatitis, cirrhosis, hepatic metastases, Gilbert syndrome), and post-hepatic (e.g. gallstones, malignancy) causes.

Cerebral oedema is the commonest cause of morbidity and mortality in acute liver failure.

The most important aspect of treatment in acute liver failure is good supportive care.

13.8 Alcoholic liver disease/withdrawal syndromes

13.8.1 Introduction

Alcoholic liver disease is a major cause of liver failure in the UK. It arises from excessive alcohol consumption over a prolonged period. It can result in a spectrum of disease:

- Fatty liver (steatosis)—is the accumulation of fat in the liver cells. It is an asymptomatic and reversible condition. Other causes include diabetes, obesity, and malnutrition.
- Alcoholic hepatitis—is an acute inflammatory reaction of the liver cells. It results in fever, jaundice, and vomiting; 80% progress to cirrhosis.
- Cirrhosis—is irreversible and may progress to liver failure.

13.8.2 Complications of excess of alcohol

The complications of excess alcohol are manifold. Table 13.12 details complications according to the system they affect.

13.8.3 Alcohol withdrawal

Alcohol withdrawal involves a spectrum of presenting symptoms

Minor withdrawal occurs 6–24 hours after the last drink. Clinical features include tremor, sweating, anxiety and panic, headache, nausea, vomiting, and insomnia, restlessness, and transient auditory hallucinations.

Table 13.12 Complications of chronic alcohol excess

Gastrointestinal	Gastritis
	Upper GI bleed (ulcer and variceal)
	Cirrhosis
	Fatty liver
	Alcoholic hepatitis
	Pancreatitis
Neurological	Withdrawal seizures
	Wernicke's encephalopathy
	Korsakoff's psychosis
	Peripheral neuropathy
Cardiac	Cardiomyopathy
	Arrhythmias
	Hypertension
Haematological	Raised MCV
	Anaemia
	Marrow depression
Orthopaedic	Head injuries
	Fractures and lacerations
Systemic	Alcoholic ketoacidosis
	Electrolyte disturbance
	Hypoglycaemia

Major withdrawal occurs 10–72 hours after the last drink. Patients may experience visual or auditory hallucinations, whole body tremors, vomiting, sweating, and hypertension.

- Withdrawal seizures can occur 6–48 hours after the last drink. Patients have a generalized tonic–clonic seizure, which is usually brief and self-terminating. Around 30–40% of these patients will progress to delirium tremens.
- Delirium tremens occur 3–10 days after the last drink. Patients are severely agitated, confused, disorientated, and experience delusions and hallucinations (usually visual but may be tactile). They are feverish and have autonomic instability (↑ heart rate, ↑ blood pressure). There is significant mortality usually from arrhythmias (secondary to acidosis, electrolyte imbalance, or cardiomyopathy), infection, or cardiovascular collapse. Management is mainly supportive with airway maintenance, intravenous fluids, monitoring and treatment of hypoglycaemia, parenteral thiamine, and sedation with parenteral benzodiazepines.

13.8.4 Alcoholic ketoacidosis

This is an uncommon complication of alcoholism. It occurs when patients stop drinking, vomit repeatedly, and are unable to take anything orally. This results in the breakdown of fatty acids to ketones and dehydration. Patients have a metabolic acidosis with a raised anion gap. It usually occurs one to two days after the last alcoholic drink.

Treatment is intravenous fluids and bicarbonate, if the acidosis fails to correct with rehydration. Thiamine is given parenterally to prevent the onset of Wernicke's encephalopathy. Benzodiazepines are given if the patient shows signs of withdrawal.

13.8.5 Wernicke's encephalopathy and Korsakoff's psychosis

Thiamine deficiency can result in Wernicke's encephalopathy and/or Korsakoff's psychosis.

The classic triad of Wernicke's encephalopathy is ataxia, ophthalmoplegia, and confusion.

Korsakoff's psychosis is a permanent disturbance of memory. Long-term alcohol abuse is the commonest cause but it can also be due to starvation, malnutrition, hyperemesis gravidarum, and chronic renal failure.

Clinical features of Wernicke's encephalopathy

- Confusion
- Ataxia
- Ophthalmoplegia
- Short-term memory loss
- Nystagmus
- Polyneuropathy

Clinical features of Korsakoff's psychosis

- Anterograde amnesia
- Retrograde amnesia
- Confabulation
- Lack of insight
- Apathy
- Meagre content of conversation

Treatment of Wernicke's encephalopathy

Any patient with long-term alcoholism/malnutrition presenting with confusion or an altered mental state should be treated with parenteral thiamine.

Thiamine must be given prior to any carbohydrate load (e.g. intravenous glucose) because there is a risk of precipitating or exacerbating the encephalopathy if not.

KEY POINTS

Chronic alcohol abuse can have multiple complications, including withdrawal syndromes, GI bleeding, liver cirrhosis, and pancreatitis.

Delirium tremens is a life-threatening condition caused by alcohol withdrawal. Patients present severely agitated, confused, disorientated, and experience delusions and hallucinations. Autonomic instability is common and there is the risk of arrhythmias and cardiovascular collapse.

Wernicke's encephalopathy is a triad of ataxia, ophthalmoplegia, and confusion due to thiamine deficiency.

Korsakoff's psychosis is a permanent disturbance of memory due to thiamine deficiency.

Any patient with long-term alcoholism/malnutrition presenting with confusion or an altered mental state should be treated with parenteral thiamine.

13.9 SAQs

13.9.1 Upper GI bleed

A 55-year-old man is brought to the ED by ambulance after vomiting large quantities of fresh blood. He is conscious, has high-flow oxygen and two intravenous cannulae. Old notes reveal a history of oesophageal varices. Observations are: HR 130 bpm, BP 80/40 mmHg, CRT 3 s, RR 20 bpm, SpO$_2$ 96%, BM 4.2.

a) List three important steps in the immediate management of this patient. (3 marks)
b) (i)   List four features specific to the examination of the hand that would suggest chronic liver disease? (2 marks)
b) (ii) List two indicators of chronic liver disease that you may see in the blood results (other than deranged liver function tests)? (1 mark)

Another patient presents, with a non-variceal upper GI haemorrhage.

c) (i)   What scoring system is commonly used to risk stratify such patients? (1 mark)
c) (ii) What components make up the initial score for this system? (3 marks)

Suggested answer

a) List three important steps in the immediate management of this patient. (3 marks)
   IV fluids
   Cross match 4–6 units
   IV antibiotics
   Vasoactive drug (e.g. terlipressin)
   FFP
   Urgent endoscopy
   (1 mark each)
b) (i)   List four features specific to the examination of the hand that would suggest chronic liver disease? (2 marks)
   Palmar erythema
   Leuconychia
   Liver flap
   Dupuytren's contracture
   Clubbing
   (Not spider naevi, telangiectasia, anaemia, oedema, jaundice—not in the hand)
   (½ mark each)
b) (ii) List two indicators of chronic liver disease that you may see in the blood results (other than deranged liver function tests)? (1 mark)
   Abnormal clotting
   Low albumin
   Low platelets/WCC
   Macrocytosis
   Low urea
   (½ mark each)
c (i)   What scoring system is commonly used to risk stratify such patients? (1 mark)
   Rockall score

c) (ii) What components make up the initial score for this system? (3 marks)
Age, co-morbidities, shock

13.9.2 Liver failure

A patient presents to the department with jaundice.

a) List four important factors to ask in the history. (2 marks)
b) (i) You perform a urine dipstick which is positive for bilirubin. What does this result mean? (1 mark)
b) (ii) Other than gallstones, list four causes of post-hepatic jaundice. (2 marks)
A patient well-known to the ED for alcohol-related injuries presents with acute confusion, agitation, and fever. His observations are: HR 140 bpm, BP 180/100 mmHg, RR 28 bpm, SpO$_2$ 93%, blood glucose 2.0 mmol/L.
c) (i) What is the most important differential diagnosis? (1 mark)
c) (ii) What are your first four intravenous treatments going to be? (4 marks)

Suggested answer

a) List four important factors to ask in the history. (2 marks)
Alcohol intake
Transfusion of blood products
Sexual contact with a person known to have hepatitis or promiscuous sexual activity
Intravenous drug misuse
Recent tattoos or body piercing
Recent foreign travel
Accidental needle stick injury
(½ mark each)
b) (i) You perform a urine dipstick which is positive for bilirubin. What does this result mean? (1 mark)
The patient has a conjugated hyperbilirubinaemia and a post-hepatic cause for the jaundice is likely.
b) (ii) Other than gallstones, list four causes of post-hepatic jaundice. (2 marks)
Pancreatic carcinoma
Primary sclerosing cholangitis
Biliary atresia
Bile duct strictures
Cholangiocarcinoma
Pancreatitis
Pancreatic pseudocyst
(½ mark each)
c) (i) What is the most important differential diagnosis? (1 mark)
Delirium tremens
c) (ii) What are your first four intravenous treatments going to be? (4 marks)
Benzodiazepines
Thiamine
Fluids
Glucose

Further reading

National Institute for Health and Care Excellence, June 2012. NICE clinical guideline 141. Acute upper gastrointestinal bleeding in over 16s: management. Available at: https://www.nice.org.uk/Guidance/CG141 [Online].

Scottish Intercollegiate Guideline Network, September 2008. SIGN guideline No. 105. Management of acute upper and lower gastrointestinal bleeding. Available at: http://www.sign.ac.uk/guidelines/fulltext/105 [Online].

CHAPTER 14

Endocrine emergencies

CONTENTS

14.1 Diabetic ketoacidosis

14.1.1 Introduction

Diabetes mellitus results from a lack of, or diminished effectiveness of, endogenous insulin and is characterized by hyperglycaemia.

- Type I diabetes (formerly known as insulin-dependent diabetes or juvenile onset diabetes) results from autoimmune destruction of insulin-producing beta cells of the pancreas.
- Type II diabetes (formerly known as non-insulin-dependent diabetes or adult-onset diabetes) results from insulin resistance or relative insulin deficiency.

Diabetic ketoacidosis (DKA) is an acute metabolic complication of diabetes caused by absolute or relative insulin deficiency. It commonly occurs in patients with type I diabetes but also occurs in some patients with type II diabetes, often of Afro-Caribbean or Hispanic origin; this is known as ketosis-prone type II diabetes.

DKA, though preventable, remains a frequent cause of morbidity and mortality in diabetic patients. Most hospitals have guidelines for the management of DKA but these often vary between hospitals. This section summarizes the main emergency department (ED) management from the Joint Diabetes Societies guideline.

14.1.2 Pathophysiology of diabetic ketoacidosis

DKA is a complex disordered metabolic state characterized by hyperglycaemia, acidosis, and keto-naemia (see Box 14.1).

Lack of insulin is accompanied by an increase in counter-regulatory hormones (i.e. glucagon, cortisol, growth hormone, and adrenaline), which results in enhanced hepatic gluconeogenesis and glycogenolysis, leading to severe hyperglycaemia.

Enhanced lipolysis increases serum-free fatty acids, which are metabolized to ketones and cause a metabolic acidosis.

Box 14.1 Diagnostic criteria for DKA

The diagnostic criteria for DKA are:

Ketonaemia (beta-hydroxybutyrate) (>3 mmol/L) or significant ketonuria (>2+ on urine
  dipstick)
Blood glucose >11 mmol/L or known diabetes mellitus
Bicarbonate <15 mmol/L and/or venous pH <7.3

Fluid depletion occurs via osmotic diuresis due to hyperglycaemia, vomiting, and ultimately a reduced oral intake due to a reduced level of consciousness.

14.1.3 Clinical features of diabetic ketoacidosis

- Hyperglycaemia typically results in thirst, polyuria, and polydipsia.
- Cardiovascular—hypotension and tachycardia due to dehydration.
- Gastrointestinal—abdominal pain, nausea, and vomiting.
- Respiratory—Kussmaul's breathing (respiratory compensation for metabolic acidosis) and the smell of acetone on the breath.
- Neurological—altered conscious level, confusion, focal neurology, and coma.

14.1.4 Investigations for diabetic ketoacidosis

Patients with DKA should be managed in an ABCDE manner and investigations should be performed concurrently with assessment and initial resuscitation.

- Blood ketone level—is now the recommended method of detecting ketonaemia using bedside meters rather than urinary testing. Measurement of blood ketones is considered best practice to monitor and guide treatment because the resolution of DKA depends on the suppression of ketonaemia. Glucose, bicarbonate, and pH are only surrogate markers of the underlying metabolic abnormality (ketonaemia) and therefore are only recommended to guide treatment in the absence of blood ketone levels.
- Glucose—should be checked using a bedside meter and confirmed with a laboratory venous plasma sample. Some patients can present with a 'normal' range glucose (euglycaemic ketoacidosis): liver disease; food deprivation with little carbohydrate intake; excessive vomiting with continued insulin administration.
- Venous blood gas—is appropriate to assess acid-base status. An arterial blood gas is no longer routinely recommended unless indicated to assess respiratory gas exchange. The difference between arterial and venous pH and bicarbonate are not significant enough to change the diagnosis or management of DKA.
- Blood tests—urea and electrolytes, FBC, chloride, and bicarbonate.
- Infective screen—blood cultures, urinalysis and culture, and CXR.
- Electrocardiogram (ECG) and cardiac monitoring—to assess for evidence of arrhythmias due to hypo- or hyperkalaemia.

14.1.5 Management of DKA

- Airway and breathing

Ensuring patency and maintenance of the airway is paramount. High-flow oxygen should be given if hypoxaemic. If the patient is unconscious advanced airway management and intubation will be required. A nasogastric tube will be required if the patient is vomiting or unconscious.

- Circulation/fluids

Table 14.1 Fluid management in diabetic ketoacidosis (DKA)

Resuscitation fluid	500 ml 0.9% sodium chloride over 10–15 min
(if systolic BP<90 mmHg)	Repeated if necessary
Replacement fluid	0.9% sodium chloride 1L over 1 h*
(once systolic BP >90 mmHg)	0.9% sodium chloride 1L with KCL over 2 h
	0.9% sodium chloride 1L with KCL over 2 h
	0.9% sodium chloride 1L with KCL over 4 h
	0.9% sodium chloride 1L with KCL over 4 h
	0.9% sodium chloride 1L with KCL over 6 h

* KCL may be required if more than 1 L of normal saline has been given as resuscitation fluid.

Identification of shock and fluid resuscitation is vital in patients with DKA. Normal saline (0.9% sodium chloride) is the recommended resuscitation fluid. Table 14.1 details the rate of fluid resuscitation as recommended by the Joint British Diabetes Societies.

If the glucose level falls below 14 mmol/L, then 10% glucose should be given at a rate of 125 ml/h alongside the 0.9% sodium chloride. The insulin infusion must not be stopped, because it is required to switch off ketone production.

Bicarbonate is not recommended to correct metabolic acidosis which should resolve with adequate fluid and insulin therapy.

- Insulin

Weight-based fixed-rate intravenous insulin infusion is now recommended rather than a sliding scale. The rate of insulin infusion is 0.1 unit/kg/hour (i.e. 7 units/hour if the patient weighs 70 kg). An initial bolus dose of insulin is no longer recommended

When blood glucose falls below 14 mmol/L, 10% dextrose should be added in addition to the saline at a rate of 125 ml/hr to allow continuation of the fixed-rate insulin, preventing hypoglycaemia while allowing continued suppression of ketogenesis by insulin.

If the level of ketones does not fall by at least 0.5 mmol/L/hour the infusion rate should be increased by 1 unit/hour increments until ketones are falling at the target rate.

If the patient usually takes long-acting insulin (e.g. detemir or glargine) this should be continued at the usual dose and time.

- Potassium chloride (KCL)

Potassium levels are often high on admission but fall precipitously upon treatment with insulin. Regular monitoring is mandatory. Table 14.2 details the recommended rate of potassium replacement.

- Monitoring

Patients should have continual cardiac monitoring and pulse oximetry. Regular observations and Early Warning Score should be recorded.

Fluid balance should be monitored, aiming for a urine output >0.5 ml/kg/hr.

Capillary ketones and glucose should be measured hourly. The method of choice for monitoring response to treatment is bedside measurement of capillary ketones using a portable ketone meter. If blood ketone measurement is not available, venous pH and bicarbonate should be used in conjunction with bedside blood glucose monitoring to assess treatment response.

Table 14.2 Potassium management in DKA

Potassium level (mmol/L)	Potassium replacement in infusion fluid
Over 5.5	Nil
3.5–5.5	40 mmol/L
Below 3.5	60–80 mmol/L (HDU support required)

A venous blood gas for pH, bicarbonate, and potassium should be checked at one hour, two hours, and then at two-hourly intervals thereafter.

- Adjuncts—consider urinary catherization and a nasogastric tube.
- Low molecular weight heparin should be considered.
- Any infective cause should be treated.

14.1.6 Complications of diabetic ketoacidosis

- Hypokalaemia and hyperkalaemia—are potentially life-threatening complications during the management of DKA. Careful monitoring and replacement are required to avoid these developing.
- Hypoglycaemia—may develop very rapidly once insulin is commenced and can cause a rebound ketosis driven by counter-regulatory hormones. Once the blood glucose falls below 14 mmol/L intravenous glucose 10% should be commenced to prevent hypoglycaemia.
- Cerebral oedema—is more common in children and adolescents with DKA. The exact cause is unknown but overaggressive fluid resuscitation may play a part. Therefore, fluid resuscitation in children and adolescents is more cautious than in adults (see DKA management in children and adolescents Chapter 19, section 19.7).
- Pulmonary oedema—is a rare complication but may result from overaggressive fluid resuscitation. In elderly patients and those with impaired cardiac function, central venous pressure monitoring should be considered to guide fluid resuscitation.
- Aspiration pneumonia—may occur in patients with a reduced level of consciousness. A nasogastric tube and/or intubation should be considered in such patients.

KEY POINTS

DKA is a complex disordered metabolic state characterized by hyperglycaemia, acidosis, and ketonaemia.

Blood ketone monitoring is recommended over urinary testing.

Fixed-rate insulin is now recommended in DKA (0.1 units/kg/hour).

If the blood glucose is <14 mmol/L, then 10% glucose should be given alongside normal saline.

Venous blood gas monitoring is acceptable; samples do not have to be arterial.

Potassium levels should be closely monitored and levels supplemented accordingly.

14.2 Hyperosmolar hyperglycaemic state

14.2.1 Introduction

Hyperosmolar hyperglycaemic state (HHS) is characterized by hyperglycaemia and high plasma osmolality, therefore it is also known as hyperglycaemic hyperosmolar state. Ketonaemia is absent and acidosis if present is mild.

14.2.2 Pathophysiology of hyperosmolar hyperglycaemic state

HHS usually develops gradually (over days or weeks) in patients with type II diabetes due to a combination of illness, dehydration, and relative insulin deficiency. In most cases there is enough circulating insulin to prevent ketogenesis, and therefore acidosis; however, if the patient is very ill, lactic acidosis may supervene.

14.2.3 Clinical features and investigation of hyperosmolar hyperglycaemic state

Clinical features in HHS are similar to DKA and the investigations required are the same.

A laboratory glucose is essential because levels are often very high (>30 mmol/L) and do not read accurately on bedside testing kits.

Serum osmolality should be calculated and measured in the laboratory (see Box 14.2). An osmolar gap >10 mosmol/kg suggest the presence of another solute, for example alcohol, which can be a precipitant for both DKA and HHS.

Characteristic features of HHS allowing differentiation from other hyperglycaemic states include:

- Hypovolaemia
- Marked hyperglycaemia (30 mmol/L or more), without significant hyperketonaemia (<3 mmol/L) or acidosis (pH >7.3, bicarbonate >15 mmol/L)
- Hyperosmolar state: osmolality usually 320 mosmol/kg or more

14.2.4 Management of hyperosmolar hyperglycaemic state

Management of HHS is similar to DKA (see section 14.1).

- Fluid and electrolytes—a similar fluid regime to DKA can be used; however, patients with HHS are generally elderly and may have poor cardiac function, so there should be a low threshold for central venous pressure monitoring to guide fluid resuscitation. If the initial serum sodium is greater than 155 mmol/L, then 0.45% sodium chloride can be used instead of 0.9% sodium chloride. Fluid should be changed to 5% glucose once the blood glucose is less than 14 mmol/L. Potassium should be monitored and replaced as per DKA guidance.
- Osmolality should be measured or calculated frequently to monitor response to treatment.
- Insulin—low-dose fixed-rate insulin (0.05 units/kg/hour) should only be commenced once the blood glucose is no longer falling with intravenous fluids alone or if there is significant ketonaemia (>1 mmol/L or urine ketone >2 +).
- The fall in blood glucose should be no more than 5 mmol/L/hour.
- Metformin should be stopped to prevent the development or worsening of lactic acidosis.
- Prophylactic anticoagulation with low molecular weight heparin is required in most patients for the full duration of admission because of the increased risk of arterial and venous thromboembolism.

Box 14.2 Calculating serum osmolality

Calculated serum osmolality = $(2\,Na^+ + urea + glucose)$

Osmolar gap = Measured osmolality − Calculated osmolality

Normal osmolar gap < 10mosmol kg

For further details see Chapter 10, section 10.8.

KEY POINTS

HHS is characterized by hyperglycaemia and high plasma osmolality.

It usually develops over days or weeks, often associated with an intercurrent illness (e.g. infection).

Investigations and management are similar to DKA. Fluid resuscitation may have to be more cautious due to the risk of pre-existing cardiac disease.

If the initial serum sodium is greater than 155 mmol/L, then 0.45% sodium chloride can be used instead of 0.9% sodium chloride.

Insulin can be given as a fixed-rate infusion (0.1 units/kg/h) or as a sliding scale.

14.3 Hypoglycaemia

14.3.1 Introduction

Hypoglycaemia is the commonest side effect of insulin and sulphonylureas in the treatment of diabetes, and is potentially fatal.

Hypoglycaemia results from an imbalance between glucose supply, glucose utilization, and current insulin levels.

It is defined as a blood glucose level less than 4 mmol/L. Cognitive function deteriorates at levels <3.0 mmol/L, but symptoms are uncommon >2.5 mmol/L.

14.3.2 Causes of hypoglycaemia

The commonest cause of hypoglycaemia is the relative imbalance of administration versus required insulin or oral hypoglycaemic agent, in a diabetic patient. This may result from undue or unforeseen exertion, insufficient or delayed food, or excessive insulin administration.

Other causes of hypoglycaemia include:

- Alcohol-induced hypoglycaemia—which particularly affects chronic alcoholics and children. It can also occur in binge drinkers who develop alcoholic ketoacidosis. Hypoglycaemia can occur during intoxication and up to 24 hours after.
- Addison's disease—see section 14.4.
- Pituitary insufficiency—see section 14.9.
- Post-gastric surgery.
- Liver failure.
- Malaria.
- Insulinomas.
- Extrapancreatic tumours.
- Overdose of insulin or oral hypoglycaemic agents.

14.3.3 Clinical features of hypoglycaemia

Hypoglycaemia can mimic any neurological presentation including seizures, acute confusion, or hemiparesis.

Patients may or may not have awareness that they are developing hypoglycaemia.

- Autonomic symptoms include sweating, palpitations, shaking, hunger, and nausea.
- Neurological symptoms include confusion, drowsiness, odd behaviour, in-coordination, irritability, speech difficulty, focal neurological deficits, and seizures.

14.3.4 Investigation of hypoglycaemia

Blood glucose should be checked in any patient with coma, altered behaviour, or neurological symptoms or signs.

A bedside blood glucose level should be checked and a confirmatory level sent to the laboratory. Treatment should not be delayed pending the laboratory result.

An insulin or sulfonylurea overdose can also lead to hypokalaemia and a serum potassium level and ECG should be checked.

Liver function tests should be checked if liver failure or alcohol-induced hypoglycaemia is suspected.

In recurrent, unexplained hypoglycaemia rarer causes should be considered such as an insulinoma. If suspected, blood should be sent for glucose, insulin, and C-peptide levels.

14.3.5 Management of hypoglycaemia

The treatment required depends on the conscious level, the suspected underlying cause, and degree of cooperation of the patient.

If the patient is conscious:

- Quick-acting carbohydrate (e.g. Lucozade or GlucoGel®).
- Followed by a long-acting carbohydrate (e.g. biscuits or toast).

If the patient has a reduced level of consciousness:

- Glucagon 1 mg intramuscularly. Glucagon is not suitable for treatment of hypoglycaemia due to sulphonylurea drugs, liver failure, or in chronic alcoholism because there is little glucagon available for mobilization.
- Intravenous 10% glucose should be given in 50-ml boluses, until the blood glucose and level of consciousness improve.

In patients whose hypoglycaemia is secondary to a long-acting insulin or suphonylurea, admission will be required and a continual infusion of 10% glucose (100 ml/hour) should be given.

Octreotide may be helpful in recurrent hypoglycaemia due to an overdose of sulphonylurea. Octreotide blocks the pancreatic release of insulin.

Patients who have a decreased awareness of hypoglycaemia must be advised to stop driving and inform the DVLA.

Diabetic patients, with hypoglycaemia, can be discharged when they have returned to their normal level of function, have no evidence of concurrent illness, and blood glucose is greater than 4 mmol/L.

KEY POINTS

Hypoglycaemia can mimic any neurological presentation including seizures, acute confusion, or hemiparesis. Blood glucose should be checked in all such patients.

Hypoglycaemia is the commonest side effect of insulin and sulfonylureas.

Other causes of hypoglycaemia include alcohol, Addison's disease, pituitary insufficiency, post-gastric surgery, liver failure, malaria, insulinoma, extrapancreatic tumours, and overdose of insulin or oral hypoglycaemic agents.

Patients who have taken an insulin or sulfonylurea overdose are at risk of hypokalaemia.

Treatment options for hypoglycaemia depend on the cause and level of consciousness. In a conscious patient, oral carbohydrate can be given. In the unconscious patient, 10% glucose IV is necessary.

Glucagon IM is suitable for patients with hypoglycaemia due to insulin excess but not in sulfonylurea overdose.

Patients who have a decreased awareness of hypoglycaemia must be advised to stop driving and inform the DVLA.

14.4 Newly diagnosed diabetes mellitus

Diabetes may be first diagnosed in the ED. Most adult patients have type 2 diabetes mellitus.

14.4.1 Diagnostic criteria

- Diabetes symptoms (e.g. polyuria, polydipsia, unexplained weight loss and excessive tiredness for type 1 diabetes mellitus) plus random venous plasma glucose 11.1 mmol/L or greater.
- In the absence of symptoms, diagnosis should not be based on a single capillary blood glucose determination but requires confirmatory plasma venous measurement.

14.4.2 Management

- Children and young people with suspected type 1 diabetes should be referred immediately to a multidisciplinary paediatric diabetes team

14.5 Acute adrenocortical insufficiency

14.5.1 Physiology of the adrenal gland

The adrenal gland is divided into the cortex and medulla. The cortex is divided into three zones:

- Zona glomerulosa—this is underregulation by the renin–angiotensin system and produces and secretes mineralocorticoids, mainly aldosterone.
- Zona fasiculata—this is under regulation by the hypothalamic–pituitary axis. It produces and secretes glucocorticoids, mainly cortisol, in response to adrenocorticotropic hormone (ACTH) from the anterior pituitary.
- Zona reticularis—this produces and secretes androgens.

The adrenal medulla receives input from the sympathetic nervous system and secretes catecholamines, mainly adrenaline and noradrenaline.

14.5.2 Causes of adrenal insufficiency

In primary adrenocortical insufficiency, glucocorticoid and mineralocorticoid functions are lost.

In secondary adrenocortical insufficiency, mineralocorticoid function is preserved because the insufficiency is due to disease or suppression of the hypothalamic–pituitary axis (Table 14.3).

Acute adrenocortical insufficiency (adrenal crisis) may result from an acute insult in a patient with chronic insufficiency or more commonly from the sudden withdrawal of exogenous steroids. Precipitants of an adrenal crisis include:

- Infection
- Trauma
- Myocardial infarction
- Stroke
- Asthma
- Hypothermia
- Alcohol
- Exogenous steroid withdrawal/reduction

14.5.3 Clinical features of adrenocortical insufficiency

Onset is usually insidious with features including weight loss, lethargy, weakness, vague abdominal pain, nausea, and oligomenorrhoea.

Table **14.3** Causes of adrenocortical insufficiency

Primary adrenocortical insufficiency (Addison's disease)

Anatomic destruction of the adrenal gland:
- Idiopathic—probably autoimmune
- Infective—TB, AIDS, disseminated fungal infection
- Haemorrhage—anticoagulant therapy, Waterhouse–Friderichsen syndrome (haemorrhage into the adrenal gland secondary to fulminant meningococcal septicaemia)
- Infiltration—carcinoma, lymphoma, sarcoidosis, amyloidosis

Metabolic failure of the adrenal gland:
- Congenital adrenal hyperplasia
- Drugs (e.g. ketoconazole, etomidate)

Secondary adrenocortical insufficiency

Disease of the hypothalamic–pituitary axis:
- Tumour
- Apoplexy
- Granulomatous disease

Suppression of the hypothalamic–pituitary axis:
- Exogenous steroids

In primary adrenocortical insufficiency, the level of ACTH is elevated resulting in pigmentation of the buccal mucosa, palmar creases, elbows, and knees. Vitiligo is also a feature of primary adrenocortical insufficiency.

In adrenal crisis, the patient can be profoundly shocked (tachycardic, hypotensive, vasoconstricted, oliguric) and hypoglycaemic.

14.5.4 Investigation of adrenocortical insufficiency

Glucocorticoid deficiency results in:

- Hyponatraemia
- Hyperkalaemia
- Elevated urea and creatinine
- Hypoglycaemia
- Metabolic acidosis

Other investigations should be directed at identifying the cause of the acute insufficiency (e.g. infective screen) or complications (e.g. ECG due to risk of hyperkalaemia).

Serum cortisol and plasma ACTH levels should be sent, but should not delay treatment with hydrocortisone (see Box 14.3).

Box 14.3 Interpretation of the cortisol and ACTH results

These results will not usually be available in the ED, but their interpretation may appear in a SAQ.

Low serum cortisol (<200 nmol/L)—indicates adrenal insufficiency. A raised ACTH in this context suggests primary adrenal insufficiency and a low ACTH suggests secondary.

High serum cortisol (>550 nmol/L)—excludes adrenal insufficiency.

Intermediate serum cortisol (200–550 nmol/L)—requires further investigation with a Synacthen® (tetracosactide) test.

14.5.5 Management of acute adrenocortical insufficiency

Treatment of a suspected adrenal crisis should not be delayed pending the results of cortisol and ACTH.

Patients should be managed in an ABCDE manner:

- Hydrocortisone 100 mg IV should be given as soon as an adrenal crisis is suspected.
- Fluctrocortisone is only required in primary adrenocortical insufficiency and is not commonly given in the ED.
- Fluid resuscitation should be directed by cardiovascular status.
- Patients should be monitored for hypoglycaemia and treated with 10% glucose IV if it develops.
- Any underlying infection should be treated with appropriate antibiotics.

KEY POINTS

The most common cause of adrenal crisis in the ED is sudden withdrawal of chronic steroid therapy.

An adrenal crisis may also be precipitated by intercurrent illness in patients on long-term steroids, which increases steroid requirements.

The majority of Addison's disease in the United Kingdom is idiopathic (autoimmune).

Patients with adrenal crisis can be profoundly shocked (tachycardic, hypotensive, vasoconstricted, oligouric) and hypoglycaemic.

Patients without known adrenal insufficiency should have blood sent for cortisol and ACTH.

Hydrocortisone 100 mg IV should be given as soon as an adrenal crisis is suspected.

14.6 Cushing's syndrome

14.6.1 Introduction

The zona fasiculata of the adrenal cortex produces glucocorticoids in response to ACTH. The anterior pituitary is stimulated to release ACTH by corticotrophin-releasing factor (CRF), produced by the hypothalamus.

Cushing's syndrome is the result of chronic glucocorticoid excess. This is most commonly caused by patients taking exogenous steroids for other medical conditions (e.g. COPD, asthma, rheumatoid arthritis).

Cushing's disease refers to a specific cause of Cushing's syndrome, which is a pituitary tumour, producing excess ACTH, which leads to adrenal hyperplasia and excess glucocorticoid production.

14.6.2 Causes of Cushing's syndrome

The causes of Cushing's syndrome can be classified as ACTH-dependent and ACTH-independent (see Table 14.4).

14.6.3 Clinical features of Cushing's syndrome

- Weight gain
- Menstrual irregularity
- Amenorrhoea
- Hirsutism
- Impotence
- Depression
- Muscle weakness

Table 14.4 Causes of Cushing's syndrome

ACTH-dependent	ACTH-independent
Cushing's disease—adrenal hyperplasia due to excess ACTH production from a pituitary tumour	Iatrogenic—pharmacological doses of steroids (common)
Ectopic ACTH production (e.g. small cell carcinoma of the lung, carcinoid tumours)	Adrenal adenoma or carcinoma
Iatrogenic—ACTH administration	Alcohol
Ectopic CRF production (rare)	

- Fractures (osteoporosis)
- Tissue wasting
- Myopathy
- Thin skin
- Purple abdominal striae
- Bruising
- Buffalo hump—growth of fat pads along clavicles and back of neck
- Hypertension

14.6.4 Investigations for Cushing's syndrome

Diagnosis of iatrogenic Cushing's syndrome is usually possible based on the clinical appearance of the patient and the use of long-term steroids.

If Cushing's syndrome is suspected, in a patient not taking long-term steroids, a dexamethasone suppression test and/or 24-hour urinary free cortisol should be measured. Once Cushing's syndrome is confirmed, imaging (e.g. abdominal CT, pituitary MRI) is performed to try and localize the source.

Laboratory findings that are supportive of a diagnosis of Cushing's syndrome include:

- Hyperglycaemia
- Hypokalaemia
- Hypercalcaemia

14.6.5 Treatment of Cushing's syndrome

Cushing's syndrome does not require acute treatment in the ED. However, patients with Cushing's syndrome are more prone to fractures, infections, and poor wound healing, so may present with complications that require treatment.

If the cause of Cushing's syndrome is exogenous steroids, these may be gradually tapered off and eventually stopped, if possible.

Definitive treatment for Cushing's disease is selective removal of the pituitary adenoma. If the source cannot be located, bilateral adrenalectomy may be required.

KEY POINTS

Cushing's syndrome is the result of chronic glucocorticoid excess.

Cushing's syndrome is most commonly caused by patients taking exogenous steroids for other medical conditions (e.g. COPD, asthma, rheumatoid arthritis).

Cushing's disease is adrenal hyperplasia due to excess ACTH from a pituitary tumour.

Patients may present to the ED with complications of their Cushing's syndrome (e.g. fractures, poor wound healing, infections).

14.7 Phaeochromocytoma

14.7.1 Introduction

Phaeochromocytomas are functional tumours that arise from chromaffin cells in the adrenal medulla. They account for 0.1–0.2% of cases of systemic hypertension.

A phaeochromocytoma crisis may be triggered by exercise, trauma, surgery, drugs (e.g. naloxone, tricyclic antidepressants), abdominal palpation, or occur spontaneously. It results in high levels of catecholamines being released into the circulation acting at adrenoreceptors; α-receptors cause vasoconstriction and increased blood pressure; β-receptors cause positive inotropic and chronotropic effects. Release of catecholamines may be episodic, resulting in acute hypertension and tachycardia.

14.7.2 Clinical features of phaeochromocytoma

- Hypertension
- Palpitations
- Sweating
- Pallor
- Headache
- Anxiety
- Pulmonary oedema
- Nausea and vomiting
- Altered level of consciousness (hypertensive encephalopathy)

14.7.3 Diagnosis of phaeochromocytoma

- 24-hour urinary free catecholamines level is the initial screening test.
- Further testing involves imaging (CT/MRI) and radio-labelled catecholamine precursors to localize the tumour.
- ED investigations should look for evidence of hypertensive end organ damage (e.g. renal failure, proteinuria, left ventricular hypertrophy, retinopathy, and papilloedema).

14.7.4 Emergency department management of phaeochromocytoma

Blood pressure control is the mainstay of ED management.

Phenoxybenzamine (α-blocker) is the drug of choice.

It is important that α-blockade precedes β-blockade to avoid exacerbating a crisis through unopposed action of catecholamines at α-receptors. Once α-blockade is achieved, propranolol can be used to treat the tachycardia.

The use of labetalol is not recommended as this has a relatively greater β-blocking action compared to its α-blocking action.

KEY POINTS

Phaeochromocytomas are functional tumours that arise from chromaffin cells in the adrenal medulla.

A phaeochromocytoma crisis may be triggered by exercise, trauma, surgery, drugs, abdominal palpation, or occur spontaneously. It results in high levels of catecholamines being released into the circulation.

ED investigations should focus on detecting hypertensive end organ damage (e.g. renal function, urinalysis, ECG, CXR, fundoscopy).

Blood pressure control is the mainstay of ED management. Phenoxybenzamine (α-blocker) is the drug of choice.

14.8 Thyroid emergencies

14.8.1 Introduction

The thyroid gland is under the control of the hypothalamic–pituitary axis. The hypothalamus releases thyrotropin-releasing hormone (TRH), which stimulates the anterior pituitary to release thyroid stimulating hormone (TSH). In response to this the thyroid produces thyroid hormones, predominantly thyroxine (T4) and some triidothyronine (T3); these exert negative feedback on the anterior pituitary. Most T3 is produced by peripheral conversion from T4, and is five times more active than T4.

14.8.2 Hyperthyroidism

Hyperthyroidism is the hyperfunctioning of the thyroid gland leading to thyrotoxicosis. Symptoms of thyrotoxicosis include weight loss, heat intolerance, sweating, diarrhoea, tremor, irritability, emotional lability, psychosis, fatigue, and oligomenorrhoea. Signs may include fever, congestive heart failure, goitre, exophthalmos (see Box 14.4), tachycardia, AF, myopathy, and a fine tremor.

Causes of hyperthyroidism

Autoimmune

- Graves' disease—is typically seen in women aged 30–50 years. Antibodies against TSH-receptors cause diffuse thyroid enlargement (goitre) and increased T4 and T3 production. TSH levels are suppressed. It is associated with other autoimmune conditions such as type 1 diabetes and pernicious anaemia.
- Hashimoto's thyroiditis—is the primary cause of hypothyroidism, however the disease process occasionally presents initially with thyrotoxicosis.

Drug-induced

- Iodine-induced hyperthyroidism—occurs after the administration of either supplemental iodine to those with prior iodine deficiency or pharmacologic doses of iodine (e.g. contrast media, medications) in those with an underlying nodular goitre.
- Amiodarone—has a high iodine content which is primarily responsible for producing a hyperthyroid state. Amiodarone may also induce autoimmune thyroid disease.

Infectious

- Subacute thyroiditis (De Quervain thyroiditis)—causes diffuse, painful inflammation of the thyroid producing a transient leakage of stored hormone, probably secondary to a viral infection.
- Suppurative thyroiditis—is often bacterial and results in a painful gland, commonly seen in those with underlying thyroid disease or in immunocompromized individuals.

Box 14.4 Thyroid eye disease

Thyroid eye disease is an autoimmune condition, which results in retro-orbital inflammation and lymphocyte infiltration. The patient may be eu-, hypo-, or hyperthyroid at the time of presentation.

Swelling of the orbital contents leads to exophthalmos, proptosis, diplopia, ophthalmoplegia, papilloedema, corneal ulceration, and conjunctival oedema. The development of reduced colour vision or decreased visual acuity suggests optic nerve compression and necessitates urgent ophthalmological assessment for decompression.

Idiopathic

- Toxic multinodular goitre—is the second most common cause of hyperthyroidism, characterized by functionally autonomous nodules, typically in patients over the age of 50.

Iatrogenic

- Thyrotoxicosis factitia—is a psychiatric condition in which high quantities of exogenous thyroid hormone are consumed.
- Surgical manipulation—of the thyroid gland during thyroidectomy can cause a flood of hormone release. This is now uncommon due to preventative measures taken prior to surgery.

Malignancy

- Toxic adenoma—is a single, hyperfunctioning nodule within a normally functioning thyroid gland.
- Thyrotropin-producing pituitary tumours (rare).

    ■ Struma ovarii—is an ovarian teratoma with ectopic thyroid tissue.

14.8.3 Thyroid storm

Previous MRCEM question

A thyroid storm occurs when there is a decompensated state of thyroid hormone-induced hyper-metabolism. It is often precipitated by a physiological stressor (Table 14.5).

Cardinal features of a thyroid storm

These include:

- Cardiovascular—severe tachycardia, atrial fibrillation, congestive heart failure, hypertension
- Neurological—agitation, confusion, delirium, coma
- Gastrointestinal dysfunction—vomiting, diarrhoea, acute abdomen
- Fever
- Biochemical—hyperglycaemia, leucocytosis, hypercalcaemia, abnormal LFTs

Patients usually have a history of thyrotoxic symptoms over several months, with poor or absent therapeutic control. Precipitants are typically systemic illness/injury or a direct insult to the thyroid gland.

Investigations of a thyroid storm

- Bloods—renal function, glucose, calcium, FBC, thyroid function tests
- Infective screen—urine, CXR, blood cultures, sputum
- ECG—to look for arrhythmias

Table 14.5 Precipitating factors of a thyroid storm

General	Thyroid specific
• Infection • Non-thyroidal trauma or surgery • Parturition, pre-eclampsia • Major acute medical conditions (e.g. myocardial infarction, DKA, HHS, hypoglycaemia)	• Radioiodine or high-doses of iodine-containing compounds (e.g. contrast media, amiodarone) • Discontinuation of antithyroid medication • Thyroid hormone overdose • Thyroid injury (infarction of an adenoma, neck trauma)

Emergency department management of thyroid storm

In addition to supportive therapy, there are three main treatment aims in a thyrotoxic crisis: inhibition of thyroid hormone synthesis and release; inhibition of the peripheral effects of thyroid hormone; and treatment of the underlying cause.

Inhibition of thyroid hormone synthesis and release

- Antithyroid treatment—propylthiouracil and carbimazole both inhibit thyroid hormone synthesis and release. Propylthiouracil is preferred because it has a quicker onset of action and also inhibits the peripheral conversion of T4 to T3.
- Iodide is given once the thyroid is blocked (at least one hour after antithyroid treatment). It blocks thyroid hormone release but if given before the thyroid is blocked, it may stimulate increased hormone production.

Inhibition of peripheral effects of thyroid hormone

- Beta-blockers (e.g. propranolol 80 mg PO—inhibits the peripheral conversion of T4 to T3 and is an antiadrenergic).
- Sedation with benzodiazepines (e.g. diazepam 5–20 mg PO/IV).
- Glucocorticoid (hydrocortisone 100 mg IV or dexamethasone 4 mg PO) decreases peripheral conversion of T4 to T3. It also prevents any relative adrenal insufficiency.

Treat underlying cause

- Broad-spectrum antibiotics should be given if an infection is the precipitant.
- Any precipitating medical condition should be treated (e.g. DKA, HONK, MI, hypoglycaemia, and so on).

Supportive management

- Assess the airway and breathing and provide supplemental oxygen if required.
- Give intravenous fluids cautiously due to the risk of pulmonary oedema.
- Monitor glucose—hyper- or hypoglycaemia may occur and should be managed appropriately.
- A nasogastric tube should be placed if the patient is vomiting.
- Antipyretics/external cooling techniques should be tried if the patient is pyrexial. Aspirin should be avoided because it displaces thyroxine from thyroid-binding globulin, which can increase the severity of the thyroid storm.
- Colestyramine may be considered. It binds thyroid hormone in the gut and interrupts the modest enterohepatic circulation.

14.8.4 Myxoedema coma

Myxoedema coma is a rare condition typically found in elderly patients with undiagnosed or under-treated hypothyroidism. It is usually precipitated by a concurrent medical emergency (e.g. myocardial infarction, stroke, infection, hypothermia, or trauma).

The three main features are:

- Altered mental state ranging from poor cognitive function to coma
- Hypothermia or the absence of fever despite severe infection
- The presence of a precipitating event

Patients often look hypothyroid and may have respiratory depression, bradycardia, hypotension, abdominal pain, and constipation.

Management of myxoedema coma

- Thyroid hormone replacement—advice varies as to whether this should be with T4 or T3, and given orally or intravenously. If given too rapidly, it can cause cardiac ischaemia.
- Treat the underlying precipitant.
- Hydrocortisone 100 mg IV—should be given eight-hourly because there is usually a degree of adrenal suppression.
- Supportive therapy—oxygen and ventilatory support should be given as required. Fluids should be given cautiously due to the risk of precipitating pulmonary oedema. Blood glucose should be regularly monitored to detect hypoglycaemia and 10% glucose IV given as required. Patients should be passively rewarmed.

KEY POINTS

A thyroid storm occurs when there is a decompensated state of thyroid hormone-induced hypermetabolism.

There are three main treatment aims in a thyrotoxic crisis:

- Inhibition of thyroid hormone synthesis and release, for example propylthiouracil, iodide (after thyroid blocked)
- Inhibition of the peripheral effects of thyroid hormone (e.g. propranolol, diazepam, hydrocortisone)
- Treatment of the underlying cause (e.g. antibiotics)

Aspirin should be avoided in a thyroid storm because it displaces thyroxine from thyroid-binding globulin, which can increase the severity of the attack.

Myxoedema coma is a rare condition typically found in elderly patients with undiagnosed or undertreated hypothyroidism.

Supportive management is the mainstay of treating a patient in a myxoedemic coma. T4/T3 replacement should be guided by an endocrinologist. Hydrocortisone should be given because there is usually a degree of adrenal suppression.

14.9 Pituitary disease

14.9.1 Introduction

The pituitary is an endocrine gland located in the sella turcica in the skull base. Superior to it is the hypothalamus and the optic chiasm, laterally is the cavernous sinus through which run the III, IV, V, and VI cranial nerves.

   The pituitary is divided into anterior and posterior parts. The anterior pituitary produces and secretes hormones; it is regulated by hypothalamic hormones and negative feedback from target organs (Table 14.6). The posterior pituitary is mainly a neuronal extension of the hypothalamus and secretes hormones made in the hypothalamus.

14.9.2 Pituitary apoplexy

Pituitary apoplexy is caused by acute haemorrhage or infarction of the pituitary gland. An existing pituitary adenoma is usually present. The anterior pituitary gland has an unusual vascular supply being perfused by a portal venous system, making it an area prone to infarction.

Predisposing factors for pituitary apoplexy

- Head trauma.
- Anticoagulation.

Table 14.6 Hormones secreted by the anterior and posterior pituitary

Anterior pituitary	Posterior pituitary
Adrenocorticotropic hormone (ACTH)	Antidiuretic hormone (ADH)
Growth hormone (GH)	Oxytocin
Follicle-stimulating hormone (FSH)	
Luteinizing hormone (LH)	
Thyroid stimulating hormone (TSH)	
Prolactin (PRL)	

- Pituitary radiotherapy.
- Endocrine stimulation tests.
- Drugs (e.g. oestrogens, bromocriptine).
- Sheehan's syndrome—during pregnancy the pituitary hypertrophies, however the blood supply from the low pressure portal venous system remains unchanged. If major haemorrhage or hypotension occurs during the peripartum period the anterior pituitary may infarct. The posterior pituitary is usually spared due to its direct arterial blood supply.

Clinical features of pituitary apoplexy

Clinically patients may present similar to a subarachnoid haemorrhage:

- Severe headache.
- Nausea, vomiting.
- Photophobia.
- Loss of consciousness.
- Meningism.
- Visual field defect—bitemporal hemianopia.
- Cranial nerve palsies—III (unilateral dilated pupil, ptosis, and a globe deviated inferiorly and laterally), IV (inability to look down and in, resulting in vertical diplopia), V (facial pain or sensory loss), VI (unable to abduct eye, resulting in horizontal diplopia).
- Patients may have a history suggestive of pre-existing endocrine dysfunction (e.g. amenorrhoea, hypogonadism, decreased libido, obesity, lethargy, constipation, and so on).

Investigations for pituitary apoplexy

- The definitive diagnosis is achieved by either an urgent MRI scan or a dedicated pituitary CT scan if MRI is contraindicated or not possible.
- Blood should be taken to measure pituitary hormones (ACTH, TSH, FSH, LH, and prolactin) and the effects these hormones have on target organs (oestradiol—women, testosterone—men, T4, T3, cortisol).
- Electrolytes and glucose should be monitored.

Management of pituitary apoplexy

- Hydrocortisone 100 mg intravenously six-hourly
- Supportive therapy (ABCDE)
- Urgent neurosurgical opinion

14.9.3 Diabetes insipidus

Diabetes insipidus (DI) is due to impaired water resorption by the kidney because of reduced secretion of antidiuretic hormone (ADH) from the posterior pituitary (cranial DI) or impaired response of the kidney to ADH (nephrogenic DI). See Table 14.7.

Table 14.7 Causes of diabetes insipidus

Cranial DI	Nephrogenic DI
Head injury	Low potassium
Hypophysectomy	High calcium
Meningitis	Drugs (e.g. lithium)
Pituitary tumour	Pyelonephritis
Metastases	Hydronephrosis
Craniopharyngioma	Polycystic kidney disease
Vascular lesion	Inherited
Idiopathic (50%)	

Clinical features of diabetes insipidus

- Polyuria
- Polydipsia
- Dilute urine
- Dehydration

Investigation of diabetes insipidus

- Plasma osmolality—high
- Urine osmolality—low
- Serum sodium—high
- Check serum potassium and calcium as potential causes
- CT head if a cranial cause suspected
- Measure pituitary function (TSH, ACTH, LH, FSH, prolactin)

Emergency treatment of diabetes insipidus

- Cranial DI—desmopressin 1 mcg intranasally
- Nephrogenic DI—treat the cause
- Rehydrate—match input to fluid losses and aim to gradually reduce the serum sodium

14.9.4 Syndrome of inappropriate antidiuretic hormone secretion (SIADH)

Excess ADH results in inappropriate water retention by the kidneys leading to hyponatraemia. The diagnosis requires concentrated urine (sodium >20 mmol/L and osmolality >500 mosm/kg) in the presence of hyponatraemia (<125 mmol/L) or low plasma osmolality (<260 mmol/kg), and the absence of hypovolaemia, oedema, or diuretics.

Causes of SIADH

- Central nervous system (CNS)—meningitis, encephalitis, abscess, stoke, subarachnoid haemorrhage, subdural haemorrhage, head injury
- Malignancy—small cell lung cancer, pancreatic cancer, prostate cancer, lymphoma
- Respiratory—pneumonia, aspergillosis
- Metabolic—porphyria
- Drugs—opiates, psychotropics
- Trauma

Management of SIADH

- Treat the underlying cause
- Fluid restriction
- Demeclocycline (rarely used)
- Urgent review by a renal consultant

KEY POINTS

Pituitary apoplexy is caused by acute haemorrhage or infarction of the pituitary gland.

Pituitary apoplexy may present clinically like a subarachnoid haemorrhage.

Sheehan's syndrome is infarction of the anterior pituitary due to hypovolaemia in the peripartum period.

Pituitary apoplexy is managed in an ABCDE manner with good supportive therapy. Patients should be given 100 mg IV hydrocortisone and referred urgently to a neurosurgeon.

Diabetes insipidus is due to impaired water resorption by the kidney because of reduced secretion of ADH from the posterior pituitary (cranial DI) or impaired response of the kidney to ADH (nephrogenic DI).

Cranial diabetes insipidus is treated with desmopressin.

SIADH causes excess ADH, which results in inappropriate water retention by the kidneys leading to hyponatraemia. Treatment is of the underlying cause and fluid restriction.

14.10 Calcium disorders

14.10.1 Calcium homeostasis

Calcium and phosphate homeostasis are linked. They are controlled by a variety of factors (Figure 14.1):

- Parathyroid hormone (PTH) is released in response to low calcium. It is also released in response to hyperphosphataemia and decreased vitamin D levels. PTH results in increased reabsorption of calcium from the bone and kidneys, and enhances vitamin D formation.
- Hypercalaemia and raised vitamin D levels switch off PTH release via negative feedback.
- Hypomagnesaemia prevents PTH release and therefore may cause hypocalcaemia.
- Vitamin D promotes calcium and phosphate absorption from the gastrointestinal (GI) tract.
- Calcitonin produced by the thyroid decreases calcium levels.
- Bone stores of calcium buffer the serum changes.

14.10.2 Hypercalcaemia

Causes of hypercalcaemia

- Malignancy—hypercalcaemia occurs in 10–20% of cases. The mechanisms include osteolytic metastases, tumours secreting parathyroid-related protein, or tumours producing vitamin D. Multiple myeloma also causes hypercalcaemia via osteolytic lesions.
- Endocrine—hyperparathyroidism (primary or tertiary)—see Table 14.8.
- Thyrotoxicosis—10% of patients have elevated calcium.
- Granulomatous disease (e.g. sarcoid, TB).
- Drugs (e.g. lithium, thiazide diuretics, theophylline toxicity, and calcium carbonate).

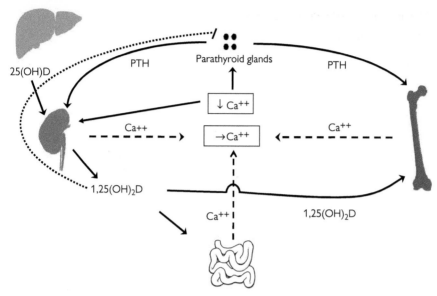

Figure 14.1 Parathyroid hormone (PTH) and vitamin D control calcium (as shown) and phosphate homoeostasis. A fall in extracellular calcium concentration triggers PTH secretion. PTH directly acts on the kidney to promote renal calcium reabsorption and conversion of 25-hydroxyvitamin D (25(OH)D) to 1,25-dihydroxyvitamin D (1,25(OH)2D). 1,25(OH)2D increases intestinal absorption of calcium (and phosphate) and, with PTH, mobilizes calcium (and phosphate) from bone. Thus, extracellular fluid (ECF) calcium is restored to normal, neutralizing the signal initiating PTH release. PTH inhibits renal phosphate reabsorption, promoting phosphaturia.

Reproduced from John A.H. Wass, and Paul M. Stewart, with Diabetes Section edited by Stephanie A. Amiel, and Melanie J. Davies, *Oxford Textbook of Endocrinology and Diabetes*, 2011, Figure 4.1.4, p. 638, with permission from Oxford University Press.

Table 14.8 Types of hyperparathyroidism

	Cause	Biochemical results
Primary hyperparathyroidism	Parathyroids produce excess PTH usually due to a single adenoma.	↑ PTH level ↑ calcium level ↓ phosphate level ↑ alkaline phosphatase
Secondary hyperparathyroidism	PTH level appropriately raised due to low calcium levels (e.g. secondary to renal failure, or dietary deficiency of vitamin D).	↑ PTH levels ↓ or normal calcium
Tertiary hyperparathyroidism	Prolonged 2° hyperparathyroidism results in hypertrophy of the parathyroids which then act autonomously even when calcium is not low (typically seen in patients with chronic renal failure or after renal transplantation).	↑PTH level ↑ calcium

Clinical features of hypercalcaemia

- Polyuria, polydipsia
- Bone pain
- Abdominal pain, renal stones, constipation
- Anorexia, depression, confusion

Investigation of suspected hypercalcaemia

- Serum corrected calcium—levels >3 mmol/L require urgent treatment.
- Albumin—levels are required to calculate the corrected calcium.
- PTH level—should be sent before treatment starts because once the serum calcium is lowered the PTH will rise and make interpretation of the result difficult.
- ECG—hypercalcaemia can lead to shortened QT interval, prolonged QRS, flat T waves, and atrioventricular block (AV) block.
- Serum total protein with electrophoresis of immunoglobulins—should be sent to look for evidence of myeloma.
- Phosphate—levels will be low in 1° and 3° hyperparathyroidism and raised in conditions which infiltrate bone.
- Magnesium—low levels inhibit PTH release.
- Renal function—to look for evidence of renal failure.
- Alkaline phosphatase—levels will be elevated in bony metastases.

Management of hypercalaemia

- Any precipitating drugs should be stopped.
- Intravenous fluids (0.9% sodium chloride)—diuresis will decrease calcium reabsorption from the kidney; 4 L are usually needed over the first 24 hours.
- Loop diuretics—furosemide has a calciuretic effect. It blocks sodium and calcium transport and thereby decreases calcium reabsorption.
- Intravenous bisphophonates (e.g. pamidronate)—inhibit osteoclasts and reduce bone turnover and calcium release.
- Prednisolone—is useful if myeloma or sarcoidosis is known to be the cause but should not be given blindly.

14.10.3 Hypocalcaemia

Causes of hypocalcaemia

- Thyroid or parathyroid surgery
- Chronic kidney disease
- Acute pancreatitis
- Rhabdomyolysis
- Hypoparathyroidism
- Calcium channel blocker overdose
- Hypomagnesaemia

Clinical features of hypocalcaemia

- Tetany
- Perioral anaesthesia
- Carpopedal spasm
- Depression
- Seizures

Investigation of hypocalcaemia

- Serum calcium and albumin—calcium may be spuriously low if the albumin is low. Therefore corrected calcium should always be checked.
- Renal function.
- Amylase.
- Creatine kinase.
- Magnesium.
- Phosphate.
- ECG—hypocalcaemia can lead to prolonged PT and QT, inverted T waves, and AV block.

Management of hypocalcaemia

- If the patient has evidence of ECG changes or is symptomatic, calcium chloride or gluconate 10 ml of 10% IV should be given.
- Correction of hypocalcaemia is difficult if magnesium levels are not also corrected, therefore magnesium 2 g intravenously should be given if there is concurrent hypomagnesaemia.

14.11 Sodium disorders

14.11.1 Hyponatraemia

Hyponatraemia is diagnosed as a serum sodium concentration <130 mmol/L. Symptoms are predominantly gastrointestinal at levels between 125–130 mmol/L and predominantly neuropsychiatric at levels below 125 mmol/L.

Management is guided by:

1) Rate of onset:
   - Acute: develops within 48 hours following normal serum sodium concentration
   - Chronic: slow development and persisting for greater than 48 hours
2) Severity of hyponatraemia:
   - Mild: 130-135 mmol/L
   - Moderate: 125-129 mmol/L
   - Severe: < 125 mmol/L
3) Extracellular fluid volume status
   - Hypovolaemic: signs of dehydration
   - Euvolaemic
   - Hypervolaemic: peripheral or pulmonary oedema

Cause of hyponatraemia

The differential diagnosis of hyponatraemia is dependent on the extracellular fluid status. Calculating urinary sodium and serum and urine osmolality can aid diagnosis.

Serum osmolality: 2x (Na) + Urea + Glucose (normal range: 275–295 mOsm/kg [mmol/kg])

- **Isotonic hyponatraemia** (normal plasma osmolality)

Rare cause of hypnatraemia known as Pseudohyponatraemia which is caused Hypertriglyceridaemia; hyperparaproteinaemia; post-transurethral resection of prostate or bladder tumour. Tretament is not usually required.

- **Hypertonic hyponatraemia** (> 295 mOsm/kg)

Table 14.9 Causes of hyponatraemia

Renal losses Urinary Na >20 mmol/l	Extrarenal losses Uriary Na <20 mmol/l
Diuretics: thiazide diuretics; loop diuretics; potassium-sparing diuretics; combined diuretics	**Gastrointestinal losses:** vomiting; diarrhoea; fistula; stoma
Mineralocorticoid deficiency: adrenocortical insufficiency	**Third space losses:** bowel obstruction; pancreatitis; burns
Salt-losing nephropathy	
Diuretic phase of acute kidney injury	
Osmotic diuresis: DKA; renal tubular acidosis	
Cerebral salt wasting (hypovolaemia): neurosurgery; CNS trauma, especially subarachnoid haemorrhage	

Is a form of redistributive hyponatraemia causes include hyperglycaemia, mannitol, azotaemia, and alcohol ingestion.

• **Hypotonic hyponatraemia** (<280 mOsm/kg)

The causes of hypotonic hypovolaemia are dependent on overall fluid status of the individual, see below.

Hypovolaemic hyponatraemia

This is loss of sodium and water leading to a depletional hyponatraemia (decrease in total body water with a greater decrease in total body sodium). See Table 14.9.

Hypervolaemic hyponatraemia

This is caused by a total body water rise greater than the total body sodium rise (dilutional hyponatraemia). Individuals will have signs of volume overload such as peripheral/pulmonary oedema (see Table 14.10).

Euvolaemic hyponatraemia
Occurs when there is a mild increase in total body water, but not enough to cause oedema, with normal total body sodium (see Table 14.11).

Treatment of hyponatraemia

Depends on the cause and fluid status of the indvidual (see Table 14.12).

Table 14.10 Causes of hypervolaemic hyponatraemia

Urinary Na >20 mmol/l AND Urinary osmolality <100 mOsm/kg	Urinary <20 mmol/l AND Urinary osmolality >100 mOsm/kg
Acute kidney injury	Nephrotic syndrome
Chronic kidney disease	Cirrhosis of the liver
	Congestion heart failure

Table 14.11 Causes of euvolaemic hyponatraemia

Urinary Na >20 mmol/l AND Urinary osmolality <100 mOsm/kg	Urinary <20 mmol/l AND Urinary osmolality >100 mOsm/kg
Glucocorticoid deficiency; secondary adrenocortical insufficiency	Psychogenic polydipsia (water intake >10 litres/day; associated with acute psychosis)
Postoperative	Beer potomania
ADH analogues	Replacement of isotonic gastrointestinal and third space fluid losses with hypotonic fluids
Severe hypothyroidism	
Syndrome of inappropriate ADH secretion	
Exercise-induced hyponatraemia	

14.11.2 Hypernatraemia

Hypernatraemia is classified as serum sodium >145 mmol/L and is related to net water loss or sodium gain. The clinical significance depends on severity, rapidity of onset, and underlying cause. The majority of cases are due to water loss and serum osmolality is usually increased.

Causes of hypernatraemia

Normal body sodium (urine sodium variable):

- Reduced water intake: lack of environmental water; altered mental state (critical illness, sedation)
- Water with solute loss (hypotonic fluid (water) loss more than solute loss)
- Skin losses: insensible and sweat losses-heat stroke/exhaustion, exercise; burns
- Gastrointestinal losses: diarrhoea
- Renal losses: central (pituitary) or nephrogenic diabetes insipidus; renal medullary disease (reflux nephropathy; polycystic disease); drugs: aminoglycosides, amphotericin.B

Table 14.12 Treatment options for hyponatraemia

Causes of hypovolaemia	Treatment optiona
Hypovolaemia (depletional) hyponatraemia	• Mild acute: isotonic saline (1 mmol/L/ hour or 8-10 mmol/L/day) • Severe acute: hypertonic (3%) saline (2 mmol/L/hour or 12 mmol/L/day) • Chronic: water restriction (0.5 mmol/L/ hour or 4–6 mmol/L/day)
Euvolaemic (dilutional) hyponatraemia	• Treat underlying cause • Fluid restriction • Salt supplementation • Vaptans (vasopressin receptor antagonists): tolvaptan • Demeclocyline • Diphenylhydantoin
Hypervolaemic (dilutional) hyponatraemia	• Treat underlying cause: discontinue hypotonic fluids) • Water restriction (50–60% of daily fluid requirements) • Vaptans • 3% saline with loop diuretics

(Diagnosis, evaluation, and treatment of hyponatraemia: expert panel recommendations Am J Med, 2013, 126: 510–542).

Low total body sodium

- Urine sodium> 20 mmol/L: renal losses: diuretics, renal parenchymal disease
- Urine sodium < 20 mmol/L: extrarenal losses: diarrhoea

High total body sodium

- Solute gain (iatrogenic sodium overload); for example, infusion of hypertonic sodium solute
- Increased mineralocorticoid: primary aldosteronism
- Increased glucocorticoid: Cushing's syndrome

Treatment of hypernatraemia

Hypovolaemic hypernatraemia

- Acute: free water replacement (2 mmol/L/hour or 12 mmol/L/day)
- Chronic: free water replacement (0.5 mmol/L/hour or 4–6 mmol/L/day); pitressin 5–10 units 6–12 hourly IM; desmopressin 1–2 mcg 12 hourly SC/IV

Isovolaemic hypernatraemia

- Water replacement
- Loop diuretics

Hypervolaemic hypernatraemia

- Water replacement
- Loop diuretics
- Dialysis

KEY POINTS

Hyponatraemia may be categorized clinically based on extracellullar fluid volume status as normovolaemic (or euvolaemic), hypovolaemic, or hypervolaemic.

Hypernatraemia is associated with raised serum osmolality and the majority of cases are due to reduced total body water.

14.12 SAQs

14.12.1 Diabetic emergencies

An 18-year-old female, who is a type 1 diabetic, presents to the department drowsy, vomiting, and dehydrated. She is well-known to the department and frequently presents having not used her insulin. Her observations are: HR 110, BP 80/40, RR 30, SpO2 100% on oxygen. She has a bedside blood glucose reading high and ketones in her blood.

Her initial blood results reveal pH 7.1, pO2 36.9, pCO2 2.5, HCO^{3-} 21, BE −8, Na^+ 137, K^+ 5.0, Cl^- 90.

a) You diagnose DKA. What three criteria are required to diagnose DKA and what are their cut-off levels? (3 marks, ½ mark criteria, ½ mark level)

b) (i) Calculate her anion gap (show your workings). (2 marks)

b) (ii) Apart from DKA, what else could have caused her metabolic acidosis with a raised anion gap. (½ mark per answer; total 3 marks)

c) What rate of insulin would you start this patient on? She weighs 50 kg. (1 mark)

d) She is receiving fluid resuscitation with normal saline. After three hours of treatment, her blood glucose level is 12 mmol/L. What change would you make to her fluid management? (1 mark)

Suggested answer

a) You diagnose DKA. What three criteria are required to diagnose DKA and what are their cut-off levels? (3 marks, ½ mark criteria, ½ mark level)

Ketonaemia (>3 mmol/L) or ketonuria (>2 + on urine dipstick)

Blood glucose >11 mmol/L or known diabetes

Bicarbonate <15 mmol/L and/or venous pH <7.3

b) (i) Calculate her anion gap (show your workings). (2 marks)

$$(K + Na) - (HCO_3 + Cl)$$

Normal <18

$$(5 + 137) - (21 + 90) = 31$$

(b) (ii) Apart from DKA what else could have caused her metabolic acidosis with a raised anion gap. (½ mark per answer; total 3 marks)

Methanol/metformin

Uraemia

Paraldehyde/propylene glycol

Isoniazid

Lactic acid

Ethanol or ethylene glycol

Salicylate

Acetazolamide

c) What rate of insulin would you start this patient on? She weighs 50 kg. (1 mark)

5 units per hour

d) She is receiving fluid resuscitation with normal saline. After three hours of treatment her blood glucose level is 12 mmol/L. What change would you make to her fluid management? (1 mark)

Continue fluid resuscitation with normal saline and give 10% glucose at a rate of 125 ml/h

14.12.2 Thyroid storm

Your F2 doctor asks you to review a patient in the resuscitation room. The patient is a 35-year-old lady who was discharged from a neighbouring hospital the previous day following an elective laparoscopic cholecystectomy. The F2 has also established a history of weight loss over the past few months as well as experiencing 'panic attacks' and palpitations.

After assessing the lady you think she is having a thyroid storm.

She has high-flow oxygen, full monitoring, and intravenous access with fluids running.

a) Other than surgery list four precipitants of a thyroid storm. (2 marks)

Observations: temp. 38.5°C, HR 130, BP 120/70, RR 32, SpO2 100% on 15 L oxygen.

b) Supportive management has been instituted. List the three main treatment aims in a thyroid storm and the drugs you would use to achieve this. (6 marks)

The F2 has prescribed Lugol's iodine and the staff nurse wants to check the prescription with you.

c) When should iodide be given and why? (2 marks)

Suggested answer

a) Other than surgery, list four precipitants of a thyroid storm. (2 marks)

Infection

Trauma

Parturition

MI, DKA, HONK (or other medical emergency)

Radioiodine

Discontinuation of thyroid medication

Thyroid injury

Drugs –amiodarone, levothyroxine OD

(½ mark per answer)

b) Supportive management has been instituted. List the three main treatment aims in a thyroid storm and the drugs you would use to achieve this. (6 marks)

Inhibition of thyroid hormone synthesis and release (e.g. propylthiouracil).

Inhibition of peripheral effects of thyroid hormone (e.g. propranolol, diazepam, hydrocortisone).

Treatment of any precipitating illness (e.g. antibiotics for post-op infection).

(1 mark for treatment aim and 1 mark for drug)

c) When should iodide be given and why? (2 marks)

Give at least one hour after antithyroid treatment, when the thyroid is blocked, because if given earlier it may stimulate increased hormone production.

Further reading

Joint British Diabetes Societies Inpatient Care Group, August 2012.

National Institute for Health and Care Excellence, August 2015. NICE guidline 18. Diabetes (type 1 and type 2) in children and young people: diagnosis and management. Available at: https://www.nice.org.uk/guidance/ng18 [Online].

Rajasekaran S, Vanderpump M, Baldeweg S, et al. 2011. UK Guidelines for the Management of Pituitary Apoplexy. *Clin Endocrinol* **74**:9–20.

Savage ML, Dhatariya KK, Kilvert A, et al. 2011. Diabetes UK Position Statements and Care Recommendations Joint British Diabetes Societies guideline for the management of diabetic ketoacidosis. *Diabet Med* **28**:508–15.

Spasovski G, Vanholder R, Allolio B, *et al.* 2014. Clinical practice guideline on diagnosis and treatment of hyponatraemia. *Eur J Endocrinol* **170**(3):G1–47.

Joint British Diabetes Societies Inpatient Care Group. The management of the hyperosmolar hyperglycaemic state (HHS) in adults with diabetes. Available at: https://www.diabetes.org.uk/Documents/Position%20statements/JBDS-IP-HHS-Adults.pdf [Online].

Infectious diseases

CONTENTS

15.1 Sepsis

15.1.1 Introduction

Sepsis is a life-threatening condition that arises when the body's response to an infection injures its own tissues and organs. Sepsis leads to shock, multiple organ failure, and death, especially if not recognized early and treated promptly. It remains the primary cause of death from infection despite advances in modern medicine, including vaccines, antibiotics, and acute care.

EXAM TIP

Sepsis is one of the major presentations covered in the ACCS curriculum. The Surviving Sepsis Campaign Guidelines are recognized nationally and internationally. Sepsis is also one of the College of Emergency Medicine published clinical standards for EDs, produced by the Clinical Effectiveness Committee.

This makes sepsis a prime topic for the FRCEM Intermediate examination and previous MRCEM Part B SAQs have included the subject.

There are multiple online resources available about the management of sepsis including the Surviving Sepsis Campaign (https://www.survivingsepsis.org) and the UK Sepsis Trust website (https://sepsistrust.org/).

Worldwide, sepsis kills well over 1400 people every single day. In the United Kingdom alone, it is estimated that over 37,000 people die annually. This equates to more people dying each year from sepsis than from lung cancer, and from breast and bowel cancer combined.

15.1.2 Definitions used in sepsis

Severe sepsis is part of a spectrum of disease, ranging from a minor localized infection with no systemic complications through to multiple organ failure.

The diagnosis of severe sepsis was first facilitated by an international consensus conference of the Society of Critical Care Medicine and American College of Chest Physicians on sepsis and organ failure in 1992. This defined a small number of acceptable terms in reference to infective processes and systemic effects, which were refined following a second consensus conference and developed to give a precise set of diagnostic criteria for sepsis, severe sepsis, and septic shock (see Table 15.1).

Infection

An infection is defined as the inflammatory response to the presence of a micro-organism, or the presence of micro-organisms (bacteria, viruses, fungi, parasites, and prions) in normally sterile tissues.

Table 15.1 Definitions used in sepsis

	Definition	Mortality
Infection	Inflammatory response to a micro-organism OR The presence of micro-organisms in normally sterile tissues	
SIRS	Two or more of: • Temperature >38.3°C or <36°C • Hear rate >90 beats per minute • Respiratory rate >20 breaths per minute • White cell count <4 or >12 × 10⁹/L	
Sepsis	SIRS due to an infection	~10%
Severe sepsis	Sepsis plus evidence of organ dysfunction: • Respiratory: new or increased oxygen requirement to maintain saturations >90% • Renal: creatinine >177 µmol/L or urine output <0.5 ml/kg/h for 2 h • Hepatic: bilirubin >34 µmol/L • Coagulation: Platelets <100 × 10⁹/L or INR >1.5 or APTT >60 s OR Sepsis plus evidence of tissue hypoperfusion: • BP: Systolic <90 mmHg or mean arterial pressure (MAP) <65 mmHg • A reduction of >40 mmHg from the patient's normal systolic BP • Lactate >2 mmol/L A single organ dysfunction criterion or a single hypoperfusion criterion is sufficient to define severe sepsis	~35% (7 times higher than acute coronary syndrome)
Septic shock	Evidence of ongoing hypoperfusion despite initial fluid challenges (20 ml/kg bolus of crystalloid): • MAP <65 mmHg or systolic BP <90 mmHg • A reduction >40 mmHg of the patient's normal systolic BP • Lactate >4 mmol/L	~50%

Data from Levy MM, Fink MP, Marshall JC, et al: 2001 SCCM/ ESICM/ ACCP/ ATS/ SIS International Sepsis Definitions Conference. Critical Care Medicine 2003; 31: 1250–1256.

The systemic inflammatory response syndrome

The systemic inflammatory response syndrome (SIRS) is the systemic response to a variety of clinical insults including infection, trauma, burns, pancreatitis, surgery, massive blood transfusion, and so on.

The diagnostic criteria for SIRS are two or more of:

- Temperature >38.3°C or <36°C.
- Heart rate >90 beats per minute.
- Respiratory rate >20 breaths per minute.
- White cell count <4 or >12 × 10⁹/L.

Sepsis = SIRS + infection

Sepsis is the systemic response to infection, manifested by two or more of the SIRS criteria caused by an infection.

Severe sepsis = sepsis + organ dysfunction

Severe sepsis is defined as sepsis with dysfunction of one or more organs, or the presence of tissue hypoperfusion.

Septic shock

Septic shock is reserved for those who remain hypoperfused following initial fluid challenges.

15.1.3 Pathophysiology of sepsis

Severe sepsis can occur as a result of infection at any site in the body. Bacteria are the pathogens most commonly associated with the development of sepsis, although fungi, viruses, and parasites can cause sepsis.

The main processes involved in the pathophysiology of severe sepsis are increased vascular permeability, myocardial dysfunction, disseminated intravascular coagulation, and impaired oxygen delivery/extraction.

Increased vascular permeability

The systemic response to infection can be initiated by the outer membrane component of gram-negative organisms (e.g. lipopolysaccharide) or gram-positive organisms (e.g. lipoteichoic acid, peptidoglycan), as well as fungal, viral, and parasitic components.

White cells try to engulf the micro-organisms to overcome the infection, releasing a flood of pro-inflammatory cytokines, including Interleukin-1 (IL-1), IL-6, and tumour necrosis factor (TNF). This damages the endothelial lining of the blood vessels.

One of the main functions of the endothelium is regulation of vascular permeability, and disturbance of this function causes the endothelial lining to become 'leaky', allowing increased passage of protein and water from the intravascular to extravascular compartments, causing a 'capillary leak syndrome'. Capillary leak in the lungs leads to pulmonary oedema and hypoxia. Loss of fluid from the intravascular space results in hypovolaemia and a reduced cardiac output.

Myocardial dysfunction

Cardiac output is determined by the heart rate and stroke volume.

The body can initially increase cardiac output by increasing heart rate. Increasing the heart rate to approximately 150 beats per minute will roughly double the cardiac output in most people. However, rates above this result in decreased cardiac filling time and a subsequent decrease in cardiac output. Further increases in cardiac output depend on an increased stroke volume.

Stroke volume is determined by preload, myocardial contractility, and afterload. In the early stages of sepsis, the stroke volume often increases in an attempt to maintain blood pressure. However, as sepsis progresses these compensatory mechanisms often become exhausted and cardiac output falls.

Preload is decreased in sepsis due to increased vascular permeability causing loss of fluid from the intravascular space and hypovolaemia. In addition, nitric oxide and other vasoactive mediators cause vasodilatation and a 'vasoparesis' leading to poor response to inotropes.

Myocardial contractility is decreased due to reduced filling of the heart, hypoxaemia, and acidosis. This is in addition to inflammatory mediators and other poorly defined 'myocardial depressant factors', which directly reduce myocardial contractility in sepsis.

Afterload, which is related to systemic vascular resistance, is reduced in sepsis. In the absence of heart failure this leads to an increase in cardiac output, but reduced preload and contractility often negate this effect.

Disseminated intravascular coagulation

Endothelial damage activates the coagulation cascade and anti-clotting pathways (e.g. activated protein C) are down-regulated, leading to a pro-coagulant state. Platelets rush to the site of damage to repair the endothelium. Clots start to form. This widespread clotting causes consumption of platelets, clotting factors, and fibrinogen. Clotting times are prolonged and thrombocytopenia occurs.

Disseminated intravascular coagulation can cause bleeding, large vessel thrombosis, and haemorrhagic tissue necrosis. Microthrombi formation in the kidneys, lungs, and other organs can lead to multiple organ failure and death.

Oxygen demands/extraction in sepsis

The immune and inflammatory response to sepsis causes an increased oxygen demand from the tissues (up to 12-fold).

Oxygen delivery depends on the oxygen content of the blood and cardiac output. The oxygen content of the blood depends on haemoglobin concentration, oxygen saturation, and partial pressure of oxygen in arterial blood.

The body tries to improve oxygen content by increasing respiratory rate. Therapies attempt to maximize oxygen content by correcting any anaemia with blood transfusions and optimizing arterial haemoglobin saturation with supplemental oxygen.

Even if oxygen delivery is maintained, most patients have poor peripheral uptake of oxygen. The cause of this phenomenon remains unclear. However, it is postulated that damage to the vascular endothelium and mitochondrial dysfunction may be responsible. The vascular endothelium normally produces vasoactive substances that regulate microvascular blood flow to ensure all organs are adequately oxygenated. Endovascular damage results in disruption of this microvascular blood flow and tissue hypoxia. In addition, inflammatory mediators impair intracellular mechanisms, including mitochondrial function, which regulate oxygen uptake and use.

Once the oxygen demands of the tissues are not met, anaerobic metabolism occurs. Lactate is the product of anaerobic metabolism of glucose by the tissues. This process is less efficient than aerobic metabolism in terms of adenosine triphosphate (ATP) production per unit of substrate. Raised lactate indicates a failure of peripheral perfusion, oxygen delivery, and uptake. Increased lactate causes a metabolic acidosis leading to an increased respiratory rate, cardiac depression, and altered mental state. Ultimately, tissue hypoxia leads to cell death and multiple organ failure.

15.1.4 Causes of sepsis

The College curriculum includes knowledge of common gram-positive and gram-negative infections, which can cause sepsis (Table 15.2).

Table 15.2 Common gram-positive and gram-negative infections

	Examples of infection
Gram-positive	
Cocci	
Staphylococcus	Staphylococcus can cause a wide variety of diseases through either toxin production or penetration. Staphylococcal toxins are a common cause of food poisoning.
Streptococcus	Streptococcus can cause a wide variety of diseases including pharyngitis, meningitis, pneumonia, endocarditis, erysipelas, and necrotizing fasciitis. Streptococcus species can be classified based on their haemolytic properties: alpha haemolytic (e.g. Streptococcus pneumonia and Streptococcus viridans) and beta haemolytic (e.g. group A and group B Streptococcus).
Enterococcus	Enterococcus can cause urinary tract infections, bacterial endocarditis, diverticulitis, and meningitis.
Bacilli	
Bacillus	Bacillus anthracis causes anthrax.
Listeria	Listeria monocytogenes can cause sepsis and meningitis.
Clostridium	Clostridium botulinum produces botulinum toxin and can cause botulism. Clostridium difficile can flourish in the gut when other bacteria are killed by antibiotic therapy, leading to pseudomembranous colitis. Clostridium perfringens causes a range of symptoms from food poisoning to gas gangrene. It may be part of the polymicrobial infection causing necrotizing fasciitis. Clostridium tetani is the causative agent of tetanus.
Corynebacterium	Corynebacterium diphtheriae is the pathogen responsible for diphtheria.
Gram-negative	
Cocci	
Neisseria	Neisseria gonorrhoea can cause sexually transmitted disease. Neisseria meningitidis can cause meningitis.
Moraxella	Moraxella catarrhalis can cause pneumonia.
Bacilli	
Escherichia coli	E. coli primarily cause urinary tract infections. Serotype 0157:H7 can cause serious food poisoning through the production of Shiga toxin.
Haemophilus influenzae	H. influenzae mainly causes respiratory tract infections.
Legionella pneumophila	Legionella pneumophila causes pneumonia (Legionnaires disease).
Pseudomonas aeruginosa	P. aeruginosa is characteristically an opportunistic infection of immunocompromized patients. It typically infects the pulmonary tract, urinary tract, burns and/or wounds. It can be the cause of sepsis in neutropenic patients.
Helicobacter pylori	H. pylori can cause chronic low grade inflammation of the stomach and is strongly linked to the development of peptic ulcers and stomach cancer.
Salmonella	Salmonellae cause illnesses like typhoid fever (S. typhi), paratyphoid fever (S. paratyphi), and food poisoning.
Campylobacter jejuni	C. jejuni is the commonest cause of food poisoning.

Toxin-producing bacteria

The ACCS curriculum includes knowledge of common toxin-producing bacteria that can cause sepsis.

The ability to produce toxins is the underlying mechanism by which many bacterial pathogens cause disease. There are two main types of bacterial toxins: endotoxins and exotoxins. Endotoxins are components of the cell wall of gram-negative bacteria (e.g. lipopolysaccharides). Exotoxins are usually proteins secreted by bacteria that act enzymatically or through direct interaction with host cells to stimulate a variety of host responses. Most exotoxins act at tissue sites distant to the site of bacterial growth.

The following conditions are well-recognized toxin-mediated diseases:

● Staphylococcal scalded skin syndrome

Staphylococcal scalded skin syndrome (SSSS) is a toxin-mediated type of exfoliative dermatitis. *Staphylococcus aureus* produces an exotoxin, which causes separation of the outer layers of the epidermis. It can range from localized bulla to extensive flaccid blisters and erosions.

ED management involves treatment with flucloxacillin (IV or orally depending on severity) and supportive management (IV fluids, analgesia, and wound care).

SSSS is discussed in more detail in Chapter 16, section 16.2.

● Toxic shock syndrome

Toxic shock syndrome is a potentially fatal toxin-mediated disease. The causative bacteria include *Staphylococcus aureus* or *Streptococcus pyogenes*. Toxic shock syndrome is classically known to be caused by a retained tampon, but it can also occur after trauma, burns, surgery, or local infections.

Clinical features include high fever, a generalized erythematous rash, malaise, confusion, diarrhoea, myalgia, and hypotension. After approximately two weeks, the rash desquamates, particularly on the palms and soles.

Treatment is the same as for severe sepsis with fluid resuscitation and antistaphylococcal antibiotics (e.g. flucloxacillin and benzylpenicillin). If a tampon is the cause, it should be removed.

● Necrotizing fasciitis

Necrotizing fasciitis is a rare and severe bacterial infection of soft tissues. It is usually a polymicrobial infection, often involving aerobic and anaerobic organism. The most important cause is *Streptococcus pyogenes* (also known as Group A *Streptococcus*).

Necrotizing fasciitis may occur with or without obvious trauma or breach of the skin. Infection involves the fascia and subcutaneous tissues with gas formation and development of gangrene. Infection may spread to adjacent muscles, causing myonecrosis or pyogenic myositis.

Initial clinical features may be vague, with severe pain but little on examination, except tenderness of the affected area. There may be slight swelling or erythema at the site. Patients usually have a fever and are systemically unwell with malaise, lethargy, diarrhoea, and vomiting. The disease often progresses rapidly leading to marked soft tissue swelling with discoloration, haemorrhagic blisters, and skin necrosis. Septic shock may develop and the mortality rate is high.

Necrotizing fasciitis is a clinical diagnosis but X-rays may show gas in the soft tissues. A CT scan of the affected area may give more detailed information.

Treatment involves intravenous antibiotics (e.g. piperacillin-tazobactam and clindamycin) and supportive management with fluid resuscitation. Patients require prompt surgery to debride the affected area and excise necrotic tissues.

Fournier's gangrene is necrotizing fasciitis of the external genitalia and perineum. It is due to a polymicrobial, synergistic infection of the subcutaneous tissues. Fournier's gangrene is covered in more detail in Chapter 6, section 6.16.

15.1.5 Risk factors for sepsis

Although everyone is at potential risk of developing sepsis from common infections (e.g. flu, urinary tract infection, gastroenteritis, and so on), sepsis is more likely in certain patient groups including:

- Extremes of age (e.g. premature infants, neonates, elderly)
- Immunocompromized (e.g. active chemotherapy, long-term steroids, HIV, and so on)
- Associated injuries (e.g. burns, trauma, large areas of devitalized tissue, and so on)
- Indwelling medical devices (e.g. intravenous catheters, wound drains, urinary catheters, and on)
- Concurrent medical conditions (e.g. recent surgery, malnutrition, alcoholism, IVDU, diabetes, and so on)
- Recent or repeated antibiotic treatment increasing the risk of colonization with bacteria with multiple resistance patterns
- Genetics (e.g. genetic polymorphism of a receptor known as the Toll-like receptor predisposes individuals to overwhelming infections with gram-negative organisms)

15.1.6 Clinical features of sepsis

There is a spectrum of disease severity in the presentation of sepsis, ranging from a minor localized infection with no systemic symptoms through to full-blown failure of multiple organ systems.

The criteria for identifying SIRS are described in Table 15.1. Once SIRS has been identified a potential infective cause must be sought. The diagnosis of infection cannot be delayed until an organism is identified because unnecessary and dangerous delays in treatment would occur. Initially infection has to be identified based on clinical features alone (see Table 15.3).

15.1.7 The Surviving Sepsis Campaign

The Surviving Sepsis Campaign (SSC) was developed as a collaboration of the European Society of Critical Care Medicine, the International Sepsis Forum, and the Society of Critical Care Medicine. The initial aim was to reduce the mortality from sepsis by improving its management, diagnosis, and treatment.

In March 2004, recommendations drawn from research, clinical trials, and expert opinion were collated and published as the 'Surviving Sepsis Campaign guidelines for the management of severe sepsis and septic shock'. These were subsequently revised in 2008 and 2012.

Early goal-directed therapy

The Surviving Sepsis Guidelines were initially drawn from the term 'early goal-directed therapy' (EGDT), which refers to the manipulation of physiology to achieve pre-determined goals.

EGDT in sepsis relates to a paper by Rivers et al., in which 263 patients presenting to an ED with severe sepsis or septic shock were randomly assigned to receive either EGDT or standard therapy during the first six hours of their care. In-hospital mortality for the EGDT group was 30.5%, as compared with 46.5% for the control group ($P = 0.009$).

The resuscitation strategy in the Rivers study was to enhance oxygen delivery to the tissues by optimizing cardiac output. The aim was to initiate resuscitation and treatment early, before the onset of organ failure.

Sepsis is a time-sensitive disease and early intervention helps prevent a catastrophic and irreversible decline. If resuscitation is delayed until after cell dysfunction and death are present, then strategies to provide the cells with more oxygen will not work.

Rivers et al. described four main goals in an effort to improve oxygen delivery.

Goal 1: CVP>8 mmHg

Patients with sepsis that continue to be hypotensive (or have high lactate >4 mmol/L) despite an initial fluid bolus of 20 ml/kg of crystalloid have septic shock. Such patients should have a central

Table 15.3 Clinical features suggesting particular infective sites

Site of infection	Clinical features	Frequency
Respiratory (e.g. pneumonia)	Productive cough Dyspnoea Focal signs on respiratory examination (e.g. crepitations) (CXR—if a pneumonia is suspected clinically, completion of a CXR should not delay treatment)	Accounts for 50–70% of severe sepsis cases
Abdominal infection (e.g. appendicitis, diverticulitis, perforated viscus, ischaemic bowel)	Abdominal pain Abdominal distension Diarrhoea	20–25% of cases
Urinary tract infection	Dysuria Offensive urine Loin pain Haematuria (Ideally a urine sample should be obtained prior to antibiotic therapy. A positive dipstick result may confirm the source of infection)	7–10% of cases
Soft tissue and bone/ joint infection (e.g. cellulitis, septic arthritis, fasciitis, wound infections)	Redness Heat Pain Swelling Pus on aspiration of a collection or joint	<10% of cases
Device related (e.g. indwelling vascular catheters, urinary catheter)	Assess patient for any indwelling medical devices and consider removal	
Other infections (e.g. meningitis, endocarditis)	Meningitis—non-blanching petechial rash, neck stiffness, headache, etc (see section 15.4) Endocarditis—history of valvular heart disease or prosthetic valve, new murmur, vascular or immunological phenomenon (see Chapter 9, section 9.11)	

venous catheter inserted and their CVP measured. Fluid resuscitation should continue with 500–1000 ml boluses every 30 minutes to achieve and maintain a CVP>8 mmHg.

Giving fluid increases cardiac preload and improves cardiac output. The volume of venous blood returned to the heart determines the degree of ventricular filling and the length of myocardial muscle fibres. Muscle fibre length is related to the contractile properties of the myocardium (Frank–Starling law). Increased muscle fibre length results in a greater stroke volume. The Frank–Starling law is covered in more detail in Chapter 2, section 2.8.

By optimizing preload, cardiac output improves, which increases oxygen delivery to the tissues.

Goal 2: MAP>65 mmHg or systolic BP>90 mmHg

If the CVP is greater than 8 mmHg, the patient can be considered adequately 'filled'. If the mean arterial pressure (MAP) remains less than 65 mmHg or systolic BP less than 90 mmHg despite this, then a vasopressor is required. The recommended vasopressor is noradrenaline, which should be started to maintain a MAP of at least 65 mmHg.

The aim of this intervention is to ensure adequate perfusion of the organs.

Goal 3: urine output >0.5mls/kg/hr

Goal 4: $ScvO_2$>70%

Central venous oxygen saturation ($ScvO_2$) is measured by taking blood in a heparinized syringe (e.g. a normal blood gas syringe) from the central venous line and measuring the oxygen saturation using a blood gas analyser. The result is the oxygen saturation of central venous blood.

$ScvO_2$ can be considered a surrogate marker for measuring the balance between oxygen delivery and demand. If low (<70%), the tissues are extracting 'too much' oxygen for each ml of blood that passes. This may be due to very high oxygen demands or insufficient oxygen delivery.

Mixed venous oxygen saturation (SvO_2) measured from a pulmonary artery catheter is the measurement which most accurately reflects the imbalance between oxygen supply and demand. However, very few patients will have a pulmonary artery catheter *in situ* and it has been shown, and is widely accepted, that $ScvO_2$ gives a good approximation of SvO_2.

If the $ScvO_2$ is low, then interventions to improve the oxygen content of the blood and increase cardiac output are required.

Improving the oxygen content of the blood

The oxygen content of the blood may be improved through the administration of high-flow oxygen and/or mechanical ventilation. In addition, if the patient is anaemic a blood transfusion may be considered to improve the oxygen carrying capacity of the blood. Rivers et al. transfused patients with a low $ScvO_2$ to a haematocrit >30% (approximating to a haemoglobin concentration >10 g/dl). Concerns have be raised about the need to transfuse patients to such a level and the Surviving Sepsis Guidelines recommend transfusing patients when the haemoglobin is less than 7 g/dl to a target haemoglobin of 7–9 g/dl.

Improve myocardial contractility

If the patient is not anaemic, or repeat $ScvO_2$ levels remain low after transfusion, the next strategy to redress the imbalance between oxygen delivery and demand is to increase the cardiac output, by improving myocardial contractility. To achieve this, an infusion of the inotrope dobutamine is recommended.

Dobutamine like noradrenaline should be given via a central line. The dobutamine infusion should be increased incrementally until the $ScvO_2$ >70% or the maximum dose is reached (20 mcg/kg/minute).

15.1.8 Surviving Sepsis Campaign bundles

Two 'bundles' or packages of care for the treatment of patients with severe sepsis were developed based on EGDT. The surving sepsis bundles were revised in 2014, following the publication of three key trails in 2014 and 2015 on the management of sepsis. The multicentre trials revealed no superiority with the use of central venous pressure monitoring and central venous saturations (as previously described in Rivers et al.) in patients with septic shock or a lactate >4, who received timely antibioctics and fluids resuscitation.

- Bundle 1: to be completed within three hours of the time of presentation.
- Bundle 2: be completed within six hours of the time of presentation.

(Time of presentation is is described as the time of triage in the emergency department or, if presenting from another care venue, from the earliest identification of severe sepsis or septic shock.)

15.1.9 The Surviving Sepsis Campaign bundle 1

The firt bundle comprises four tasks designed to be completed within three hours following the onset of severe sepsis (Box 15.1).

Serum lactate

Serum lactate is the product of anaerobic metabolism of glucose by the tissues and used as a marker of tissue hypoperfusion. There is good evidence that lactate carries prognostic value, and a higher lactate suggests a poorer prognosis. Lactate is particularly useful measured serially, to guide the response to resuscitation and fluid therapy.

Blood cultures

Two or more blood cultures are recommended: one drawn percutaneously and one through each vascular access device if it has been in for longer than 48 hours. The majority of ED patients will not have a vascular access device *in situ*, however some patients may have an indwelling vascular catheter (e.g. a Portacath or Hickman line).

A blood culture taken from the access device may be positive earlier than a percutaneous sample and indicate the device as the source of infection.

Consideration should also be given to sampling and culturing other sites, if clinical signs suggest a possible source of infection (e.g. cerebrospinal fluid, sputum, urine, synovial fluid, pleural fluid, and so on). Imaging studies to identify sources of infection should be considered.

Antibiotic administration

Antibiotics should be given as early as possible, and always within the first hour of recognizing severe sepsis or septic shock. There is ample evidence to support early and appropriate antibiotic administration; such that it can be argued that this is one of the most important aspects of the care bundle.

In the first instance, one or more broad-spectrum antibiotics should be administered, which are active against the likely bacterial/fungal pathogens (see Table 15.4) and with good penetration into the presumed infective site. The recommended antimicrobial regime will vary between hospitals depending on local resistance patterns and organisms. Table 15.4 gives examples of possible empirical antibiotic regimes.

The antimicrobial regimen should be reviewed daily to optimize efficacy, prevent resistance, avoid toxicity, and minimize costs. Once the causative organism has been isolated, the antibiotic(s) should be changed to a narrower spectrum.

In addition to antibiotics, patients may require control of the source of the infection (e.g. drainage of an abscess, tissue debridement, removal of infected intravascular devices, and so on).

Box 15.1 Severe sepsis—bundle 1

Severe sepsis—bundle 1

1. Measure serum lactate.
2. Obtain blood cultures prior to antibiotic administration.
3. Administer broad-spectrum antibiotic within 1 h of the recognition of severe sepsis and septic shock.
4. Adminster 30 ml/kg of crystalloid for the management of hypotension and/or serum lactate >4 mmol/L.

Data from Surviving Sepsis Campaign—updated Bundles in response to new evidence. www.survivingsepsis.org/Guidelines/Pages/default.aspx

Table 15.4 Possible empirical antibiotic regimes in severe sepsis

Presumed site of infection	Empirical antibiotic regime	Alternative regime if penicillin allergy
Community-acquired pneumonia	Co-amoxiclav 1.2 g tds IV PLUS Clarithromycin 500 mg bd IV (PLUS Metronidazole 500 mg tds IV if aspiration suspected)	Teicoplanin 10 mg/kg bd IV PLUS Clarithromycin 500 mg bd IV
Intra-abdominal sepsis	Piperacillin-tazobactam 4.5 g tds IV PLUS Gentamicin 5 mg/kg od IV	Teicoplanin 10 mg/kg bd IV PLUS Metronidazole 500 mg tds IV PLUS Gentamicin 5 mg/kg od IV
Urinary tract infection	Gentamicin 5 mg/kg od IV OR Piperacillin-tazobactam 4.5 g tds IV	Gentamicin 5 mg/kg od IV
Soft tissue infections/cellulitis	Flucloxacillin 2 g qds IV PLUS Benzylpenicillin 1.2 g qds IV (If necrotizing fasciitis is suspected Piperacillin-tazobactam 4.5 g tds IV plus Clindamycin 900 mg qds IV) (If MRSA suspected, teicoplanin 10 mg/kg bd IV plus sodium fusidate 500 mg tds PO)	Clindamycin 900 mg qds IV PLUS Ciprofloxacin 400 mg qds IV PLUS Metronidazole 500 mg tds IV
Bacterial meningitis	Ceftriaxone 2 g bd IV OR Cefotaxime 2 g qds IV (If age >55 years or immunocompromized, add ampicillin 2 g IV)	Chloramphenicol 25 mg/kg qds IV (If age > 55 years or immunocompromized, add co-trimoxazole 1.44 g bd IV)
Endocarditis	Co-amoxiclav 1.2 g tds IV PLUS Gentamicin 5 mg/kg od IV	Vancomycin 1 g bd IV PLUS Gentamicin 5 mg/kg od IV PLUS Ciprofloxacin 500 mg bd PO
Neutropenic sepsis	Piperacillin-tazobactam 4.5 g tds IV PLUS Gentamicin 5 mg/kg od IV	Aztreonam 2 g bd IV PLUS Teicoplanin 10 mg/kg bd IV PLUS Gentamicin 5 mg/kg od IV
Sepsis of unknown origin	Piperacillin-tazobactam 4.5 g tds IV ± Gentamicin 5 mg/kg od IV ± Teicoplanin 10 mg/kg bd IV	Aztreonam 2 g bd IV PLUS Teicoplanin 10 mg/kg bd IV PLUS Gentamicin 5 mg/kg od IV

Fluid challenges

Fluid boluses of 500–1000 ml crystalloid or 300–500 ml colloid should be used. There is little evidence to the support the use of colloids over crystalloids. Colloids have a smaller volume of distribution than crystalloids and therefore less volume is required to achieve the same degree of intravascular volume expansion.

Patients with severe sepsis frequently require large volumes of fluids for adequate resuscitation. In hypoperfused patients, a minimum volume of 20 ml/kg crystalloid is recommended as an initial bolus. Patients with shock will frequently require volumes up to 60 ml/kg in resuscitation. Patients should be monitored closely and frequently reassessed for signs of fluid overload and pulmonary oedema.

15.1.9 The Surviving Sepsis Campaign bundle 2

The second bundle consists of a set of three tasks to be completed within six hours of identification of severe sepsis (see Box 15.2).

The management guidline focuses on the reassessment and documentation of volume statuts and tissue perfusion. This can be achieved by either:

- Repeat focused examination including vital signs, cardiopulmonary and capillary refill

OR two of the following:

- Measure CVP
- Measure ScvO2
- Bedside cardiovascular ultrasound
- Dynamic assessment of fluid resposivness with passive leg raise or fluid challenge

Low-dose steroids

There is some evidence that steroids administered at physiological doses (e.g. hydrocortisone 50 mg qds) to patients with shock resistance to fluid resuscitation, and requiring the administration of vasopressors, are of benefit. Other studies have not supported these conclusions. Therefore, the guidelines stipulate that steroids be considered in patients with shock unresponsive to fluids and vasopressors, according to local policy.

ACTH stimulation testing does not appear to predict steroid-responsiveness and is not recommended.

Box 15.2 Severe sepsis—bundle 2

Severe sepsis—bundle 2

1. Apply vasopressors (for hypotension that does not respond to initial fluid resuscitation) to maintain a mean arterial pressure (MAP) ≥65 mmHg.

2. In the event of persistent hypotension after initial fluid administration (MAP <65 mmHg) or if initial lactate was ≥4 mmol/L, reassess volume status and tissue perfusion and document findings according to Table 15.1.

3. Remeasure lactate if initial lactate elevated. Consider low-dose steroid for patients with septic shock, which is refractory to fluids and vasopressors.

Data from Surviving Sepsis Campaign—updated Bundles in response to new evidence. https://www.survingsepsis.org

15.1.10 The Sepsis Six

Surviving Sepsis (https://www.survivingsepsis.org) is a UK-developed educational resource approved by the Surviving Sepsis Campaign nationally and internationally. The education programme has introduced the concept of the Sepsis Six: six tasks to be completed by non-specialist staff within the first hour. It enables the non-specialist to start completing the bundles while liaising with the critical care team. Implementation of the Sepsis Six has been shown to independently improve outcome.

The Sepsis Six are:

1. Give high-flow oxygen—via a facemask with a reservoir bag.
2. Take blood cultures (at least two sets)—and consider source control.
3. Give IV antibiotics—according to local protocol.
4. Start IV fluids—Hartmann's or equivalent (up to 60 ml/kg in divided boluses of 500–1000 ml boluses. Minimum 20 ml/kg in shock).
5. Check lactate.
6. Monitor hourly urine output—consider catheterization (urine output in the early stages of sepsis is a useful assessment of cardiac output).

15.1.11 Complications of sepsis

If sepsis is not recognized early and treated promptly, it can lead to shock, multiple organ failure, and death.

Complications for individual organs include:

- Lung injury—increased vascular permeability in pulmonary capillaries causes pulmonary oedema and infiltrates, including proteins and activated neutrophils. Surfactant production is reduced. Interstitial fibrosis may develop. These changes lead to arterial hypoxaemia, reduced respiratory compliance, and increased work of breathing. This syndrome is known as acute lung injury or in more severe forms, ARDS.
- Cardiovascular injury—myocardial dysfunction results from reduced preload, hypoxia, acidosis, and inflammatory mediators reducing myocardial contractility. In addition, a myocardial cytotoxic process causes myocardial cell necrosis, which can result in permanent damage.
- Acute kidney injury is a common complication of severe sepsis. This results from hypoperfusion of the kidneys due to hypovolaemia and hypotension. In addition, nitric oxide and other inflammatory mediators have been postulated to impair mitochondrial oxygen transport resulting in renal dysfunction. The early use of haemofiltration to correct fluid imbalance and (possibly) remove circulating inflammatory mediators has been advocated, but the benefits are unproven. It is essential to restore circulating volume and achieve an adequate blood pressure and cardiac output to prevent and treat acute renal failure.
- Gastrointestinal (GI) tract—the bowel is particularly susceptible to ischaemic insults and the GI tract is thought to help propagate the injury of sepsis. The normal barrier of the gut may be affected, allowing translocation of bacteria and endotoxins into the systemic circulation and extending the septic response. Severe sepsis can cause paralytic ileus which may be exacerbated by the use of opiates and muscle relaxants. This may lead to a delay in instituting enteral feeding at a time when the patient has high protein and calorie requirements.
- Liver failure—is common in septic patients, possibly resulting from a reduced blood flow relative to an increased metabolic demand. It can manifest as elevation of liver enzymes and bilirubin, coagulation defects, and failure to excrete toxins such as ammonia, which can lead to encephalopathy.

KEY POINTS

The diagnostic criteria for SIRS are two or more of:

- Temperature >38.3°C or <36°C
- Heart rate >90 beats per min
- Respiratory rate >20 breaths per min
- White cell count <4 or >12 × 10^9/L

Sepsis = SIRS + infection

Severe sepsis = sepsis + organ dysfunction

Septic shock = evidence of ongoing hypoperfusion despite initial fluid challenges

The Surviving Sepsis Campaign developed two 'bundles' for the treatment of those with severe sepsis:

- Bundle 1 —to be completed within three hours
- Bundle 2 —to be completed within six hours

Based on the sepsis bundles, the 'Sepsis Six' was developed. These are six tasks to be completed by non-specialist staff within the first hour.

1. Give high-flow oxygen.
2. Take blood cultures.
3. Give IV antibiotics.
4. Start IV fluid.
5. Check lactate.
6. Monitor hourly urine output.

15.2 Fever (including neutropenic sepsis)

15.2.1 Pathophysiology of fever

Body temperature is usually maintained at 36.8°C ± 0.7°C in order to maintain normal enzyme and cell function.

Temperature is controlled by the hypothalamus. The hypothalamus monitors body temperature and balances heat production with heat loss.

Under normal circumstances heat is generated internally during metabolic processes or when external environmental temperatures exceed those of the body. Heat can also be produced by increased skeletal muscle activity (e.g. shivering).

Heat loss occurs predominantly from the skin via evaporative losses which can be increased by vasodilatation of cutaneous blood vessels and sweating. The hypothalamus also affects behavioural influences in humans, with individuals changing clothes and/or seeking appropriate shelter to maintain body temperature.

Fever is a temporary elevation in the body's thermoregulatory set point. Temperature is regulated by the hypothalamus in response to prostaglandin E$_2$ (PgE$_2$). PgE$_2$ release is triggered by pyrogens.

There are two types of pyrogens: endogenous and exogenous. Exogenous pyrogens are microbial products and toxins, such as gram-negative endotoxins. Exogenous pyrogens bind to macrophages causing the release of endogenous pyrogens which are cytokines such as IL-1, IL-6, and

TNF. These cytokines stimulate production of the enzyme cyclooxygenase, which results in the production of PgE$_2$. PgE$_2$ resets the hypothalamic thermal set point elevating the body temperature.

15.2.2 Causes of fever

Infection is the commonest cause of fever; however, there are many other causes.

Causes of fever include:

- Infection—the commonest cause of fever.
- Malignancy (paraneoplastic fever), for example Hodgkin's lymphoma, acute leukaemia, lymphoma, renal cell carcinoma, phaeochromocytoma, and so on.
- Allergic reactions.
- Hypersensitivity reaction to drugs—drug-associated fever is an ill-defined syndrome in which fever is the predominant manifestation of an adverse drug reaction. Drugs that modify biological response are more likely to cause fever (e.g. amphotericin B or bleomycin). Other commonly implicated drugs include antibiotics, anticonvulsants, and cytotoxics.
- Blood transfusions—due to the presence of antibodies to antigens on the donor's white blood cells.
- Graft-versus-host disease.
- Thrombosis (e.g. pulmonary embolism or deep vein thrombosis).
- Central nervous system (CNS) haemorrhage—the local production of cytokines in the CNS following haemorrhage may account for the fever.
- Connective tissue disorders (e.g. rheumatoid arthritis, systemic lupus erythematous, polyarteritis nodosum, and so on).
- Inflammatory (e.g. inflammatory bowel disease, thyroiditis, sarcoidosis, pancreatitis, and so on).

15.2.3 Clinical evaluation of fever

Assessment of fever requires careful history taking, medication review, and a thorough physical examination.

Key elements in the history include:

- Onset and duration of fever—the pattern of fever may sometimes give a clue to diagnosis (e.g. daily spikes in malaria, abscess, or schistosomiasis; or continuous fever in pneumonia, urinary tract infection, or typhoid).
- Associated symptoms—may indicate the source of fever (e.g. respiratory symptoms, genitourinary symptoms, GI symptoms, and so on).
- Chronic symptoms (e.g. cough, recurrent infections, weight loss, lymphadenopathy, and so on may suggest causes such as tuberculosis, malignancy, or HIV).
- Past medical history (e.g. malignancies or implanted medical devices/prostheses).
- Travel history—dates of travel, places visited (which countries, rural versus urban), vaccinations, and chemoprophylaxis.
- Sexual history—number of sexual partners in last three months (men, women, homosexual, heterosexual), last sexual intercourse, use of protection, previous history of sexually transmitted infections, current partner (and any knowledge of their sexual health/history).
- Intravenous drug use (past and present).
- Animal contacts, for example birds (*Chlamydia psittaci*), cats (*toxoplasmosis*), farm animals (*E. coli*), and so on.
- Medication history—current prescribed medications, any recent alterations, and use of over the counter medications.
- Vaccination history.

15.2.4. Fever in the returning traveller

Medical history in returning traveller should include:

- Severity of illness (severe respiratory syndrome; signs of haemorrhagic fever)
- Travel itinerary (countries visited/ transited through) and duration of travel
- Timing of onset of illness in relation to international travel
- Past medical history and medications
- History of pre-travel consultation: travel immunizations; adherence to malaria chemoprophylaxis

Individual exposures:

- Type of accommodation
- Insect precautions taken: repellent, bed nets, window screens
- Source of drinking water
- Ingestion of raw milk or seafood or unpasteurized dairy products
- Insect or arthropod bites
- Freshwater exposure (swimming, rafting) in schistosomiasis-endemic areas
- Animal bites and scratches
- Body fluid exposure (tattoos, piercings, intravenous drug use, sexual activity, sexual tourism)
- Medical care while overseas (injections, transfusions, and so on)

A thorough examination of the main systems (e.g. respiratory, cardiovascular, abdominal, and nervous system) should be performed.
Key elements include:

- Vital signs: relative bradycardia
- Lymphadenopathy
- Jaundice
- Skin—evidence of rash or cellulitis
- Musculoskeletal examination—evidence of arthropathy (erythema, warmth, pain, and/or swelling), spinal, or sternal tenderness
- Genitalia—presence of ulcers (syphilitic chancre), vesicles (herpes), and/or discharge (gonorrhoea)
- Mouth and oropharynx—mucosal ulcers, oral candidiasis, teeth, gingivitis, tonsillar enlargement
- Eyes—subconjunctival haemorrhage, conjunctivitis, uveitis
- Abdominal examination—hepatomegaly, splenomegaly
- Cardiovascular system—new diastolic murmur, change in existing murmur

There are numerous different causes for an individual presenting with a fever in first two weeks after travel (see Table 15.5).

15.2.5 Investigation of fever of unknown origin

Fever of unknown origin is defined as a febrile illness lasting more than three weeks, with temperatures exceeding 38.3°C on several occasions, and lacking a definitive diagnosis after one week of evaluation in hospital. Therefore, by definition, fever of unknown origin is not an ED diagnosis. However, the initial investigations will be performed in the ED.
ED investigations should include:

- Blood tests—FBC and white cell count differential, U&E, LFT, clotting, ESR, and CRP
- Blood cultures—at least two sets from different sites
- Sputum culture and microscopy

Table 15.5 Causes of fever in the first two weeks of travel

Symptoms	Disease
Systemic febrile illness with mild non-specific symptoms	Malaria, dengue, typhoid fever, rickettsial disease, acute HIV infection, leptospirosis
Fever + CNS involvement	Meningococcal meningitis, malaria, arboviral encephalitis (Japanese encephalitis), East African trypanosomiasis, angiostrongyliasis, rabies
Fever with respiratory complications	Influenza, bacterial pneumonia, acute histoplasmosis, or cocciodomycosis, *Legionella* pneumonia, malaria, tularaemia, pneumonic plague
Fever + skin rash:	Dengue, measles, varicella, viral haemorrhagic fever, spotted fever, or typhus group rickettsial diseases, typhoid fever, parvovirus B19, mononucleosis, acute HIV infection, schistosomiasis (urticarial rash-Katayama fever)
Fever + gastroenteritis	*E. coli*, *Campylobacter*, *Salmonella*, *Shigella*
Fever + jaundice	Leptospirosis, viral hepatitis, viral haemorrhagic fever, yellow fever

- Chest X-ray (CXR)
- ECG
- Urinary dipstick, microscopy, and culture
- Stool culture

Other investigations depend on the clinical picture and may include:

- Thick and thin films (plus falciparum antigen testing if available)—if travel to a malarial area in the last year
- Glandular fever screen (monospot test)
- HIV serology after appropriate counselling and consent (this may be more appropriate via the genitourinary clinic)
- Syphilis serology (this may be more appropriate via the genitourinary clinic)
- Echocardiography if endocarditis a possibility
- Further imaging (e.g. CT chest and abdomen if the source remains occult)
- Autoantibodies (e.g. rheumatoid factor, anti-nuclear antibodies, and so on)
- Hepatitis screen

15.2.6 Emergency department management of fever of unknown origin

The specific management of fever is determined by the underlying aetiology. However, there are general interventions that can be performed in the ED to manage fever.

- Empirical antibiotics—if an infective source is suspected, empirical antibiotics should be commenced once appropriate samples and cultures are obtained. Table 15.4 gives examples of possible empirical antibiotic regimes.
- Antipyretics.
- Increase fluid intake—patients are at risk of dehydration and may require IV fluids.
- Remove excess clothing and bed linen.
- Bath or sponge with tepid water.

Antipyretics

Antipyretic agents, such as paracetamol or non-steroidal anti-inflammatory drugs (NSAIDs), act by lowering the elevated thermal set point by inhibiting cyclooxygenase. Inhibition of cyclooxygenase impairs the production of PgE_2.

There is evidence that fever may be useful in aiding host defence. Some immunological reactions are sped up by higher temperatures and some pathogens with strict temperature preference may be hindered. However, fever is associated with potential metabolic consequences including dehydration, increased oxygen consumption, and increased metabolic rate. In addition, fever often results in constitutional symptoms of fatigue, myalgia, diaphoresis, and chills. Therefore, it is appropriate to manage fever with antipyretics in the ED.

15.2.7 Malaria

Malaria should be suspected in the presence of a flu-like illness (fever, chills, sweating, anorexia, headache, myalgia, arthralgia, nausea, abdominal pain, vomiting, diarrhoea) in anyone who has visited a malaria endemic zone within the preceding three months.

- Malaria is endemic in sub-Saharan, central and west Africa, south and central Asia, the Middle East, Korea, central (including Mexico) and South America, Haiti and the Dominican Republic (Hispaniola), Oceania, and Papua New Guinea.
- The minimum incubation period for naturally acquired infection is six days. Most patients with falciparum infection present in the first three months after exposure, with almost all presenting within six months.
- Leukopenia, anaemia, and thrombocytopenia are common.

Malaria is caused by the parasite plasmodium which is spread by mosquitos. There are many different types of plasmodium, however the five species that cause human disease are: *P. vivax, P. ovale, P. knowlesi, P. malariae,* and *Pf. alciparum,* with the latter being thos most severe.

Falcipirum malaria is a potentially fatal condition—the Hospital of Tropical Disease classifies it as either severe or non-severe (see Table 15.6) based on the parasataemia count and presence of complications.

Complicated malaria is classified as the presence of one or more of the following:

- Cerebral malaria (unrousable coma with peripheral plasmodium falciparum parasitaemia after exclusion of other causes of encephalopathy)
- Severe normocytic anaemia (haemoglobin<5 g/dl)
- Acute kidney injury (serum creatinine > 265 μmol/L)
- Acute pulmonary oedema/adult respiratory distress syndrome
- Hypotension/shock (systolic blood pressure <80 mmHg)
- Spontaneous bleeding and/or laboratory evidence of disseminated intravascular coagulation

Table 15.6 Classification of severity of falciparum malaria

Severity	Parasataemia
Uncomplicated	Parasataemia <2%, with no shizonts AND No complications
Severe	Paracetaemia >2% OR paracetaemia <2% with shizonts OR paracetaemia <2% with complications

- Generalized convulsions—more than two episodes in 24 hours
- Jaundice
- Hyperpyrexia
- Hypoglycaemia (blood glucose < 2.5 mmol/L)
- Metabolic acidosis (plasma bicarbonate <15 mmol/L)
- Hyperlactataemia (lactate >5 mmol/L)
- Macroscopic haemoglobinuria

Investigations

- Examination of thick and thin blood slides by microscopy. In the presence of a clinical suspicion of malaria, repeat films should be examined after 12–24 hours and again after a further 24 hours.
- Rapid diagnostic tests based upon detection of parasite antigens or enzymes are also commonly used.

Management

Uncomplicated falciparum malaria or non-falciparum malaria can generally be treated with oral antimalarial treatment according to local guidelines.

Severe malaria is a medical emergency and requires immediate management and high-dependency unit care. Treatment should include:

- Parenteral antimalarial therapy: intravenous quinine dihydrochloride 20 mg/kg loading dose in 5% glucose over four hours, followed by 10 mg/kg infusion over four hours every eight hours or intravenous artesunate 2.4 mg/kg at 0, 12, and 24 hours.
- Careful management of fluid balance, guided by CVP monitoring.
- Regular monitoring for hypoglycaemia.
- Consider broad-spectrum antibiotics if evidence of shock or secondary bacterial infection is present.
- Haemofiltration for acute kidney injury.
- Seizure management with anti-epileptic drugs.
- Exchange transfusion in patients with hyperparasitaemia.

15.2.7 Neutropenic sepsis

Approximately 50–60% of febrile neutropenic patients prove to have infections and approximately 20% have a bacteraemia. Fever is commonly due to gram-positive cocci (e.g. coagulase negative staphylococci, *Staphylococcus aureus*, and *Streptococcus viridans*) or gram-negative bacilli (e.g. *E. coli*, *Klebsiella*, *Pseudomonas aeruginosa*). Fungal infections tend to occur after patients have received broad-spectrum antibiotics and have had prolonged periods of neutropenia but may occur as primary infections.

A diagnosis of neutropenic sepsis is made in the presence of infection in patients who have a neutrophil count of $<1.0 \times 10^9$/L and systemic signs of sepsis.

Neutropenic sepsis can occur in any patient with a low neutrophil count, but is often more severe when the neutropenia is part of a generalized pancytopenia resulting from systemic anti-cancer treatment (e.g. chemotherapy or monoclonal antibody treatment). This is thought to be due to two factors: first, chemotherapeutic agents are cytotoxic and cause damage to the mucous membranes of the GI tract, allowing the passage of large numbers of organisms into the bloodstream; second, in pancytopenia there is a decrease in the number of functioning monocytes in addition to neutrophils, both of which are required for a functioning immune system.

Fever may not always be present in infected neutropenic patients who are dehydrated, or taking steroids or NSAIDs. The possibility of infection must always be considered in any neutropenic patient who is unwell.

504 Chapter 15 Infectious diseases

Causes of neutropenia include:

- Bone marrow failure (e.g. chemotherapy, aplastic anaemia, myelodysplasia)
- Bone marrow infiltration (e.g. acute leukaemia or metastases from solid tumours)
- Drugs (e.g. sulfonamides, carbimazole, carbamazepine, clozapine)
- Infections (e.g. influenza, Epstein–Barr virus, HIV, bacterial sepsis)
- Immunological (e.g. systemic lupus erythematous, Felty's syndrome)

Emergency department management of neutropenic sepsis

Neutropenic sepsis is initially treated in an identical manner to non-neutropenic severe sepsis and septic shock (see section 15.1).

The patient should be fully examined and a detailed history taken as for any patient with a fever. A per rectum examination should be avoided in a neutropenic patient because this may disrupt the mucous membranes of the rectum, resulting in a bacteraemia.

Patients should be nursed in a single room and infection control procedures should be employed: hand washing, apron, and gloves.

The recommended antibiotic regime depends on local pathogens and resistance patterns. The management of neutropenic patients should be discussed with a consultant microbiologist. Piperacillin-tazobactam plus gentamicin is a reasonable initial regime. Once the source of infection and organism is identified, antibiotic therapy can be adjusted.

Patients with evidence of lesions suspicious of herpes simplex or varicella zoster should also receive IV aciclovir.

15.2.8 Hyperthermia

An elevated body temperature usually represents a fever in the vast majority of patients; however, an elevated temperature can also be the results of hyperthermia, which has a different pathophysiology to fever.

Fever results from elevation of the hypothalamic thermal set point due to the actions of PgE_2. The thermoregulatory mechanisms remain intact, resulting in behavioural and physiological responses to control body temperature.

Hyperthermia results from uncontrolled increases in body temperature. The setting of the thermoregulatory centre in the hypothalamus remains unchanged but the body's ability to lose heat is overwhelmed by disease, drugs, or excessive external or internal heat.

Causes of hyperthermia include:

- Heat-stroke syndromes—see Chapter 2, section 2.2.5.
- Metabolic disorders (e.g. hyperthyroidism).
- Drugs (e.g. ecstasy, cocaine, amphetamines, and so on).
- Neuroleptic malignant syndrome—an idiosyncratic drug reaction to antipsychotics (e.g. haloperidol—see Chapter 18, section 18.5).
- Malignant hyperthermia—a rare autosomal dominant condition related to the use of suxamethonium or inhaled anaesthetic agents (see Chapter 3, section 3.3.5). It results in uncontrolled skeletal muscle oxidative metabolism.
- Prolonged muscular activity—seizures, marathon running, excessive dancing secondary to recreational drugs (e.g. ecstasy).

Distinguishing fever from hyperthermia is important because the management of these syndromes differs. Hyperthermia is often diagnosed based on the history of heat exposure or the use of certain drugs that interfere with normal thermoregulation.

Management of hyperthermia includes:

- External cooling, (e.g. removing the patient from the hot environment, removing bed clothes, evaporative cooling—spraying with tepid water and fans), surface cooling devices, and ice packs.

- Cold intravenous fluids.
- Gastric, peritoneal, pleural, or bladder lavage with cold fluids.
- Benzodiazepines to suppress shivering and endogenous heat production.
- Dantrolene, a non-specific skeletal muscle relaxant, may be used in the management of malignant hyperthermia.

Antipyretics are of no use in the management of hyperthermia. Antipyretics act by lowering the elevated thermal set point in fever, but in hyperthermia the set point is normal so they have no effect on the body temperature.

KEY POINTS

Fever results from elevation of the hypothalamic thermal set point due to the actions of prostaglandin E_2.
Causes of fever include:

- Infection
- Malignancy
- Hypersensitivity reaction to drugs
- Blood transfusions
- Graft-versus-host disease
- Thrombosis
- CNS haemorrhage
- Connective tissue disorders
- Inflammatory

Fever of unknown origin is defined as a febrile illness lasting more than three weeks, with temperatures exceeding 38.3°C on several occasions, and lacking a definitive diagnosis after one week of evaluation in hospital.
Assessment of fever requires careful history taking, medication review, and a thorough physical examination.
Antipyretic agents act by lowering the elevated thermal set point by inhibiting cyclooxygenase. Inhibition of cyclooxygenase impairs the production of prostaglandin E_2.
Neutropenic sepsis is the presence of infection in patients who have a neutrophil count of $<1.0 \times 10^9/L$ and systemic signs of sepsis.
Neutropenic sepsis is initially treated in an identical manner to non-neutropenic severe sepsis and septic shock.
Hyperthermia has a different pathophysiology to fever and is the result of uncontrolled increases in body temperature. The body's ability to lose heat is overwhelmed by disease, drugs, or excessive external or internal heat production.

15.3 Central nervous system infections

15.3.1 Introduction

Central nervous system infections are relatively rare but are an important differential diagnosis in the unwell ED patient. Delayed treatment can result in significant increases in morbidity and mortality.

The CNS is an area of relative immunodeficiency with lower levels of complement and immunoglobulin. The choroid plexus is a common portal of entry for haematogenous spread into the cerebrospinal fluid (CSF).

The text which follows here covers meningitis, encephalitis, cerebral abscess, and cerebral malaria. Section 15.4 covers meningococcal meningitis and septicaemia in more detail.

15.3.2 Causes and clinical features of meningitis

Meningitis may be caused by bacterial, viral, fungal, or tuberculous infection. Most cases of meningitis in the United Kingdom are bacterial or viral. The key discriminators between bacterial and viral meningitis are the speed of onset and severity of symptoms. Bacterial meningitis tends to have a much more rapid onset and more severe symptoms.

When patients present to the ED with a potential CNS infection the cause is unknown and clinical features have to be used to determine the most likely pathogen and direct treatment appropriately. Table 15.7 details causes of meningitis and clinical features that may help differentiate them.

Bacterial meningitis

Bacterial meningitis can affect anyone of any age, but mainly affects babies, young children, and adolescents. Risk factors include season (with more cases occurring in the winter months), exposure to smoke, recent influenza A infection, and living in 'closed' communities, such as university halls of residence and military barracks.

The epidemiology of bacterial meningitis in the United Kingdom has changed dramatically in the past two decades following the introduction of vaccines to control *Haemophilus influenzae* type b (Hib), serogroup C meningococcus, and some types of pneumococcus. As no vaccine is currently licensed against serogroup B meningococcus, this pathogen is now the most common cause of bacterial meningitis (and septicaemia) in children and young people aged three months or older (see Table 15.8).

15.3.3 Encephalitis

Encephalitis is inflammation of the brain parenchyma. Clinical features include fever, altered level of consciousness, headache, psychiatric symptoms, seizures, vomiting, focal neurological signs, and memory loss.

Encephalitis is usually caused by a viral infection, the most severe of which is herpes simplex virus (HSV). Other infections that may cause encephalitis include mumps, measles, varicella, rubella, adenovirus, cytomegalovirus, Lyme's disease, syphilis, and tuberculosis (TB).

15.3.4 Brain abscesses

Brain abscesses usually arise as a consequence of the direct spread of infection from chronic sinusitis, otitis media, dental abscess, neurosurgical procedures, or penetrating head injury. They can also occur via haematogenous seeding from remote sources.

Streptococcus viridans is the commonest pathogen.

Inflammation and oedema around the site of the abscess lead to signs of a space-occupying lesion (e.g. headache, vomiting, reduced level of consciousness, and focal neurological signs). The classic triad is headache, fever, and focal neurological signs.

15.3.5 Cerebral malaria

The definition of cerebral malaria is coma in a patient with a *Plasmodium falciparum* infection, and no other cause for the coma.

Patients with malaria usually have a non-specific and irregular fever, rigors, headache, and malaise.

Table 15.7 Causes and clinical features of meningitis

Type of meningitis	Cause	Clinical features	Morbidity and mortality
Bacterial meningitis	Meningococcal (commonest cause of meningitis in the UK) More prevalent in winter months	Acute onset illness Headache Nausea and/or vomiting Neck stiffness Focal neurological signs Altered level of consciousness A petechial rash may be seen in meningococcal septicaemia	Mortality 19–25% in meningococcal septicaemia Lowest risk of neurological sequelae compared to pneumococcal and *H. influenzae* meningitis
	Pneumococcal (second commonest cause of meningitis in the UK)	As for meningococcal disease except no petechial rash	20% mortality 40% have long-term sequelae (e.g. deafness, seizures, functional impairment)
	Haemophilus (uncommon since introduction of Hib vaccine)	As for meningococcal disease except no petechial rash	Mortality rate <5% 20% have long-term neurological sequelae
Viral meningitis	More common in the summer Causes include enteroviruses (commonest), HSV, VZV, and mumps (rare since the introduction of MMR vaccine) 50% of cases no cause found HIV and EBV are important causes of viral meningitis in immunocompromized patients	Subacute illness of 1–7 days High fever Headache	Usually self-limiting Those with HSV infections have a risk of developing HSV encephalitis heralded by increasing confusion and worsening fever HSV encephalitis has a 70% mortality rate

(continued)

Table 15.7 Continued

Type of meningitis	Cause	Clinical features	Morbidity and mortality
Cryptococcal meningitis	*Cryptococcus neoformans* is a fungal infection acquired by inhaling dust containing the fungus Usually seen in immunocompromised hosts. Cryptococcal meningitis is an AIDS-defining illness	Chronic or subacute symptoms Fever of unknown origin Chronic headaches Personality change Confusion Lethargy	It is not possible to cure cryptococcal meningitis in patients with AIDS Mortality rate 25–30%. 40% of survivors have significant neurological sequelae (e.g. loss of vision, cranial nerve palsies, hydrocephalus)
Tuberculous meningitis	Usually seen in immunocompromised hosts Patients who have not received a BCG vaccine are at greater risk Common secondary infection in patients with HIV	More indolent presentation than bacterial meningitis Non-specific prodrome of headache, lethargy, photophobia, and fever Most cases present within 2 weeks of symptom onset Symptoms of meningism are rare in the immunocompromized	Significant mortality in patients with HIV

Table 15.8 Causes of bacterial meningitis

Age group	Commonest causes of bacterial meningitis
Neonates (<28 days old)	*Streptococcus agalactiae* (Group B *Streptococcus*), *Escherichia coli*, *Streptococcus pneumoniae*, and *Listeria monocytogenes*
Infants	*Neisseria meningitidis* (meningococcus), *Streptococcus pneumoniae* (pneumococcus), and *Haemophilus influenzae* type b (Hib)
Children	*Neisseria meningitidis*, *Streptococcus pneumoniae*
Adults	*Streptococcus pneumoniae*, *Neisseria meningitidis*, and *Mycobacteria*

Patients with cerebral malaria have additional features, which may be predominantly cortical signs (drowsiness, confusion, seizures, and/or decorticate rigidity) or brainstem signs (decerebrate rigidity, pupillary abnormalities, abnormal respiratory patterns, and/or gaze palsies).

15.3.6 Investigations for central nervous system infections

The initial ED diagnosis of a CNS infection is a clinical one. Investigations should be performed to guide and inform subsequent management.

If a patient is unwell with suspected CNS infection, treatment should not be delayed pending results. A third-generation cephalosporin (e.g. IV ceftriaxone) should be given immediately.

The following investigations should be performed:

- FBC and CRP—a raised white cell count (WCC) and CRP are supportive of infection but normal values do not rule it out. Patients with septicaemia are at risk of thrombocytopenia.
- U&E and calcium and magnesium—metabolic derangement is common in septicaemia and may contribute to myocardial dysfunction. Renal failure is a common complication of septicaemia.
- LFTs and clotting—patients are at risk of disseminated intravascular coagulation (DIC) and liver failure.
- Group and save—patients may require blood products for the treatment of DIC.
- Blood glucose—hypoglycaemia is common, particularly in children.
- Arterial blood gas—probably the most useful initial blood test in the ED. The ABG provides information about the acid-base state and ventilatory status.
- Microbiology—blood cultures, throat swab, clotted blood for serology, and ethylenediaminetetraacetic acid (EDTA) sample for polymerase chain reaction (PCR) should be sent.

Lumbar puncture

Lumbar puncture is an important investigation for suspected meningitis, particularly if the clinical diagnosis is in doubt (Table 15.9). Even if there are obvious meningeal symptoms, microbiological confirmation is valuable for determining the duration of treatment, decisions about prophylaxis and public health management, disease surveillance, and follow-up care for those with neurological sequelae.

Lumbar puncture must not be performed when there are contraindications and should never delay treatment. With modern PCR techniques, CSF samples may still be positive after antibiotics.

Contraindications to lumbar puncture:

- Signs and symptoms of raised intracranial pressure
- Shock

Table 15.9 CSF findings in meningitis of different aetiologies

	Bacterial	Viral	Tuberculous
Appearance	Often turbid	Usually clear	Often fibrin web
Predominant cell	Polymorphs (neutrophilic)	Mononuclear	Mononuclear
Cell count/mm^3	100—5000	50–1000	50–300
Glucose	<½ plasma	>½ plasma	<½ plasma
Protein (g/L)	>1.5	<1	1–5
Organisms	In smear and culture	Not in smear or culture	Often absent in smear

- Extensive or spreading purpura
- After convulsions until stabilized
- Coagulation abnormalities
- Platelet count <100 × 10^9/L
- Anticoagulant therapy
- Local superficial infection at the lumbar puncture site
- Respiratory insufficiency

CSF examination should include white blood cell count and examination, total protein and glucose concentrations, gram stain, and microbiological culture. The opening pressure should be noted.

CT scan

A CT scan is not recommended to exclude raised intracranial pressure prior to a lumbar puncture. Clinical assessment is the recommended method of assessing whether there is raised intracranial pressure. A CT may be normal and the patient can still have raised intracranial pressure and be at risk of herniation.

A CT is recommended to detect other intracranial pathology if the level of consciousness is reduced or fluctuating, or if there are focal neurological signs (e.g. suspected HSV encephalitis, brain abscess, etc.).

CT should not delay treatment and the patient should be stabilized prior to performing the scan.

15.3.7 Emergency department management of central nervous system infections

Patients with a suspected CNS infection should receive a third-generation cephalosporin (e.g. ceftriaxone) urgently.

All patients should be assessed in an ABCDE manner and receive good supportive care. Hypoglycaemia is a potential cause of neurological signs and a common complication of CNS infections. The blood glucose level must be regularly monitored and hypoglycaemia treated with 10% glucose IV if present.

Further management of CNS infection depends on the suspected cause (e.g. bacterial meningitis, viral meningitis, HSV encephalitis, cerebral malaria, and so on—see Table 15.10).

A more detailed discussion of the management of meningococcal meningitis and septicaemia is included in section 15.4.

Corticosteroids

The Meningitis Research Foundation and NICE recommend administration of corticosteroids to:

Table 15.10 Empirical treatment of CNS infections

Suspected diagnosis	Host factors	Additional organism to cover	Third-generation cephalosporin plus
Bacterial meningitis	Adult		Nil
	Age >55 years	Gram-negative L. monocytogenes	Ampicillin
	Neonate	Enterococcus L. monocytogenes	Ampicillin
Viral meningitis		Enteroviruses Herpes virus Mumps	Aciclovir
High risk of abscess	Recent surgery or ventriculopertioneal shunt	Strep. epidermidis	Vancomycin Amikacin
Fungal meningitis	Immunocompromized		Amphotericin B, flucytosine
TB meningitis	Immunocompromized Alcoholics	Cryptococcus	Rifampicin, isoniazid, and pyrazinamide for 2 months Rifampicin plus isoniazid for 4–7 months
	Without HIV	Cryptococcus	Amphotericin B alone for 6–10 weeks or flucytosine for 2 weeks then fluconazole for at least 10 weeks
Cerebral malaria			Quinine IV (can be given orally once patient able to swallow)

- Adults with suspected bacterial meningitis, particularly when pneumococcus is suspected.
- Children who have lumbar puncture results that suggest bacterial meningitis.

The recommended agent and dose is dexamethasone 0.15 mg/kg qds for four days. Dexamethasone should be given with, or just before, the first dose of antibiotics in adults. In children dexamethasone can be given if fewer than 12 hours have elapsed since the first dose of antibiotics.

Corticosteroids are not recommended acutely if the patient is septicaemic or shocked with their CNS infection.

Neurosurgical intervention

Neurosurgical intervention (e.g. catheter drainage or excision of the abscess) is indicated in the following circumstances:

- Abscess with mass effect
- Abscess lying in close proximity to the ventricular system
- Hydrocephalus

KEY POINTS

Bacterial meningitis is, typically, an acute and rapid disease process. Classic symptoms include headache, nausea or vomiting, and neck pain.

The epidemiology of bacterial meningitis in the United Kingdom has changed dramatically in the past two decades following the introduction of the Hib, serogroup C meningococcus, and pneumococcus vaccines.

In September 2015 a new vaccine against serogroup B meningococcus was introduced for the under ones, as it is now the most common cause of bacterial meningitis (and septicaemia) in children and young people aged three months or older.

Viral meningitis is generally less severe than bacterial and often resolves without specific treatment.

Cryptococcal and TB meningitis are most commonly seen in immunocompromized patients. Clinical features can be very non-specific.

Patients with suspected meningitis should receive a third-generation cephalosporin (e.g. ceftriaxone) urgently. Treatment should not be delayed to perform a lumbar puncture or CT.

Adults with suspected pneumococcal meningitis should receive dexamethasone with or before their first dose of antibiotics.

15.4 Meningococcal meningitis and septicaemia

15.4.1 Introduction

Meningitis is a disease caused by the inflammation of the meninges. The inflammation is usually caused by an infection of the cerebrospinal fluid, but may also result from physical injury, cancer, or drugs.

This section focuses on *Neisseria meningitidis* (meningococcus) the commonest cause of bacterial meningitis in the United Kingdom.

Meningococcal disease can kill within hours of the first symptoms and is the leading infectious cause of death in UK children. It is associated with a significant risk of mortality and long-term morbidity.

The following section is based on the guidance from the Meningitis Research Foundation, which is endorsed by the Royal College of Emergency Medicine. The guidance from the Meningitis Research Foundation incorporates and is consistent with the NICE Guideline on Bacterial Meningitis and Meningococcal Septicaemia in Children and Young People.

15.4.2 Pathophysiology of meningococcal infection

Meningococci commonly colonize the human nasopharynx. About 1 in 10 people carry them in their nose and throat, and usually this is harmless. However, in some people, the bacteria are able to penetrate the defensive mucosal lining of the nose and throat to enter the bloodstream. Once in the bloodstream, meningococci multiply rapidly, doubling their numbers every 30 minutes.

Meningococcal disease has two main clinical presentations: meningitis (15% of cases) and septicaemia (25% of cases). However, it most commonly presents as a combination of the two syndromes (60% of cases). Septicaemia is more dangerous and most likely to be fatal when it occurs without meningitis.

Pathophysiology of meningococcal septicaemia

Meningococci in the bloodstream cause septicaemia. As they multiply, they shed endotoxin from their outer coat. Endotoxin is the prime initiator of gram-negative bacterial septic shock. Levels of circulating endotoxin correlate with disease severity.

The main processes involved in the pathophysiology of septicaemia are increased vascular permeability, myocardial dysfunction, and disseminated intravascular coagulation (see section 15.1 pathophysiology of sepsis).

Endothelial damage allows blood and other fluid to haemorrhage out into the surrounding tissues. This occurs in all small vessels in the body but is most obvious in skin, hence the hallmark non-blanching rash. Widespread clotting and haemorrhaging in small vessels in fingers, toes, and sometimes entire limbs can lead to necrosis and eventual amputation.

Death in this group of patients is from shock and multiple organ failure.

Pathophysiology of meningococcal meningitis

Meningococcal meningitis generally has a better prognosis than septicaemia.

Meningococci reach the brain from the bloodstream, implying that the patient's immune response has prevented bacterial proliferation in the blood and not suffered overwhelming sepsis. This is because organisms are handled differently in these patients, which is probably due to differences in their inflammatory response to infection, as well as different bacterial characteristics.

Deaths do occur, however, due to the severity of the inflammatory process within the brain. Once bacteria penetrate the blood–brain barrier, endotoxin and inflammatory mediators initiate a CSF inflammatory response, causing leakage of protein and fluid out of the cerebral vasculature. This results in cerebral oedema and an increase in intracranial pressure.

In addition, endothelial damage activates the coagulation cascade and platelets rush to the site of damage leading to clot formation and cerebral vascular thrombosis.

Both the increased pressure and thrombosis may lead to a reduction in cerebral perfusion, and consequently cerebral infarction, and sometimes brain death.

15.4.3 Clinical features of meningococcal disease

Meningococcal disease is extremely unpredictable. The presentation can be very varied and patients may be difficult to differentiate from those with viral illnesses during the early stages.

Prodromal phase

Initially the clinical features of meningitis and septicaemia may be very non-specific and impossible to distinguish from someone with a milder self-limiting illness. For this reason it is important to provide a 'safety net' if patients with a non-specific febrile illness are discharged from the ED.

Prodromal symptoms include:

- Fever
- Nausea, vomiting
- Lethargy
- Malaise

Differentiating meningococcal disease

Over time, the symptoms and signs of meningococcal disease develop and patients may show features that suggest a predominantly meningitic picture or a predominantly septicaemic picture. However, most patients will have a mixed picture (Table 15.11).

The clinical features may vary depending on the age of the patient. Young babies may have very non-specific features including:

- Poor feeding
- Irritability
- High pitched or moaning cry
- Abnormal tone or abnormal posturing
- Vacant staring, poorly responsive, or lethargic

Table 15.11 Clinical features that help differentiate meningococcal septicaemia and meningitis

Clinical features suggestive of septicaemia	Clinical features suggestive of meningitis
• Limb/joint pain • Cold hands and feet and prolonged capillary refill • Pale or mottled skin • Tachycardia • Tachypnoea • Rigors • Oliguria/thirst • Rash anywhere on the body (may not be an early symptom) • Abdominal pain (sometimes with diarrhoea) • Drowsiness/confusion/impaired consciousness (late sign in children) • Hypotension (very late, pre-terminal sign in children)	• Severe headache • Neck stiffness (not always present in young children) • Photophobia (not always present in young children) • Drowsiness/confusion/impaired consciousness • Seizures (late sign)

• Tense fontanelle
• Cyanosis

Management of the feverish child is covered in more detail in Chapter 19, section 19.16.

The rash

A non-blanching haemorrhagic rash is characteristic of meningococcal disease, and a rapidly evolving purpuric rash is a feature of severe disease, requiring urgent, aggressive treatment. However, in the early stages the rash may be absent, scanty, atypical (e.g. macular or maculo-papular), or blanching. A rash is more common in patients with meningococcal septicaemia than those with pure meningitis and by the time a rash appears, the underlying disease may be very advanced.

The rash can be more difficult to see on dark skin, but may be visible in paler areas, especially the soles of the feet, palms of the hands, abdomen, or on the conjunctivae or palate.

Once the rash is advanced, purpuric areas can look like bruises and be confused with injury or abuse. Extensive purpuric areas are called 'purpura fulminans'. When this occurs, tissues may be irreversibly destroyed due to thrombosis within the microvasculature, combined with vasocon-striction and ischaemia in the peripheries. The extremities are normally worst affected; often the feet and hands, and sometimes the ears, nose, or lips.

Clinical warning signs

During the assessment of a patient with suspected meningococcal disease, warning signs for septic shock and raised intracranial pressure should be looked for. These signs predict severe disease, the need for urgent senior medical involvement, and guide the subsequent management of the patient.

Signs of septic shock:

• Tachycardia or bradycardia
• Prolonged capillary refill time (>2 seconds)
• Cold hands/feet; pale or blue skin
• Respiratory distress (tachypnoea or bradypnoea)/oxygen saturation <95% in air
• Altered mental state/decreased conscious level
• Decreased urine output (<1 ml/kg/hour)
• Hypotension (late sign)

- Hypoxia
- Acidosis (base deficit worse than -5 mmol/L or pH <7.3)
- Increased lactate (>2 mmol/L)

Signs of raised intracranial pressure:

- Reduced (GCS <12) or fluctuating level of consciousness
- Relative bradycardia and hypertension
- Focal neurological signs
- Abnormal posture or posturing
- Seizures
- Unequal, dilated, or poorly responsive pupils
- Papilloedema (late sign)
- Abnormal 'doll's eye' movements

15.4.4 Investigations for suspected meningococcal disease

The initial ED diagnosis of meningococcal disease is a clinical one. Investigations should be performed to guide and inform subsequent management as discussed in section 15.3.

If a patient is unwell with suspected meningococcal disease, treatment should not be delayed pending results and IV ceftriaxone or cefotaxime should be given immediately.

15.4.5 Emergency department management of meningococcal disease

The recommended management for meningococcal disease depends on the age of the patient (adult or child) and whether the patient has predominantly meningitic or septicaemic clinical features. Therefore, the following text covers the management of meningococcal disease in children and adults separately.

15.4.6 Emergency department management of meningococcal disease in children and young people

Initial management

The most important initial management step in a child or young person with suspected meningococcal disease is antibiotics.

A third-generation cephalosporin should be given immediately to children and young people with a petechial rash if any of the following occur at any point during the assessment (these children are at high risk of having meningococcal disease):

- Petechiae start to spread.
- The rash becomes purpuric.
- There are signs of bacterial meningitis.
- There are signs of meningococcal septicaemia.
- The patient appears ill.

Empirical antibiotics for meningococcal meningitis or septicaemia

- Age >3 months—intravenous ceftriaxone 80 mg/kg.
- Age <3 months—intravenous cefotaxime 80 mg/kg (ceftriaxone may exacerbate hyperbilirubinaemia especially if the infant is premature, or has jaundice, hypoalbuminaemia, or acidosis). In addition, infants should receive ampicillin or amoxicillin to cover for listeria monocytogenes.
- If herpes simplex meningoencephalitis is part of the differential diagnosis an antiviral should also be given (e.g. aciclovir).

Table 15.12 Antibiotics for confirmed meningitis

Specific infection	Recommended antibiotic
H. influenza	Ceftriaxone
S. pneumoniae	Ceftriaxone
Group B Strep.	Cefotaxime
L. monocytogenes	Amoxicillin or ampicillin
Gram-negative bacilli	Cefotaxime

Once the specific infection is identified, the antibiotic regime can be adjusted. The recommended antibiotics for specific infections are detailed in Table 15.12.

Supportive management

Patients with suspected meningococcal meningitis and/or septicaemia should be managed in an ABCDE manner.

- **Airway and breathing**—ensure an adequate and maintained airway. Patients should receive high-flow oxygen to optimize tissue oxygenation. Intubation and ventilation should be undertaken for the following indications:
  - Threatened or actual loss of airway patency.
  - The need for any form of assisted ventilation (e.g. bag–mask ventilation).
  - Increasing work of breathing.
  - Hypoventilation or apnoea.
  - Features of respiratory failure, including irregular respiration, hypoxia, or hypercapnea.
  - Continuing shock following infusion of a total of 40 ml/kg of resuscitation fluid.
  - Signs of raised intracranial pressure.
  - Impaired mental status (reduced or fluctuating level of consciousness—GCS <9 or a drop of ≥3).
  - Moribund state.
  - Control of intractable seizures.
  - Need for stabilization and management to allow brain imaging or transfer to the intensive care unit or another hospital.
- **Circulation and fluid management**—the goal of circulatory support is the maintenance of tissue perfusion and oxygenation. Intravenous or intraosseous access should be secured.

The recommended fluid management depends on whether the patient has signs of shock, dehydration, or raised intracranial pressure (see Table 15.13).

- **Disability and raised intracranial pressure**—patients may have raised intracranial pressure, seizures, and/or hypoglycaemia.

Raised intracranial pressure

- The main objective of managing patients with raised intracranial pressure is to maintain oxygenation and perfusion of the brain.
- Patients with a reduced or fluctuating level of consciousness should have their airway secured by tracheal intubation and mechanical ventilation. Ventilation should be optimized to ensure normocapnea and avoid hypoxia.

Table 15.13 Fluid resuscitation in meningococcal disease

Patients with signs of shock	Patients with bacterial meningitis without signs of shock	Patients with signs of raised intracranial pressure
Immediate bolus of 20 ml/kg of 0.9% sodium chloride over 5–10 min. If signs of shock persist then a second bolus of 20 ml/kg of 0.9% sodium chloride or 4.5% human albumin should be given. If signs of shock continue then a third 20-ml/kg bolus of 0.9% sodium chloride or 4.5% human albumin should be given. Patients requiring >40 ml/kg fluid resuscitation require the following: • Rapid intubation and ventilation due to the risk of pulmonary oedema. • Peripheral inotropes (dopamine IV or adrenaline IO). • Central venous access • Urinary catheter • Nasogastric tube Large volumes of fluid may be required (>60 ml/kg in the first hour) and should be guided by the clinical signs.	Correction of dehydration—enteral fluids or feeds, or IV isotonic fluids (e.g. 0.9% sodium chloride with 5% glucose). Maintenance fluids to avoid hypoglycaemia and maintain electrolyte balance.	Cautious fluid resuscitation is required (but co-existing shock should be corrected). Fluid management should be discussed with and guided by a paediatric intensivist. Fluid restriction may be required. Mannitol or 3% saline (hypertonic) should be considered.

• The goal of fluid management is to maintain circulating volume and adequate blood pressure. Overzealous fluid resuscitation will exacerbate cerebral oedema. Only patients with shock require aggressive fluid resuscitation to ensure cerebral perfusion. Patients without shock require close monitoring and judicious fluid replacement depending on heart rate, blood pressure, urine output, and metabolic acidosis.
• Mannitol or hypertonic saline should be considered for acute rises in intracranial pressure suggested by pupillary changes or sudden hypertension and bradycardia.
• Patients should be nursed 30° head up.
• CVP line insertion should be avoided in the internal jugular as this may impede venous drainage of the head and insertion requires a head-down position, which may exacerbate raised intracranial pressure.

Seizures

Seizures should be managed in a stepwise manner with benzodiazepines and phenytoin as for status epilepticus (see Chapter 11, section 11.6).

Hypoglycaemia

Hypoglycaemia is common and should be corrected with boluses of 2 ml/kg of 10% glucose IV. Blood glucose should be checked hourly.

Further management

The focus of a SAQ on the management of meningococcal disease is likely to be the initial interventions such as early antibiotics, airway management, and fluid resuscitation. However, questions may require knowledge of some of the further management steps which might occur on paediatric intensive care.

- Corticosteroids—are not usually indicated in the ED for the management of bacterial meningitis in children and young people. Dexamethasone may be indicated if the results of the lumbar puncture suggest bacterial meningitis. However, lumbar punctures are rarely performed on children in the ED and the results are seldom available while the patient is still being managed in the ED.
- Metabolic problems—may develop and should be monitored for and corrected if present (e.g. hypoglycaemia, acidosis, hypokalaemia, hypocalcaemia, hypomagnesaemia, anaemia, and coagulopathy).
- Hyperthermia—should be managed with antipyretics.
- Inotropes—may be changed once a central route is available. Options include dopamine, noradrenaline, and adrenaline.

15.4.7 Emergency department management of meningococcal disease in adults

The management of meningococcal meningitis and septicaemia in adults follows a very similar format to the management in children. The main differences are:

- Antibiotics—2 g IV ceftriaxone or cefotaxime should be given immediately in suspected meningococcal septicaemia. In patients with suspected bacterial meningitis, a lumbar puncture may be performed first, provided there are no signs of raised intracranial pressure, shock, or respiratory failure. If the lumbar puncture will delay antibiotics by more than 30 minutes, these should be given first. In patients over the age 55 years, ampicillin 2 g IV should be given as well to cover for *Listeria monocytogenes*.
- Fluid management—is not as prescriptive in the adult guideline as in the paediatric. However, a stepwise approach similar to the paediatric guidance is appropriate. Caution is required in patients with a history of heart failure and CVP monitoring may be required to guide fluid resuscitation.
- Corticosteroids—should be considered for adults with predominantly meningitic symptoms, particularly where pneumococcal meningitis is suspected. The recommended dose of dexamethasone is 0.15 mg/kg qds for four days and should be given with or just before the first dose of antibiotics. Corticosteroids should not be given unless there is confidence that the correct antimicrobial is being used. Corticosteroids are not recommended acutely for patients with predominantly septicaemic symptoms; however, they may be considered, at physiological doses, for refractory shock on intensive care.

15.4.8 Public health issues

Notification

Bacterial meningitis and meningococcal septicaemia are notifiable diseases. The consultant in communicable disease control (CCDC) must be informed of suspected cases. This is the legal duty of the doctor who makes or suspects the diagnosis.

Prophylaxis

Prophylaxis is required for close contacts living in the same household as the patient in the seven days before disease onset, or kissing contacts.

Healthcare staff only require prophylaxis if their mouth or nose has been splattered with large particle droplets/secretions from the respiratory tract of the patient.

The CCDC arranges for prophylactic antibiotics to be prescribed, as necessary. Rifampicin, ciprofloxacin, and ceftriaxone are all recommended for use in preventing secondary cases of meningococcal disease.

Antibiotic prophylaxis should eliminate carriage, but if the contact is already incubating the bacteria, s/he can still get the disease. Therefore, contacts should be counselled about the risk and alerted to the symptoms to look out for.

The CCDC will arrange for close contacts to have immunizations, if required. They will also ensure information is disseminated to appropriate schools, work places, and general practitioners.

15.4.9 Complications of meningococcal disease

One in five survivors of meningococcal disease experiences reduced quality of life and approximately one in seven has neurological or sensory disability, amputation or tissue loss, or other lifelong sequelae.

Complications include:

- Multiple organ failure and death
- Amputation or tissue loss
- Limb deformities
- Loss of hearing or sight
- Intellectual impairment
- Motor and coordination deficits
- Epilepsy
- Psychological disorders

KEY POINTS

Meningococcus serogroup B is now the most common cause of bacterial meningitis and septicaemia in the United Kingdom. Meningococcal B vaccine was introduced in the United Kingdom in September 2015, initially for all babies born on or after 1 July 2015.

Meningococcal disease has two main clinical presentations: meningitis (15% of cases) and septicaemia (25% of cases). However, it most commonly presents as a combination of the two syndromes (60% of cases).

Meningococcal septicaemia has a higher mortality that meningococcal meningitis, and is most likely to be fatal when it occurs without concurrent meningitis.

The clinical features of meningococcal disease can be very non-specific (e.g. fever, malaise, nausea, lethargy) during the early stages. As the disease progresses, clinical features may suggest a predominantly septicaemic or meningitic picture.

Features suggestive of septicaemia include:

Limb/joint pain	Cold hands and feet and prolonged capillary refill
Pale or mottled skin	Tachycardia
Tachypnoea	Rigors
Oliguria/thirst	Rash anywhere on the body
Abdominal pain	Drowsiness/confusion/impaired consciousness
Hypotension	

Features suggestive of meningitis include:

Severe headache	Neck stiffness
Photophobia seizures	Drowsiness/confusion/impaired consciousness

The most important initial management step in a patient with suspected meningococcal disease is intravenous antibiotics (e.g. ceftriaxone or cefotaxime).

Supportive management should follow an ABCDE structure.

Corticosteroids (e.g. dexamethasone 0.15 mg/kg) should be considered for adults with predominantly meningitic symptoms, particularly where pneumococcal meningitis is suspected. They are only indicated in children and young people if the lumbar puncture result suggests bacterial meningitis.

Corticosteroids are not recommended acutely for adult patients with predominantly septicaemic symptoms.

Bacterial meningitis and meningococcal septicaemia are notifiable diseases. The consultant in communicable disease control must be informed of suspected cases.

Prophylaxis is required for household and kissing contacts.

15.5 Viral haemorrhagic fever

Viral haemorrhagic fevers (VHFs) are severe, life-threatening viral diseases which are endemic in parts of Africa, South America, the Middle East, and Eastern Europe. The viruses are geographically restricted to the areas of their animal or insect host species. Environmental conditions do not allow any natural reservoirs or vectors of haemorrhagic fever viruses in the United Kingdom.

VHF should be considered in any patient with the following clinical presentation:

- Acute onset of fever (<3 weeks duration) in a severely ill patient
- Haemorrhagic manifestations—at least two of the following: haemorrhagic or purpuric rash, epistaxis, haematemesis, haemoptysis, blood in stool, or other bleeding
- No conditions predisposing for haemorrhagic illness
- No alternative diagnosis

Viral haemorrhagic fevers can spread rapidly within a hospital setting, can be difficult to recognize rapidly, have a high case-fatality rate, and no effective treatment.

The main transmission routes are direct contact through broken skin or mucous membranes, with blood or body fluids (during invasive, aerosolizing or splash procedures), or indirect contact with environments, surfaces, equipment, or clothing contaminated with splashes or droplets of blood or body fluids. There is no circumstantial or epidemiological evidence of aerosol transmission risk.

15.5.1 Viral haemorrhagic fever risk assessment

- **Fever** (>38 C) or history of fever in previous 24 hours
- **AND a travel history** (return from, or currently residing in VHF endemic country)
- **OR epidemiological exposure** (cared for/came into contact with body fluids of/handled clinical specimens –blood, urine, faeces, tissues, laboratory cultures) from an individual or laboratory animal known or strongly suspected to have VHF) within 21 days

Additional questions with a positive travel history:

- Travel to any area with a current VHF outbreak
- Lived and worked in basic rural conditions where lassa fever is endemic
- Visited caves or mines, or had contact with primates, antelopes or bats in a Marburg/Ebola endemic area
- Travel in an area where Crimean-Congo haemorrhagic fever is endemic and sustained tick bite or crushed tick with bare hands or had close involvement with animal slaughter

Isolation and infection risk

Minimal risk:

- Standard precautions apply: hand hygiene, gloves, plastic apron
- Eye protection and fluid repellent surgical facemask for splash-inducing procedures

Staff at risk:

- Hand hygiene
- Gloves
- Plastic apron
- Fluid repellent surgical face mask
- Eye protection (goggles or face shield-full face visor)
- FFP3 respirator (light weight, contoured fit, single use respirator with exhalation valve and low breathing resistance), or EN certified equivalent for aerosol generating procedures

Patients with extensive bruising, active bleeding, uncontrolled diarrhoea, uncontrolled vomiting:

- Hand hygiene
- Double gloves
- Fluid repellent disposable gown or suit
- Disposable shoe covers
- Eye protection
- FFP3 respirator or EN certified equivalent

Staff at high risk:

- Hand hygiene
- Double gloves
- Fluid repellent disposable gown or suit
- Plastic apron (over disposable gown or suit)
- Eye protection
- FFP3 respirator or EN certified equivalent

Reassess VHF risk if patient with relevant exposure history fails to improve or develops:

- Nose bleed
- Bloody diarrhoea
- Sudden rise in AST
- Sudden fall in platelets
- Clinical shock
- Rapidly increasing oxygen requirements in the absence of other diagnoses

Viral haemorrhagic fevers screening

- Contact **Imported Fever Service** (0844 778 8990)

- **Rare and Imported Pathogens Laboratory** (RIPL), PHE Porton, Porton Down, Salisbury, Wiltshire SP4 0JG (01980 612 100)
- If RIPL not available, **Microbiology Services Division**-Colindale, 61 Colindale Avenue. Colindale, London NW9 5HT (020 8200 4400/6868)

15.6 Needlestick injuries

15.6.1 Introduction

The main group of workers at risk from needlestick injuries are those within the healthcare sector. Out of hours, most EDs act as the site of advice and treatment for needlestick injuries.

Knowledge of the management of needlestick injuries is included as one of the additional acute presentations in the CT3 year. The management of needlestick injuries has appeared in previous SAQs.

15.6.2 Risks from needlestick injuries

The main risk posed from a needlestick injury is exposure to blood-borne viruses (Table 15.14). The principle blood-borne viruses of concern are hepatitis B (HBV), hepatitis C (HCV), and HIV.

The factors to be considered when determining whether a needlestick injury is high risk include: the mechanism of injury; the bodily fluid involved; and the characteristics of the donor patient (Table 15.15).

Factors that reduce the risk of transmission of a blood-borne virus include:

- Recipient wearing gloves
- Wound immediately bled and irrigated
- Skin intact
- No blood visible on device
- Bodily fluid was urine, faeces, or saliva (not bloodstained)
- Recipient has confirmed immunity against HBV
- Donor not known to have any risk factors for blood-borne viruses

15.6.3 Emergency department management of needlestick injuries

Patients should be seen urgently following a needlestick injury so that HIV post-exposure prophylaxis, where indicated, can be started promptly, and if possible within one hour of injury.

Table 15.14 Risk of transmission after exposure to infected blood

Blood-borne virus	Risk of transmission following a percutaneous injury
Hepatitis B	30%
Hepatitis C	3%
HIV	0.3% (mucocutaneous <0.1%)

Data from Department of Health. HIV Post-exposure prophylaxis: Guidance from the UK Chief Medical Officers' Expert Advisory Group on AIDS. London: Department of Health, September 2008.

Table 15.15 High-risk factors for blood-borne viral transmission following a needlestick injury

Mechanism of injury	Bodily fluid	Donor
• Hollow, wide-bore needle • Visible blood on the device • Gloves not worn • Deep puncture wound • Injury with needle that had been placed in the donor's artery or vein • Contaminated material injected • Exposure through broken skin or mucous membranes	• Blood • Peritoneal fluid • Pleural fluid • Pericardial fluid • Cerebrospinal fluid • Synovial fluid • Amniotic fluid • Vaginal secretions or semen • Human breast milk • Bloodstained saliva	• HCV, HBV, or HIV positive • Terminal HIV-related illness • Acute liver disease • IVDU (past or present) • Recipient of blood products or organ • From a country with a high prevalence of blood-borne viral disease • Homosexual men

The ED management should involve:

- First aid—patients who have sustained a puncture wound or cut should gently encourage bleeding of the wound and wash the area with soap and running water. Those with contamination of a mucous membrane should irrigate it copiously with water.
- Risk assessment—the recipient (i.e. the healthcare professional) should be asked about the nature of the injury, particularly focusing on high-risk factors as detailed in Table 15.15. A risk assessment should be made of the donor, which may be most appropriately performed by the ward doctor.
- Immunization status of recipient—the recipient should be asked about their hepatitis B immunization status.
- Blood tests—the recipient should have blood sent to determine their hepatitis B antibody titre and serum saved for possible future baseline HIV/HCV testing. The donor's blood should be sent for hepatitis B antigen, hepatitis C, and HIV testing. Informed consent must be obtained from the donor before the sample can be taken.
- Post-exposure prophylaxis—the risk assessment should determine the need for hepatitis B immunization and HIV post-exposure prophylaxis.
- Follow-up—should be arranged with occupational health the following day.

Hepatitis B vaccination

All healthcare workers in the NHS who perform exposure-prone procedures are required to have a course of hepatitis B vaccination and should have their immunity confirmed with a blood test showing a hepatitis B antibody titre (anti-HBs) >10 mIU/L.

Following a significant exposure, the immunization status of the recipient should be determined. The recipient may already know this or it may be available from previous laboratory results.

The treatment required depends on the immunization status of the recipient and the status of the donor (see Table 15.16).

Post-exposure prophylaxis for HIV

Post-exposure prophylaxis (PEP) should be recommended to healthcare workers if they have had a significant exposure to blood or another high-risk body fluid from a patient known to be HIV infected, or considered to be at high risk of HIV infection.

PEP should not be offered after exposure to low-risk materials (e.g. urine, vomit, faeces, or saliva) unless they are visibly blood stained. PEP should not be offered where testing has shown the donor is HIV negative, or the risk assessment has concluded that HIV infection of the donor is highly unlikely.

Table 15.16 Prophylaxis for hepatitis B following a needlestick injury

Pre-exposure HBV status of recipient	Hepatitis B positive donor	Unknown donor	Hepatitis B negative donor
≤1 dose of hepatitis B vaccine	Hepatitis B immunoglobulin plus accelerated course of hepatitis B vaccine (dose at 0, 1, and 2 months)	Accelerated course of hepatitis B vaccine	Initiate course of hepatitis B vaccine
≥2 doses of hepatitis B vaccine but anti-HB level unknown	One dose of hepatitis B vaccine (followed by a second dose one month later)	One dose of hepatitis B vaccine	Finish course of hepatitis B vaccine
Known responder to hepatitis B vaccine (anti-HB >10 mIU/L)	Consider booster of hepatitis B vaccine	Consider booster of hepatitis B vaccine	Consider booster of hepatitis B vaccine
Known non-responder to hepatitis B vaccine (anti-HB <10 mIU/L)	Hepatitis B immunoglobulin plus consider booster of hepatitis B vaccine	Hepatitis B immunoglobulin plus consider booster of hepatitis B vaccine	Consider booster of hepatitis B vaccine

Following exposure, for which PEP is considered appropriate, the healthcare worker should be given the opportunity to discuss the risks and benefits of PEP.

PEP reduces the risk of transmission of HIV by about 80%. However, knowledge about the efficacy and long-term toxicity of PEP is limited. Side effects with PEP are common, including gastrointestinal disturbance (e.g. nausea, vomiting, and diarrhoea), dizziness, and headache. PEP can also have significant interactions with other medications, which should be checked in the British National Formulary.

Prior to commencing PEP, the recipient's medical history, drug history, and in females pregnancy status, must be determined. They should be advised to use barrier contraception for sexual intercourse and not to give blood until subsequent HIV seroconversion has been ruled out.

PEP is recommended for four weeks; however it may be discontinued earlier if HIV testing of the donor is negative or if further information is gained about the donor making HIV unlikely.

Hepatitis C

There is no effective post-exposure prophylaxis for hepatitis C.

A baseline serum should be obtained from the recipient and stored for two years.

Hepatitis C testing of the donor should be performed, if possible. Most results will be available within 24–48 hours. If negative, the recipient can be reassured. If the donor is hepatitis C positive, then the recipient will require further blood tests at 6, 12, and 24 weeks after exposure. If the donor is unknown, the recipient will require a blood test at 24 weeks.

KEY POINTS

The risk of blood-borne virus transmission after percutaneous exposure to infected blood is:

- Hepatitis B, 30%
- Hepatitis C, 3%
- HIV, 0.3%

ED management should comprise:

- First aid.
- Risk assessment.
- Blood tests (recipient: anti-HB titre and serum save; donor: hepatitis B, C, and HIV testing).
- Post-exposure prophylaxis, if indicated.
- Occupation health follow-up.
- The requirement for hepatitis B prophylaxis is determined by the immunization status of the patient and infection status of the donor.

Post-exposure prophylaxis for HIV should be offered if there has been a significant exposure to blood or another high-risk body fluid from a patient known to be HIV infected, or considered to be at high risk of HIV infection. Post-exposure prophylaxis reduces the risk of transmission of HIV by about 80%.

There is no effective prophylaxis against hepatitis C.

15.7 SAQs

15.7.1 Sepsis

A 58-year-old man presents to the ED unwell with a history of cough, shortness of breath, myalgia, and fever. He has no significant past medical history. His initial observations are: pulse 110; BP 95/50; respiratory rate 28; saturations 89% on air; GCS 15; temperature 39°C; and blood glucose 10.1 mmol/L.

You suspect he has pneumonia.

a) List three of the diagnostic criteria for SIRS and their cut-off values? (3 marks: ½ for criteria, ½ for cut-off value)

b) After assessing the patient you think he has severe sepsis. According to the 'Sepsis Six' guidance, what six interventions (three investigations and three treatments) should be initiated in the first hour? (3 marks: ½ mark per intervention)

Suggested answer

a) List three of the diagnostic criteria for SIRS and their cut-off values? (3 marks: ½ for criteria, ½ for cut-off value)

Temperature >38.3°C or <36°C
Hear rate >90 beats per minute
Respiratory rate >20 breaths per minute
White cell count <4 or >12 × 10⁹/L

b) After assessing the patient you think he has severe sepsis. According to the 'Sepsis Six' guidance, what six interventions (three investigations and three treatments) should be initiated in the first hour? (3 marks: ½ mark per intervention)

Investigations: Treatments:
Take blood cultures Give high-flow oxygen
Check lactate Give IV antibiotics
Monitor hourly urine output Start IV fluids

15.7.2 Meningococcal disease

A six-year-old boy is brought to the ED by his mother. He has become unwell over the last few hours and has developed a non-blanching purpuric rash.

His initial observations are: pulse 160; BP 65/40; capillary refill 5 s; respiratory rate 40; saturations 99% (on high-flow oxygen); temperature 39.5°C; GCS 14 (E3, V5, M6).

a) What is the most likely causative organism for the presentation? (1 mark)

b) (i) The patient is protecting his airway and is receiving high-flow oxygen. What are your two initial treatments (give volume/doses)? (2 marks)

b) (ii) What additional antibiotic would you give if the child was 2 months old and why? (2 marks)

c) List four blood tests you would perform on this patient in the ED and a reason why. (4 marks: ½ mark for test, ½ mark for reason)

d) Name two groups who should receive prophylaxis if the child has confirmed meningococcal disease? (1 mark)

Suggested answer

a) What is the most likely causative organism for the presentation? (1 mark)
    Neisseria meningitidis

b) (i)   The patient is protecting his airway and is receiving high-flow oxygen. What are your
          two initial treatments (give volume/doses)? (2 marks)
          IV ceftriaxone 80 mg/kg or IV cefotaxime 80 mg/kg (1.6g)
          IV fluids 20 ml/kg (400 ml)
          (Estimated weight (6 + 4) × 2 = 20kg)

b) (ii) What additional antibiotic would you give if the child was 2 months old and why?
          (2 marks)
          Ampicillin or amoxicillin to cover for Listeria monocytogenes

c) List four blood tests you would perform on this patient in the ED and a reason why.
    (4 marks: ½ mark for test, ½ mark for reason)
    FBC—raised WCC is supportive of meningococcal disease. Patients are at risk of
       thrombocytopenia
    U&E—renal failure is a common complication of septicaemia
    Calcium, phosphate, and magnesium—metabolic derangement is common in septicaemia and
       may contribute to myocardial dysfunction
    LFTs and clotting—patients are at risk of DIC and liver failure
    Group and save—patients may require blood products for the treatment of DIC
    Blood glucose—hypoglycaemia is common particularly in children.
    Venous or capillary blood gas—provides information about the acid-base state and lactate (an
       arterial blood gas is not appropriate in a conscious six year old)
    Blood cultures and EDTA blood for PCR for N. Meningitidis

d) Name two groups who should receive prophylaxis if the child has confirmed meningococcal
    disease? (1 mark)
    Household contacts—those living in the same household as the patient in the seven days
       before disease onset.
    Kissing contacts
    Healthcare staff—if their mouth or nose has been splattered with large particle droplets/
       secretions from the respiratory tract of the patient

Further reading

Johnson V, Stockley JM, Dockrell D, et al. 2009. Fever in returning travellers presenting in
    the United Kingdom: recommendations for investigation and initial management. *J Infect*
    59(1): 1–18.
Lalloo DG, Shingadia D, Pasvol G, et al. 2007. UK malaria treatment guidelines. *J Infect* **54**:111–21.
National Institute for Health and Care Excellence, June 2010. NICE clinical guidline 102. Bacterial
    meningitis and meningococcal septicaemia: management of bacterial meningitis and meningococ-
    cal septicaemia in children and young people younger than 16 years in primary and secondary
    care. Available at: https://www.nice.org.uk/Guidance/CG102 [Online].
Rivers E, Nguyen B, Havstad S, et al. 2001. Early goal-directed therapy in the treatment of severe
    sepsis and septic shock. *New Engl J Med* **345**(19):1368–77.

Sprung CL, Annane D, Keh D, *et al*. CORTICUS Study Group, 2008. Hydrocortisone therapy for patients with septic shock. *New Engl J Med* **358**(2):111–24.

Surviving Sepsis Campaign. 2013. International Guidelines for Management of Severe Sepsis and Septic Shock: 2012. *Crit Care Med* **41**(2):580–637.

UCLH, The Hospital for Tropical Diseases Trust wide Guideline. Malaria Diagnosis and Treatment Guidline. June 2013. Available at: https://www.thehtd.org [Online].

Dermatology

CONTENTS

16.1 Describing rashes

16.1.1 Introduction

Dermatology questions commonly appear in the FRCEM Intermediate exam. There are several reasons for this: first, images of dermatological conditions are easy to obtain and therefore structure questions around; second, they tend to be quite discriminating questions; finally, dermatological conditions are more difficult to exam as an objective structured clinical examination (OSCE) and therefore often appear in the SAQ paper.

16.1.2 Describing rashes

The first stem of a dermatology question will often ask for a description of the rash shown. This is an opportunity to gain marks, even if you are uncertain of the diagnosis. Unfortunately, candidates who know the diagnosis often lose marks because they write the diagnosis down rather than describing the rash. It is, therefore, important to read the question carefully to ensure the correct answer is given.

The main descriptive terms for describing rashes are:

- Macule—flat, coloured lesion <1 cm diameter
- Patch—flat, coloured lesion >1 cm diameter
- Papule—raised, discrete lesion <1 cm diameter
- Nodule—raised, discrete lesion >1 cm diameter
- Plaque—raised, flat-topped lesion >1 cm diameter
- Vesicle—fluid-filled lesion <1 cm diameter
- Bulla—fluid-filled lesion >1 cm diameter
- Pustule—pus-filled lesion
- Scales—heaped up accumulations of horny epithelium
- Crusts—dried serum, blood, or pus
- Erosions—open areas of skin resulting from loss of part or all of the epidermis
- Ulcers—loss of the epidermis and at least part of the dermis
- Purpura—non-blanching lesions due to haemorrhage into the skin

- Petechiae—small (<2 mm), non-blanching areas of haemorrhage into the skin
- Ecchymosis—larger (>2 mm), non-blanching areas of haemorrhage into the skin
- Telangiectasia—focus of small permanently dilated blood vessels

---

KEY POINTS

If the question asks for a description, remember to describe the rash and do not immediately jump to the diagnosis. Look at the mark breakdown carefully to ensure you gain all the marks. For example, if three marks are allocated, then three descriptive terms will usually be required.

16.2 Life-threatening skin conditions

16.2.1 Erythema multiforme

Erythema multiforme (EM) encompasses a disease spectrum from a mild cutaneous syndrome (EM minor) to a severe life-threatening systemic illness (Steven-Johnson syndrome/toxic epidermal necrolysis) (Figure 16.1). The following is an accepted definition of the condition:

- EM minor—patients have target lesions located mainly on distal extremities.
- EM major—patients have more extensive target lesions with involvement of one or more mucous membranes.
- Steven-Johnson Syndrome (SJS)—patients have widespread blisters mainly on the trunk and face with epidermal detachment involving <10% of the body surface area. One or more mucous membranes are involved.
- Toxic epidermal necrolysis (TEN)—patients have sheet like erosions involving >30% of the body surface area and severe involvement of several mucous membranes.

Aetiology of erythema multiforme

EM appears to involve a hypersensitivity reaction that can be triggered by a variety of stimuli. Infections, particularly herpes simplex, seem to be the main cause of EM, whereas drugs are a more common trigger for SJS/TEN (see Table 16.1).

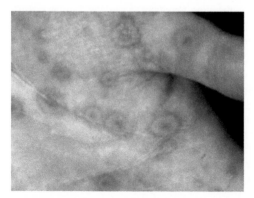

Figure 16.1 Typical target lesions of erythema multiforme.

Reproduced from Chantal Simon, Hazel Everitt, and Francoise van Dorp, *Oxford Handbook of General Practice*, 2010, plate 1 'Typical target lesions of erythema multiforme', with permission from Oxford University Press.

Table 16.1 Causes of erythema multiforme

Infection	Drugs	Other
Viral—herpes simplex, adenovirus, Coxsackie	Antibiotics—sulfonamides, penicillin, cephalosporins	Malignancy—leukaemia, non-Hodgkin's lymphoma
Bacterial—mycoplasma, TB, proteus, streptococcus	Anticonvulsants—phenytoin, barbiturates, carbamazepine	Autoimmune—sarcoidosis, vasculitides
Fungal—histoplasmosis	NSAIDs—piroxicam, diclofenac	Physical factors—tattooing, radiotherapy
	Others—allopurinol	Idiopathic

Clinical features of erythema multiforme

- Target lesions—are pathognomonic of EM. They are round with three zones: a central dusky erythema/purpura; a middle paler zone; and an outer ring of erythema with a well-defined edge. The lesions first appear on extensor surfaces peripherally and gradually extend centrally. The palms are often involved. In SJS/TEN, the target lesions often coalesce forming extensive blisters and erosions.
- Mucous membranes—oral lesions are common, but the genitalia may also become involved. In severe disease, mucosal involvement may lead to bronchitis and pneumonitis.
- Systemic symptoms—there is often a prodrome of fever, malaise, myalgia, arthralgia, headache, sore throat, and nausea.

Investigations for erythema multiforme

The diagnosis of EM is clinical and no specific investigations are indicated. A skin biopsy may be performed by dermatologists in equivocal cases.

Investigations may be used in severe cases to direct management (e.g. renal function in patients with significant fluid losses).

Management of erythema multiforme

In mild cases of EM, only symptomatic treatment is required and, if a drug is thought to be responsible, it should be stopped.

SJS and TEN can be life-threatening and should be treated in a similar manner to thermal burns.

- Volume repletion with intravenous fluids—estimate the percentage of skin involved and manage like a burn using the Parkland formula (see Chapter 4, section 4.7).
- Respiratory support—suction, positioning, and ventilation should be instituted as required.
- Nasogastric or nasojejunal feeding.
- Intravenous opiates—should be given to manage pain.
- Meticulous wound care and dressings are necessary.
- Patients should be monitored for secondary infection and given antibiotics if present (antibiotics are not given empirically).
- Isolation should be considered for infection control.
- Mouth washes with warm water or xylocaine should be used for oral lesions.
- Topical eye lubricants and topical antibiotics (preservative-free) for eye involvement.
- Steroid use is controversial and not routinely recommended.
- Aciclovir may be used in patients with herpes-induced EM.
- Refer patients to a dermatologist, and ophthalmologist if ocular involvement is present. Patients may need admission to a high-dependency area.

The SCORTEN score is a Severity of Illness Score for TEN, which can be used to assess the mortality rate for individuals with TEN, based on seven independent high-risk features.

- Age >40 years
- Malignancy
- Heart rate >120/minute
- Initial percentage of epidermal detachment >10%
- Serum urea >10 mmol/L
- Serum glucose >14 mmol/L
- Bicarbonate level <20 mmol/L*

Complications of erythema multiforme

- Acute kidney injury
- Adult respiratory distress syndrome (ARDS)
- Disseminated intravascular coagulation (DIC)
- Secondary infection or sepsis
- Oesophageal strictures
- Ocular complications, including corneal ulceration, anterior uveitis, blindness
- Death (SJS 5% mortality, TEN 30% mortality)

16.2.2 Staphylococcal scalded skin syndrome

Staphylococcal scalded skin syndrome (SSSS) is a toxin-mediated type of exfoliative dermatitis. *Staphylococcus aureus* produces an exotoxin, which causes separation of the outer layers of the epidermis. It can range from localized bulla to extensive flaccid blisters and erosions.

SSSS occurs most commonly in children under five years of age. The source of the *S. aureus* infection is often the nasopharynx, but may also originate from the umbilicus, eyes, urinary tract, or blood.

Clinical features of SSSS

- Prodrome of fever, irritability, and cutaneous tenderness.
- The rash often starts as multiple, widespread, red papules, which then progress to blistering eruptions, with flaccid bullae. Sheets of epidermis are shed leaving large raw areas that resemble a scald. The rash often begins in flexural areas, including the axillae and groins. Sloughing of the skin within one to two days is followed by complete re-epithelialization within two weeks.
- Nikolsky's sign is positive (slippage of the superficial layer of epidermis on gentle pressure).
- Circumoral erythema evolving to crusting.

Investigations for SSSS

The diagnosis of SSSS is confirmed by skin biopsy. The main differential is TEN, which produces full thickness epidermal necrosis.

Cultures obtained from bullae are usually sterile, which is consistent with haematogenous spread of toxin produced by a distant focus of staphylococcal infection.

A culture obtained from the source of infection (e.g. nasopharynx) confirms the causative organism and antibiotic sensitivities.

---

* Reprinted from *Journal of Investigative Dermatology*, volume 115, issue 2, Nathalie Fouchard, M. Bertocchi, Jean-Claude Roujeau, Jean Revuz, Pierre Wolkenstein, Sylvie Bastuji-Garin, SCORTEN: A Severity-of-Illness Score for Toxic Epidermal Necrolysis, pp.149–153, Copyright (2000), with permission from Elsevier.

Management of SSSS

- Supportive management is the mainstay of treatment—intravenous fluids, analgesia, and wound care.
- Antibiotics (e.g. flucloxacillin) should be given. The route (IV or oral) depends on the severity.

16.2.3 Erythroderma

Erythroderma is any inflammatory skin disease with erythema and scaling that affects >90% of the body surface.

Aetiology of erythroderma

- Exacerbation of an underlying skin disease (e.g. psoriasis, eczema, dermatitis, pityriasis rubra pilaris)
- Drug reaction—multiple drugs have been implicated including NSAIDs, penicillin, ACEI, and so on
- Malignancy, for example lymphoma (cutaneous T cell) and leukaemia
- Idiopathic

Clinical features of erythroderma

- Rapidly extending erythema with scales appearing after a few days
- Fever, malaise, lethargy
- Pruritus
- Lymphadenopathy
- Thickened skin and nails, which may eventually be shed

Management of erythroderma

Patients with erythroderma are at risk of hypothermia, fluid loss, protein and electrolyte imbalance, and haemodynamic compromise. Management is directed at preventing and correcting these.

Unnecessary medications should be stopped.

Steroids may be helpful, depending on the underlying cause, but should only be given in consultation with a dermatologist.

16.2.4 Necrotizing fasciitis

Necrotizing fasciitis is a rare and severe bacterial infection of soft tissues. It is usually a polymicrobial infection, often involving aerobic and anaerobic organism. The most important cause is *Streptococcus pyogenes* (also known as Group A streptococcus).

Initial clinical features may be vague, with severe pain but little on examination, except tenderness of the affected area. There may be slight swelling or erythema at the site. Patients usually have a fever and are systemically unwell with malaise, lethargy, diarrhoea, and vomiting. The disease often progresses rapidly leading to marked soft tissue swelling with discoloration, haemorrhagic blisters, and skin necrosis.

Necrotizing fasciitis is covered in more detail in Chapter 15, section 15.1.

16.2.5 Urticaria and angioedema

Urticaria and angioedema are different manifestations of the same pathological process. In urticaria there is swelling of the upper dermis resulting in well-circumscribed wheals. In angioedema the swelling is subdermal, resulting in well-demarcated, non-pitting oedema. Angioedema typically affects the periorbital region, lips, tongue, and oropharynx. Urticaria and angioedema can occur together or separately.

Angioedema can be classified as allergic, hereditary, acquired, drug-induced, or idiopathic.

- Allergic angioedema—is the most common cause presenting to the emergency department (ED), mediated by Immunoglobulin E (IgE), after exposure to an antigen, usually food substances or drugs. The management of allergic angioedema and urticaria is discussed in Chapter 2, section 2.3.
- Hereditary angioedema—results from a qualitative or quantitative deficiency of C1-esterase inhibitor, which is involved in the regulation of bradykinin. It is characterized by recurrent attacks that do not respond to antihistamines, corticosteroids, or adrenaline. It is treated with C1-esterase inhibitor concentrate, which the patient may carry with them if they are a known sufferer. If this is not available, fresh frozen plasma can be used as an alternative.
- Acquired angioedema—is the result of autoantibodies that act on C1-esterase inhibitor and increase its consumption. Clinically it presents like hereditary angioedema and is initially treated in the same way. It is associated with B-cell proliferative disorders and autoimmune diseases.
- Drug-induced angioedema—is associated with ACE inhibitors and angiotensin II receptor blockers. These drugs inhibit the degradation of bradykinin, thereby potentiating its biological effects. The implicated drug should be stopped.
- Idiopathic angioedema—the cause is usually unknown, but may be due to direct mast-cell releasing agents in certain compounds (e.g. contrast media and opiates).

16.2.6 Bullous disorders

Bullous disorders are primary blistering disorders of the skin and involve fluid collection between two layers of the skin. Clinical presentation and diagnosis depends on the depth of the blister and the pathophysiology (see Tables 16.2 and 16.3). Skin biopsy for microscopy and imunoflourescence are thus often required.

The two comonest types of immunobulous disorders are pemphigus vulgaris and bullous pemphigoid which differ in pathophysiology and presentation (see Table 16.4).

Previous MRCEM question

Pemphigus vulgaris

Pemphigus vulgaris is a potentially fatal skin condition caused by the development of antibodies against the desmosomal proteins leading to an intraepidermal split and the development of intraepidermal flaccid blisters. The blisters are Nikolsky sign positive and mucous membranes are commonly involved. Diagnosis is by immunoflourescence confirming IgG within the epidermis.

Bulous pemphigoid

Bulous pemphigold is commoner than pemphigus and results in the formation of deeper blisters at the subepidermal space caused by autoantiboides against the hemidesmosomal proteins at the

Table 16.2 Classification of bullous disorders according to depth

Subcorneal (very thin roof)	Intracorneal/epidermal (thin roof)	Subepidermal (tense roof, often intact)
Bullous impetigo	Acute eczema	Bullous pemphigoid
Pustular psoriasis	Herpes simplex	Dermatitis herpetiformis
Staphylococcal scalded skin syndrome	Herpes zoster	Erythema multiforme
	Varicella	Toxic epidermal necrolysis
	Pemphigus	Cold and thermal injury: burns
		Dystrophic epidermolysis bullosa

Table 16.3 Differential diagnosis of bullous disorders

Causes	Disorder
Immunological	Bullous pemphigoid
	Pemphigus
	Dermatitis herpetiformis
	Lichen planus
Genetic	Epidermolysis (EB)
Inflammatory	Infection (SSSS, strep, heprpes, fungale)
	Alergic (insect bite)
	Dermatitis
	EM/SJS
Physical	Heat/cold
	Friction
	Chemical
	Oedema
Drug Reaction	Fixed drug reaction
	EM
	TEN
	Photosensitie eruption
Systemic	Porphyria cutanae tarda
	Carcinoma

Table 16.4 Pemhigoid and pemphigus

	Pemphigoid	Pemphigus
Age of onset	>60 yrs	Wide range
		Peak in middle age
Clinical features	Large tense blisters of variable size on an erythematous base	Small superficial blsiters on the trunk
	Classically on flexor surfaces and Trunk	
	Associated pruritus	
Nikolsky sign	Negative	Positive
Mucosal imvolvement	Rare	Common (may never recover)
Histology	Autoantibodies against hemidesmosomal proteins at the basement membrane	Autoantibodies against desmosomal protiens
	Subepidermal	Intraepidermal
Immunofluorescene	Linear IgG deposits along the basement membrane	Intraepidermal IgG between cells
Management	Steroids (oral then topical)	Hign-dose oral steroids, azathioprine, and immunomodulatory drugs
	Azathioprine occasionaly used	
Prognosis	Remits after 2–5 years	15–30% mortality (100% without treatment)

basement membrane. Immunoflourescence shows IgG at the basement membrane. In contrast to pemphigus, mucous membranes are rarely affected and blisters are described as Nikolsky sign negative.

KEY POINTS

The mainstay of ED management of patients with life-threatening skin conditions is good supportive care. Patients often require management in a high-dependency area.

Erythema multiforme may be triggered by a variety of stimuli (e.g. viral infections, drugs, autoimmune conditions, and malignancy). Target lesions are pathognomonic.

Steven-Johnson syndrome and toxic epidermal necrolysis are severe, life-threatening conditions believed to be part of the erythema multiforme spectrum. Patients with SJS and TEN are systemically unwell. They have large areas of blistering and erosions, along with mucous membrane involvement.

Staphylococcal scalded skin syndrome is a toxin-mediated exfoliative dermatitis usually seen in children. Treatment is supportive therapy and flucloxacillin.

Erythroderma is erythema and scaling affecting >90% of the body surface.

Necrotizing fasciitis is a rare and severe bacterial infection of soft tissues, which can lead to septic shock. Initially there may be little to see on examination except slight swelling or erythema, and tenderness of the affected area.

Urticaria/angioedema may be allergic, hereditary, or idiopathic. Early recognition of anaphylaxis and treatment with adrenaline 0.5 mg IM is paramount.

16.3 Rashes in multisystem diseases

16.3.1 Dermatitis herpetiformis

Dermatitis herpetiformis is an autoimmune disorder associated with coeliac disease. It is characterized by groups of vesicles and papules on the extensor surfaces of the elbows, knees, and buttocks. It is very pruritic, resulting in excoriations. It is treated with dapsone and a gluten-free diet.

16.3.2 Erythema chronicum migrans

Erythema chronicum migrans is the rash associated with Lyme disease (Figure 16.2). It can appear anywhere on the body starting as a red papule that spreads to produce an erythematous ring, with central fading. The rash classically looks like a 'Bull's-eye'.

Lyme disease is a multisystem disorder resulting from a tick-borne infection, *Borrelia burgdorferi*. It occurs in temperate regions of North America, Asia and Europe, including the United Kingdom. Most cases occur in the summer or early autumn and are transmitted by ticks from deer or sheep.

In addition to the rash, patients may report fever, lethargy, headache, arthralgia, and myalgia. Left untreated, patients may develop joint, cardiac, and neurological complications over weeks to months. These include myocarditis, heart block, meningitis, encephalitis, cranial nerve palsies, and peripheral nerve palsies.

Diagnosis is based on clinical signs and symptoms, and confirmed by blood serology. Treatment is with doxycyline or ceftriaxone.

16.3.3 Erythema marginatum

Erythema marginatum occurs in 20% of cases of rheumatic fever. The rash is transient and consists of pink macules with well-demarcated, sometimes raised, edges and central clearing. The rash is predominantly on the trunk and proximal limbs.

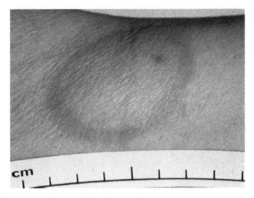

Figure 16.2 Lyme disease—erythema chronicum migrans.

Reproduced from Chris Johnson, Sarah Anderson, Jon Dallimore, Shane Winser, and David A. Warrell, *Oxford Handbook of Expedition and Wilderness Medicine*, 2008, plate 4, with permission from Oxford University Press.

Rheumatic fever is a non-infectious immune disease which follows a Group A β-haemolytic streptococcal infection. Symptoms appear between one and five weeks after a throat infection. Diagnosis is based on the Revised Jones Criteria (see Table 16.5):

- Evidence of a recent streptococcal infection (e.g. history of scarlet fever, positive throat swab, or increased anti-streptolysin O titre).
- Plus two major criteria or one major and two minor criteria.

Treatment is bed rest, aspirin, intravenous benzylpenicillin, splintage for arthritis, and diazepam or haloperidol for chorea.

16.3.4 Scarlet fever

Scarlet fever is due to a streptococcal throat infection, leading to a sore throat and fever. It is usually only seen in children.

The rash of scarlet fever is diffuse, bright red (scarlet) erythema, with raised hair follicles making the skin feel rough. Approximately 10–14 days after the rash the skin may peel away, predominantly on the hands and feet.

The tongue has a white coating with red papillae protruding through giving a 'white strawberry tongue' appearance. Over time the white coating goes, leaving a 'red strawberry tongue'.

Treatment is aimed at speeding recovery and preventing complications (e.g. rheumatic fever, glomerulonephritis). Penicillin or erythromycin is given for 14 days.

Table 16.5 Revised Jones criteria for rheumatic fever

Major criteria	Minor criteria
Polyarthritis	Fever
Carditis	ECG changes (↑ PR)
Sydenham chorea	↑ ESR/CRP
Subcutaneous nodules	Arthralgia
Erythema marginatum	History of previous rheumatic fever

Data from Ferrieri P; Jones Criteria Working, Group (2002). 'Proceedings of the Jones Criteria workshop'. Circulation 106 (19): 2521–2523.

16.3.5 Erythema nodosum

Erythema nodosum is inflammation of the fat cells under the skin resulting in tender red nodules that usually appear on the shins. It is usually associated with systemic symptoms of lethargy, fever, arthralgia, and myalgia.

There are numerous causes of erythema nodosum:

- Infective—streptococcal infection, TB, mycoplasma, EBV
- Drugs—oral contraceptive pill, sulphonamides
- Inflammatory bowel disease—ulcerative colitis and Crohn's disease
- Autoimmune (e.g. Behcet's disease)
- Sarcoidosis
- Pregnancy
- Idiopathic (>50% cases)

Treatment is directed at the underlying cause and symptomatic relief with analgesia. The nodules tend to resolve spontaneously.

16.3.6 Kawasaki disease

Kawasaki disease is also known as mucocutaneous lymph node syndrome and is believed to be related to a viral infection. Most cases are in children <5 years old.

The rash of Kawasaki disease is a polymorphous, erythematous rash on the trunk, plus erythema and desquamation of the hands, feet, and genitalia.

Kawasaki disease is diagnosed clinically based on the following criteria:

- Five days of fever

Plus four of the five principle characteristics:

- Eye involvement—conjunctivitis, uveitis
- Cervical lymphadenopathy
- Rash—polymorphous erythema on the trunk
- Oral involvement—red cracked lips, diffuse erythema of oropharynx, 'strawberry tongue'
- Erythema of the hands and feet followed by desquamation

Patients should have a full blood count check looking for leucocytosis and thrombocytosis, plus an erythrocyte sedimentation rate (ESR), and viral titres sent.

The main complication is coronary artery aneurysms and patients should have an echocardiogram two weeks after onset. Early treatment reduces the risk of aneurysms and consists of high-dose aspirin, intravenous immunoglobulin, and corticosteroids in resistant cases.

Patients should be admitted under the paediatricians and cardiologists.

16.3.7 Viral exanthems

Exanthems are widespread rashes occurring as a symptom of a systemic disease. They are usually caused by a viral infection, however some may be due to drugs (e.g. antibiotics, NSAIDs) or bacterial infections (e.g. scarlet fever, staphylococcal scalded skin syndrome).

Viral exanthems are common rashes seen in children.

- **Measles** causes a maculopapular rash, which develops several days after the fever starts. It starts on the face and spreads to cover most of the body. Koplik's spots, if seen, are pathognomonic of measles, and are small white spots on the buccal mucosa.
- **Rubella** results in a macular rash on the face and trunk.
- **Fifth disease** (erythema infectiosum, slapped-cheek syndrome) is caused by parvovirus B19 and results in a distinctive red rash on the face which makes the child appear to have 'slapped cheeks'. The rash then spreads down the trunk and limbs. The rash typically appears a few days after the febrile illness has resolved.

- **Roseola infantum** (exanthema subitum, sixth disease) is caused by human herpes viruses (human herpes virus 6 and 7). It results in a sudden, high fever, and children may present with a febrile convulsion. As the child appears to be recovering from the illness a fine red rash appears, usually on the trunk which then spreads to the legs and neck.
- **Hand-foot-mouth disease** is usually caused by Coxsackie A virus. Children have a prodrome of fever, malaise, loss of appetite, and a sore mouth. After one to two days, ulcers develop in the mouth and papules develop on the palms and soles.
- **Chicken pox** is caused by varicella zoster. It results in a pruritic, vesicular rash most densely on the trunk and face. The vesicles appear in crops and crust over after three to five days. Reactivation of the herpes zoster virus in later life results in shingles causing a vesicular rash affecting one dermatome.

EXAM TIP

A common mistake in exams is for candidates to assume the diagnosis based on a characteristic finding. For example, not all purpuric rashes are caused by a meningococcal infection.

It is useful to know a differential diagnosis for conditions that can cause purpuric rashes, desquamation, pruritus, and skin and mouth ulceration.

Causes of a purpuric rash:

- Meningococcal septicaemia (see Chapter 15, section 15.4)
- Henoch–Scholein purpura—characteristically concentrated on the buttocks and extensor surfaces (see Chapter 19, section 19.12)
- Thrombocytopenia (ITP, leukaemia, septic shock, aplastic anaemia)
- Bacterial endocarditis
- Enteroviral infections
- Trauma
- Forceful coughing or vomiting
- Rocky Mountain spotted fever

Causes of desquamation:

- Staphylococcal scalded skin syndrome
- Kawasaki's disease
- Scarlet fever
- TEN/SJS
- Pemphigus/pemphigoid

Causes of pruritus:

- Allergic reaction (e.g. urticaria)
- Infections (e.g. varicella zoster, herpes, scabies, lice, insect bites)
- Dermatological (e.g. psoriasis, eczema, sunburn, xerosis (dry skin), dermatitis herpetiformis)
- Medical disorders (e.g. jaundice, diabetes, iron-deficiency anaemia, polycythaemia), malignancy (e.g. lymphoma, Hodgkin's disease), thyroid disease, hyperparathyroidism, pregnancy, and so on
- Medications (e.g. opiates, chloroquine)

Causes of ulceration of the skin and mouth:

- Mouth—EM, SJS, TENs, pemphigus, Kawasaki disease, hand-foot-mouth disease, herpes simplex virus, minor trauma, immunodeficiency, Behcet's disease, Crohn's disease
- Skin—skin malignancies, chronic venous insufficiency, arterial insufficiency, pressure sores, neuropathic ulcers, bullous pemphigoid, impetigo

---

KEY POINTS

Rashes are common in multisystem diseases and could appear in the MRCEM examination.

Dermatitis herpetiformis—is an autoimmune disorder associated with coeliac disease, characterized by groups of vesicles and papules on the extensor surfaces of the elbows, knees, and buttocks.

Erythema chronicum migrans—is the rash associated with Lyme disease. The classic finding is a 'bull's eye', which can appear anywhere on the body.

Erythema marginatum—occurs in 20% of cases of rheumatic fever. The rash consists of pink macules with well-demarcated, sometimes raised, edges and central clearing.

Erythema nodosum—results in tender red nodules that usually appear on the shins.

Kawasaki disease (mucocutaneous lymph node syndrome)—results in a polymorphous, erythematous rash on the trunk, plus erythema and desquamation of the hands, feet, and genitalia.

Scarlet fever—results in a diffuse, bright red (scarlet) erythema, with raised hair follicles making the skin feel rough (sometimes likened to 'bumpy sunburn'). Approximately 10–14 days after the rash the skin may peel away, predominantly on the hands and feet.

Common viral exanthems include chicken pox, fifth disease, hand-foot-mouth disease, roseola infantum, measles, and rubella.

16.4 Cellulitis, erysipelas, and impetigo

Cellulitis, erysipelas, and impetigo are all the consequence of bacterial skin infections.

16.4.1 Cellulitis

Cellulitis is usually caused by streptococcus and occasionally staphylococcus. A minor breach in the skin (e.g. insect bite) may act as the portal for infection, but it may occur in patients without any obvious breach of the skin. Infection develops within the dermis and subcutaneous tissues.

Cellulitis results in warm, erythematous skin, which has a poorly defined edge. Patients may have associated lymphangitis and lymphadenopathy.

Treatment is with antibiotics, which may be oral or intravenous depending on the severity. Patients who are systemically unwell or have spreading infection (e.g. lymphangitis extending above the knee from cellulitis on the foot) should be treated with intravenous antibiotics (e.g. benzylpenicillin and flucloxacillin). Patients with facial cellulitis are at risk of significant intracranial complications (e.g. cavernous sinus thrombosis) and should be treated with intravenous antibiotics.

16.4.2 Erysipelas

Erysipelas is a superficial bacterial skin infection that characteristically extends into the cutaneous lymphatics. It is caused by a streptococcal infection, the source of which is often the nasopharynx.

Erysipelas begins as a small erythematous patch, which progresses rapidly to a fiery-red, indurated, tense, and shiny plaque. The lesion classically has clearly defined, raised margins, distinguishing it from cellulitis. Lymphatic involvement leads to erythematous tracks in the overlying skin and regional lymphadenopathy.

Treatment is with penicillin and/or a macrolide, as for cellulitis.

16.4.3 Impetigo

Impetigo is a staphylococcal or streptococcal infection, which develops due to a breach in the skin (e.g. eczema, nappy rash). It affects the superficial layers of the skin and is highly contagious.

Non-bullous impetigo is the commonest form. Lesions begin as vesicles or pustules, which rapidly burst and therefore are rarely seen. The burst lesions evolve into gold-crusted plaques, typically 2 cm in diameter. The area around the mouth and nose is most commonly affected. Systemic symptoms are uncommon unless the infection is widespread.

Bullous impetigo is less common, and usually affects neonates. It presents as flaccid, fluid-filled vesicles and blisters. When the blisters burst, raw areas of skin are left, which eventually form brown-golden crusts. The face is less commonly affected; instead the axillae, neck, and nappy folds are usually affected. Unlike non-bullous impetigo, lesions tend to be painful and systemic symptoms are more common.

If the infection is localized and the patient is well, impetigo can be treated with topical antibiotic cream (e.g. fusidic acid). If the infection is more extensive, oral or intravenous antibiotics (e.g. penicillin and flucloxacillin) are required.

KEY POINTS

Cellulitis is an infection of the dermis and subcutaneous tissues usually caused by streptococcus or staphylococcus.

Erysipelas is a superficial streptococcal skin infection that characteristically extends into the cutaneous lymphatics.

Impetigo is a staphylococcal or streptococcal infection which affects the superficial layers of the skin and is highly contagious. It results in ulcerated erythematous areas which from a golden crust.

Cellulitis, erysipelas, and impetigo are all treated with antistreptococcal/staphylococcal antibiotics (e.g. penicillin, flucloxacillin). The route is determined by the severity of the disease.

16.5 Eczema

Eczema is an inflammatory disorder of the epidermis. The clinical features include redness, itching, scaling, oedema, cracking, crusting, and bleeding.

16.5.1 Types of eczema

- Atopic eczema—is the most common form of eczema. It has a hereditary element and often occurs in those with a history of atopy (e.g. asthma, hayfever). The age of onset is usually between two and six months, with improvement during childhood. The flexural sites are commonly affected.
- Contact dermatitis—may be allergic or irritant. Allergic results from a delayed reaction to an allergen (e.g. nickel). Irritant is due to a direct reaction to a substance (e.g. a detergent).
- Seborrhoeic dermatitis—is probably an inflammatory reaction to a yeast called *Malassezia* (formerly known as Pityrosporum ovale). The red, scaly rash appears on the scalp, face, and upper trunk.
- Pompholyx—is characterized by itchy vesicles occurring on the palms and soles.

16.5.2 Treatment of eczema

- Avoidance of triggers—contact dermatitis is curable provided the offending substance can be avoided. Dietary restrictions may help if a food substance is the trigger.
- Moisturize—soaps and detergents should be avoided and emollients (e.g. aqueous cream) should be used regularly.
- Steroids—are commonly used in the treatment of eczema. They do not provide a cure but are highly effective in suppressing symptoms. The strength and route (topical or oral) depends on the severity of the condition.
- Symptomatic relief—antihistamines may be useful for pruritus.
- Other therapies—dermatologists may prescribe phototherapy. Immunosuppressants may be given in resistant cases of eczema.

16.5.3 Complications of eczema

- Secondary bacterial infection—commonly staphylococcal or streptococcal.
- Eczema herpeticum—caused by herpes simplex virus. Typically heralded by areas of rapidly worsening painful eczema, which fail to respond to antibiotics and topical steroids. Patients may have clusters of blisters (which look like early cold sores) and punched-out erosions which may coalesce.
- Erythroderma.

KEY POINTS

Eczema is an inflammatory disorder of the epidermis. The clinical features include redness, itching, scaling, oedema, cracking, crusting, and bleeding.

Atopic eczema and contact dermatitis are the two most common presentations.

Eczema herpeticum is a potentially life-threatening complication of eczema caused by herpes simplex virus.

Treatment options in eczema include: avoidance of triggers, emollients, steroids, symptomatic relief (e.g. antihistamines), phototherapy, and immunosuppressants.

16.6 SAQs

16.6.1 Eczema herpeticum

A three-year-old presents to the emergency department with a five-day exacerbation of his eczema. Flucloxacillin was started three days earlier by the GP but has not helped. You suspect the patient may have eczema herpeticum.

a) (i) List four clinical features of eczema herpeticum. (4 marks)

a) (ii) What are the two most important treatments to start in the ED for eczema herpeticum? (2 marks)

b) Another child presents with an itchy rash and you suspect atopic eczema. Give four potential trigger factors. (2 marks)

c) Atopic eczema has a number of different treatment options—list four of them. (2 marks)

Suggested answer

a) (i) List four clinical features of eczema herpeticum. (4 marks)

Failure of eczema to respond to oral antibiotics and topical steroids

Areas of rapidly worsening, painful eczema

Clustered blisters consistent with early-stage cold sores

Punched-out erosions (circular, depressed, ulcerated lesions) usually 1–3 mm that are uniform in appearance (these may coalesce to form larger areas of erosion with crusting)

Systemic symptoms (e.g. fever, lethargy)

(a) (ii) What are the two most important treatments to start in the ED for eczema herpeticum? (2 marks)

Systemic aciclovir

Systemic antibiotic active against *Staph. aureus* and Strep (e.g. flucloxacillin and benzylpenicillin)

b) Another child presents with an itchy rash and you suspect atopic eczema. Give four potential trigger factors. (2 marks)

Irritants (e.g. soaps or detergents)

Skin infections

Contact allergens

Food allergens

Inhaled allergens

c) Atopic eczema has a number of different treatment options—list four of them. (2 marks)

Emollients

Topical steroids

Symptomatic therapy (e.g. antihistamines)

Bandages and dressings

Phototherapy

Immunosuppressants (e.g. tacrolimus)

16.6.2 Kawasaki disease and erythema multiforme

A four-year-old presents with a polymorphous rash on her chest and a high fever. A junior colleague asks you whether this could be Kawasaki disease.

a) List four of the diagnostic criteria for Kawasaki disease. (4 marks)

b) What is the main complication of Kawasaki disease and what investigation is required to monitor for it? (2 marks)

Another patient presents with a rash on their trunk that look like 'target lesions'. They also have oral ulceration. You diagnose erythema multiforme.

c) List four potential causes of erythema multiforme. (2 marks)
d) Name four potential complications of erythema multiforme. (2 marks)

Suggested answer

a) List four of the diagnostic criteria for Kawasaki disease. (4 marks)

Five days of fever, plus four of the five principle characteristics:
Eye involvement—conjunctivitis, uveitis
Cervical lymphadenopathy
Rash—polymorphous erythema on the trunk
Oral involvement—red cracked lips, diffuse erythema of oropharynx, 'strawberry tongue'
Erythema of the hands and feet followed by desquamation

b) What is the main complication of Kawasaki disease and what investigation is required to monitor for it? (2 marks)

Coronary artery aneurysm
Echocardiogram

c) List four potential causes of erythema multiforme. (2 marks)
See Table 16.6

Table 16.6 Causes of erythema multiforme

Infection	Drugs	Other
Viral—herpes simplex, adenovirus, Coxsackie	Antibiotics—sulfonamides, penicillin, cephalosporins	Malignancy—leukaemia, non-Hodgkin's lymphoma
Bacterial—mycoplasma, TB, proteus, streptococcus	Anticonvulsants—phenytoin, barbiturates, carbamazepine	Autoimmune—sarcoidosis, vasculitides
Fungal—histoplasmosis	NSAIDs—piroxicam, diclofenac	Physical factors—tattooing, radiotherapy
	Others—allopurinol	Idiopathic

d) Name four potential complications of erythema multiforme. (2 marks)

Renal failure
ARDS
DIC
Secondary infection or sepsis
Oesophageal strictures
Ocular complications, including corneal ulceration, anterior uveitis, blindness
Death (SJS 5% mortality, TEN 30% mortality)

Further reading

Bastuji-Garin S, Rzany B, Stern RS. 1993. Clinical classification of cases of toxic epidermal necrolysis, Stevens-Johnson syndrome, and erythema multiforme. Arch Dermatol 129(1):92–6.

CHAPTER 17

Toxicology

CONTENTS

17.1 Introduction

A toxicology question usually appears in every diet of the FRCEM intermediate examination. Poisoning is a common emergency department (ED) presentation and there is well-established guidance for the management of many substances, which makes it an ideal SAQ. TOXBASE (https://www.toxbase.org/) is the primary clinical toxicology database for the UK National Poisons Information Service and is a very useful resource both for revision and work purposes.

EXAM TIP

Toxicology is a very common SAQ. Make sure you are happy with the management of drugs commonly used in overdose, or those that are particularly toxic.

17.2 General principles of poisoning management

General principles apply when managing a patient who presents with poisoning. Candidates often jump straight to the specific antidote required for certain poisons and forget that the vast majority of poisoning management is good symptomatic and supportive care.

Poisoning management can be broken down into the following components:

- ABCDE assessment and supportive management
- Decontamination
- Elimination
- Antidotes
- Psychiatric assessment (see Chapter 18)

17.2.1 ABCDE and supportive management

All patients presenting with poisoning require a thorough ABCDE assessment and appropriate supportive management.

Often the stem of the question will include details of management the patient is already receiving; for example, the patient may already be in the resuscitation room and receiving high-flow oxygen. Repetition of this in the answer is unlikely to gain marks, so it is very important to read the question carefully.

- **A**—assess the adequacy of the airway and provide protection with endotracheal intubation if necessary. Patients who are not intubated should be nursed in the recovery position to minimize the risk of aspiration should vomiting occur.
- **B**—monitor breathing and ventilate if necessary. Patients may be at risk of ventilatory failure leading to hypoxia and hypercarbia.
- **C**—manage hypotension according to the cause (e.g. hypovolaemia, arrhythmias, cardiac depression). Patients with hypotension (systolic BP <90 mmHg) should be given a fluid bolus, for example 500 ml crystalloid or colloid repeated as necessary. Occasionally patients will require inotropic support. Arrhythmias are uncommon in poisoning and should initially be treated with correction of hypoxia, hypercarbia, acidosis, and electrolyte abnormalities. Antiarrhythmics are rarely needed.
- **D**—prolonged convulsions should be treated with benzodiazepines. Hypoxia and hypoglycaemia should be excluded as potential causes.
- **E**—ensure normoglycaemia and normothermia. Check for any other injuries, particularly to the head.

17.2.2 Decontamination

The aim of decontamination is to stop the substance being absorbed. There are various forms of decontamination including:

- Skin decontamination.
- Activated charcoal.
- Gastric lavage—is rarely indicated and only considered in life-threatening overdoses presenting within one hour. The airway must be protected by a cuffed endotracheal tube or the patient should have a strong cough reflex.
- Whole bowel irrigation—Klean-Prep® is the only preparation available in the United Kingdom suitable for whole bowel irrigation. It is an osmotically balanced polyethylene glycol electrolyte solution, which is given orally or via a nasogastric tube. The solution is continued until the rectal effluent runs clear. Treatment may be required for up to 12 hours. Renal function should be checked at the end of treatment. It should only be used on expert advice. It may be used for sustained-release drug formulations, or poisons which are not absorbed by activated charcoal.
- Induced emesis is not recommended.

Activated charcoal

Previous MRCEM question

Activated charcoal absorbs substances onto its surface by weak electrostatic forces thereby preventing absorption of the ingested drug ('gut decontamination').

The dose of activated charcoal is 50 g orally and should be given within one hour of the overdose.

EXAM TIP

Previous MRCEM questions have expected candidates to know the dose and route of activated charcoal (50 g orally).

There are certain drugs for which activated charcoal is resistant and others for which repeated doses may be useful.

Substances that do not bind to activated charcoal include:

- Lithium
- Boric acid
- Iron
- Petroleum distillates
- Ethanol
- Methanol
- Ethylene glycol
- Strong acids and alkalis
- Cyanide
- Organophosphates

Repeated dose activated charcoal (usually four doses taken at four-hour intervals) may be beneficial in the following poisonings:

- Carbamazepine
- Digoxin
- Phenobarbital
- Quinine
- Theophylline
- Dapsone
- Salicylate (NB A second dose may be indicated if plasma salicylate levels continue to rise, suggesting delayed gastric emptying, or when an enteric-coated formulation has been taken.)

17.2.3 Elimination

Active elimination is rarely required in poisoning. It can be achieved by several techniques depending on the poison:

- Urinary alkalinization, which enhances urinary excretion of weak acids (e.g. moderate salicylate poisoning). This is achieved with a sodium bicarbonate infusion (1.5 L of 1.26% over two hours).
- Haemodialysis (e.g. severe salicylate poisoning, ethylene glycol, methanol, lithium, phenobarbital).
- Haemoperfusion (e.g. barbiturates, theophylline, choral hydrate).

17.2.4 Antidotes

Table 17.1 details antidotes to poisons.

17.2.5 Psychiatric assessment

A focused history should be taken to identify the likely toxin, plus the amount, and time of ingestion. Concurrent medications and a past medical history should be sought to identify any risk factors that may compound the poisoning (e.g. enzyme inducing drugs in paracetamol poisoning).

Table 17.1 Antidotes to poisons

Poison	Antidote
Paracetamol	Acetylcysteine, methionine
Opiates	Naloxone
Benzodiazepines	Flumazenil (should not be given in a mixed overdose)
β-blockers	Glucagon
	(Patients may also require treatment with atropine for bradycardia and salbutamol for bronchospasm. Patients with hypotension resistant to glucagon may require insulin-glucose infusion, lipid emulsion, and/or inotropes.)
Tricyclic antidepressants	Sodium bicarbonate (see section 17.6)
Iron	Desferrioxamine
Calcium-channel blockers	Calcium gluconate or calcium chloride
	(Patients with resistant hypotension may require an insulin-glucose infusion, lipid emulsion, inotropes, and/or glucagon. Patients with bradycardia may require atropine and/or pacing.)
Carbon monoxide	Oxygen (hyperbaric) (see section 17.7)
Digoxin	Digoxin-specific antibodies
Ethylene glycol, Methanol	Ethanol, fomepizole
Organophosphates	Atropine, pralidoxime
Cyanide	Dicobalt edetate, hydroxocobalamin, sodium nitrite/thiosulfate
Sulphonylurea	Glucose, octreotide
Warfarin	Vitamin K, FFP, prothrombin complex concentrate

The physical examination should look for signs providing clues to the cause of the poisoning and particular features suggestive of a toxidrome (see section 17.3).

Once the patient has been assessed for the medical consequences of poisoning, and treatment initiated, a psychiatric assessment can be started (see Chapter 18, section 18.3).

KEY POINTS

Poisoning management can be broken down into the following components:

- ABCDE assessment and supportive management
- Decontamination
- Elimination
- Antidotes
- Psychiatric assessment

With all poisoning, the mainstay of management is good supportive therapy.

Activated charcoal absorbs substances onto its surface by weak electrostatic forces, thereby preventing absorption of the ingested drug. The dose of activated charcoal is 50 g orally and it should be given within one hour of the overdose.

Active elimination is rarely required in poisoning. It can be achieved by urinary alkalinization, haemodialysis, or haemoperfusion.

17.3 Toxidromes

Toxidromes are clinical syndromes that suggest a specific class of poisoning.

EXAM TIP

A SAQ may describe a constellation of signs and symptoms suggestive of a particular toxidrome, but not specifically state the substance involved. It is then necessary to recognize the particular toxidrome in order to instigate the correct management.

The most common clinical toxidromes are:

- Sympathomimetic
- Anticholinergic
- Cholinergic
- Opiate

17.3.1 Sympathomimetic toxidrome

Table 17.2 details the causes, pathophysiology, clinical features, and management of sympathomimetic toxidrome.

17.3.2 Anticholinergic toxidrome

Table 17.3 details the causes, pathophysiology, clinical features, and management of anticholinergic toxidrome.

17.3.3 Cholinergic toxidrome

Table 17.4 details the causes, pathophysiology, clinical features, and management of cholinergic (muscarubuc) toxidrome.

Table 17.2 Sympathomimetic toxidrome—causes, pathophysiology, clinical features, and management

Causative drugs	Pathophysiology	Clinical features	Treatment
Cocaine	Stimulation of α- and β-adrenergic receptors.	Sweating	Supportive.
Amphetamines		Hyperthermia	Intravenous fluids.
Gamma-hydroxybutyrate	Indirect release of presynaptic norepinephrine.	Anxiety	Benzodiazepines for agitation or seizures.
Decongestants	Prevention of presynaptic uptake of noradrenaline.	Hypertension	Intravenous glyceryl trinitrate (GTN) or phentolamine for hypertension that does not respond to benzodiazepines.
Caffeine		Chest pain	
Theophylline	Prevention of noradrenaline metabolism.	Agitation	
		Hyperreflexia	
		Seizures	
		Rhabdomyolysis	Aspirin, benzodiazepines, and GTN for chest pain.
		Intracerebral bleeds	Cooling (if resistant hyperthermia consider dantrolene).

Table 17.3 Anticholinergic toxidrome—causes, pathophysiology, clinical features, and management

Causative drugs	Pathophysiology	Clinical features	Treatment
Tricyclic antidepressants Antihistamines Antipsychotics Selective serotonin reuptake inhibitors Anti-parkinsonian Atropa belladonna (deadly nightshade)	Inhibition of cholinergic transmission at muscarinic receptors. Predominantly at peripheral parasympathetic muscarinic receptors. The degree of CNS disturbance depends on the ability of the drug to cross the blood-brain barrier.	Mad as a hatter (confusion, delirium). Hot as a hare (hyperthermia). Blind as a bat (mydriasis). Red as a beet (flushing). Dry as a bone (dry mouth and skin). Urinary retention. Sinus tachycardia. Functional ileus (reduced bowel sounds, constipation). Hypertension.	Supportive. Intravenous fluids. Benzodiazepines for agitation or seizures. Cooling.

Table 17.4 Cholinergic (muscarinic) toxidrome—causes, pathophysiology, clinical features, and management

Causative drugs	Pathophysiology	Clinical features	Treatment
Organophosphates Physostigmine Carbamate insecticides	Inhibition of acetylcholinesterase results in increased levels of acetylcholine Stimulation of muscarinic receptors results in excessive parasympathetic activity Stimulation of nicotinic receptors results in persistent muscle depolarization	Parasympathetic symptoms: **D**iarrhoea **U**rination **M**iosis and muscle weakness **B**ronchorrhoea **B**radycardia **E**mesis **L**acrimation **S**weating, salivation Nicotinic symptoms: weakness, fasiculations, and paralysis CNS symptoms: drowsiness, seizures	Decontamination Supportive Atropine (titrate until secretions dry up) Pralidoxime

Table 17.5 Opiate toxidrome—causes, pathophysiology, clinical features, and management

Causative drugs	Pathophysiology	Clinical features	Treatment
Morphine Heroin	Stimulation of opioid receptors in the peripheral and central nervous system.	Miosis Respiratory depression Reduced level of consciousness Coma Hypotension	Supportive. Naloxone (indose 400 mcg IV/IM, which may need repeating up to a dose of 10 mg.

17.3.4 Opiate toxidrome

Table 17.5 details the causes, pathophysiology, clinical features, and management of opiate toxidrome.

> **KEY POINTS**
>
> Toxidromes are clinical syndromes that suggest a specific class of poisoning.
>
> Sympathomimetic toxidrome is caused by drugs such as cocaine and amphetamines. It results in sweating, hyperthermia, hypertension, chest pain, and agitation. Treatment is supportive. Benzodiazepines are used to control hypertension, agitation, chest pain, and seizures. Patients may require cooling.
>
> Anticholinergic toxidrome is caused by drugs such as tricyclic antidepressants and antipsychotics. The clinical features can be remembered by the saying 'Mad as hatter, hot as a hare, blind as a bat, red as a beet, and dry as a bone'. Treatment is supportive. Benzodiazepines are used to treat agitation and seizures. Cooling may be required.
>
> Cholinergic toxidrome is caused by drugs such as organophosphates. Clinical features can be recalled using the mnemonic DUMBBELS. Patients must be decontaminated prior to treatment and high doses of atropine may be required until the patient is atropinized (dry skin and tachycardia). Pralidoxime is required for moderate and severe poisoning.
>
> Opiate toxidrome results in respiratory depression, reduced level of consciousness, miosis, and hypotension. Treatment is naloxone and supportive therapy.

17.4 Paracetamol poisoning

Previous MRCEM question

Paracetamol poisoning is a common ED presentation and has appeared in several previous SAQ papers.

17.4.1 Pathophysiology of paracetamol poisoning

Paracetamol in therapeutic doses is conjugated in the liver to inactive substrates (Figure 17.1). A small amount (~1%) is metabolized by the cytochrome P450 system producing a toxic metabolite, N-acetyl-p-benzoquinoneimine (NAPQI), which is inactivated by conjugation with glutathione.

In paracetamol overdose, the normal pathway of conjugation is saturated and a greater proportion of the paracetamol is metabolized by the cytochrome P450 system (Figure 17.2). Once the reserves of glutathione are depleted, the toxic metabolite (NAPQI) causes hepatic necrosis.

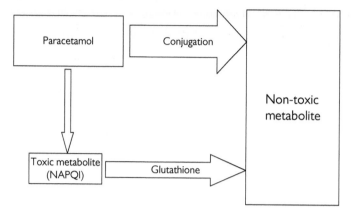

Figure 17.1 Therapeutic paracetamol metabolism.

Severe liver damage may occur if greater than 75 mg/kg is taken. Patients taking medications that induce the cytochrome P450 system or those with glutathione depletion are at increased risk of hepatic toxicity, however, these factors are no longer used to guide choice of treatment.

17.4.2 Clinical features of paracetamol poisoning

Most patients presenting acutely with a paracetamol overdose are asymptomatic. Patients with a delayed presentation may have more apparent clinical features.

Clinical features evolve depending on the time of presentation:

- Under 12 hours—asymptomatic or nausea, vomiting and/or abdominal discomfort
- 12–24 hours—vomiting, hepatic tenderness
- 2–3 days—jaundice, hypoglycaemia
- 4–5 days—hepatic encephalopathy, loin pain due to renal failure, hyperventilation due to metabolic acidosis, bleeding due to coagulopathy

17.4.3 Investigations for paracetamol poisoning

- Paracetamol levels—blood paracetamol level should be checked four hours after ingestion. There is no value in checking a level prior to this. Patients presenting greater than four hours after ingestion should have their level checked immediately.

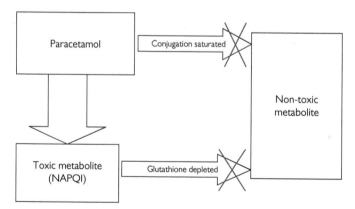

Figure 17.2 Paracetamol metabolism in overdose.

- Liver function tests (LFTs)—all patients should have their LFTs checked, however they may not be abnormal until >18 hours after the overdose. ALT and AST may reach >10,000 units/L at three to four days and are the most sensitive markers of liver damage.
- International normalized ratio (INR)—is a very sensitive marker of liver damage and the best prognostic parameter.
- Renal function—creatinine is a useful prognostic marker and a low urea may suggest malnutrition and therefore glutathione depletion.
- Glucose—patients are at risk of hypoglycaemia.
- Blood gas (venous or arterial)—metabolic acidosis is a poor prognostic sign.

17.4.4 Antidotes for paracetamol poisoning

There are two available antidotes for paracetamol toxicity in the United Kingdom: acetylcysteine and methionine. They work by binding to the toxic metabolite (NAPQI) and preventing hepatic necrosis.

Acetylcysteine is the most commonly used antidote and is give intravenously. The dosing schedule is:

- 150 mg/kg in 200 ml 5% glucose over 1 hour.
- 50 mg/kg in 500 ml 5% glucose over 4 hours.
- 100 mg/kg in 1000 ml 5% glucose over 16 hours.

Weight-based dosing tables have been introduced for adults and children.

Acetylcysteine can cause side effects, the most common being erythema and urticaria around the infusion site. It can also cause nausea, generalized urticaria, angioedema, bronchospasm, and hypotension. During infusion of the first two bags of acetylcysteine, up to 5% of patients develop an anaphylactoid reaction, mediated by histamine, and dependent on blood acetylcysteine concentrations, associated with flushing and wheezing.

If an anaphylactoid reaction occurs, temporarily stop the infusion for at least 30 minutes, and administer an antihistamine such as chlorpheniramine and nebulized salbutamol as needed. The entire dose of acetylcysteine may then be administered, possibly at a slower rate of infusion (e.g. at a rate of 50 mg/kg/hour).

Methionine is an oral formulation that can be used if intravenous access is not possible. TOXBASE now recommend giving the intravenous acetylcysteine formulation orally, instead of methionine, if intravenous access cannot be gained. The dosage of orally acetylcysteine is available on the TOXBASE website, but knowledge of the dosage is highly unlikely to be asked for in a SAQ.

17.4.5 Treatment of paracetamol toxicity

The treatment for a paracetamol overdose depends upon the timing of the overdose (Table 17.6). The measured blood level should be interpreted using the paracetamol treatment graph (Figure 17.3).

17.4.6 Criteria for liver transplantation in paracetamol poisoning

Selected patients with severe paracetamol-induced liver injury require urgent liver transplantation. It is vital that such patients are identified early after paracetamol ingestion.

The Kings College Criteria for paracetamol toxicity is used to identify patients that may require transplantation, it includes the following criteria:

- pH <7.3
- PT >100 seconds (INR >6.5)
- Creatinine >300 µmol/L

Table 17.6 Management of paracetamol poisoning according to timing

Less than 4 h	• If the patient presents less than 1 h since the overdose activated charcoal (50 g orally) should be given. • Paracetamol levels should be checked at 4 h and treatment guided by the level.
4–8 h	• Paracetamol levels should be checked immediately. • If the result is available before 8 h, treatment should be guided by the result. • If the result is not available before 8 hours and a potentially toxic amount (>75 mg/kg) has been taken acetylcysteine, should be started empirically until the paracetamol level is known.
8–24 h	• Paracetamol levels should be checked immediately. • Acetylcysteine should be started immediately if a potentially toxic amount has been taken (>75 mg/kg). • The acetylcysteine can be stopped if the laboratory levels are below the treatment line, the INR, liver transaminases, and creatinine are normal and the patient is asymptomatic. If any of these criteria are not met the acetylcysteine should continue.
24–36 h	• Paracetamol levels should be checked immediately. • Acetylcysteine should be started immediately if a potentially toxic amount has been taken. The paracetamol level is unlikely to be detectable. A measurable level suggests a very large overdose, inaccurate timing, or a staggered overdose. • A full course of acetylcysteine should be given if paracetamol is detected or if there is any evidence of liver injury (abnormal LFTs, INR, creatinine, or symptomatic). Bloods should be initially monitored every 8 h to assess progression of liver injury and need for referral to a liver unit.
Greater than 36 h	• Paracetamol levels should be checked immediately. • There is no evidence that starting acetylcysteine immediately in this group of patients confers any benefit. Therefore, the result should be known before commencing treatment. • If paracetamol is detected, a full course of acetylcysteine should be given. • If the patient is asymptomatic with normal liver transaminases, INR, and creatinine, and with no detectable paracetamol, then treatment is not required. • If the patient has mildly deranged INR and/or transaminases consult the National Poisons service or TOXBASE for further guidance.
Staggered overdose	• Paracetamol levels should be checked immediately. • The paracetamol level cannot be used on the treatment graph but may confirm ingestion. • If greater than 75 mg/kg has been taken in 24 h, then acetylcysteine should be considered. • If the patient is asymptomatic and has normal liver transaminases, INR, and creatinine at 24 h after the last ingestion then acetylcysteine can be stopped.

• Lactate >3.5 mmol/L on admission or >3.0 mmol/L, 24 hours post-paracetamol ingestion, or after fluid resuscitation
• Grade 3 or 4 hepatic encephalopathy*

* Reprinted from *Gastroenterology*, volume 97, issue 2, John G. O'Grady, Graeme J.M. Alexander, Karen M. Hayllar, Roger Williams, Early indicators of prognosis in fulminant hepatic failure, pp.439-445, Copyright (1989), with permission from Elsevier.

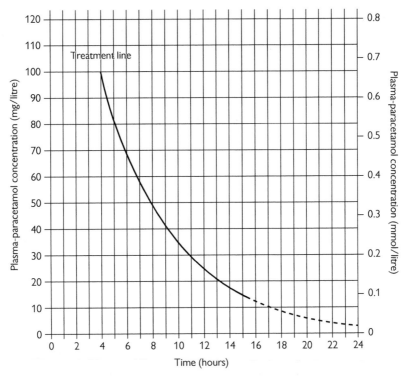

Figure 17.3 Paracetamol treatment graph.

Reproduced with the kind permission of the Royal College of Emergency Medicine http://www.rcem.ac.uk/Shop-Floor/Clinical%20Guidelines/College%20Guidelines/Paracetamol%20Overdose.

KEY POINTS

The toxic dose of paracetamol is >75 mg/kg.

ALT and AST may reach >10,000 units/L at three to four days after overdose and are the most sensitive markers of liver damage.

There are two available antidotes in the United Kingdom; acetylcysteine and methionine. TOXBASE now recommend that acetylcysteine be used orally rather than methionine if intravenous access is not possible.

The treatment of paracetamol overdose depends on the time of presentation and the paracetamol level.

Allergic reactions are quite common with acetylcysteine. The infusion should be stopped and the patient given chlorphenamine. Once the reaction settles, the infusion can be restarted at the slowest infusion rate.

17.5 Salicylate poisoning

Previous MRCEM question

17.5.1 Pathophysiology of salicylate toxicity

Aspirin is a derivative of salicylic acid. It is metabolized in the liver and excreted in the urine. In overdose, the high concentration of salicylates directly stimulate the respiratory centre, causing a respiratory alkalosis. The accumulation of metabolites and salicylate derivatives results in a metabolic acidosis. The respiratory effects usually dominate in adults, however in children the acidosis can predominate.

17.5.2 Toxic dose of aspirin

Table 17.7 details the toxic dose of aspirin.

17.5.3 Clinical features of salicylate poisoning

Common clinical features in mild poisoning include:

- Nausea
- Vomiting
- Tinnitus
- Lethargy
- Dizziness

Features of moderate to severe poisoning include:

- Sweating
- Hyperventilation
- Warm extremities and bounding pulses
- Dehydration
- Hyperpyrexia
- Confusion, disorientation
- Convulsions
- Coma

17.5.4 Severity of salicylate poisoning

The severity of salicylate poisoning is not determined by plasma levels alone. Severe poisoning is indicated by a combination of neurological features, metabolic acidosis, and high salicylate levels.
  Risk factors for death in severe poisoning include:

- Age over 70 or less than 10 years
- Central nervous system (CNS) features (confusion, convulsions, reduced GCS)
- Metabolic acidosis
- Hyperpyrexia
- Pulmonary oedema
- Salicylate concentration >700 mg/L (5.1 mmol/L)

17.5.5 Investigations for salicylate overdose

- Salicylate levels—should be checked at two hours after ingestion in symptomatic patients and four hours in asymptomatic patients. If salicylate is detected, a further level should be checked

Table 17.7 Aspirin toxicity

Aspirin dose	Likely toxicity
>125 mg/kg	Mild
>250 mg/kg	Moderate
>500 mg/kg	Severe

after two hours because of the possibility of continuing absorption. This should be continued every three hours until the peak is reached and levels are falling. This can take up to 12 hours with enteric-coated preparations.

- Renal function—patients are at risk of hypokalaemia and renal failure.
- Glucose—risk of hypoglycaemia.
- Arterial blood gas—to determine the presence of respiratory alkalosis and metabolic acidosis.
- INR—risk of coagulopathy.
- FBC—risk of thrombocytopenia.
- Electrocardiogram (ECG)—patients may develop arrhythmias due to hypokalaemia or acidosis.

17.5.6 Treatment of salicylate poisoning

Table 17.8 details the management of salicylate toxicity.

Table 17.8 Management of salicylate toxicity

Activated charcoal	• 50 g orally, if the patient presents within 1 h of ingestion. • This may need repeating if plasma levels continue to rise or an enteric-coated preparation has been taken.
Gastric lavage	• Consider if >500 mg/kg has been ingested and the patient presents within 1 hour of the overdose.
Rehydration	• This can be achieved orally or intravenously depending on the degree of toxicity. • It may be all that is required for patients with mild-moderate toxicity (<500 mg/L in adults and <350 mg/L in children).
Urinary alkalinization	• Increases the elimination of salicylates. • Target urine pH 7.5–8.5. • Indicated when levels are >500 mg/L (3.6 mmol/L) in adults and >350 mg/L (2.5 mmol/L) in children. • The dose in adults is 1.5 L of 1.26% (or 225 ml of 8.4%) sodium bicarbonate. Repeat doses may be required to maintain the urinary pH 7.5–8.5. • Effective alkalinization may be complicated by hypokalaemia and the potassium level should be checked every 1–2 h. • Forced alkaline diuresis is no longer recommended because it does not increase salicylate excretion and may cause pulmonary oedema.
Sodium bicarbonate	• Is recommended to correct metabolic acidosis (50–100 ml 8.4% over 30 minutes). • Sodium bicarbonate reduces transfer of salicylate into the central nervous system thereby reducing toxicity.
Haemodialysis	• Indicated in severe poisoning: • Salicylate levels >900 mg/L (consider if >700 mg/L); • Renal failure; • Congestive cardiac failure; • Non-cardiogenic pulmonary oedema; • Convulsions; • Coma; • CNS effects not resolved by correction of acidosis; • Severe metabolic acidosis (pH <7.2); • Persistently elevated salicylate levels despite urinary alkalinization.

KEY POINTS

Salicylate poisoning can result in a combined metabolic acidosis, due to the accumulation of salicylate derivatives and metabolites, and respiratory alkalosis, due to stimulation of the respiratory centre.

Salicylate levels should be checked at 2 h after ingestion in symptomatic patients and 4 h in asymptomatic patients. If salicylate is detected, a further level should be checked after 2 h because of the possibility of continuing absorption. This should be continued every 3 h until the peak is reached and levels are falling.

TOXBASE do not recommend measuring salicylate levels in conscious overdose patients who deny taking them and have no symptoms suggestive of toxicity.

Activated charcoal, rehydration, and sodium bicarbonate are the mainstay of treating salicylate toxicity.

Haemodialysis is the treatment of choice in severe poisoning.

17.6 Tricyclic antidepressant poisoning

17.6.1 Pathophysiology of tricyclic antidepressant poisoning

Tricyclic antidepressants (TCAs) are very toxic by ingestion. Overdose of greater than 15 mg/kg can result in severe, life-threatening poisoning.

Toxicity is due to a combination of anticholinergic effects at autonomic nerve endings and in the brain; blockade of cardiac sodium channels; and blockade of α_1 adrenergic receptors.

TCAs are metabolized by the liver and excreted by the kidney. They are highly protein-bound and the amount of unbound (i.e. active) TCA increases in acidosis.

The anticholinergic action prevents reuptake of norepinephrine into nerve terminals at noradrenergic and serotonergic sites. This can result in urinary retention, dilated pupils, pyrexia, confusion, convulsions, and a dry mouth.

Blockade of cardiac sodium channels causes prolongation of the PR, QRS, and QT intervals on the ECG.

Blockade of α_1-adrenergic receptors results in vasodilatation, which leads to hypotension and reflex tachycardia.

17.6.2 Clinical features of tricyclic antidepressant poisoning

- Anticholinergic—dry mouth, hot dry skin, urinary retention, ileus, dilated pupils, pyrexia, confusion, and convulsions.
- Cardiovascular—hypotension, sinus tachycardia, prolonged PR, QRS and QT, atrioventricular block.
- CNS—drowsiness, ataxia, divergent squint, hyperreflexia, hypertonia, extensor plantars, seizures, coma, and respiratory depression.
- Serotonin syndrome—may occur. Features include CNS effects (agitation, confusion, seizures, coma), neuromuscular hyperactivity (tremor, teeth grinding, hyperreflexia), and autonomic instability (tachycardia, labile blood pressure, hyperpyrexia). Chapter 18, section 18.5 includes further details on the features and management of serotonin syndrome.

17.6.3 Investigations for tricyclic antidepressant overdose

- ECG—to assess the PR, QRS, and QT length. The QRS duration is a useful marker of toxicity. QRS >120 ms may indicate cardiotoxicity and >160 ms suggests severe cardiotoxicity with a high risk of arrhythmias.

- Arterial blood gas—looking for hypoxia, hypercapnea, and metabolic acidosis.
- Renal function and CK—patients are at risk of rhabdomyolysis, especially if unconscious.
- Glucose—risk of hypoglycaemia.

17.6.4 Treatment of TCA poisoning

- Supportive therapy—as with all poisoning, an ABCDE approach and supportive therapy should be instituted. Any hypoxia should be corrected with supplemental oxygen and patients who are hypercapnic should receive assisted ventilation. Often correction of hypoxia, hypercapnea, and fluid resuscitation will be sufficient to correct the acidosis and any arrhythmias.
- Activated charcoal—should be considered if the patient presents within one hour of ingestion and is able to protect their airway.
- Sodium bicarbonate—is indicated if the patient has a metabolic acidosis which persists, despite correction of hypoxia and fluid resuscitation. Rapid correction is required if the patient is acidotic with a prolonged QRS or QT. The dose of sodium bicarbonate is 50 mmol (50 ml of 8.4%), which may need repeating, aiming for pH 7.5. Even in the absence of acidosis, alkalinization with sodium bicarbonate should be considered in patients with:
  - QRS>120 ms
  - Arrhythmias
  - Hypotension resistant to fluid resuscitation

Alkalinization by sodium bicarbonate reduces TCA toxicity by increasing protein binding, thereby reducing the available active substrate; antagonizing cardiac sodium channel blockade; and improving myocardial contractility by correcting the acidosis.

- Benzodiazepines—are used to control convulsions (e.g. lorazepam 4 mg IV) or sedate agitated patients. Phenytoin is contraindicated in TCA overdose because it also blocks sodium channels and increases the risk of cardiac arrhythmias.
- Arrhythmias—are best treated with correction of hypoxia and acidosis. Class Ia (quinidine, procainamide) and Ic (flecanide, propafenone) antiarrhythmics are contraindicated because they may worsen sodium channel blockade and exacerbate arrhythmias.
- Hypotension—should be treated with intravenous fluids and correction of acidosis with sodium bicarbonate. If hypotension persists despite this, then lipid emulsion may be considered. Inotropes may be required for resistant hypotension. Glucagon is also a treatment option for severe hypotension, heart failure, or cardiogenic shock.
- Cardiac arrest—may respond to prolonged resuscitation and efforts should be continued for at least one hour.

KEY POINTS

TCA toxicity is due to a combination of anticholinergic effects at autonomic nerve endings and in the brain; blockade of cardiac sodium channels; and blockade of α_1 adrenergic receptors. Clinical features include:

- Anticholinergic (see Table 17.3)
- Cardiovascular—hypotension, sinus tachycardia, prolonged PR, QRS and QT, atrioventricular block
- CNS—drowsiness, ataxia, divergent squint, hyperreflexia, hypertonia, extensor plantars, seizures, coma, and respiratory depression

Indications for sodium bicarbonate include:

- Persistent acidosis despite correction of hypoxia and fluid resuscitation
- QRS >120 ms
- Arrhythmias
- Hypotension resistant to fluid resuscitation

Lipid emulsion, inotropes, and/or glucagon may be required for resistant hypotension.

17.7 Carbon monoxide poisoning

17.7.1 Introduction

Carbon monoxide (CO) is a colourless, odourless gas produced by the incomplete combustion of any hydrocarbon (gas, coal, charcoal, petrol, diesel, paraffin) or carbohydrate (wood, paper) fuel. Carbon monoxide can also be generated by methylene chloride, a constituent of some paint strippers and sprays.

The Chief Medical Officer published a letter in 2010 to encourage health professionals to raise awareness of the risks of CO poisoning. There are approximately 50 accidental deaths per year from CO poisoning in England and Wales and this is likely to be an underestimate.

17.7.2 Pathophysiology of carbon monoxide poisoning

Carbon monoxide binds approximately 240 times more strongly than oxygen to haemoglobin and results in the oxyhaemoglobin dissociation curve being shifted to the left (Figure 17.4 and Table 17.9).

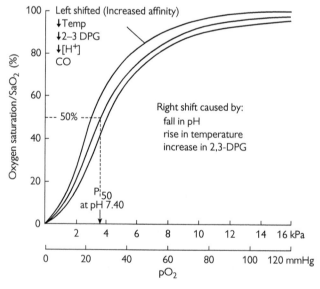

Figure 17.4 Oxyhaemoglobin dissociation curve.

Reproduced from Stephen Chapman, Grace Robinson, John Stradling, and Sophie West, *Oxford Handbook of Respiratory Medicine*, 2009, Figure A1.5, p. 802, with permission from Oxford University Press.

Table 17.9 Causes of left or right shift of the oxyhaemoglobin dissociation curve

Left shift (increased affinity of Hb for O2)	Right shift (decreased affinity of Hb for O2)
Increased pH (alkalosis)	Decreased pH (acidosis)
Decreased 2,3-diphosphoglycerate (DPG)	Increased DPG
Decreased temperature	Increased temperature
CO	Increased pCO_2

Haemoglobin can bind four oxygen molecules and the presence of CO on one of the four haem sites causes oxygen to bind with greater affinity. The result is that oxygen is less readily released to the tissues. Therefore, a patient can suffer hypoxia despite a normal PaO_2. Carbon monoxide also inhibits cytochrome oxidase thereby preventing cells from using the reduced amounts of oxygen they receive.

Recent studies have shown that CO may function as a local transmitter substance in the body playing a role in controlling the permeability of the microvasculature and increasing adhesion of inflammatory cells and platelets to the capillary endothelium. CO poisoning leads to leakage of fluid across cerebral capillaries leading to cerebral oedema. In those who have been exposed to enough CO to produce unconsciousness, delayed damage due to leukoencephalopathy may occur. Damage tends to be focused on 'watershed' areas such as the basal ganglia. Neurological damage seems to be the result of free radical generation and lipid peroxidation.

The half-life of CO is five to six hours when breathing room air (21%), approximately 1½ hours when breathing 100% oxygen, and approximately 23 minutes when breathing oxygen at 2 atmospheres (hyperbaric oxygen).

17.7.3 Clinical features of carbon monoxide poisoning

Acute features include:

- Headache, nausea, vomiting, and malaise
- Neurological features—ataxia, in-coordination, agitation, impaired conscious level, retinal haemorrhages, hyperreflexia, weakness, extensor plantars, and convulsions
- Respiratory features—hyperventilation, pulmonary oedema, respiratory failure
- Cardiac features—chest pain, MI, arrhythmias
- Dermatological features—rarely cherry red skin, blisters

The symptoms from chronic CO exposure are very non-specific, including headache, nausea, dizziness, lethargy, subjective weakness, and flu-like symptoms. Therefore CO poisoning is frequently undiagnosed. Patients may go on to develop neuropsychiatric features, including memory impairment, disorientation, apathy, personality change, Parkinsonism, and gait disturbance.

Clues to the diagnosis of CO poisoning are:

- More than one person in the house, including pets, are affected.
- Symptoms are better when away from the house.
- Symptoms are related to cooking (i.e. when the stove is in use).
- Symptoms are worse in the winter, with the heating in use.

17.7.4 Indicators of severity of CO poisoning

One or more the following features suggest higher level carbon monoxide poisoning:

- Any new objective acute neurological signs, including blindness, deafness, and extrapyramidal effects

- Impaired mini-mental state examination
- Vertigo and ataxia
- Breathlessness and tachycardia
- Chest pain related to angina
- Coma
- Seizure(s)
- Need for ventilation
- ECG indication of infarction or ischaemia
- Clinically significant acidosis
- Initial carboxyhaemoglobin level >30%

17.7.5 Investigations for CO poisoning

- Measuring COHb level—the two main ways to measure COHb levels are a breath analyser or a blood test, on either venous or arterial blood. The breath test is a useful screening tool and should be confirmed with an anticoagulated blood test if elevated. The level measured will depend on the time since exposure, whether the patient is a smoker, and what percentage of oxygen the patient has been breathing prior to the test. A normal carboxyhaemoglobin level does not exclude carbon monoxide poisoning, however a raised level increases the likelihood of diagnosis. A level of up to 5% can be expected in people smoking up to 20 cigarettes a day, non-smokers living in urban areas, and pregnant women. Heavy smokers may have levels up to 13%. Carboxyhaemoglobin levels have a weak correlation with clinical signs and symptoms, especially of neurological origin. However, in general terms levels <2% are not associated when any adverse features, levels at 20–30% are associated with neurological symptoms and 50% is associated with seizures, respiratory arrest, and death.
- Oxygen saturations—read falsely high in CO poisoning due to the similar light absorbency of carboxyhaemoglobin and oxyhaemoglobin. Therefore, saturations should not be used to guide the need for supplemental oxygen.
- ECG—risk of infarction and arrhythmias.
- Arterial blood gases (ABG)—looking for evidence of metabolic acidosis.
- CK—risk of rhabdomyolysis.
- Renal function—risk of renal failure.

17.7.6 Management of CO poisoning

- 100% oxygen therapy, which reduces the half-life of carboxyhaemoglobin from 320 to 80 minutes.
- Supportive therapy with fluid resuscitation.
- Sodium bicarbonate should only be considered if metabolic acidosis persists despite oxygen and fluid resuscitation.
- Assessment and management of hypoxic injury, especially to the heart and central nervous system.
- Mannitol should be given if cerebral oedema is suspected (1 g/kg over 20 minutes).
- Arrange checking of appliances and flues, and measurements of CO levels in the patient's house before letting anyone back in. Social services should be contacted if necessary.
- TOXBASE and the National Poisons Information Service no longer recommend hyperbaric oxygen therapy. The evidence base is insufficient to support transport of patients over long distances to hyperbaric units.

KEY POINTS

Carbon monoxide is a colourless, odourless gas produced by the incomplete combustion of any hydrocarbon or carbohydrate fuel.

Carbon monoxide binds approximately 240 times more strongly than oxygen to haemoglobin and results in the oxyhaemoglobin dissociation curve being shifted to the left.

Carbon monoxide also inhibits cytochrome oxidase, thereby preventing cells from using the reduced amounts of oxygen they receive.

Clinical features of carbon monoxide poisoning are very non-specific and may be dismissed as flu or food poisoning.

Clues to the diagnosis of CO poisoning are:

- More than one person in the house is affected.
- Symptoms are better when away from the house.
- Symptoms are related to cooking (i.e. when the stove is in use).
- Symptoms are worse in the winter, with the heating in use.

Treatment for carbon monoxide is high concentration oxygen. TOXBASE no longer recommend hyperbaric oxygen due to a lack of evidence of efficacy.

17.8 SAQs

17.8.1 Salicylate poisoning

A 60 kg, 45-year-old woman presents to the ED 30 minutes after taking 12 × 300 mg aspirin tablets. She is tearful but alert. She has no significant past medical history, takes no regular medication, and has no allergies.

a) (i) List three early symptoms associated with salicylate poisoning. (3 marks)

a) (ii) Give two blood tests, other than paracetamol and salicylate levels, that you should do and what abnormality you would be looking for? (2 marks)

b) Would gastric lavage be indicated? Explain your answer. (2 marks)

c) Give three substances for which activated charcoal is ineffective. (3 marks)

Suggested answer

a) (i) List three early symptoms associated with salicylate poisoning. (3 marks)

    Tinnitus

    Hyperventilation

    Nausea, vomiting

    Dizziness

    Lethargy

    Sweating

    Restlessness

    Confusion/disorientation

    Coma

    Convulsions

    Deafness

    Hyperpyrexia

a) (ii) Give two blood tests, other than paracetamol and salicylate levels, that you should do and what abnormality you would be looking for? (2 marks)

    Glucose Hypoglycaemia

    ABG Mixed metabolic acidosis and respiratory alkalosis

    U&E Renal failure and/or hypokalaemia

    Clotting Coagulopathy

    (½ mark for test, ½ mark for reason)

b) Would gastric lavage be indicated? Explain your answer. (2 marks)

    No (1 mark)

    Patient has not taken enough (1 mark)

    (Gastric lavage should be considered in patients who have ingested >500 mg/kg (or >4.5 g) and present less than one hour after the overdose (OD); this patient has taken approximately 60 mg/kg.)

c) Give three substances for which activated charcoal is ineffective. (3 marks)

    Lithium

    Boric acid

    Iron

    Petroleum distillates

    Ethanol

    Methanol

Ethylene glycol
Strong acids and alkalis
Cyanide
Malathion
Organophosphates

17.8.2 Tricyclic antidepressants

A 45-year-old man is brought to the ED by ambulance. He was found by his partner with empty packets of amitriptyline tablets by him. There was an empty whisky bottle beside him.

a) (i) Name four abnormal neurological signs you may find in overdose of drugs of this type? (2 marks)

a) (ii) An ECG is performed. Other than a tachycardia, what key features may be apparent? (2 marks)

You ensure he has a clear airway and adequate ventilation. Oxygen is administered and he is appropriately monitored. An ABG is done. It demonstrates a metabolic acidosis.

b) (i) What drug would you now give? (Name the drug, dose, and route) (2 marks)

b) (ii) Name two other indications for this drug in a TCA overdose. (2 marks)

c) Name two other drugs that can be used in the treatment of amitriptyline overdose. (2 marks)

Suggested answer

a) (i) Name four abnormal neurological signs you may find in overdose of drugs of this type? (2 marks)

   Dilated pupils

   Ataxia

   Nystagmus

   Divergent squint

   Drowsiness

   Coma

   Increased tone

   Hyperreflexia

   Extensor plantars

   Absent reflexes (in deep coma)

   Convulsions

   Seizures

a) (ii) An ECG is performed. Other than a tachycardia, what key features may be apparent? (2 marks)

   Prolongation of PR, QRS, and QT intervals

   Non-specific ST segment and T-wave changes

   Atrioventricular block

b) (i) What drug would you now give? (Name the drug, dose, and route) (2 marks)

   50 ml of 8.4% sodium bicarbonate IV

   (1.26% sodium bicarbonate is an alternative in the haemodynamically stable patient)

b) (ii) Name two other indications for this drug in a TCA overdose. (2 marks)

   QRS duration prolonged (>120 ms)

   Arrhythmias

   Hypotension resistant to fluid resuscitation

c) Name two other drugs that can be used in the treatment of amitriptyline overdose.

Sodium bicarbonate (if not mentioned in a previous answer)
Activated charcoal
Lorazepam or diazepam
Lipid emulsion
Inotropes (e.g. dobutamine)
Vasopressors (e.g. noradrenaline)
Glucagon

Further reading

Royal College of Emergency Medicine, December 2009. Guideline for the Management of Tricyclic Antidepressant Overdose, (GemNet). Available at: https://www.rcem.ac.uk [Online].

Royal College of Emergency Medicine, September 2012. Paracetamol overdose: new guidance on the use of intravenous acetylcysteine. Available at: https://www.rcem.ac.uk [Online].

Royal College of Emergency Medicine, December 2013. College of Emergency Medicine and National Poisons Information Service Guideline on Antidote Availability for Emergency Departments. Available at: https://www.rcem.ac.uk [Online].

Psychiatric emergencies

CONTENTS

18.1 Introduction

Psychiatry frequently appears in short-answer questions (SAQs) in a variety of manners. Most SAQ papers will include a question on toxicology, which may have a section on mental health law or the Mental Capacity Act.

NICE have produced guidance on the management of self-harm and the management of the violent patient. The pertinent points from these NICE guidelines are covered in this chapter.

Chapter 21 covers the Mental Capacity Act 2005 and the Mental Health Act 2007.

18.2 Types of mental disorder

18.2.1 Introduction

A mental disorder is a psychological or behavioural pattern associated with distress or disability that occurs in an individual and is not a part of normal development or culture. Disorders may be of two main types:

- Neuroses—these can be regarded as extreme forms of normal experience (e.g. anxiety, depression). Most mental health illnesses are of this type.
- Psychoses—these are more severe and involve the distortion of a person's perception of reality, often accompanied by delusions (fixed, false belief) and/or hallucinations (false perception due to sensory distortion or misinterpretation). Examples of psychotic disorders include schizophrenia and manic depression.

The aetiology of mental health disorders can be divided into two categories:

- Functional disorder—not due to a simple structural abnormality of the brain.
- Organic disorder—resulting from an identifiable impairment of the brain.

18.2.2 Functional disorders

Most mental health illness lies within this category (Table 18.1). Emergency department (ED) management involves careful assessment of the patient to identify any underlying organic cause for the disorder and if so appropriately managing it.

If the condition is felt to be functional, an assessment should be made of the severity of the condition. In milder disease, follow-up with the GP may be appropriate or the mental health team as an outpatient. Patients with severe exacerbations of their condition, suicidal ideation, or psychotic features should be assessed by the mental health team in the ED before discharge.

Consent should always be gained from the patient for such an assessment. If the patient is felt to lack capacity, the Mental Health Act should be used to guide management (see Chapter 21, section 21.4).

18.2.3 Organic disorders

Organic disorders that can result in mental illness include dementia, delirium, head injury, chronic substance misuse/withdrawal, temporal lobe epilepsy, intracranial tumours, encephalitis, and metabolic disturbances (e.g. hypoglycaemia, hypo/hyperthyroidism).

Patients presenting with an acute confusional state should have a thorough physical and mental state examination. The history may have to be gained from relatives, carers, and/or the GP. Investigations should be directed according to the clinical picture and to exclude potentially reversible causes.

Delirium/acute confusional state

Delirium is characterized by:

- Acute and rapid onset.
- Impairment of/clouding of consciousness: reduced awareness of the environment and inability to maintain attention (perseveration in answer to a question; wandering off during a conversation) and shortened attention span. The alertness or arousal to the surrounding environment fluctuates between falsely increased alertness and a lowered awareness of the surroundings.
- Global disturbance of cognition affecting multiple cognitive domains-memory, attention, concentration, orientation.
- Disorganized thinking (e.g. rambling or incoherent speech, constructional apraxia (impaired ability to copy geometrical figures), dysnomia.)
- Fluctuating clinical state with lucid intervals.
- Confusion worse at night with morning lucid interval; increased severity at evening or night-time (sun-downing) when environmental stimulation is lowered.
- Psychomotor disturbance: agitation, reduced activity.
- Disturbance of sleep-wake cycle; for example, frequent daytime naps (daytime drowsiness); night-time agitation (insomnia at night); sleep fragmentation.
- Emotional lability: anxiety; fear; depression; tearfulness; elation; fatuousness.
- Perceptual abnormalities; illusions; hallucinations especially visual (also tactile, auditory, olfactory).
- Paranoid ideas/delusions.
- Disturbance of memory: short-term, immediate, and working memory are commonly affected but long-term memories can also be disturbed.
- Reversibility.

Table 18.1 Causes of functional mental illness and recognized clinical features

Depression	• Low mood • Suicidal ideation • Poor concentration • Change in normal sleep pattern • Social withdrawal • Feelings of guilt • Loss of interest or enjoyment (anhedonia) • Loss of libido • Lethargy • Losing/gaining appetite/weight
Anxiety	• Headache • Tachycardia, increased respiratory rate • Giddiness/fainting • Chest pain • Tension • Sweating
Manic depression (bipolar affective disorder)	• Disinhibition • Over activity—physical and mental • Pressure of speech • Flight of ideas • Poor judgement • Excessive spending/gambling • Extreme mood swings • Ideas of grandeur • Insomnia • Promiscuity • Hallucinations • Delusions (mood-congruent)
Schizophrenia	No single symptom is pathognomonic: the presence of hallucinations or delusions simply confirms psychosis. The WHO ICD-10 classification is based on the evidence of present or previous psychosis for >1 month and the absence of predominant affective symptoms. Schneider's first rank symptoms were originally used to diagnose schizophrenia but can also occur in other causes of psychosis: • Auditory hallucinations (usually abusive or critical) • Thought withdrawal, insertion, broadcasting • Somatic passivity (sensation, emotions, or actions are externally controlled) • Delusional perception • Gedankenlautwerden (voices repeating the subject's thoughts out loud) Other features of schizophrenia include: • Excessive fear • Disturbed behaviour • Believing someone is following/persecuting them • Preoccupation with religion

It is often misdiagnosed as functional psychosis or dementia, but the following symptoms make delirium more likely:

• Non-auditory hallucinations
• Dysarthria
• Ataxia
• Gait disturbance
• Incontinence
• Focal neurological signs

Delirium can occur at any age but is more common in the elderly. Predisposing factors for delirium include:

- Increasing age
- Pre-existing cognitive decline (e.g. dementia)
- Polypharmacy
- Hypertension
- Alcohol-related health concerns
- Poor physical health
- Depression
- Visual impairment
- Hearing impairment
- Abnormal sodium level
- Use of an indwelling catheter

Delirium may be caused by many different conditions including:

- Intracranial infections (e.g. encephalitis, meningitis)
- Extracranial infections (e.g. urinary infections or pneumonia, especially in the elderly)
- Head injury—causing intracranial bleeds
- Strokes
- Epilepsy
- Metabolic disturbance (e.g. hypo- or hyperglycaemia, hypo- or hyperthyroidism, hyponatraemia, hypercalcaemia, renal failure)
- Drugs—particularly anticholinergics, benzodiazepines, steroids, and opiates
- Alcohol intoxication or withdrawal
- Carbon monoxide poisoning

Patients with delirium should have the following investigations:

- Blood glucose—to exclude hypoglycaemia or DKA.
- FBC, lactate, and blood cultures—to look for evidence of sepsis.
- Arterial blood gas—to exclude hypercapnoea and look for evidence of an acid-base disturbance (e.g. renal failure).
- Urea and electrolytes—to look for evidence of an electrolyte abnormality and/or renal failure.
- Thyroid function test—to look for evidence of thyroid disease.
- Clotting—if the patient is taking anti-coagulants to exclude a coagulopathy.
- ECG—to exclude an acute MI or arrhythmia.
- Urine dipstick and culture—to look for evidence of infection.
- CXR—to look for evidence of pneumonia or malignancy.
- CT head—if no other cause is found or if clinical features suggest a stroke, intracranial bleed, or malignancy.
- Lumbar puncture—should be considered if an intracranial infection is suspected and the patient has no contraindications.

The management of delirium depends on the underlying cause and usually requires a medical admission for further investigation and management.

Dementia

Dementia is defined as an acquired, progressive decline in intellect, behaviour, and personality. It is irreversible and typically occurs with a normal level of consciousness. Patients with dementia are at risk of delirium resulting from an acute infection or metabolic abnormality. Such patients may present with a sudden deterioration in their mental state.

Dementia can present with:

- Loss of memory, especially short term

(Memory disorder typically affects the registration, storage, and retrieval of new information, which is forgotten more quickly and learnt more slowly. Later in the course, memory of familiar and previously learnt material is also lost. The patient tries to cover any memory impairment).

- Episodes of increasing confusion
- Falls, with or without head injury
- Wandering and getting lost, especially at night
- Insomnia
- Weight loss
- Slow recovery and mobilization from injury (hip fracture) or illness (myocardial infarct, pneumonia)
- Incontinence
- Difficulty dressing (parietal lesion of dressing dyspraxia)
- Behavioural disinhibition (frontal lobe sign)
- Severe extrapyramidal reaction to dopamine antagonists (Lewy body dementia)
- Apraxia; agnosia: inability to recognize objects; aphasia-are associated with cortical dementias

End-stage disease is characterized by:

- Near-mutism
- Inability to sit up, hold the head, or track objects with the eyes
- Difficulty with eating and swallowing and associated weight loss
- Bladder or bowel dysfunction
- Recurrent respiratory or urinary infections

KEY POINTS

Functional mental health disorders are those that are not due to a simple structural abnormality of the brain. Examples include depression, anxiety, manic depression, and schizophrenia.

Organic mental health disorders are due to an identifiable impairment of the brain. Examples include dementia, delirium, head injury, chronic substance misuse/withdrawal, temporal lobe epilepsy, intracranial tumours, encephalitis, and metabolic disturbances (e.g. hypoglycaemia, hypo/hyperthyroidism).

Delirium is characterized by rapid onset, global disturbance of cognition, and disturbed conscious level.

Dementia is defined as an acquired, progressive decline in intellect, behaviour, and personality. It is irreversible and typically occurs with a normal level of consciousness.

18.3 Self-harm

18.3.1 Introduction

Self-harm is a complex behaviour that can be thought of as a maladaptive response to acute and chronic stress, often but not exclusively linked with thoughts of dying.

Patients presenting with self-harm usually have current psychosocial difficulties, are likely to be suffering from mental health problems, and are at significant risk of further self-harm and suicide.

18.3.2 **NICE guidance on the management of self-harm**

NICE (CG133) 2011 produced guidance on the management of self-harm. The key priorities identified in the guideline are summarized here:

- People who have self-harmed should be treated with the same care, respect, and privacy as any patient.
- Clinical and non-clinical staff should have appropriate training to understand and care for people who have self-harmed.
- Activated charcoal should be immediately available when appropriate.
- Patients should have a preliminary psychosocial assessment at triage. Assessment should determine a person's mental capacity, willingness to stay for (psychosocial) assessment, level of distress, and presence of any possible mental illness.
- Patients who have to wait for treatment should be offered an environment which is safe, supportive, and minimizes any distress.
- Treatment should be offered for the physical consequences of self-harm, regardless of the willingness to accept psychosocial assessment.
- Adequate analgesia/anaesthesia should be offered.
- Patients should be provided with full information about treatment options to enable them to give informed consent before any treatment is initiated.
- Patients should be offered an assessment of needs, to include social, psychological, and motivational factors specific to the act of self-harm, current suicidal intent, and hopelessness, as well as a full mental health and social needs assessment. Ideally this should be performed by a specialist mental health professional.
- All patients should be assessed for risk, including identification of the main clinical and demographic features known to be associated with the risk of further self-harm or suicide and identification of the key psychological characteristics associated with risk, in particular depression, hopelessness, and continued suicidal intent.
- Psychosocial assessment should not be delayed until after medical treatment, unless life-saving treatment is required, the patient is unconscious, or incapable of assessment (e.g. intoxicated).

Mental capacity should always be assessed with the assumption that the patient has capacity unless there is evidence to the contrary. Fully informed consent should be gained before each treatment or procedure. If the patient lacks capacity, then management should be in the patient's best interests, even if against their wishes.

18.3.3 **Assessing suicide risk**

There are many different risk assessment tools in use. Probably, the most commonly used is the SAD PERSONS scale. The accuracy of these scales in predicting future self-harm and suicide is poor.

NICE does not recommend the use of risk assessment tools in assessing the risk of suicide/future self-harm or in considering treatment eligibility or discharge. They do recommend however that tools can be used to aid and structure risk assessment.

When assessing an individual's risk of future self-harm, NICE recommends discussion with the individuals who self-harm and identifying and agreeing on specific personal risks/triggers. Box 18.1 lists the risks for self-harm that should be taken into account.

KEY POINTS

Self-harm is a complex behaviour that can be thought of as a maladaptive response to acute and chronic stress, often but not exclusively linked with thoughts of dying.

NICE no longer recommends the use of risk assessment tools. Risk factors should be identified and agreed with the self-harmer.

Box 18.1 Factors associated with self-harm

- Methods and frequency of current and past self-harm
- Current and past suicidal intent
- Depressive symptoms and relationship to self-harm
- Psychiatric illness and relationship to self-harm
- Personal and social context
- Specific risk factors and protective factors
- Coping strategies
- Significant relationships that are supportive or may represent a threat
- Immediate and longer-term risks

Adapted from NICE, CG133, Self-harm in over 8s: long-term management, (November, 2011), https://www.nice.org.uk/guidance/cg133/resources/selfharm-in-over- 8s-longterm-management- 35109508689349

18.4 Managing the violent patient

18.4.1 Introduction

Disturbed or violent behaviour by a patient in the ED poses a serious risk to the individual, other patients, visitors, and staff. The management of a disturbed or violent patient is covered by a multifaceted legal framework. The management of such patients frequently involves interventions to which the patient does not or cannot consent. Any actions must be a reasonable and proportionate response to the risk it seeks to address.

18.4.2 NICE guidance on the management of the disturbed/ violent patient

NICE produced guidance on the management of a disturbed/violent patient in 2015. The main points from this guideline are summarized here:

- Staff should receive appropriate training in the recognition of acute mental illness and awareness of organic differential diagnoses. Staff should have ongoing training in the management of disturbed/violent behaviour.
- A system should be in place to alert staff to patients known to pose a risk of disturbed/violent behaviour.
- If after the initial ED assessment a mental health assessment is required, specialist advice should be sought.
- Every ED should have a designated room for mental health assessments.
- Staff interviewing a patient should always inform a senior member of the ED nursing staff before commencing the interview. Ordinarily, a chaperone should be present.
- Appropriate psychiatric assessment should be available within one hour of alert from the ED.
- De-escalation techniques should be used.
- If rapid tranquilization is considered necessary, lorazepam should be considered the first-line drug.

18.4.3 Rapid tranquilization

- The aim of rapid tranquilization is to achieve a state of calm sufficient to minimize the risk posed to the patient and others.
- Prior to the use of drugs to provide rapid tranquilization, de-escalation techniques should be tried.

- Physical intervention should be avoided if at all possible but may be required to enable rapid tranquilization. The level of force applied must be justifiable, appropriate, reasonable, and proportionate to the situation, and applied for the shortest possible time.
- Resuscitation equipment should be immediately available.
- Flumazenil must be available in case of oversedation. An anticholinergic (e.g. procyclidine) must be available in case of an acute dystonic reaction to antipsychotics.
- Oral medication should be offered before parenteral.
- If parenteral medication is required then intramuscular is preferred over intravenous. Intravenous medication should only be used in exceptional circumstances.
- Vital signs must be monitored after parenteral medication.
- Choice of drug (e.g. lorazepam, or haloperidol and promethazine) should depend on patient specific factors such as past medical history, intoxication, previous response to medication, and possible drug interactions. If insufficient information is available, lorazepam should be used as first line.
- If there is partial response to lorazepam, a repeat dose can be administered and if there is no response, haloperidol and promethazine should be used.
- Olanzapine is not recommended by NICE for rapid tranquilization.

KEY POINTS

The aim of rapid tranquilization is to achieve a state of calm sufficient to minimize the risk posed to the patient and others.

Lorazepam is the drug of choice for rapid tranquilization.

Intravenous medication should only be used in exceptional circumstances.

Resuscitation equipment must be immediately available.

Flumazenil and procyclidine must be available to treat complications of rapid tranquillization.

18.5 Complications of psychiatric medications

There are some well-recognized syndromes that patients may present with when taking antidepressants or antipsychotics.

18.5.1 Serotonin syndrome

Serotonin syndrome is a potentially life-threatening adverse drug reaction due to excess serotonergic activity in the central nervous system and at peripheral serotonin receptors. The syndrome is more likely to occur if the patient has been exposed to two or more drugs that increase the effect of serotonin in serotonergic synapses.

Serotonin syndrome may be caused by:

- Overdose of selective serotonin reuptake inhibitors (SSRIs).
- Concomitant use of SSRIs and monoamine oxidase inhibitors (MAOIs), often when there is insufficient time between stopping one and starting the other.
- Concomitant use of SSRIs and tricyclic antidepressants (TCAs).
- Concomitant use of SSRIs and any of the following: tramadol, serotonin noradrenaline reuptake inhibitors (SNRIs), triptans, linezolid, St John's wort.
- Use of stimulant drugs of abuse (e.g. ecstasy, amphetamines, cocaine), especially if taken in conjunction with a SSRI.

Clinical features of serotonin syndrome

Serotonin syndrome may occur insidiously over a period of minutes to hours after exposure. It is characterized by a triad of altered mental status, neuromuscular hyperactivity, and autonomic instability.

Altered mental status—occurs in 40% of patients and includes:

- Agitation
- Confusion
- Delirium
- Hallucinations
- Drowsiness
- Coma
- Seizures (in severe cases)

Neuromuscular hyperactivity—occurs in ~50% of patients and includes:

- Tremor
- Shivering
- Teeth grinding
- Myoclonus
- Hyperreflexia

Autonomic instability—occurs in ~50% of patients and includes:

- Tachycardia
- Hyperthermia
- Hyper or hypotension
- Flushing
- Diarrhoea and vomiting

Investigations for serotonin syndrome

Serotonin syndrome is a clinical diagnosis. The following investigations should be performed to identify complications and guide therapy:

- Urea and electrolytes—risk of acute kidney injury
- Creatine kinase—risk of rhabdomyolysis; may need to be performed serially
- ABG—to detect any hypoxia or acid-base disturbance
- Clotting—risk of coagulopathy
- Urine for myoglobin—screen for rhabdomyolysis
- Blood glucose
- ECG—risk of arrhythmias

Management of serotonin syndrome

- Stop all potentially offending drug(s).
- Airway and breathing—any hypoxia should be corrected with supplemental oxygen. Patients who are unable to maintain and/or protect their airway should be intubated and ventilated. Patients with inadequate respiratory effort should be intubated and ventilated.
- Circulation—intravenous fluids should be given to correct hypotension and ensure adequate hydration, especially if the patient has increased insensible losses due to hyperthermia. Urine output should be monitored.
- Disability—single, brief seizures do not require treatment. Frequent or prolonged seizures should be controlled with intravenous benzodiazepines (e.g. lorazepam 4 mg IV). If seizures

persist despite benzodiazepines, then consider phenobarbital. An alternative is phenytoin but caution is required if the patient has taken a sodium channel blocking agent (e.g. TCAs) because this may worsen cardiotoxicity. If seizures persist then the patient will require intubation and ventilation under general anaesthesia. Thiopental is recommended as the induction agent for such cases.

- Hyperthermia—mild hyperthermia should be controlled with external cooling (e.g. tepid sponging, fans). Temperatures >39°C require urgent cooling with ice baths and sedation (e.g. diazepam 10–20 mg). If hyperthermia persists then dantrolene may be considered. Such patients should be discussed with the National Poisons Information Service.
- Rhabdomyolysis—patients should be given intravenous volume replacement and considered for urinary alkalinization. Urinary alkalinization is achieved with sodium bicarbonate; the dose in adults is 1.5L of 1.26% (or 225 ml of 8.4%). Repeat doses may be required to maintain the urinary pH >7.5. In severe cases of rhabdomyolysis haemodiafiltration may be required.
- Cyproheptadine—is a 5HT antagonist and has been successfully used to treat serotonin syndrome. It should be given on advice from the National Poisons Information Service.

Complications of serotonin syndrome

- Seizures
- Hyperthermia
- Rhabdomyolysis
- Acute kidney injury
- Coagulopathy
- Death—usually due to hyperpyrexia induced multiorgan failure

18.5.2 Neuroleptic malignant syndrome

Neuroleptic malignant syndrome is an idiosyncratic drug reaction to antipsychotics (e.g. haloperidol, thioridazine, clozapine, risperidone, and chlorpromazine). It usually occurs within three to nine days of starting the drug but can occur in long-term use. It is thought to be due to central dopaminergic blockade.

The differential diagnosis of neuroleptic malignant syndrome includes:

- Serotonin syndrome
- Malignant hyperthermia (if recent anaesthesia)
- CNS infection
- Vasculitis
- Heat stroke
- Drug toxicity—MAOI, lithium, cholinergic

Clinical features of neuroleptic malignant syndrome

- Triad—hyperthermia, muscle rigidity, and disturbed consciousness (encephalopathy)
- Autonomic instability—labile blood pressure, tachycardia, and hyperthermia
- Dyskinesia

Investigations for neuroleptic malignant syndrome

- Creatine kinase—risk of rhabdomyolysis.
- Urine myoglobin (dipstick positive for blood)—screen for rhabdomyolysis.
- Urea and electrolytes—risk of renal failure, hyperkalaemia, and hypo- or hypernatraemia.
- FBC and clotting—risk of disseminated intravascular coagulation (DIC) and thrombocytopenia. Often patients have a raised white cell count.

Management of neuroleptic malignant syndrome

- Discontinue the antipsychotic drug.
- Cooled intravenous fluids should be given to correct for insensible losses and help reduce any hyperthermia.
- Cooling techniques should be employed, such as tepid sponging and use of fans. If these fail to reduce temperature, and there is muscle rigidity, then dantrolene may be of benefit.
- Bromocriptine (dopamine agonist) may be considered on advice from the National Poisons Information Service. Bromocriptine may cause a recurrence of psychotic symptoms.
- Patients with resistant symptoms may require paralysing and ventilating.
- Patients with rhabdomyolysis should be given intravenous volume replacement and considered for urinary alkalinization. Urinary alkalinization is achieved with sodium bicarbonate; the dose in adults is 1.5 L of 1.26% (or 225 ml of 8.4%). Repeat doses may be required to maintain the urinary pH>7.5. In severe cases of rhabdomyolysis, haemodiafiltration may be required.

Complications of neuroleptic malignant syndrome

- Mortality 12–20%
- Renal failure
- Rhabdomyolysis
- DIC
- Thrombocytopenia
- Electrolyte disturbances—hyperkalaemia, hyponatraemia, hypernatraemia

EXAM TIP

Confusion can sometimes exist about the difference between serotonin syndrome, neuroleptic malignant syndrome, and malignant hyperthermia. All can cause hyperpyrexia and cardiovascular instability.

- Serotonin syndrome—is due to an overdose of SSRIs, or a combination of SSRI and MAOI/TCA.
- Neuroleptic malignant syndrome—is an idiosyncratic drug reaction to antipsychotics.
- Malignant hyperthermia—is a rare autosomal dominant condition related to general anaesthesia (suxamethonium, gaseous agents). It causes uncontrolled skeletal muscle oxidative metabolism. Treatment is supportive management and dantrolene.

18.5.3 Acute dystonic reaction

Acute dystonic reactions may occur following the ingestion of antipsychotic medications (e.g. phenothiazine, haloperidol) or other drugs such as metoclopramide. Reactions can occur up to one week after ingestion.

Clinical features of an acute dystonic reaction:

- Grimacing
- Facial and masseter spasm which may cause trismus and/or cause jaw dislocation
- Deviated gaze (oculogyric crisis)
- Torticollis
- Orolingual dyskinesia
- Limb rigidity
- Behavioural disturbance
- May be mistaken as malingering, because symptoms can be briefly interrupted for voluntary actions

Management of an acute dystonic reaction

- Discontinue the offending drug.
- Benzatropine 2 mg intravenously or procyclidine 5 mg intravenously (doses may need repeating).
- Dramatic resolution of symptoms should occur within minutes.
- Patients should be discharged with oral procyclidine 5 mg total dissolved solid (TDS) because symptoms may recur.

KEY POINTS

Serotonin syndrome is caused by excess serotonergic activity in the central nervous system and at peripheral serotonin receptors.

Serotonin syndrome is more likely to occur if the patient has been exposed to two or more drugs that increase the effect of serotonin in serotonergic synapses (e.g. SSRI and TCA or MAOI).

Serotonin syndrome is characterized by a triad of altered mental status, neuromuscular hyperactivity, and autonomic instability.

Treatment of serotonin syndrome involves stopping the offending drug(s), intravenous fluids, external cooling, and benzodiazepines for seizures. Urinary alkalinization may be required if the patient develops rhabdomyolysis. Dantrolene and cyproheptadine may be required on advice of the National Poisons Information Service.

Neuroleptic malignant syndrome is an idiosyncratic drug reaction to antipsychotics (e.g. haloperidol). It is thought to be due to central dopaminergic blockade. It usually occurs within three to nine days of starting the drug, but can occur in long-term use.

Neuroleptic malignant syndrome usually results in a triad of hyperthermia, disturbed consciousness, and muscle rigidity. Autonomic instability is common.

The initial treatment of neuroleptic syndrome is very similar to that for serotonin syndrome. Dantrolene and bromocriptine may be required in more severe cases on advice of the National Poisons Information Service.

Acute dystonic reactions may occur following the ingestion of antipsychotic medications (e.g. phenothiazine, haloperidol) or other drugs such as metoclopramide. Reactions can occur up to one week after ingestion.

Symptoms of acute dystonic reaction include grimacing, trismus, oculogyric crisis, torticollis, muscle rigidity, orolingual dyskinesia, and behavioural disturbance.

Treatment of acute dystonic reaction is with procyclidine or benzatropine.

18.6 SAQs

18.6.1 Psychiatry

You are pre-alerted to the arrival of an agitated and aggressive patient. He is a patient who is well-known to the department and has a diagnosis of manic depression. He has been found in the centre of town shouting that he is invincible and the Risen Son. He has wounds to both palms and feet which are bleeding. He is being brought in by ambulance with the police in attendance.

a) Give two features in his history which suggests he is having an episode of mania? (2 marks)

   He arrives in the department and is being restrained by four police officers. He is shouting that he has to die in order that he can rise again.

b) You decide he needs rapid tranquilization. What monitoring do you want the nurse to get ready (2 marks) and what drug(s) do you need? (2 marks)

c) The nurse is concerned that the patient is being treated against his wishes. Which piece of legislation permits treatment of this patient and why? (2 marks)

d) The patient develops a temperature after the sedation—what two conditions should you be concerned that the patient may have? (2 marks)

Suggested answer

a) Give two features in his history which suggests he is having an episode of mania? (2 marks)

   Disinhibition
   Grandiosity
   Delusions
   Impaired judgement
   Preoccupation with religion

b) You decide he needs rapid tranquilization. What monitoring do you want the nurse to get ready (2 marks) and what drug(s) do you need (2 marks)?

   Equipment—cardiac monitor, saturation probe, BP monitor, BM machine.
   Drugs—lorazepam and haloperidol to sedate. Flumazenil and procyclidine/benzatropine in case of complications.
   (Must have lorazepam to get marks)

c) The nurse is concerned that the patient is being treated against his wishes. Which piece of legislation permits treatment of this patient and why? (2 marks)

   Mental Capacity Act.
   Patient lacks capacity to consent to treatment and therefore can be treated in his best interests.

d) The patient develops a temperature after the sedation what two conditions should you be concerned that the patient may have? (2 marks)

   Neuroleptic malignant syndrome
   Serotonin syndrome
   Underlying infection causing delirium

Further reading

Juhnke GA. 1994. SAD persons scale review. *Measurement and Evaluation in Counselling and Development* **27**(1):325–7.

National Institute for Health and Care Excellence, November 2011. NICE clinical guideline 133. Self Harm in over 8s: Long Term Management. Available at: https://www.nice.org.uk/guidance/cg133 [Online].

National Institute for Health and Care Excellence, May 2015. NICE guideline 10. Violence and Aggression: Short-term management in mental health, health and community settings. Available at: https://www.nice.org.uk/guidance/ng10 [Online].

Paediatric emergencies

CONTENTS

19.1 Introduction

This chapter relates to the Paediatric Emergency Medicine curriculum published in 2015 and follows a symptom-based approach. Inevitably with a symptom-based approach, a particular condition may be relevant to several different sections. Therefore, this chapter is cross-referenced to other sections and chapters where applicable.

This chapter is divided into major and acute paediatric presentations.

19.2 Anaphylaxis

Anaphylaxis is a severe, life-threatening, systemic, type 1 hypersensitivity reaction to ingested, inhaled, or topical substances. Anaphylaxis may present as respiratory distress and/or shock. The pathophysiology and clinical features of anaphylaxis are similar in adults and children and are discussed in Chapter 2, section 2.3.

19.2.1 Management of anaphylaxis

The management of anaphylaxis in children follows an ABCDE approach, treating life-threatening problems as they are recognized. Initial treatments should not be delayed by the lack of a complete history or definite diagnosis. If possible, the trigger should be removed (e.g. stop any drug or fluid infusions).

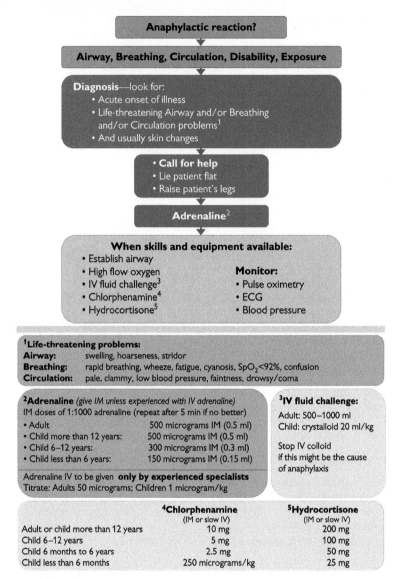

Figure 19.1 Anaphylaxis algorithm.
Reproduced with the kind permission of the Resuscitation Council (UK)

The anaphylaxis algorithm (Figure 19.1) details the Resuscitation Council guidance for adults and children.

The main difference in the management of children with anaphylaxis is the drug dosages as detailed in Table 19.1.

Table 19.1 Paediatric doses for the treatment of anaphylaxis

Drug	Dose			
	Age >12 years	>6–12 years	6 months–6 years	<6 months
Adrenaline	500 mcg IM (0.5 ml of 1:1000 adrenaline)	300 mcg IM (0.3 ml)	150 mcg IM (0.15 ml)	150 mcg IM (0.15 ml)
	IM adrenaline should be repeated at 5-min intervals if there is no improvement in the patient's condition.			
Chlorphenamine	10 mg IM or slowly IV	5 mg	2.5 mg	250 mcg/kg
Hydrocortisone	200 mg IM or slowly IV	100 mg	50 mg	25 mg
Fluids	20 ml/kg bolus of IV crystalloid			

KEY POINTS

Patients who have an anaphylactic reaction have life-threatening airway and/or breathing and/or circulation problems usually associated with skin and mucosal changes.

Early recognition of anaphylaxis and treatment with adrenaline is essential.

IM adrenaline should be repeated at five-minute intervals if there is no improvement in the patient's condition.

19.3 Apnoea, stridor, and airway obstruction

Airway obstruction is one of the main causes of cardiorespiratory arrest in children. Airway obstruction may have multiple aetiologies, including those affecting the upper and lower airways. This section focuses on pathologies affecting the upper airway; those affecting the lower airways are discussed in section 19.13.

19.3.1 Causes of airway obstruction

There are numerous causes of upper airway obstruction in children, the details of which are covered in Table 19.2.

19.3.2 Clinical features

Clinical features of airway obstruction include:

- Stridor—a monophasic, harsh, high-pitched inspiratory noise due to laryngeal or tracheal obstruction (compared with stertor or snoring, which is a lower-pitched inspiratory noise suggestive of poor airway positioning or pharyngeal obstruction).
- Chest wall recession.
- Accessory muscle use.
- Drooling of saliva.
- Hoarse or altered voice.
- Cyanosis.
- Dyspnoea.
- Drowsiness.
- Feeding problems in infants.

Table 19.2 Causes of upper airway obstruction in children

Causes of airway obstruction	Examples
Infective (covered in section 19.12)	Epiglottis
	Croup
	Bacterial tracheitis
	Diptheria
	Whooping cough
	Retropharyngeal abscess
Allergic (section 19.2)	Anaphylaxis (angioedema)
Obstructive	Foreign body
	Post-tonsillectomy bleed
	Burns
	Facial or laryngeal trauma (e.g. compressive haematomas)
	Tongue (in an obtunded patient)

The clinical presentation may suggest the likely cause of airway obstruction.

There may be a clear history of foreign body inhalation; if not, other clues include a sudden onset of respiratory compromise in a previously well child, associated with coughing, gagging, and stridor.

An infective cause is more likely in a child who has been unwell in the last few days and has a fever.

Anaphylaxis is suggested by a sudden onset of respiratory distress with associated urticaria and angioedema.

Table 19.3 details some the clinical features which may help differentiate the cause.

19.3.3 Management of airway obstruction

In a child with a compromised but functioning airway, it is important not to worsen the situation by upsetting the child. Crying and struggling may quickly convert a partially obstructed airway into a completely obstructed one.

Partial airway obstruction

Management of a child with a partially obstructed airway depends on the cause. Senior airway support should be sought early.

- *Infective*. A child with an infective cause of obstruction will often position themself sitting upright and very still. If possible supplemental oxygen should be administered, but this must not distress the child further. Employing the parents' assistance will often help alleviate the child's anxieties. The management of different causes of infective airway obstruction are discussed in section 19.13.
- *Allergic*. The management of anaphylaxis is discussed in section 19.2.
- *Obstructive*. Patients with a partially obstructed airway due to secretions or a depressed level of consciousness should have their airway supported using basic airway manoeuvres (e.g. chin lift or jaw thrust) and/or suction. Further maintenance may be accomplished with basic airway adjuncts (e.g. oropharyngeal or nasopharyngeal airways).

Table 19.3 Clinical presentations of upper airway obstruction

	Croup	Epiglottis	Bacterial tracheitis	Anaphylaxis	Foreign body
Age	Commonest in second year of life (may occur age 6 months to 5 years)	Young adults (Hib vaccine has virtually eradicated it in young children)	Throughout childhood	Throughout childhood	Throughout childhood
Onset	1–2 days	<24 h	<24 h	Sudden	Sudden
History	Coryza, barking cough	Sore throat, dysphagia	Rattling cough, sore throat	Known trigger (e.g. wasp sting, eating nuts)	Playing with a small object or onset during eating
Signs	Temperature <38.5°C, not toxic, harsh stridor, hoarse voice	Temperature >38.5°C, toxic, upright position, very still, drooling	Temperature >38.5°C, toxic, mucopurulent secretions, soft/absent stridor	Facial swelling, urticarial rash, cardiovascular compromise	Afebrile, coughing, gagging, distressed

Children with a foreign body obstructing their airway and an effective cough should be encouraged to cough. A spontaneous cough is more effective at relieving an obstruction than any externally imposed manoeuvre.

If a foreign body is easily visible and accessible in the mouth, then a careful attempt to remove it is acceptable, being careful not to push it further into the airway. Blind finger sweeps of the mouth or upper airway should not be performed.

The choking algorithm

The management of a choking child depends on whether they are conscious with an ineffective cough or unconscious. Figure 19.2 details the Resuscitation Council Guidelines on the management of a choking child.

In conscious patients with an ineffective cough, five back blows should be followed by five thrusts, if the object has not been expelled. The cycle continues until the object is expelled or the patient becomes unconscious. Infants (age <1 year) should not receive abdominal thrusts due to the risk of intra-abdominal injury. Therefore, chest thrusts are performed using the same landmarks as for cardiopulmonary resuscitation (CPR), but the thrusts are sharper and performed more slowly at a rate of one per second.

In the unconscious patient with foreign body airway obstruction, the airway is opened, and any obvious object removed. Five rescue breaths are given followed by CPR at a ratio of 15:2. Each time breaths are attempted, the mouth should be checked for the presence of a foreign body.

Complete airway obstruction

Patients with complete airway obstruction should be managed in a step-wise manner:

- Basic airway-opening manoeuvres (chin lift, head tit, or jaw thrust).
- Secretions should be cleared with suction and/or airway position (recovery position).
- Any obvious foreign body should be removed under direct revision with Magill's forceps.
- If obstruction persists, an airway adjunct (e.g. oropharyngeal, nasopharyngeal airway, or laryngeal mask airway (LMA)) may be used.

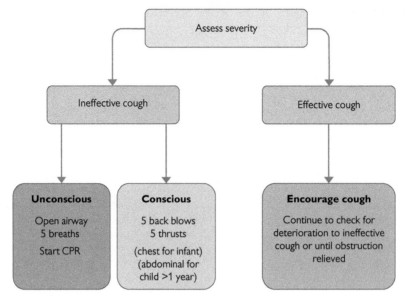

Figure 19.2 Paediatric choking treatment algorithm.
Reproduced with the kind permission of the Resuscitation Council (UK)

- If obstruction persists and ventilation is not possible, intubation should be attempted.
- If intubation is impossible or unsuccessful, a surgical airway is required.
- Once an airway is achieved, the patient should receive high-concentration oxygen and assisted ventilation if not breathing or breathing inadequately.

Paediatric surgical airways

Occasionally it is impossible to ventilate an apnoeic patient with a bag-valve mask, or to pass a tracheal tube or other airway device. In these circumstances a surgical airway below the level of the obstruction is required. The management options are a needle cricothyroidotomy or a surgical cricothyroidotomy.

Surgical airway management is discussed in Chapter 3, section 3.4.3. In children under the age of 8 years, needle cricothyroidotomy is preferred to surgical cricothyroidotomy. In adolescents either technique can be used. The advantages and disadvantages of the two techniques are discussed in Chapter 3.

The technique for needle cricothyroidotomy in a child is the same as an adult (section 3.4.3.), however the oxygen flow rate is different. In an adult, a flow rate of 15 L is used, in a child it is set at the child's age in years (e.g. a 5-year-old child will have a starting flow rate of 5 L/minute).

The technique for a surgical cricothyroidotomy is the same for a child as an adult, however a smaller tracheal or tracheostomy tube will be required.

KEY POINTS

Airway obstruction is one of the main causes of cardiorespiratory arrest in children.

The main causes of airway obstruction are:
- Infective
- Allergic

- Obstructive

Clinical features of airway obstruction include:

- Stridor
- Chest wall recession
- Accessory muscle use
- Drooling of saliva
- Hoarse or altered voice
- Cyanosis
- Dyspnoea
- Drowsiness
- Feeding problems in infants

Needle cricothyroidotomy is the recommended surgical airway technique in children under the age of eight years. The oxygen flow rate should be set at the child's age in years (e.g. a six-year-old child should have a flow rate of 6 L/min)

19.4 Cardiopulmonary arrest

19.4.1 Introduction

Cardiopulmonary arrest in children is fortunately rare and gaining competence managing such situations is often most easily achieved by attendance at a paediatric resuscitation course; for example, a European Paediatric Life Support (EPLS) or Advanced Paediatric Life Support (APLS) course.

EXAM TIP

The Resuscitation Council website (https://www.resus.org.uk) has the adult and paediatric guidelines available to download. The website also has details of any recent updates to the guidelines which are worth checking prior to the examination

Section 19.4.2 is based on the 2015 Resuscitation Council Guidelines. It includes the paediatric advance life-support algorithm, the important drug dosages, and calculations to remember. This section, although based on the Resuscitation Council guidance, is not a verbatim reproduction of it, and if further detail is required, this should be sought from EPLS or APLS manuals, or the Resuscitation Council website.

19.4.2 Causes of cardiopulmonary arrest in children

Cardiopulmonary arrest in children is most frequently caused by either respiratory or circulatory failure (see Table 19.4). Cardiac arrest is rarely due to primary cardiac disease. The outcome from cardiopulmonary arrests in children is poor and identification of the antecedent stages of cardiac or respiratory failure is a priority, as effective early intervention may be life-saving.

19.4.3 The paediatric advanced life-support algorithm

See Figure 19.3.

19.4.4 Main changes in the 2015 guidelines for paediatric advanced life support

Table 19.5 details the main changes in the 2015 Resuscitation Council Paediatric Advanced Life-Support Guidelines.

Table 19.4 Causes of cardiac arrest in childhood

Mechanism	Respiratory failure		Circulatory failure	
	Respiratory obstruction	Respiratory depression	Fluid loss	Fluid maldistribution
Examples of underlying causes	Foreign body	Convulsions	Blood loss	Sepsis
	Asthma	Poisoning	Burns	Anaphylaxis
	Croup	Head injury	Vomiting	Cardiac failure

19.4.5 Drug doses and calculations required in paediatric cardiopulmonary arrest

Chapter 2, Table 2.2 includes details of the drugs commonly used in cardiac arrest, their indications, and mechanism of action.

Table 19.6 includes the commonly used paediatric formulas in paediatric resuscitation and drug dosages for cardiac arrest and peri-arrest scenarios which may be appear in a short-answer question (SAQ) paper.

19.4.6 Newborn life support

Newborn life support is a rare event in the emergency department (ED), but is included in the paediatric curriculum. The guidelines are specifically intended for resuscitation at birth. Therefore, these guidelines are only required for neonates delivered in the ED (Figure 19.4). A baby who has successfully adapted to extrauterine life and has subsequently collapsed and presented to the ED should be resuscitated according to the paediatric life-support algorithms with a 15:2 compression to ventilation ratio.

The initial management in the newborn guidelines is warming, drying, and assessment of the baby. Resuscitation is rarely required and, if necessary, is mainly concerned with the initial inflation of the lungs and establishing stable respiration. Almost all babies needing help at birth will respond to successful lung inflation with an increase in heart rate, followed quickly by normal breathing. However, in some cases chest compressions are needed. Chest compressions should only be started when there is certainty oversuccessful aeration of the lungs. The ratio of compressions to ventilations is 3:1.

KEY POINTS

Cardiopulmonary arrest in children is rare. The outcome from cardiopulmonary arrest in children is poor.
Cardiac arrest is usually due to respiratory or circulatory failure and rarely due to primary cardiac disease.

The main 2015 guideline changes are:

- Interruptions to chest compressions should be kept to a minimum and pauses should only occur briefly to enable specific planned interventions (e.g. defibrillation, intubation).
- Intraosseous infusion (IO) is the recommended technique for circulatory access in cardiac arrest.

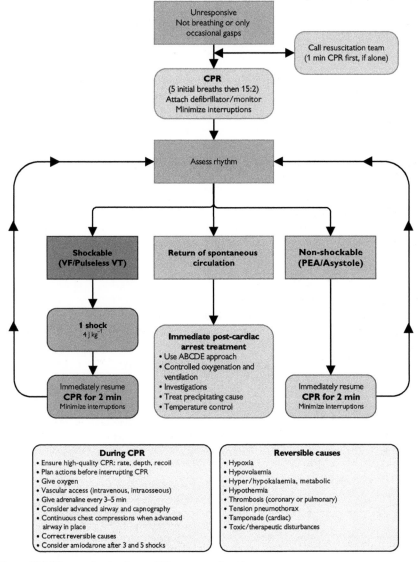

Figure 19.3 The paediatric advanced life-support algorithm.
Reproduced with the kind permission of the Resuscitation Council (UK)

- Adrenaline 10 mcg should be given as soon as IV/IO access is gained in asystole/PEA and after the third shock in VF/VT.
- Amiodarone 5 mg/kg IV is given after the third shock in VF/VT.
- Capnography should be used, if available, in an intubated patient to confirm and continually monitor tube placement, quality of CPR, and to provide an early recognition of return of spontaneous circulation (ROSC).
- Therapeutic hypothermia should be considered in comatose survivors of shockable and non-shockable rhythms.

Table 19.5 Main changes in the 2015 Resuscitation Council Paediatric Advance Life-support Guidelines

BLS	• If there are no 'signs of life' CPR should be commenced unless there is definitely a pulse >60 beats/min within 10 s (unchanged from 2005 guidance).
	• Chest compressions should be to at least a depth 1/3 of the chest and at a rate of 100–120 per min. The ratio is 15:2 (unchanged).
	• For all children the lower half of the sternum should be compressed. In infants use two fingers or two thumbs (encircling technique) to compress the chest. In children over 1 year, use one or two hands, as needed, to achieve an adequate depth of compression.
Automated external defibrillators	• Automated external defibrillators (AEDs) with paediatric pads or programmes are recommended for children aged 1–8 years. If no such system is available an unmodified adult AED may be used.
	• For infants in a shockable rhythm, the risk:benefit ratio favours the use of an AED (ideally with an attenuator) if a manually adjustable model is not available.
Defibrillation	• Interruptions to chest compressions should be kept to a minimum and pauses should only occur briefly to enable specific planned interventions (e.g. defibrillation, intubation).
	• Chest compressions should continue during charging of the defibrillator to reduce the pre-shock pause to less than 5 s.
Drugs	• Intraosseous (IO) access is the recommended technique for circulatory access in cardiac arrest if intravenous IV access is not present.
	• In the shockable (VF/VT) algorithm, adrenaline 10 mcg/kg is given after the third shock, once chest compressions have resumed. Adrenaline is then given every 3–5 min (alternate cycles).
	• Amiodarone 5 mg/kg is given after the third shock in VF/VT cardiac arrests.
Airway	• Bag-valve mask ventilation is the recommended first-line method for achieving airway control and ventilation however the LMA is an acceptable airway device for providers trained in its use.
	• Early tracheal intubation has been de-emphasized. It should only be attempted by highly skilled individuals with minimal interruption to chest compressions (<10 s).
	• If the child is intubated, a cuffed endotracheal tube is now considered acceptable in children less than 8 years of age (except neonates).
	• The use of capnography is recommended to confirm and continually monitor tracheal tube placement, quality of CPR, and to provide an early indication of return of spontaneous circulation (ROSC).
Post-resuscitation care	• Hyperoxia may be harmful after ROSC therefore oxygen should be titrated to maintain saturations of 94–98%.
	• Hyper and hypoglycaemia should be avoided following ROSC.
	• A child who regains a spontaneous circulation but remains comatose after CPR may benefit from a period of therapeutic hypothermia.

19.5 Major trauma

19.5.1 Introduction

Trauma management in adults is discussed in Chapter 4. The advanced trauma life support (ATLS) method, detailed in Chapter 4, is the internationally accepted approach to major trauma and these same principles apply to children. The underlying concepts of ATLS are:

Table 19.6 Paediatric formulas and drug doses for arrest and peri-arrest scenarios

	Formula
Weight	1–12 months = (0.5 × age months) + 4
	1–5 years = (2 × age years) + 8
	6–12 years = (3 × age years) + 7
Endotracheal tube (ETT)	Length: Oral ETT = age/2 + 12. Nasal ETT = age/2 + 15
	Diameter: Age/4 + 4
CPR	Ratio 15:2 (5 rescue breaths first)
	Rate: 100–120 per min
	Hand positioning: lower ½ of sternum (locate as one finger-breadth above xiphisternum)
	Depth of compression: at least one-third depth of chest
	Technique: infant, two fingers (or encircling technique with two thumbs); child, one or two hands
Defibrillation	Cardiac arrest 4 J/kg (single shocks)
	Cardioversion 1 J/kg then 2 J/kg then amiodarone and repeat
	Drug doses and indications
Adrenaline	Cardiac arrest: 10 mcg/kg (0.1 ml/kg of 1:10,000)
	Anaphylaxis: Age >12 years 0.5 mg IM. Age 6–12 years 0.3 mg IM. Age <6 years 0.15 mg IM
	Croup: 5 ml of 1:1000 nebulized
Amiodarone	Shockable cardiac arrest rhythms (VF/VT) 5 mg/kg IV (after third shock)
	Pulsed VT 5 mg/kg IV
Atropine	0.02 mg/kg (min dose 0.1 mg, max 0.6 mg)
	Use pre-intubation or for bradycardia secondary to vagal stimulation (not recommended in cardiac arrest)
Budesonide	Croup: 2 mg nebulizer
Ceftriaxone or cefotaxime	Meningitis: 80 mg/kg IV (avoid ceftriaxone in neonates)
Dexamethasone	Croup: 0.15–0.6 mg/kg
Glucose	Hypoglycaemia: 2 ml/kg of 10% glucose
Fluids	Shock due to severe sepsis or dehydration: 20 ml/kg crystalloid (consider 4.5% albumin)
	Shock due to trauma: 10 ml/kg crystalloid. Blood 10 ml/kg
	Burns: % burn × weight × 4 (½ given in first 8 h, ½ given over next 16 h)
	Maintenance fluids: Based on weight of child—first 10 kg = 100 ml/kg; second 10kg = 50 ml/kg; Subsequent kg = 20 ml/kg
	Correcting fluid deficits: Base on the weight loss or percentage dehydration of the child. Add to the maintenance requirements and replace over 24–48 h
Hydrocortisone	Anaphylaxis: Age >12 years 200 mg IV. Age 6–12 years 100 mg IV. Age 6 months to 6 years 50 mg IV. Age <6 months 25 mg IV

(continued)

Table 19.6 Continued

	Drug doses and indications
Insulin	Diabetic ketoacidosis: 0.1 unit/kg/hr IV infusion
Ipratropium Bromide	Asthma: Age <5 years 125–250 mcg. Age >5 years 250–500 mcg
Lorazepam	Status epilepticus: 0.1 mg/kg IV
Paraldehyde	Status epilepticus: 0.4 ml/kg PR (dilute with equal amount of olive oil)
Phenobarbital	Status epilepticus: 20 mg/kg IV
Phenytoin	Status epilepticus: 18 mg/kg IV
Prednisolone	Asthma: 1–2 mg/kg PO (max dose 40 mg)
	Croup: 1 mg/kg PO
Salbutamol	Severe asthma: Age <5 years 2.5 mg nebulizer. Age >5 years 5 mg nebulizer
	Mild-moderate asthma: 10 puffs of inhaler via spacer
Sodium bicarbonate	Cardiac arrest due to hyperkalaemia or tricyclic overdose: 1 ml/kg of 8.4%

- Treat the greatest threat to life first.
- The lack of a definitive diagnosis should never impede the application of an indicated treatment.
- A detailed history is not essential to begin the evaluation of a patient with acute injuries.

These concepts resulted in the development of the ABCDE approach. The mnemonic defines the specific, ordered evaluations, and interventions that should be followed in all injured patients:

- **A**irway with cervical spine protection
- **B**reathing and ventilation
- **C**irculation with haemorrhage control
- **D**isability: neurological status
- **E**xposure/**E**nvironment control: completely undress the patient, but prevent hypothermia

Trauma management consists of a rapid primary survey, resuscitation, a more detailed secondary survey, and, finally, the initiation of definitive care.

19.5.2 Trauma in children

Children and adults are affected differently by major injuries—physically, physiologically, and psychologically.

Seven S's can be used to highlight some of these key differences:

- **S**ofter skeleton: bones tend to bend rather than break. Children may have significant internal injuries despite an intact overlying skeleton. The identification of skull or rib fractures suggests the transfer of a massive amount of energy and underlying organ injuries should be suspected.
- **S**urface area: the ratio of a child's body surface area to volume is greater than an adult, resulting in faster temperature loss and the potential for hypothermia to develop quickly.
- **S**ize: the size of a child affects the mechanism of injury and they are more likely to suffer multisystem trauma, and/or a higher force per unit area.
- **S**hape: children have bigger heads proportional to their body resulting in a higher frequency of blunt brain injuries.

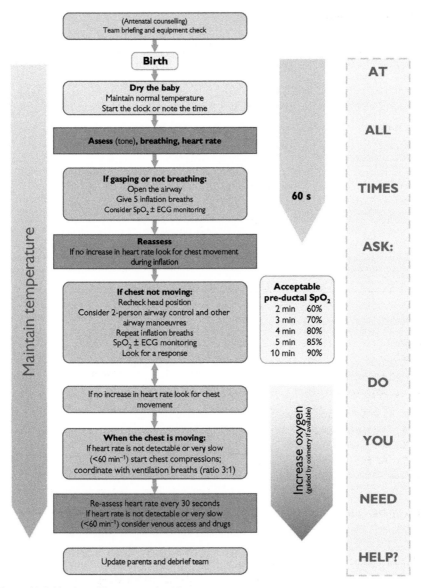

Figure 19.4 Newborn life-support algorithm.
Reproduced with the kind permission of the Resuscitation Council (UK)

- **S**equelae: trauma in children may have an effect on their subsequent growth and development. The child has to recover from the effects of the traumatic event and continue the normal growing process; consequently, long-term complications need to be considered from the outset.
- p**S**ychology: children often regress by a stage when ill or injured. This can result in communication difficulties and involvement of the parents is paramount.
- **S**tuff (equipment): different size equipment is needed and calculations for drug doses are required. An electronic medical application, length-based resuscitation tape (e.g. Broselow tape), or specific age-based resuscitation draws are useful for this.

19.5.3 Paediatric head injuries

Previous MRCEM question

The anatomy, pathophysiology, and clinical features of head injuries in adults are discussed in Chapter 4, section 4.5.

There are certain anatomical and physiological differences in children that make the clinical features and management of head injuries slightly different to that in adults. These differences are:

- Children have a relatively larger head for the size of their body, so are more likely to injure it in trauma.
- The brain reaches 80% of its adult size by age two years.
- The brain is still developing in childhood, so there is plasticity to redevelop damaged areas. However, this development means that not all areas of damage maybe identified until later in life.
- The subarachnoid space is relatively smaller, so there is less 'cushioning' around the brain.
- In young children (age 12–18 months), the cranial sutures are not closed. An open fontanelle allows more tolerance for expanding intracranial contents (e.g. haematoma, oedema). Signs of these conditions may be hidden unless a bulging fontanelle is recognized, leading to late and sudden decompensation.
- Unfused cranial sutures may allow significant volumes of extradural or subdural blood to accumulate, resulting in hypovolaemic shock.
- Children are more susceptible to secondary brain injury, especially due to hypoxia (normal cerebral blood flow increases to almost twice that in adults by age five years, and then decreases).
- Children are more likely to vomit after a head injury, which is not necessarily related to a raised intracranial pressure (ICP).
- The verbal component of the Glasgow Coma Scale (GCS) is modified for young children:

  - V5 = appropriate words or social smiles, fixes, and follows;
  - V4 = cries but consolable;
  - V3 = persistently irritable;
  - V2 = restless, agitated;
  - V1 = none.*

NICE indications for computed tomography head scanning in children (under 16)

The NICE guidance for imaging children with head injuries is slightly different to that for adults (Chapter 4). CT scanning is the recommended imaging technique in head-injured children. However, plain X-rays of the skull may be performed as part of a skeletal survey in children presenting with suspected non-accidental injury (NAI). The possibility of an associated neck injury should always be considered. A CT should be requested immediately and performed within one hour, if any of the following are present:

- Clinical suspicion of NAI.
- Post-traumatic seizure but no history of epilepsy.
- GCS less than 14 on initial emergency department assessment (for under 1s <15 on paediatric GCS).
- GCS <15 two hours after injury.
- Suspicion of open or depressed skull injury or tense fontanelle.

---

* Reproduced with permission from P. L. Reilly, Assessing the conscious level in infants and young children: a paediatric version of the Glasgow Coma Scale, *Child's Nervous System*, Volume 4, Issue 1, pp.30-33, Copyright © 1988 Springer.

- Any sign of basal skull fracture (haemotympanum, 'panda eyes', cerebrospinal fluid leakage from ears or nose, Battle's sign).
- Focal neurological deficit.
- Children aged less than 1 year: presence of bruise, swelling, or laceration >5 cm on the head.

A provisional radiologists report should be available within one hour of the scan.

Children who have presented with a head injury and **more than one** of the following risk factors should have a CT head within one hour of identifying the risk factors and a provisional report within one hour of scan.

- Witnessed LOC >5 minutes.
- Abnormal drowsiness; three or more discrete vomits (>15 minutes apart).
- Dangerous mechanism of injury (high-speed road traffic collisions), fall from height greater than 3 metres or any high-speed injury from projectile or other object.
- Amnesia (retrograde or anteriograde) >5 minutes.

Children who have sustained a head injury and only have one of these aforementioned risk factors should be observed for a minimum of four hours. During the period of observation, if any of the following risk factors occur a CT scan should be performed within one hour.

- Further vomiting
- GCS <15
- Further episode of drowsiness

In the absence of these risk factors in children who have sustained a head injury, length of observation should be under the discretion of the clinician.

Emergency department management of head injuries

- The focus of ED management is the prevention and treatment of secondary brain injury. Causes of secondary brain injury include: hypoxia; hypovolaemia and cerebral hypoperfusion; hypercapnea; intracranial haematoma with localized pressure effects and increased ICP; cerebral oedema; hyperthermia; seizures; and infection.
- The ED management of head-injured children follows the same principles as those for adults; see Chapter 4, section 4.5.

19.5.4 Spinal injuries in children

Only 5% of spinal cord injuries occur in children. They have more flexible soft tissues, but relatively larger heads which applies more force on the upper neck than in adults, so an appropriate index of suspicion should be maintained.

The anatomical differences in children to be considered include:

- More flexible interspinous ligaments and joint capsules.
- Vertebral bodies are wedged anteriorly and tend to slide forward with flexion.
- The facet joints are flat.
- Relatively larger head compared with the neck.

The radiological considerations in children are:

- Pseudo-subluxation is a common finding radiologically (40% of children age <7 years have anterior displacement of C2 on C3).
- 20% of young children have an increased distance between the peg and the anterior arch of C1 (normal gap <3 mm in adults, <5 mm in children).
- Skeletal growth plates can resemble fractures.
- Children may sustain a 'spinal cord injury without radiological abnormality' (SCIWORA). A normal cervical spine series may be found in up to two-thirds of children with a spinal cord

injury. Therefore, if a spinal cord injury is suspected, a normal spinal X-ray does not exclude significant injury.

Due to the anatomy of the neck, children are relatively at a lower risk of developing a significant spinal injury compared to adults. In addition due to the risk of ionizing radiation to the developing thymus gland, NICE has produced guidelines on cervical spine imaging in children.

19.5.5 Chest injuries in children

Chest injuries rarely occur in isolation and are frequently a component of major multisystem injury in children. The vast majority are due to blunt mechanisms, principally caused by road traffic collisions (RTCs).

The compliance of a child's chest wall allows impacting forces to be transmitted to underlying pulmonary parenchyma. The plasticity of the chest wall makes pulmonary contusion and other internal organ injuries potentially more difficult to spot because there are no rib fractures to highlight the forces involved. If rib fractures are present, they indicate a severe impacting force.

Children have relatively little respiratory reserve. Their high metabolic rate and small functional residual capacity results in rapid desaturation when oxygen supply is curtailed. Their horizontal ribs and underdeveloped musculature makes them tolerate chest wall disruption badly (e.g. flail chest).

The specific injuries caused by thoracic trauma in children are similar to those encountered in adults (Chapter 4, section 4.2), although the frequencies are different. The mobility of mediastinal structures makes children more prone to tension pneumothorax. Pulmonary contusions are common. Diaphragmatic rupture, aortic transection, major tracheobronchial tears, flail chest, and cardiac contusion are rarely encountered.

Most paediatric thoracic injuries can be successfully managed using an appropriate combination of supportive care and tube thoracostomy.

19.5.6 Abdominal injuries in children

Most paediatric abdominal injuries occur as the result of blunt trauma. The abdominal contents are very susceptible to injury in children for several reasons:

- Thin abdominal wall offering little protection to underlying organs (e.g. duodenal injury from bicycle handlebars).
- Horizontal diaphragm (compared to adults) resulting in the liver and spleen lying lower and more anteriorly.
- Plasticity of the rib cage offering less protection to the liver and spleen.
- Intra-abdominal bladder due to the shallow depth of the pelvis.

Imaging in paediatric abdominal injuries is usually CT. FAST scanning may be used but its efficacy is not as well-evidenced as in adults.

Non-operative management of blunt abdominal injuries is more frequently employed in children and the presence of free intraperitoneal blood does not mandate a laparotomy. If non-operative management is selected, the child should be under the care of a surgeon qualified in paediatric trauma surgery.

19.5.7 Burns in children

The management of burns is discussed in Chapter 4, section 4.7. The same principles apply for the management of burns in children as in adults.

The possibility of non-accidental injury must always be considered in a child with burns and appropriate safeguarding action taken. Suspicious patterns of burn include cigarette burns, immersion-type injuries (glove and stocking pattern or buttocks), or burns to the dorsum of the hands.

Scalds from pulling hot drinks off surfaces are common accidental injuries. Advice should be given about how to prevent future similar injuries occurring.

Table 19.7 Infant rule of 5's

Body area	Infant rule of 5s
Head	20%
Each arm	10%
Each leg	20%
Front of trunk	10%
Back of trunk	10%

Calculating the size of the burn

Assessing the percentage of body surface area (BSA) burnt can be done using several different techniques:

- Infant rule of 5's (Table 19.7).
- Lund–Browder charts (see Chapter 4, Figure 4.7).
- Patient's palm size (including the fingers) = approximately 1% BSA.

Size should only include those burns which are partial or full thickness; superficial burns are excluded from the estimation. Accurate estimation is important for managing fluid resuscitation and communicating with a burns centre.

Management of burns in children

The management of burns in children is the same as in adults (see Chapter 4, section 4.7).

Children with burns >10% BSA require intravenous fluids. Fluid requirements are calculated using the Parkland formula (see Box 19.1).

Maintenance fluid requirements will also need adding to the fluid calculation.

ATLS recommend the following children require referral to a burns centre:

- Partial/full thickness >10% BSA in patients <10 years
- >20% BSA in all other age groups
- Burns to 'special areas'—face, ears, eyes, hands, feet, genitalia/perineum, and major joints
- Full thickness >5% BSA
- Significant electrical and chemical burns
- Inhalation injury
- Burns in patients with pre-existing illness that could complicate treatment, prolong recovery, or affect mortality
- Patients with concomitant trauma that poses an increased risk of morbidity or mortality

Box 19.1 Parkland formula

Parkland formula:

Percentage burn (partial and full) × weight (kg) × 4 = total fluid (ml).

This calculates the total volume required for the first 24 h of resuscitation.

½ should be given over the first 8 h and ½ over the next 16 h.

Data from Baxter CR, Shires T. 'Physiological response to crystalloid resuscitation of severe burns'. Ann NY Acad Sci. 1968; 150: 874–894.

KEY POINTS

The ATLS principles of trauma management apply to children as for adults.

Children and adults are affected differently by major injuries—physically, physiologically, and psychologically.

The key differences can be summarized by seven S's:

- **S**ofter skeleton: bones tend to bend rather than break. Children may have significant internal injuries despite an intact overlying skeleton. The identification of skull or rib fractures suggests the transfer of a massive amount of energy and underlying organ injuries should be suspected.
- **S**urface area: the ratio of a child's body surface area to volume is greater than an adult, resulting in faster temperature loss and the potential for hypothermia to develop quickly.
- **S**ize: the size of a child affects the mechanism of injury and they are more likely to suffer multisystem trauma, and/or a higher force per unit area.
- **S**hape: children have bigger heads proportional to their body, resulting in a higher frequency of blunt brain injuries.
- **S**equelae: trauma in children may have an effect on their subsequent growth and development. The child has to recover from the effects of the traumatic event and continue the normal growing process; consequently, long-term complications need to be considered from the outset.
- p**S**ychology: children often regress by a stage when ill or injured. This can result in communication difficulties and involvement of the parents is paramount.
- **S**tuff (equipment): different size equipment is needed and calculations for drug doses are required. An electronic medical application, length-based resuscitation tape (e.g. Broselow tape), or specific age-based resuscitation draws are useful for this.

19.6 The shocked child

Septic shock and the management of a child with suspected meningitis or meningococcal septicaemia is covered in Chapter 15, sections 15.1 and 15.4.

19.7 The unconscious child

19.7.1 Introduction

The conscious level in children may be altered by disease, injury, or intoxication. In 95% of cases coma is caused by a diffuse metabolic insult (including cerebral hypoxia and ischaemia) with structural lesions making up the remaining 5%.

Causes of a reduced level of consciousness in children include:

- Hypoxia—following respiratory failure
- Hypotension—following circulatory failure
- Epileptic seizures (see Chapter 11, section 11.6)
- Trauma (e.g. intracranial haemorrhage, cerebral oedema)
- Infections (e.g. meningitis, encephalitis, malaria—see Chapter 15, section 15.4)
- Poisoning (e.g. opiates, carbon monoxide, alcohol—see Chapter 17)
- Metabolic (e.g. hypoglycaemia, hyperglycaemia, hypercapnea, hypothermia, renal failure, hepatic failure)
- Vascular lesions

Patients should be assessed using the standard ABCDE approach. Assessment and treatment should occur simultaneously. It is essential to ensure the patient is not hypoxic, hypercarbic, or hypotensive because these can all cause unconsciousness, and will worsen the outcome in other causes.

The curriculum specifically includes knowledge of unconscious states due to seizures, hypoglycaemia, and diabetic ketoacidosis.

19.7.2 Seizures

The management of epilepsy and status epilepticus in adults and children is covered in Chapter 11, section 11.6.

Febrile convulsion

Previous MRCEM question

A febrile convulsion is a seizure associated with fever occurring in a young child. They affect approximately 3% of children. Most occur between six months and five years of age.

Febrile convulsions arise most commonly from infection or inflammation outside the central nervous system (CNS) in a child who is otherwise neurologically normal. Seizures due to infection in the CNS (e.g. meningitis or encephalitis) are not included in the definition of febrile convulsion. Fever is defined as a temperature >38°C.

Definitions for febrile convulsions include:

- Simple febrile convulsion—isolated, generalized tonic–clonic seizure lasting less than 15 minutes, which does not recur within 24 hours or within the same febrile illness.
- Complex febrile seizures—these have one or more of the following features: a partial (focal) onset or focal feature during the seizure; duration of more than 15 minutes; recurrence within 24 hours, or within the same febrile illness; incomplete recovery within one hour.
- Febrile status epilepticus—febrile seizure lasting longer than 30 minutes.

Most febrile convulsions will have ceased by arrival in the ED. The child should initially be assessed in an ABCDE manner. The history and examination should aim to determine the cause of the fever (e.g. viral upper respiratory tract infection, otitis media, urinary tract infection, and so on). The NICE traffic light system is helpful to identify the likelihood of serious underlying illness (section 19.16).

If the child is still fitting on arrival in the ED they should be managed using the status epilepticus guidance in Chapter 11, section 11.6.

Indications for referral to the paediatric team after a febrile convulsion include:

- Children aged <18 months.
- Signs of meningism.
- Complex or prolonged seizures.
- No clear focus of infection.
- Systemically unwell.
- Parental anxiety.
- Current or recent antibiotic use.
- First febrile convulsion (this is not universal but many centres will admit children with a first febrile seizure for observation overnight).

Parents should be given clear advice following a febrile convulsion, as detailed in Box 19.2.

19.7.3 Hypoglycaemia in children

All children can become hypoglycaemic when seriously ill. Hypoglycaemia in infants, especially if recurrent, may be due to an inborn error of metabolism, congenital hypopituitarism, or

Box 19.2 Parental advice following a febrile convulsion

Advice following a febrile convulsion

Parents are understandably anxious when their child has had a febrile convulsion. Giving advice to parents following such an event has appeared in previous MRCEM examinations.
  The following advice should be given:

- Explain what a febrile convulsion is and that they are not harmful to the child, do not cause brain damage, and will not cause the child to die.
- Explain that febrile seizures are not the same as epilepsy. Epilepsy may develop later, but this is rare—the chance is about 1 in 50 for children who have had one simple febrile seizure (compared to 1 in 131 for the general population). No treatment is available to reduce this risk.
- Explain that the febrile seizure may recur—about 1 in 3 children will have another febrile seizure.
- Give advice on how to manage future fevers. Explain that controlling fever does not prevent recurrence but does make the child more comfortable if they are distressed. The aim of controlling fever is to ease symptoms and prevent dehydration. Antipyretics (paracetamol and/or ibuprofen) should not be given with the sole aim of reducing body temperature or of preventing febrile seizures. Tepid sponging, fanning, and cold baths are not recommended. An adequate fluid intake should be ensured.
- Explain how to manage recurrent febrile seizures. Parents should: place the child in the recovery position; not force anything into the child's mouth; note the time that the seizure starts and stay with the child; telephone for an urgent ambulance if the seizure lasts >5 minutes (phone the GP if the seizure resolves within 5 minutes).
- Explain that immunizations are still advised after a febrile seizure, even if, as rarely happens, the febrile seizure followed an immunization.

congenital hyperinsulinism. Hypoglycaemia in adolescents is often due to insulin use in type 1 diabetes.

Blood glucose should be checked as part of the assessment of disability and frequently rechecked.

Hypoglycaemia (blood glucose <3 mmol/L) should be treated with intravenous 10% glucose to a maximum dose of 5 ml/kg (500mg/kg). If intravenous access is not available, concentrated oral glucose can be given; or if reduced, GCS intramuscular glucagon can be administered. A dose of 1 mg glucagon should be given to children over eight years (or >25 kg) and 0.5 mg to under 8s (<25 kg).

19.7.4 Diabetic ketoacidosis in children and adolescents

Introduction

Previous MRCEM question

Diabetic ketoacidosis (DKA), though preventable remains a frequent and life-threatening complication of type 1 diabetes. There is overlap in the management of DKA in children and adults and this section should be read in conjunction with Chapter 14, section 14.1.

The management of DKA has appeared in previous SAQs.

The section 'Definition of diabetic ketoacidosis' is based on the guidance from the British Society of Paediatric Endocrinology and Diabetes (BSPED) and NICE Guidelines.

Definition of diabetic ketoacidosis

DKA is a complex disordered metabolic state characterized by hyperglycaemia, acidosis, and ketonaemia.

Diagnosis of DKA in children with diabetes includes:

- Ketonaemia (>3 mmol/L) or ketonuria (>2 + on urine dipstick)
- Bicarbonate <18 mmol/L and/or venous pH <7.3 (severe DKA is defined as pH <7.1)

DKA should be suspected in any non-diabetic child presenting with increased thirst; polyuria; recent unexplained weight loss; or drowsiness, as DKA may be their first presentation. All children should receive capillary blood glucose testing in the presence of:

- Nausea or vomiting
- Abdominal pain
- Hyperventilation
- Dehydration
- Reduced GCS

Children or young persons with a blood glucose of greater than 11 and any of these features should be treated as DKA.

Children with known diabetes may also present with DKA in the presence of a normal blood sugar level. DKA should be expected in diabetic patients with normal blood sugar levels presenting with the following:

- Nausea or vomiting
- Abdominal pain
- Hyperventilation
- Dehydration
- Reduced GCS

Investigations in DKA

Children with DKA should be managed in an ABCDE manner and investigations should be performed concurrently with assessment and initial resuscitation. The investigations are listed separately to the management section to facilitate revision for the SAQs and highlight the differences in terminology used in the exam.

The initial investigations which should be performed in the ED are:

- Blood ketones—measurement of blood ketone levels is now recommended via bedside meters rather than urinary testing. Measurement of blood ketones is considered best practice to monitor and guide treatment because the resolution of DKA depends on the suppression of ketonaemia. Glucose, bicarbonate, and pH are only surrogate markers of the underlying metabolic abnormality (ketonaemia) and therefore are only recommended to guide treatment in the absence of blood ketone levels.
- Glucose—bedside blood glucose should be checked and a venous plasma sample sent to the laboratory for confirmation.
- Venous blood gas—arterial blood gases are no longer recommended unless indicated to assess respiratory function. The difference between arterial and venous pH and bicarbonate are not significant enough to change the diagnosis or management of DKA.
- Blood tests—urea and electrolytes, full bood count (FBC), chloride, bicarbonate.
- Infective screen—blood cultures, urinalysis and culture, blood cultures, chest X-ray (CXR).
- ECG and cardiac monitoring—looking for evidence of arrhythmias due to hypo- or hyperkalaemia.

Management of diabetic ketoacidosis in children

The following guidance is for children with a diagnosis of DKA and >5% dehydration, vomiting, drowsiness, and/or clinical acidosis. Children who are less than 5% dehydrated and not clinically unwell usually tolerate oral rehydration and subcutaneous insulin.

- Airway and breathing—ensuring patency and maintenance of the airway is paramount. High-flow oxygen should be given. If the child is unconscious advanced airway management and intubation will be required. A nasogastric tube will be required if the child is vomiting or unconscious.
- Circulation/fluids—identification of shock and careful fluid management is vital in the paediatric population to avoid cerebral oedema. For the first 12 hours 0.9% sodium chloride is the recommended fluid with added potassium (40 mmol/L). If the blood glucose falls below 14 mmol/L, glucose is added to the fluid or, if available, 500 ml bags of 0.9% sodium chloride with 5% glucose and 20 mmol potassium used. Box 19.3 details the recommended method for fluid management in children with DKA.

Box 19.3 Fluid management in children with diabetic ketoacidosis

Fluid management

Fluid management should be divided into three components: resuscitation fluid; rehydration fluid; and maintenance fluid:

- *Resuscitation fluid*—if the child is shocked (weak peripheral pulses, prolonged capillary refill, with tachycardia, and/or hypotension) they should receive a fluid bolus of 10 ml/kg 0.9% sodium chloride. A second bolus should only be given after discussion with the consultant overseeing the child's care.
- *Rehydration fluid*—is calculated based on the percentage dehydration multiplied by the body weight (kg); for example, deficit = % dehydration × body weight (kg). The degree of dehydration can be estimated from the child's clinical features (see Table 19.8). Weight loss can also be used to calculate the fluid deficit if the 'normal' weight of the child is known (e.g. weight loss of 1kg = 1000 ml fluid deficit). Assume a child has a 5% fluid deficit in mild-moderate DKA and a 10% fluid deficit in sever DKA.
- *Maintenance fluid*—there are several different methods to calculate maintenance fluid requirements. The APLS formula is a well-recognized technique but tends to overestimate fluid requirements and increases the risk of cerebral oedema in DKA. Therefore, NICE recommend the maintenance volumes detailed in Table 19.9.

Once shock has been treated, fluids are calculated over a 48-hour period using the following formula:

48h fluid requirement = Maintenance + Rehydration − Resuscitation fluid already given. An example calculation of the 48-h fluid requirements in a child with DKA is as follows:

A 25 kg boy with DKA presents to the ED. He is 8% dehydrated clinically and has received 20 ml/kg normal saline as resuscitation fluid.

- Resuscitation fluid = 20 ml × 25 kg = 500 ml.
- Rehydration fluid = 8% × 25 kg = 0.08 × 25,000 ml = 2000 ml.
- Maintenance fluid = 25 kg × 55 ml = 1375 ml (24-h requirement) or 2750 ml (48-h requirement).

Therefore the boy's 48-h fluid requirement is:

- 2750 ml + 2000 ml − 500 ml = 4250 ml.
- This is an infusion rate of 89 ml/h.

Table 19.8 Estimating the degree of dehydration

Percentage dehydration	Clinical features
Mild, 3%	Only just clinically detectable
Moderate, 5%	Dry mucous membranes, reduced skin turgor
Severe, 8%	As for moderate plus sunken eyes, poor capillary refill
Shocked	Severely ill with poor perfusion, thready rapid pulse

- Potassium—once the child has been fluid resuscitated, potassium should be commenced with the fluid. Potassium levels will fall upon treatment with insulin. For the first 12 hours, 0.9% sodium chloride is the recommended fluid with added potassium (40 mmol/L). Potassium levels and renal function should be checked two hours after resuscitation has begun and then four-hourly thereafter. Cardiac monitoring should be instituted.
- Insulin—fixed-rate intravenous insulin infusion is recommended rather than a sliding scale. An initial bolus dose of insulin is no longer recommended. There is some evidence that cerebral oedema is more likely if the insulin is started early. Therefore insulin should not start until intravenous fluids have been running for at least one hour. Insulin should be given at a fixed rate of 0.05–1 unit/kg/hour. Once the blood glucose falls to 14 mmol/L, the fluid should be changed to 0.9% saline with 5% glucose and 40 mmol potassium chloride (KCL). The insulin dose must be maintained to switch off ketogenesis.
- If the child usually takes long-acting insulin (e.g. glargine), this should be discussed with the paediatric consultant who may want it continued. Children on continuous subcutaneous insulin infusion pump therapy should have the pump stopped when starting DKA treatment.
- Monitoring—patients should have continual cardiac monitoring and pulse oximetry. Regular observations and Early Warning Score should be recorded. Fluid balance should be monitored, aiming for a urine output >0.5 ml/kg/hour. Blood ketones and capillary glucose should be measured hourly. Urea and electrolytes, bicarbonate, blood pH, and laboratory glucose should be checked two hours after the start of resuscitation and then four-hourly thereafter.
- Cerebral oedema should be treated with mannitol (20%) 0.5–1 g/kg over 20 minutes or hypertonic (3%) saline 2.5–5 ml/kg over 10–15 minutes.
- Urinary catheterization is not recommended in children, but fluid balance should be closely monitored.
- Low molecular weight heparin should be considered. There is a significant risk of femoral vein thrombosis in young and very sick children with DKA who have femoral lines inserted.
- Sodium bicarbonate should not be given.
- Any infective cause should be treated.

Table 19.9 Maintenance fluid requirements

Weight (kg)	Rate
<10	2 ml/kg/hr
10–40	1 ml/kg/hr
>40	40 ml/hr fixed volume

Adapted from NICE, NG18, Diabetes (type 1 and type 2) in children and young people: diagnosis and management (Aug 2015)

Fluid management in children with diabetic ketoacidosis

NB The recommendation of the BSPED is that shock should be treated prior to fluid calculations being performed; therefore, no more than 8% dehydration should be used in managing a child with DKA. This is slightly different to the APLS technique for estimating percentage dehydration (Table 19.8), which may be used for children with dehydration from other causes (e.g. diarrhoea).

EXAM TIP

Paediatric fluid calculations have appeared in previous SAQs. The table recommended by the BSPED (Table 19.9) is difficult to memorize for the exam. If a question did appear in a SAQ on maintenance fluid in DKA, then it is likely that either the table would be provided or the APLS formula (Table 19.10) would be acceptable because it is still included in the curriculum.

The values in Table 19.9 are difficult to remember and an online tool to calculate fluid requirements is provided by the BSPED (http://www.bsped.org.uk/clinical/docs/DKACalculator.pdf).

Complications of DKA

Children can die from the complications of DKA, which include:

- Cerebral oedema
- Hypokalaemia
- Hypoglycaemia
- Aspiration pneumonia
- Systemic infections

Cerebral oedema

Cerebral oedema is much more common in the paediatric population, especially the newly diagnosed diabetic. The causes are unknown but slow correction of metabolic abnormalities aims to minimize the risk.

Clinical features of cerebral oedema include:

- Headache
- Bradycardia, hypertension
- Irritability, drowsiness, incontinence
- Seizures, abnormal posturing
- Focal neurology, papilloedema
- Respiratory depression

Management of cerebral oedema:

- Exclude hypoglycaemia.
- Restrict intravenous fluids to half maintenance and replace deficit over 72 rather than 48 hours.

Table 19.10 APLS maintenance fluid requirements

Weight (kg)	ml/kg/24 h
First 10 kg	100 ml
Second 10 kg	50 ml
Subsequent kg	20 ml

- Give hypertonic (2.7%) saline (5 ml/kg over 5–10 minutes) or mannitol (2.5–5 ml/kg of 20% mannitol over 20 minutes).
- Contact PICU.
- Once stable arrange a CT head.

KEY POINTS

Causes of a reduced level of consciousness in children include:

- Hypoxia
- Hypotension
- Epileptic seizures
- Trauma
- Infections
- Poisoning
- Metabolic
- Vascular lesions

A febrile convulsion is a seizure associated with fever occurring in a young child. They affect approximately 3% of children. Most occur between six months and five years of age.

Clear advice to the parents is vital following a febrile convulsion. This advice should include:

- What a febrile convulsion is.
- Explanation that a febrile convulsion is not the same as epilepsy.
- How to manage future fevers.
- The likelihood of recurrence and how to manage further febrile convulsions.
- Importance of future vaccinations.

DKA is a complex disordered metabolic state characterized by hyperglycaemia, acidosis, and ketonaemia; however, children with diabetes may present in DKA with a normal blood sugar level.

Careful fluid management is very important in the management of DKA in children and adolescents because of the risk of cerebral oedema.

Fluid should be replaced over 48 h once shock has been treated.

Do not routinely give fluid boluses unless there are signs of shock.

Fluid requirements = Maintenance + Rehydration—Resuscitation fluid already given.

Supplemental 5% glucose is required if the blood glucose <14 mmol/L.

Insulin is given at a fixed rate of 0.05–0.1units/kg/hr and should not be started until fluids have been running for at least one hour.

19.8 Abdominal pain

19.8.1 Introduction

Many of the common causes of abdominal pain are the same in children as in adults (e.g. acute appendicitis, Chapter 6, section 6.4). However, there are certain conditions which are characteristically only seen in the paediatric population (see Table 19.11).

The differential diagnosis for abdominal pain is extensive and includes surgical and medical conditions (see Table 19.12).

Table 19.11 Differential diagnosis of an acute abdomen based on age group

Age	Differential diagnosis
Infants	Meconium ileus
	Hypertrophic pyloric stenosis
	Intussusception
	Appendicitis
	Hernia
	Volvulus
	Testicular torsion
Adolescents	Appendicitis
	Testicular torsion
	Epididymo-orchitis
	Ectopic pregnancy
Elderly	Aortic aneurysm
	Urinary retention
	Mesenteric infarction
	Acute cholecystitis
	Bowel obstruction
	Acute pancreatitis
	Diverticular disease
	Malignancy
	Hernia

Table 19.12 Surgical and medical causes of abdominal pain in children

Surgical causes of abdominal pain	Medical causes of abdominal pain
Infective: • Acute appendicitis • Peritonitis **Obstructive:** • Meconium ileus • Hypertrophic pyloric stenosis • Intussusception • Hernias (inguinal, umbilical) • Volvulus • Oesophageal or duodenal atresia • Hirschsprung's disease **Extra-abdominal:** • Testicular torsion	• Gastroenteritis • Mesenteric adenitis • Urinary tract infection • Diabetic ketoacidosis • Lower lobe pneumonia • Upper respiratory tract infection • Sickle cell disease • Inflammatory bowel disease • Constipation • Henoch–Schönlein purpura • Infant colic

19.8.2 Hypertrophic pyloric stenosis

This is a relative common condition caused by hypertrophy of the circular muscles of the pylorus. It is four times more common in boys than girls, and more commonly affects first-borns.

The clinical features include:

- Effortless, projectile vomiting between the ages of 2 and 10 weeks.
- Vomiting within 30 minutes of a feed.
- Vomit that is not bile-stained.
- An infant who is usually hungry after vomiting.
- Dehydration and constipation.
- Gastric peristalsis may be visible moving across the epigastrium following a feed.
- An olive-sized lump may be palpable in the epigastrium (most prominent during a feed).

Diagnosis is mainly clinical but an ultrasound may help confirm the diagnosis. The child may develop hypochloraemic alkalosis and hypokalaemia due to recurrent vomiting of gastric contents.

ED management involves:

- Intravenous cannulation and fluid resuscitation/rehydration.
- Keeping the infant nil by mouth.
- Correction of electrolyte abnormalities, including hypoglycaemia. Correction of sodium and potassium abnormalities may take >24 hours.
- Referral to the paediatric surgical team for pylorotomy.

19.8.3 Intussusception

Intussusception is the invagination of one segment of bowel into an adjacent lower segment. It may affect the small or large bowel, but most cases are ileocolic. Intussusception can rapidly compromise the blood supply to the bowel, making relief of this form of obstruction urgent.

Usually no underlying cause is found, although there is some evidence that viral infection leads to enlargement of Peyer's patches, which may form the lead point of the intussusception. Occasionally a Meckel's diverticulum, polyp, or lymphoma is the lead point.

It typically affects children aged between six months and four years.

Clinical features include:

- Paroxysmal, colicky pain. During episodes the child becomes pale, very distressed, and draws up the legs.
- Vomiting.
- 'Redcurrant jelly' stool (blood-stained mucus).
- Abdominal distension and occasionally a 'sausage-shaped' mass may be visible.
- Dehydration.
- Pyrexia.
- Occasionally the child presents shock without an obvious cause.

If intussusception is suspected urgent referral to the surgical team is required. The diagnosis may be confirmed by an air or barium enema, which may also be curative, by reducing the intussusception. A barium enema characteristically reveals a 'coiled spring' sign or sudden termination of the barium. A barium enema is contraindicated if there is evidence of perforation, which requires surgical intervention.

19.8.4 Volvulus

Volvulus may be due to congenital malrotations, Meckel's diverticulum, or adhesions from previous surgery. Congenital malrotations are the most frequent and result from the abnormal movement of the intestine around the superior mesenteric artery during embryological development.

Clinical features include:

- Abdominal pain
- Vomiting
- Abdominal distension

An abdominal X-ray should be performed and the child referred on to the surgical team.

19.8.5 Hirschsprung's disease

Hirschsprung's disease is due to an absence of ganglion cells in a section of large bowel. It is usually confined to the rectosigmoid but may extend to involve the entire colon. The result is a section of bowel that is atonic.

Presentation is usually in the neonatal period with intestinal obstruction, heralded by failure to pass meconium in the first 24 hours of life. Presentation in later childhood is with chronic constipation, abdominal distension, and bile-stained vomit.

Children with suspected Hirschsprung's should be referred on to the paediatricians for further investigation. Ultimately the aganglionic section requires surgical excision.

19.8.6 Testicular torsion

Testicular torsion is a urological emergency most commonly presenting around puberty. In patients with a high attachment of the tunica vaginalis on the testis, the testis can rotate on the spermatic cord, within the tunica vaginalis, and obstruct the blood supply.

Clinical features of testicular torsion

- Sudden scrotal pain and swelling
- Vomiting
- Abdominal pain
- Elevated, swollen, tender testis
- Horizontally lying testis
- Loss of cremasteric reflex

Investigations for testicular torsion

Testicular torsion is a clinical diagnosis and unnecessary investigation delays definitive surgical treatment. The urology team may occasionally arrange a Doppler ultrasound to assess blood flow if the diagnosis is equivocal.

Emergency department management of testicular torsion

ED management involves urgently informing the urology team of the patient and providing symptomatic relief with analgesia and anti-emetics, if required.

Differential of an acutely painful scrotum

- Testicular torsion.
- Torsion of the hydatid of Morgagni—a remnant of the paramesonephric duct on the superior aspect of the testis. Necrosis of the appendage may be visible as a blue dot and is virtually diagnostic of the condition. However, if testicular torsion is suspected, then surgical exploration is warranted.
- Epididymitis.
- Orchitis.
- Trauma.
- Incarcerated hernia.

KEY POINTS

The differential diagnosis of abdominal pain in children is extensive.

Surgical causes include:

- Infections (e.g. acute appendicitis, peritonitis)
- Obstruction (e.g. meconium ileus, hypertrophic pyloric stenosis, intussusception, hernias, volvulus, Hirschsprung's disease, oesophageal or duodenal atresia)
- Extra-abdominal causes (e.g. testicular torsion)

Medical causes include:

- Gastroenteritis
- Mesenteric adenitis
- Urinary tract infection
- Diabetic ketoacidosis
- Lower lobe pneumonia
- Upper respiratory tract infection
- Sickle cell disease
- Inflammatory bowel disease
- Constipation
- Henoch–Schönlein purpura
- Infant colic

19.9 Accidental poisoning, poisoning, and self-harm

The management of poisoning and self-harm is covered in Chapters 17 and 18, and the same principles apply as in adults.

In paediatrics, poisoning may result from different causes:

- Neonatal poisoning—due to drugs taken by the mother prior to birth (e.g. opiates, benzodiazepines, alcohol).
- Accidental poisoning—usually due to toddlers or pre-school children gaining access to drugs or substances (e.g. berries, plants, household cleaners, washing tablets, and so on) in the home.
- Inadvertent self-poisoning—often with alcohol or recreational drugs when tried for the first time as a teenager.
- Iatrogenic poisoning—by accidental administration of the wrong dose or drug.
- Deliberate poisoning—may occur in older children as an act of self-harm (see Chapter 18, section 18.3).
- Intentional poisoning—by a parent or carer as a form of non-accidental injury.

19.10 Apparent life-threatening events

19.10.1 Definition of apparent life-threatening events

An apparent life-threatening event (ALTE) is defined as an episode that is frightening to the observer and is characterized by some combination of: apnoea (central or obstructive); colour change (cyanotic, pallor, erythematous, or plethoric); change in muscle tone (usually diminished); and choking or gagging.

ALTE has replaced the term 'near-miss' sudden infant death syndrome. Children suffering from ALTEs do have a greater risk of sudden infant death but most cases are benign.

It predominantly affects children younger than one year.

19.10.2 Causes of apparent life-threatening events

There are many causes of ALTE including:

- Gastro-oesophageal reflux.
- Central apnoea—occurs when there is a lack of respiratory effort due to the cessation of output from the central respiratory centres. This can be due to immaturity of the system, as seen in some preterm infants, head trauma, or toxins.
- Obstructive apnoea—occurs due to occlusion of the airways. The most common form is obstructive sleep apnoea, but it may be caused by an aspirated foreign body, nasal congestion during an upper respiratory tract infection, regurgitated gastric contents, and so on.
- Arrhythmias (e.g. long QT, SVT).
- Structural heart disease (e.g. duct-dependent lesions).
- Breath-holding attack.
- Toxins.
- Sepsis and/or meningitis.
- Lower respiratory tract infections.
- Seizures.
- Metabolic disorders.
- Non-accidental injury.

Despite the many causes of ALTE, up to 50% of cases remain unexplained following a thorough evaluation.

19.10.3 Assessment and initial investigations for apparent life-threatening events

The assessment of an infant following an ALTE is focused on a thorough history and careful examination. In most cases, the infant has recovered by the time of arrival in the ED, allowing for a systematic approach to history taking and physical examination.

Pertinent points in the history include:

- A witness account of the event—including the infant's colour, respiratory effort, and muscle tone. Any apnoea should be noted and whether this appeared to be central (lack of respiratory effort) or obstructive (respiratory effort with inadequate airflow).
- Any history of seizure-like activity.
- Whether any resuscitation was required or whether the infant recovered spontaneously.
- Whether the infant was premature and/or any complications with pregnancy or labour.
- Any symptoms suggestive of gastro-oesophageal reflux (e.g. coughing, choking, or gagging during or after feeding; frequent or excessive regurgitation; persistent nasal stuffiness or frequent hiccups; excessive irritability, arching, or straining behaviour during or following feeding).
- Any family history of seizures, metabolic disorders, arrhythmias, or sudden infant death.

A thorough examination should be performed (see Table 19.13) including a full set of observations (pulse, bilateral blood pressures, respiratory rate, oxygen saturations, temperature, and conscious level).

Investigations are directed by the findings of a thorough history and examination and may include:

- Full blood count—looking for evidence of a systemic infection
- Blood glucose

Table **19.13** Examination of a child following an apparent life-threatening event (ALTE)

Neurological examination	Responsiveness
	Muscle tone
	Reflexes
	Any focal neurological signs
	Fontanelle (i.e. normal, bulging, sunken)
	Pupillary reaction
	Fundoscopy
Cardiovascular examination	Murmurs
	Adequacy and symmetry of pulses
	Blood pressure and/or pulse oximetry readings in the arms and legs (a difference between the right arm compared with readings in the legs may suggest duct-dependent heart disease)
Respiratory examination	Respiratory rate and pattern of breathing
	Evidence of respiratory distress
	Presence of stridor, wheeze, or crackles
Abdominal examination	Distension or tenderness of the abdomen suggesting obstruction
	Hernias and testicular torsion should be excluded
Dermatological examination	Evidence of skin rashes or signs of trauma

- Urea and electrolytes—looking for evidence of hyponatraemia or hyperkalaemia
- Capillary blood gas—to assess for acidosis and lactate
- Cultures—as directed by the clinical picture (e.g. urine, stool, blood, and so on)
- ECG—for evidence of long QT or pre-excitation

19.10.4 Emergency department management of apparent life-threatening events

The main role of the ED is to identify children who have suffered an ALTE, make a thorough assessment, initiate the appropriate investigations, and refer on to the paediatric team for further evaluation.

KEY POINTS

An apparent life-threatening event (ALTE) is defined as an episode that is frightening to the observer and is characterized by some combination of:
- Apnoea
- Colour change
- Change in muscle tone
- Choking or gagging
- 50% of cases of ALTE remain unexplained following a thorough evaluation

Causes of ALTE including:
- Gastro-oesophageal reflux
- Central apnoea
- Obstructive apnoea

- Arrhythmias
- Structural heart disease
- Breath-holding attack
- Toxins
- Sepsis and/or meningitis
- Lower respiratory tract infections
- Seizures
- Metabolic disorders
- Non-accidental injury

19.11 Congenital heart disease

Congenital heart disease in particular duct-dependent lesions are a cause of ALTE and previous MRCEM questions have involved the diagnosis and management of duct-dependent lesions. Although an in-depth knowledge of the different types of congenital heart disease is not required a basic understanding is.

The majority of children presenting to the emergency department with congenital heart disease will already have a diagnosis, either made in the antenatal or neonatal period. However it is possible that an infant's first presentation and diagnosis may be in the emergency department.

9.11.1 Duct-dependent lesions

Infants presenting acutely unwell in the first few weeks of life, with previously undiagnosed congenital heart disease typically have a duct-dependent lesions. The patent ductus is able to maintain blood flow during the first few weeks of life, but as the duct begins to close the infant becomes acutely unwell due to lack of systemic circulation.

Clinical features a duct-dependent lesion include:

- Poor feeding secondary of breathlessness
- Cyanosis unresponsive to oxygen
- Respiratory cardiovascular collapse and shock

Management of an infant with a suspected duct-dependent lesion should follow the ABCDE with senior paediatric support.

- Supplemental oxygen can be delivered to achieve saturations of 75–85%. Hyperoxaemia is avoided as it can exacerbate pulmonary congestion by increasing pulmonary blood flow and reducing systemic circulation.
- Hypotension can be treated with fluid boluses of 10 ml/kg (maximum of 30 ml/kg).
- The treatment of choice is prostaglandin E1 (PGE1), which is a potent vasodilator thus dilating the patent ductus in an attempt to temporarily maintain blood flow. PGE1 infusion should be started at a rate of 5 nanograms/kg/min and titrated to response. The commonest side effects are hypotension, respiratory depression, and apnoea, for which infants may require intubation.

KEY POINTS

The first presentation of congenital heart disease may be in the emergency department in the first few weeks of life.

Infants with duct-dependent lesions can present acutely unwell and treatment includes ABCD, senior paediatric support, and a prostaglandin E1 (PGE1) infusion.

19.12 Blood disorders

19.12.1 Sickle cell anaemia

Pathophysiology of sickle cell disease

Sickle cell disease is an autosomal recessive disease caused by a genetic mutation, which results in a single amino acid substitution in one of the chains of the haemoglobin molecule (HbS). It occurs in African, Indian, Middle Eastern, Caribbean, US, and Mediterranean populations.

The normal adult haemoglobin genotype AA produces HbA.

- In heterozygote's (sickle cell trait) one gene is abnormal (HbAS) and about 40% of the patient's haemoglobin is HbS.
- In homozygote's (sickle cell anaemia), both genes are abnormal (HbSS) and >80% of the haemoglobin is HbS.

HbS molecules polymerize in deoxygenated or acidotic conditions, causing red blood cells to sickle. Sickle cells are rigid and fragile. They may rapidly haemolyse (lifespan 10–20 days compared to 120 days for a normal red blood cell) or cause vaso-occlusion leading to tissue ischaemia, infarction, and further sickling.

Clinical features of sickle cell disease

Those with sickle cell trait usually have no disability except during conditions of severe hypoxia (e.g. cardiac arrest).

Those with sickle cell anaemia will have intermittent acute sickle cell crises. These may be spontaneous or triggered by infection, cold, dehydration, tissue hypoxia, or ischaemia. Crises may include vaso-occlusive, haematological, and/or infective emergencies.

- Vaso-occlusive crises—occur due to obstruction of the microcirculation by thromboses leading to tissue hypoxia and ischaemia. The crises cause severe pain and can mimic any acute medical or surgical emergency. Vaso-occlusion can lead to bone infarction, avascular necrosis, abdominal pain, splenic autoinfarction, liver and renal failure, acute chest syndrome, TIAs, strokes, seizures, cranial nerve palsies, priapism, hand and foot swelling, and skin ulceration.
- Haematological crises—result from a sudden exacerbation of anaemia. Patients with sickle cell anaemia have chronically low haemoglobin levels (Hb 8–10 g/dL), which can suddenly deteriorate. It may be due to acute splenic sequestration or an aplastic crisis (bone marrow stops functioning and producing red blood cells). An aplastic crisis is seen most commonly in patients with a parvovirus B19 infection or folic acid deficiency.
- Infective crises—occur due to functional asplenia leading to defective immunity against encapsulated organisms (e.g. *Haemophilus influenza*, *Streptococcus*). Patients also have low levels of IgM resulting in increased susceptibility to other common infections (e.g. *Staphylococcus aureus*, *E. coli*, *Salmonella typhi*, *Mycoplasma pneumoniae*).

There are certain notable presentations in sickle cell disease, which are potential SAQ topics. These are:

- Acute chest syndrome—this is the leading cause of death in sickle cell anaemia. It is poorly understood but infection may be a precipitant. The clinical features include chest pain, hypoxia, cough, tachypnoea, and wheezing. Pulmonary infiltrates may be seen on CXR.
- Acute splenic sequestration—sudden trapping of large numbers of red blood cells in the spleen results in splenomegaly, severe anaemia, hypovolaemia, and thrombocytopenia. It occurs most commonly in young children, with patients having a 30% chance of developing acute splenic sequestration by the age of five years.

- Osteomyelitis and septic arthritis—occurs more commonly in sickle cell disease. Presentation includes fever, soft tissue swelling, and pain. *Salmonella* is frequently implicated.

Investigations in a sickle cell crisis

Patients will often be aware that they have sickle cell disease and the diagnosis of a crisis is then largely clinical. If a patient does not have a previous diagnosis then sickle testing will detect sickling in homo- and heterozygote forms. Haemoglobin electrophoresis is required to distinguish between HbSS, HbAS, and other Hb variants.

Investigations to be performed in a patient with a suspected crisis include:

- Full blood count—chronic anaemia is expected (Hb 8–10 g/dL). If there is a sudden drop in the Hb (>2 g/dL) it suggests acute haemolysis, splenic sequestration, or aplastic anaemia. If the reticulocyte count is normal, then it suggests splenic sequestration. If the reticulocyte count is low it suggests aplastic anaemia. The white cell count and platelets are usually elevated even in the absence of infection.
- Blood film—sickle-shaped red blood cells may be seen. Howell–Jolly bodies indicate the patient is asplenic.
- Liver function tests—bilirubin is usually elevated due to haemolysis.
- Renal function.
- Arterial blood gas—looking for evidence of hypoxia and/or a raised lactate due to hypoperfusion.
- ECG—should be performed if the patient has chest pain.
- Group and save/cross match.
- Infection screen—blood, urine, and stool cultures.
- CXR—looking for evidence of infection or acute chest syndrome (may be normal initially).
- Limb X-rays—looking for evidence of bone infarcts/osteomyelitis at painful sites.
- CT head—if the patient has neurological signs or symptoms.

Emergency department management of a sickle cell crisis

The key to managing a sickle cell crisis is supportive therapy.

- The patient should be kept warm and rested.
- Oxygen should be given if the patient is hypoxic (saturations <94%).
- Intravenous fluids should be given to rehydrate the patient. Careful monitoring of haemodynamic parameters and urine output is required to avoid precipitating heart failure.
- Intravenous opiates are often required to manage the pain. A patient-controlled analgesia pump should be considered.
- Blood transfusion may be needed for severe anaemia secondary to aplastic crisis, splenic sequestration, or acute haemolysis. Patients with CNS or lung complications may also require transfusion.
- Empirical antibiotics should be started if an infection is thought to be the trigger for the crisis.
- Expert help should be sought early. An exchange transfusion may be required for patients who have acute chest syndrome or a stroke. Exchange transfusion is occasionally used in patients with acute splenic sequestration or priapism that does not resolve with supportive therapy.

19.12.2 Purpura

Purpura refers to non-blanching areas of haemorrhage into the skin. Petechiae are small, non-blanching areas of haemorrhage into the skin. Petechiae and purpura have many causes, the most well-known being meningococcal disease. If a child is unwell with a purpuric rash they should be treated for meningococcal disease until proven otherwise.

Causes of purpura include:

- Meningococcal disease (see Chapter 15, section 15.4).
- Henoch–Schönlein purpura (HSP).
- Thrombocytopenia—this may be caused by idiopathic thrombocytopenia (ITP), leukaemia, septic shock, or aplastic anaemia.
- Enteroviral infection.
- Trauma.
- Forceful coughing or vomiting—petechiae localized to face and above the clavicular line.

Henoch–Schönlein purpura

Henoch–Schönlein purpura is a vasculitic condition that affects the small arteries of the kidneys, skin, and gastrointestinal tract. It usually affects children between the ages of 3 and 10 years old. It is twice as common in boys, peaks during the winter months, and is often preceded by an upper respiratory tract infection.

Clinical features include:

- Rash—erythematous macules develop into purpuric lesions, which are characteristically concentrated over the buttocks and extensor surfaces of the lower limbs.
- Arthralgia—particularly the knees and ankles.
- Peri-articular oedema.
- Abdominal pain.
- Haematuria—due to glomerulonephritis.

Useful ED investigations include urinalysis, which may reveal micro- or macroscopic haematuria, and/or proteinuria. Other factors for investigation include: renal function, because occasionally nephrotic syndrome and acute kidney injury develop; blood pressure, because hypertension is a risk factor for progressive renal disease; and full blood count, to ensure a normal platelet count and exclude thrombocytopenia as a cause.

ED management is mainly symptomatic with the provision of analgesia for any pain and referral on to the paediatric team. There is a good spontaneous recovery rate, but some patients may require a renal biopsy and immunosuppression if renal function deteriorates.

Idiopathic thrombocytopenic purpura

Idiopathic thrombocytopenic purpura (ITP) is a condition of an abnormally low platelet count with no known cause. In many cases, the origin of ITP is autoimmune not idiopathic, with antibodies against platelets being detected in approximately 60% patients. A preceding illness is the usual likely trigger.

Clinical features include:

- Purpuric rash.
- Mucous membrane bleeding.
- Conjunctival haemorrhage.
- Occasionally gastrointestinal bleeding.
- Children may be suspected of suffering from non-accidental injury due to the ease of bruising and bleeding.
- Note—the presence of lymphadenopathy, hepatomegaly, or splenomegaly suggests an alternative diagnosis (e.g. leukaemia).

The most important investigation is a full blood count. Platelets will be less than 30×10^9/L.

Children should be referred on for paediatric review. Treatment is usually expectant because most cases resolve spontaneously over three months. Occasionally life-threatening haemorrhage occurs and patients should be managed in the usual ABCDE manner and resuscitated accordingly.

> **KEY POINTS**
>
> Sickle cell disease is an autosomal recessive disease caused by a genetic mutation which results in a single amino acid substitution in one of the chains of the haemoglobin molecule (HbS).
> There are certain notable presentations in sickle cell disease:
> - Acute chest syndrome
> - Acute splenic sequestration
> - Aplastic crisis
> - Osteomyelitis and septic arthritis
>
> The key to managing a sickle cell crisis is supportive therapy.
>
> Causes of purpura include:
> - Meningococcal disease
> - Henoch–Schönlein purpura
> - Thrombocytopenia (e.g. ITP, leukaemia, septic shock, or aplastic anaemia)
> - Enteroviral infection
> - Trauma
> - Forceful coughing or vomiting
>
> Henoch–Schönlein purpura (HSP) is a vasculitic condition which affects the small arteries of the kidneys, skin, and gastrointestinal tract.
>
> The typical rash of HSP is erythematous macules developing into purpuric lesions, concentrated over the buttocks and extensor surfaces of the lower limbs. Other clinical features include arthralgia, peri-articular oedema, abdominal pain, and haematuria.
>
> Idiopathic thrombocytopenic purpura (ITP) is a condition of an abnormally low platelet count with no known cause, although in approximately 60% of cases antibodies against platelets are detected. A preceding illness is the usual trigger.

19.13 Breathing difficulties

19.13.1 Asthma in children

Asthma in children causes recurrent respiratory symptoms of wheeze, cough, breathing difficulties, and chest tightness. The diagnosis of asthma is a clinical one based on the recognition of a characteristic pattern of episodic symptoms and signs, in the absence of an alternative explanation for them. In infants and pre-school children, episodes of wheezing, cough, and difficulty breathing are common with viral upper respiratory tract infections, but between infections they have no symptoms. This is not the same as asthma and most children with viral-induced wheeze will stop having recurrent chest symptoms by school age.

Asthma in adults is covered in Chapter 10, section 10.1 and it is worth reading that section in conjunction with this. Most notably the British Thoracic Society (BTS) severity markers for children are slightly different to those in adults. Asthma in children has appeared in previous MRCEM SAQs.

Severity markers for asthma in children aged >2 years

Previous MRCEM question

Table 19.14 details asthma severity markers in children aged over two years.

Table 19.14 Asthma severity markers in children aged over two years

Severity markers for asthma in children aged >2 years	
Moderate asthma	Clinical features: • Able to talk in sentences Measurements: • Saturations >92% • PEF >50% of best or predicted • Heart rate ≤125 (age >5 years) or ≤140 (age 2–5 years) • Respiratory rate ≤30 breaths/min (age >5 years) or ≤40 (age 2–5 years)
Severe asthma	Clinical features: • Cannot complete sentences in one breath or too breathless to talk or feed Measurements: • Saturations <92% • PEF 33–50% • Heart rate >125 (>5 years) or >140 (2–5 years) • Respiratory rate >30 breaths/min (>5 years) or >40 (2–5 years)
Life-threatening asthma	Clinical features: • Hypotension • Silent chest • Exhaustion • Cyanosis • Confusion • Poor respiratory effort • Coma Measurements: • Saturations <92% • PEF <33%

Data from British Guideline on the Management of Asthma (2014). A national clinical guideline. British Thoracic Society (www.brit-thoracic.org.uk).

Investigations for asthma in children

• Pulse oximetry—is an essential part of the assessment in all children presenting with wheeze. Saturations <92% after initial bronchodilator treatment selects a more severe group of patients.
• Peak expiratory flow (PEF) rate—are useful in children who are familiar with the use of such devices. The best of three PEF measurements, ideally expressed as percentage of the patients best ever reading, can be useful in assessing the response to treatment.
• Blood gas measurements—should be considered if there are life-threatening features not responding to treatment. Arterialized ear lobe gases can be used to gain an accurate measure of pH and $PaCO_2$. If ear lobe sampling is not possible, a finger-prick sample can be an alternative. Normal or raised $PaCO_2$ levels are indicative of worsening asthma. A venous blood gas sample with a $PaCO_2$ measurement <6 kPa excludes hypercapnea.
• Chest radiographs—are not routinely recommended. They should be performed if there is subcutaneous emphysema; persisting unilateral signs suggesting a pneumothorax, lobar collapse or consolidation; and/or life-threatening features not responding to treatment.

Treatment of asthma in children

Initial treatments for acute asthma:

- **Oxygen** should be given to children with life-threatening asthma or saturations <94%. Oxygen should be given via a tight-fitting face mask or nasal cannulae at a sufficient flow rate to achieve normal saturations.
- **Inhaled β_2-agonists** are the first-line treatment for acute asthma (e.g. salbutamol). In mild to moderate asthma, a metered-dose inhaler via a spacer is the preferred method of delivery. Up to ten 100 mcg puffs of salbutamol may be required. Puffs should be given one at a time and inhaled separately with five tidal breaths via a spacer. Children with severe or life-threatening asthma should receive frequent doses of nebulized bronchodilator driven by oxygen (e.g. salbutamol 2.5 mg).
- **Ipratropium bromide** (250 mcg nebulizer) should be given if symptoms are refractory to initial β_2-agonist therapy. There is good evidence for safety and efficacy of frequent doses of ipratropium bromide (every 20–30 minutes), used in addition to a β_2 agonist, for the first two hours of a severe asthma attack.
- **Steroids** given early in the ED can reduce the need for admission and prevent a relapse in symptoms after initial presentation. Oral and intravenous steroids are of similar efficacy. Intravenous hydrocortisone (4 mg/kg) should be reserved for children unable to retain oral medication. The recommended dose of oral prednisolone is 20 mg for children aged 2–5 years and 30 mg for children aged >5 years. For children already on steroids, a dose of 1 mg/kg (maximum dose 60 mg) should be given. Treatment for three days is usually sufficient.

Second-line treatments for acute asthma

Children with continuing severe asthma despite initial treatment (frequent nebulized β_2-agonists and ipratropium bromide, and oral steroids) need urgent senior review to consider the need for transfer to a paediatric high-dependency area or intensive care unit and initiate second-line intravenous therapies.

There are three main intravenous options to consider:

- Intravenous salbutamol (15 mcg/kg over 10 minutes) should be considered early on in severe cases where the patient has not responded to initial inhaled therapy.
- Intravenous aminophylline (5 mg/kg over 20 minutes) should be considered in the HDU/PICU setting for children with severe or life-threatening asthma unresponsive to maximal doses of bronchodilators plus steroids.
- Intravenous magnesium sulfate is a safe treatment in acute asthma, although its place in paediatric management is not yet established.

Discharge planning

Children can be discharged when stable on three to four-hourly inhaled bronchodilators, have a PEF >75%, and saturations >94%.

Discharge plans should include:

- Checking the inhaler technique.
- Consideration of the need for preventive therapy.
- A written asthma action plan for subsequent exacerbations, with clear instructions about the use of bronchodilator therapy and the need to seek urgent medical attention if symptoms are not controlled by up to 10 puffs of salbutamol every four hours.
- GP follow-up arranged for within two days.

Acute asthma in children aged <2 years

The assessment of acute asthma in early childhood can be difficult. Intermittent wheezing attacks are usually due to viral infection and the response to asthma medication is inconsistent. Prematurity and low birthweight are risk factors for recurrent wheezing.

The differential diagnosis of wheezing includes:

- Pneumonitis
- Pneumonia
- Bronchiolitis
- Tracheomalacia
- Cystic fibrosis
- Congenital anomalies

If acute asthma is thought to be the cause of the wheeze, the following treatment is recommended:

- Inhaled β_2 agonist—via a metered-dose inhaler and spacer is the optimal delivery device in mild and moderate acute asthma. If inhalers have been delivered successfully but there is no improvement in symptoms, review the diagnosis and consider the use of other treatment options.
- Steroid therapy (10 mg prednisolone)—should be considered in the early management of infants with severe acute asthma.
- Inhaled ipratropium bromide—should be considered in combination with an inhaled β_2 agonist for more severe symptoms.

19.13.2 Pneumonia in children

The text that follows is based on the BTS guidance on the management of community-acquired pneumonia in children.

Aetiology of pneumonia in children

Streptococcus pneumoniae is the commonest bacterial cause of pneumonia in children, followed by *Mycoplasma*, and *Chlamydia pneumonia*. In younger children, viral pathogens are the most common cause. In a significant proportion of children (8–40%) community-acquired pneumonia is due to a mixed infection.

Clinical features of pneumonia

Bacterial pneumonia should be considered in children aged up to three years when there is a high fever (>38.5°C), chest recession, and a respiratory rate >50/min. In older children, a history of difficulty in breathing is more useful than clinical signs.

Severity assessment of pneumonia

Table 19.15 details indicators for admission in pneumonia.

Investigations for pneumonia

- Pulse oximetry must be performed on all children.
- CXR is not routinely indicated in children with uncomplicated acute lower respiratory tract infections. Radiographic findings are a poor indicator of aetiology.
- FBC and C-reactive protein (CRP) do not distinguish between bacterial and viral infections, and routine measurement is not recommended. In a severely unwell child, a baseline measurement may be useful to monitor response to treatment, if the child does not improve as expected.

Table **19.15** Indicators for admission in pneumonia

Indicators for admission in infants	Indicators for admission in older children
Oxygen saturation ≤92%, cyanosis	Oxygen saturation ≤92%, cyanosis
Respiratory rate >70 breaths/min	Respiratory rate >50 breaths/min
Difficulty in breathing	Difficulty in breathing
Intermittent apnoea, grunting	Grunting
Not feeding	Signs of dehydration
Family not able to provide appropriate observation or supervision	Family not able to provide appropriate observation or supervision

Data from BTS Guidelines for the Management of Community Acquired Pneumonia in Children Update 2011. British Thoracic Society (www.brit-thoracic.org.uk).

- Urea and electrolytes are useful to assess electrolyte imbalance, if the patient is severely ill or shows dehydration.
- Microbiological tests are not indicated for children with pneumonia managed in the community. Therefore, if the child is well enough for discharge from the ED, no investigations are required.
- Children admitted do not routinely require microbiological tests to try and establish the causative pathogen, unless they have signs of severe pneumonia requiring intensive care. Blood cultures should be performed in all suspected cases of bacterial pneumonia. A nasopharyngeal aspirate should be performed in children younger than 18 months and sent for viral antigen testing and culture. Those with a significant pleural effusion should have an aspirate sent for diagnostic purposes.

Treatment of community-acquired pneumonia

- The carers of children who are well enough for discharge from the ED should be given advice on managing pyrexia, preventing dehydration, and identifying any deterioration.
- Supplemental oxygen should be given if the child is hypoxic to maintain saturations >92%. Those receiving oxygen should have at least four-hourly observations.
- Nasogastric tubes may compromise breathing and should be avoided in severely ill children and especially in infants with small nasal passages.
- Intravenous fluids should be given if there is evidence of volume depletion; 80% of maintenance levels should be given and electrolytes monitored.
- Antipyretics and analgesics should be given as necessary to keep the child comfortable.
- Antibiotics are not required in young children with mild symptoms of a lower respiratory tract infection.
- Amoxicillin is the first-line oral antibiotic in children younger than five years. A macrolide can be added as second line if there is poor response to amoxicillin or if mycoplasma or chlamydia infection is suspected. Co-amoxiclav is recommended in pneumonia associated with influenza. Intravenous antibiotics should be used if the child is unable to absorb oral medication or is severely unwell. An appropriate intravenous antibiotic would be co-amoxiclav, cefotaxime, or cefuroxime.

19.13.3 Acute stridor in children

Stridor is a monophasic, harsh, inspiratory noise due to partial airway obstruction. The most important consideration in a child with stridor is to not upset or distress them, causing a partial to become a complete obstruction.

Causes of stridor:

- Croup
- Foreign body inhalation
- Angioedema
- Bacterial tracheitis
- Diphtheria
- Whooping cough
- Epiglottitis
- Retropharyngeal abscess
- Trauma

19.13.4 Croup

Previous MRCEM question

The commonest cause of croup is viral, also known as acute viral laryngotracheobronchitis. The peak incidence is the second year of life but ranges from six months to five years.

Causes of croup

- Parainfluenza virus (commonest)
- Respiratory syncytial virus
- Adenovirus

Clinical features of croup

- Barking cough
- Harsh stridor, usually inspiratory, but biphasic in severe disease
- Hoarseness of voice
- Preceding fever and coryza for one to three days
- Symptoms usually worse at night
- Usually a benign, self-limited disease
- No specific treatment is required for most children

Some children have repeated episodes of croup without preceding fever and coryza. Symptoms often start suddenly at night and last a few hours. This is often called spasmodic croup and may be associated with atopic disease.

Severity assessment—Westley croup score

The Westley croup score is a well-recognized severity assessment tool and has been questioned in previous SAQs. It is not necessary to memorize how many points are scored for each feature, but it is necessary to learn what the five scored features are.

Treatment of croup

- Steroids—are the main stay of treatment. Dexamethasone orally (dose varies from 0.15 to 0.6 mg/kg) or budesonide nebulizer (2 mg) or prednisolone (1 mg/kg bd orally).
- Anti-pyretic—should be given if the child is pyrexial and unwell.
- Humidified oxygen—should be given if the child is hypoxic (saturations <92%).
- Adrenaline nebulizer (5 ml of 1:1000—APLS guidance)—reduces the clinical severity acutely but has not been shown to improve blood gases, reduce length of hospital stay, or eliminate the need for intubation.
- Intubation—is required if there is increasing cyanosis, exhaustion, coma, increasing heart and respiratory rate, or marked inter- and subcostal retractions.

Discharge advice for croup

Children with mild croup may be considered for discharge from the ED. Extreme caution is needed before discharging a child at night. Parents should be given advice to return if the child develops any of the following:

- Stridor at rest
- Increasing respiratory distress
- Excessive dribbling
- Difficulty swallowing
- Reduced feeding
- Restlessness, confusion, or drowsiness

19.13.5 Bacterial tracheitis

Bacterial tracheitis (pseudomembranous croup) is an uncommon but life-threatening form of croup. It is caused by *Staph. Aureus, Streptococci*, or *H. influenza B*, which infect the tracheal mucosa. This causes copious, purulent secretions, and mucosal necrosis. The child appears toxic, with a high fever, and evidence of airway obstruction. It can be difficult to differentiate from epiglottitis—but unlike epiglottitis, drooling is absent.

Treatment is early intubation and intravenous antibiotics (cephalosporin and flucloxacillin). Septic shock can rapidly develop.

19.13.6 Epiglottitis

Epiglottitis has virtually been eradicated from children by the introduction of the Hib vaccine. It is now a disease of young adults. Further details on epiglottitis can be found in Chapter 7, section 7.4.

19.13.7 Whooping cough

Whooping cough (pertussis infection) is caused by *Bordetella pertussis* and is a notifiable disease. It is a highly infectious bacterial disease of the respiratory tract and is spread by droplet transmission. The incubation period is 7–10 days, but the infectious period can be from four days before to three weeks after the onset of typical paroxysms.

The highest incidence is in infants who are unimmunized or too young to be fully protected. School children are often the source of infection for younger siblings at home. However, infection also occurs in adolescents and adults, even if previously immunized, because immunity wanes over time.

Pertussis vaccination

Acellular pertussis vaccine is given with the primary course of diptheria, tetanus, polio, and Hib at ages two, three, and four months. A further dose is given with the pre-school boosters between the ages of three and five years.

Clinical features of whooping cough

Initial symptoms include coryza and cough. Gradually the cough progresses to severe coughing bouts, which can be prolonged. Not all children have the characteristic 'whoop' (inspiratory noise) at the end of a coughing bout, and some cough spasms may be followed by periods of vomiting.

Investigation of whooping cough

In England and Wales, whooping cough is a notifiable disease and initial notification should be made based on the clinical diagnosis. A notification certificate should be completed immediately on diagnosis of suspected whooping cough, prior to laboratory confirmation, and sent to the 'Proper Officer' of the Local Authority.

Confirmation of the diagnosis is via polymerase chain reaction and serological testing, because the viral culture lacks sensitivity.

Other investigations should be directed as for a suspected pneumonia.

ED management of whooping cough

- Infants aged less than six months should be admitted due to the risk of apnoea. Acutely unwell children should also be admitted.
- Treatment is with oral erythromycin.
- The infected child should not have contact with other children for at least five days.
- Prophylactic erythromycin should be given to any close contacts who are particularly vulnerable, unvaccinated, partially vaccinated, or less than five years of age.

Complications of whooping cough

The illness can be prolonged and complications include bronchiectasis, neurological damage, and prolonged apnoeic episodes. Severe complications and deaths occur most commonly in infants under six months of age.

19.13.8 Bronchiolitis

Bronchiolitis is the commonest serious respiratory infection of childhood. Most patients develop it between one and nine months old. There is an annual winter epidemic.

Causes of bronchiolitis include

- Respiratory syncytial virus (75% cases)
- Others—parainfluenza, influenza, adenoviruses

Clinical features of bronchiolitis

- Seasonal viral illness, characterized by fever, clear nasal discharge, and dry wheezy cough
- Preceding coryzal phase of two to three days
- Low grade fever
- Head bobbing
- Feeding difficulty
- The chest may be visibly hyperinflated
- Subcostal, intercostal, and supraclavicular recessions are common
- Fine inspiratory crackles +/- high-pitched expiratory wheeze
- In most infants, self-limiting, typically lasting three to seven days

High-risk groups for bronchiolitis

These are:

- Premature infants
- Chronic lung disease (e.g. cystic fibrosis)
- Congenital heart disease
- Immunodeficiency
- Age <6 weeks

Investigations for bronchiolitis

- Nasopharyngeal aspirate for respiratory syncytial virus.
- CXR, if there are severe symptoms—may show hyperinflation, collapse, consolidation, or perihilar infiltrates.
- Capillary blood gas analysis (if severe).
- Blood glucose.
- Other blood tests as clinically indicated (e.g. FBC, renal function, blood cultures).

Management of bronchiolitis

- Suction to clear secretions.
- Oxygen to maintain saturations >94%.
- Monitor and maintain hydration and nutrition (intravenous or nasogastric if necessary).
- Monitor for apnoea (respiratory rate, saturations, apnoea monitor).
- Ventilatory support—CPAP or intubation may be required in severe cases.
- There is no evidence of benefit from steroids, bronchodilators, or antibiotics.
- Nebulized ribavirin may be considered.

KEY POINTS

Asthma in children causes recurrent respiratory symptoms of wheeze, cough, breathing difficulties, and chest tightness.

The severity markers for asthma are different for adults and children. They can be remembered by dividing them into those that are clinical features (e.g. inability to complete sentences) and those that are measured (e.g. saturations, PEF, and so on).

The initial ED treatment of acute asthma includes:

- Oxygen
- β_2 agonist
- Ipatropium bromide
- Steroids

Second-line treatments for asthma include intravenous salbutamol or aminophylline.

Stridor is a monophasic, harsh, inspiratory noise due to partial airway obstruction. Causes include:

- Croup
- Foreign body inhalation
- Angioedema
- Bacterial tracheitis
- Diphtheria
- Whooping cough
- Epiglottitis
- Retropharyngeal abscess
- Trauma

The Westley croup score can be used to assess the severity of croup. The five components are: stridor; intercostal recession; air entry; cyanosis; and level of consciousness.

Croup is treated with steroids: either dexamethasone (0.15–0.6 mg/kg) or budesonide (2 mg nebulizer).

Whooping cough (pertussis) is a notifiable disease.

19.14 Concerning presentations in children

19.14.1 Introduction

Children may present to the ED with both the physical and psychological consequences of maltreatment.

The abuse or maltreatment of children is not a new problem; it has been recognized since Victorian times. However, it is only recently, with the enactment of the Children Act 1989, the

Human Rights Act 1998, and the Protection of Children Act 1999, that children have enjoyed legal protection from abuse.

The Royal College of Emergency Medicine has produced guidance on the best practice for safeguarding children and standards that Eds should meet. NICE produced guidance in 2009 on when to suspect maltreatment in children. The text which follows is based on this guidance.

> **EXAM TIP**
>
> All staff working permanently in the NHS are required to have Level 1 training on Safeguarding Children, and Level 2 training if they regularly care for children. Attendance at such sessions or completion of an e-learning module can be a useful way to revise the topic.
>
> The e-learning for healthcare website (https://www.e-lfh.org.uk) is free for NHS employees and provides modules for Level 1 and 2 Safeguarding Children. Doctors.net (https://www.doctors. net.uk) also has an e-learning module on child protection.

19.14.2 Types of abuse

Child abuse is described in four categories:

- Physical abuse
- Sexual abuse
- Neglect
- Emotional abuse

Many children experience more than one form of abuse. All forms of abuse, including domestic violence, result in emotional harm to the child and can be considered as emotional abuse.

Physical abuse

About 7% of children in the UK experience serious physical abuse at the hands of their parents or carers during childhood.

Physical abuse includes:

- Smacking and hitting.
- Pinching.
- Shaking, throwing, or knocking down.
- Kicking.
- Punching.
- Burning or scalding on purpose.
- Suffocating, grabbing around the neck, and choking.
- Threatening with a knife or gun, or inflicting pain or injury to a child in any other way.
- Administering harmful substances to a child, such as drugs, alcohol, or poison.
- Fabricating or inducing an illness by reporting non-existent symptoms of illness (e.g. recurrent reports of ALTEs, see section 19.10), or deliberately causing illness.

Some of the alerting features of physical abuse are:

- Bruising—especially in areas that are not usually injured (e.g. not on a bony prominence) and if in the pattern of a hand, ligature, stick, teeth marks, grip, or implement.
- Lacerations, abrasions, and scars—for which there is inadequate explanation (e.g. in an child who is not independently mobile; that are multiple; that occur in areas usually covered by clothes; or in areas that are not usually injured).
- Bite marks.
- Burns and scalds—especially on areas that would not be expected to come into contact with a hot object in an accident (e.g. back of hands, soles, buttocks); or in the shape of an implement

(e.g. cigarette, iron); or suggesting immersion (e.g. symmetrical with sharply delineated borders on the buttocks, hands, or feet).

- Fractures—that are multiple and/or of different ages without adequate explanation (i.e. no medical condition that predisposes to fragile bones, e.g. osteogenesis imperfect, osteopenia, prematurity). These include fractures of ribs or the spine. Fractures in a child who is not independently mobile. Long bone fractures in children aged <3 years old. Epiphyseal separation and metaphyseal 'chip' fractures of the knee, wrist, elbow, or ankle, which are associated with traction, rotation, and shaking.
- Intracranial injuries—in the absence of major confirmed accidental trauma or known medical cause.
- Eye trauma (e.g. retinal haemorrhages or eye injuries in the absence of confirmed major trauma or medical explanation).
- Oral injury—such as a torn frenulum, without adequate explanation.

Sexual abuse

In the United Kingdom, 1% of children experience sexual abuse by a parent or carer, 3% by another relative, 11% by people known but unrelated to them, and 5% by an adult stranger or someone they have just met.

Sexual abuse is when a child or young person, male or female, is pressurized, forced, or tricked into taking part in any kind of sexual activity with an adult or young person. This can include kissing, touching the young person's genitals or breasts, intercourse, or oral sex. Encouraging a child to look at pornographic magazines, videos, or sexual acts is also sexual abuse.

Most children who present with an allegation or a history of sexual abuse do not have any physical signs when examined. This is because the abuse may have taken place some time before the examination and injuries to the genital area heal very quickly, or because the abuse was non-penetrative (e.g. kissing or touching).

Physical signs that may be present include:

- Injury to the genitalia or anus
- Perineal pain, discharge, or bleeding
- Pregnancy
- Sexually transmitted infections

The child's behaviour may suggest sexual abuse if he or she:

- Becomes anxious about going to a particular place or seeing a particular person.
- Suddenly starts having behaviour problems, such as being aggressive.
- Suddenly starts having extreme mood swings, such as brooding, crying, or fearfulness.
- Has a sudden deterioration in school results.
- Displays unexpectedly explicit sexual knowledge for their age.
- Starts wetting the bed again, having previously been dry by night.
- Engages in risky behaviours—drug-taking, unprotected sex with numerous partners (in an adolescent).
- Starts harming him or herself.

Neglect

About 6% of children in the United Kingdom experience a serious absence of care at home during childhood.

Neglect is the persistent lack of appropriate care of a child. This includes lack of love, stimulation, safety, nourishment, warmth, education, and medical attention.

Neglect may be suspected if the mechanism of injury suggests lack of appropriate supervision.

Child neglect is not always deliberate. Sometimes, a caregiver becomes physically or mentally unable to care for a child, such as in untreated depression or anxiety. Other times, alcohol or drug abuse may seriously impair judgement and the ability to keep a child safe.

Physical signs of neglect include:

- Ill-fitting, dirty clothes and shoes.
- Not dressed warmly enough in cold weather.
- Appearing very dirty, with matted and unwashed hair, or smelling bad.
- Untreated or delayed treatment for illnesses and physical injuries.
- Failure to thrive, gain weight, and meet developmental milestones.

Emotional abuse

Parents from all types of backgrounds may emotionally abuse their children. About 6% of children in the United Kingdom experience frequent and severe emotional maltreatment during childhood.

Emotional abuse is the hardest type of abuse to define precisely, but occurs when a parent or carer behaves in a way that is likely to seriously affect their child's emotional development.

Physical abuse, sexual abuse, and neglect nearly always involve an element of emotional abuse. However, emotional abuse can be the only form of abuse a child is suffering. It can range from constant rejection and denial of affection through to continual severe criticism. It is not a one-off outburst, but continues over time.

It is not always easy to identify when a child is being emotionally abused.

Some of the ways children react to emotional abuse are:

- Having low self-confidence and a poor self-image.
- Being withdrawn, unable to trust others, and having difficulty forming relationships.
- Being delayed emotionally, socially, or academically.
- Becoming anxious, depressed, demanding, aggressive, destructive, or even cruel.

19.14.3 Risk factors for child abuse

Any child can be at risk of abuse regardless of their age, sex, ethnicity, ability, or disability. Those most at risk are babies and young children, those with learning difficulties, and physical disabilities.

Children are hurt by adults of all ages, class, sex, race, and sexual orientation. The following factors may increase the likelihood of abuse:

- Stress—possibly caused by financial problems and difficulties in the parents' relationships. This can reduce some adults' ability to control aggressive feelings towards their children or to care for their children properly.
- Social disadvantage (e.g. living on a low income in inadequate housing or being discriminated against because of ethnicity, religion, disability, or sexual orientation). All of these factors could affect parents' ability to care for their children properly.
- Mental illness, substance abuse, and domestic violence—could also have a damaging effect on their ability to meet their children's needs.
- Domestic violence—is a factor involved in the families of more than 70% of children presenting with child abuse.

19.14.4 Legal framework for child protection

Everyone who deals with children is responsible for safeguarding and has a legal obligation to raise any concerns they may have about a child's welfare.

The Children Act 1989 contains most of the relevant law relating to child protection.

Section 47 of the Children Act 1989 covers children at risk or suffering harm, from physical, sexual, or emotional abuse, or neglect. If there is significant concern that a child is at risk of harm, then social services will instigate section 47 and contact the police. Social services, the police, and the paediatricians will then formulate a joint strategy plan to decide if the child needs to be taken into care or can be discharged home. If it is felt that a child needs to be in a place of safety, the parents can voluntarily allow the child to be taken into care, which may be the hospital or a close relative (Section 20 of the Children Act). If the parents insist on taking the child out of hospital when there is concern for the child's welfare, the police should be informed. Under Section 46 of the Children Act, the police have the power to enforce a police protection order that can keep the child in a designated place of safety for up to 72 hours. The social worker can apply for an extension to this in the form of an emergency protection order (Section 44 of the Children Act).

The Children's Act 2004 requires each local authority in England and Wales to promote cooperation between different agencies involved in the welfare of children. It also requires them to establish Local Safeguarding Children Boards, of which NHS Trusts are statutory members.

Every NHS Trust will have a named doctor for child protection who is responsible for promoting and advising on safeguarding issues.

19.14.5 Emergency department assessment of a child with a concerning presentation

Doctors and nurses working in the ED need to be vigilant to abuse when assessing and treating children. Clinical features suggestive of physical, sexual, neglect, and/or emotional abuse (as previously detailed here) should be noted.

Features in the child's history that may suggest possible abuse include:

- Injuries inconsistent with the history given.
- Injuries inappropriate for the developmental age.
- Changing history—either between parents/carers/child or alterations over time.
- Vague history or lacking details.
- Delay in seeking medical attention with no adequate explanation.
- Abnormal parental attitudes (e.g. lack of parental concern).
- Frequent ED attendances—children with three or more attendances for different conditions in the past year should be referred on to the community health visitor team or social worker team within five days of attendance (College of Emergency Medicine standard).

In addition to the history of current events, a past medical history for the child should be established. For example, was the child premature, do they have any significant medical or developmental problems? This helps determine if the child has a possible medical cause for the presentation (e.g. osteogenesis imperfect) or if they have risk factors for abuse (e.g. prematurity, physical or learning disabilities).

A detailed social history should be obtained:

- Establish the family structure—which adults are at home? Are there any siblings and what are their names and ages? Does the child have a minder or attend nursery or playgroup?
- Which nursery/school does the child attend?
- Are they registered with a GP?
- Have the family had contact with social services before?
- Is there a history of domestic violence?
- Is there a history of illness in the parents/carers (e.g. postnatal depression, alcohol abuse)?

Examination of a child presenting with an injury or illness suspected of being caused by abuse should include the following:

- General appearance (e.g. underweight, dirty, unkempt, inappropriately dressed for weather, and so on).
- Social interaction (e.g. withdrawn, poor eye contact, or tearful).

- Child–parent interaction (e.g. remote and unconcerned or critical and hostile).
- Bruises (e.g. location—are they in unusual areas such as the medial aspect of upper arms or thighs?); patterns (e.g. hand marks, finger prints, and so on); ages (are they of varying ages?).
- Burn marks, lacerations, abrasions, or scars.
- Poor dentition.
- Retinal haemorrhages.

19.14.6 Emergency department management of a child with a concerning presentation

The immediate management should involve ensuring the child is pain-free and treating any injuries or illness appropriately.

Meticulous documentation is essential. Notes should be factual (e.g. 4 × 1cm round bruises found on the medial aspect of the left upper arm) and not attribute blame or causation (e.g. finger imprints found on medial aspect of left upper arm). Documenting injuries in a diagram is a useful way to capture information.

If sexual assault is suspected, a genital examination should not be pursued in the ED. This should be performed only once, by a senior clinician in child protection, in collaboration with a police surgeon (clinical forensic physician).

Further information should be gathered about the child. For example: checking whether the child or any siblings are known to social services or whether they are subject of a Child Protection Plan; looking up previous ED attendances; contacting the GP to gain a past medical history for the child and background information on the family (e.g. parental mental health or substance misuse issues).

Any suspicion of abuse should prompt early involvement of an expert senior doctor (e.g. ED consultant and/or paediatrician).

Once information has been gathered and the case has been discussed/reviewed with a senior clinician, the level of concern can be established (e.g. no concern; minor concern or unsure; more than a minor concern). The level of concern determines the ongoing management:

- No concern—a routine notification letter of the child's ED attendance should be sent to the GP. Plus, a letter of notification should be sent to the midwife if the child is <10 days old (faxed urgently); the Health Visiting Team, if the child is aged 10 days–5 years (pre-school children); or the school nurse for school children (within five days). This is the standard recommended by Lord Laming's report in 2009 (*The Protection of Children in England: A Progress Report*), the Government's report *Working together to safeguard children 2006*, and the College of Emergency Medicine Best Practice Statement for Safeguarding Children.
- Minor concern or unsure—should have a senior emergency medicine opinion and then be referred to the ED liaison health visitor the next working day.
- More than a minor concern—should be referred directly for a senior paediatric opinion and referred to social services (the local Trust's child protection policy should be followed for this).

19.14.7 Roles of other agencies in safeguarding children

The curriculum includes knowledge of the role of other agencies involved in safeguarding children. Key agencies involved in a child's life include:

- **Children's Social Care (CSC)**—commonly referred to as social services, take the lead in investigating and managing child protection cases. They will know whether or not a child and/or family have been previously involved with children's social care.
- **Police**—safeguarding children is a fundamental part of the duties of all police officers. All forces have child abuse investigation units who undertake criminal investigations in cases of suspected child abuse. The child abuse investigation team will have knowledge of any previous criminal involvement of child/parents/carers.

- **Education**—schools have a statutory responsibility, like healthcare organizations, to safeguard children and young people. School teachers will have a good knowledge of a child's day to day demeanour and developmental/academic strengths and weaknesses. The school nurse will be aware of issues relating to health and development as well as other issues, if any, affecting the parents or other children in the family.
- **Health**—all layers and elements of the health service have a statutory responsibility to safeguard children and young people. This includes health visitors, GPs, staff in secondary and tertiary healthcare (e.g. specialist hospitals, private hospitals, mental health services, genitourinary and family planning services, dentists, and professions allied to medicine).
- **CAFCASS**—The Family Justice System is a network of organizations including family courts, the Children and Family Court Advisory and Support Service (CAFCASS), the Child Support Agency, and lawyers. Safeguarding children's welfare is a key consideration for all professionals working in the Family Justice System. In all cases, the child's welfare is the court's paramount consideration and the role of the court is to make decisions which are in the best interest of children based on the evidence before it and the law.

KEY POINTS

Children may present to the ED with both the physical and psychological consequences of maltreatment.

Child abuse is described in four categories:

- Physical abuse
- Sexual abuse
- Neglect
- Emotional abuse

The immediate management of a child with a concerning presentation should involve ensuring the child is pain-free and treating any injuries or illness appropriately.

Assessment of a child in the ED should establish the level of concern: none; minor; more than a minor concern. The level of concern determines the ongoing management.

If there is more than a minor concern, the child should be referred for a senior paediatric opinion and on to social services for further investigation.

19.15 Dehydration secondary to diarrhoea and vomiting

19.15.1 Introduction

Between 70% and 80% of a child's body is made up of water. The water is distributed between the intracellular, interstitial, and intravascular spaces. The intravascular volume is approximately 80 ml/kg.

In health, fluid balance is tightly controlled by thirst, hormonal responses, and renal function. In critical in illness or injury, some or all of the mechanisms may be profoundly disrupted, and fluid therapy has to be tailored to the specific needs of the child.

Table 19.16 contains the APLS formula for normal maintenance fluid requirements in a child. The curriculum includes knowledge of this formula.

19.15.2 Dehydration and shock

Dehydration and shock are not the same condition, although they may coexist. Dehydration is a lack of water content in the body. Shock is an abnormality of the circulatory system resulting in

Table 19.16 Maintenance fluid requirements

Body weight	Fluid requirement per day (ml/kg)	Fluid requirement per hour (ml/kg)
First 10 kg	100	4
Second 10 kg	50	2
Subsequent kg	20	1

For example: The maintenance fluid requirement for a child weighing 26 kg is: 1000 + 500 + 120 = 1620 ml/day (67.5 ml/h).

inadequate tissue perfusion and oxygenation. Shock may be caused by hypovolaemia secondary to fluid losses.

Rapid loss of fluid from the intravascular space will cause shock unless the volume is replaced. Loss of 25% of the circulating volume (i.e. 20 ml/kg) will result in clinically apparent shock.

In dehydration, fluid losses are more gradual and are from all compartments (intracellular, interstitial, and intravascular). Clinical signs of dehydration are only clinically apparent when the patient is approaching 2.5–5% dehydrated; 5% dehydration implies that the body has lost 5 g/100 g body weight (i.e. 50 ml/kg).

Dehydration and shock therefore require different management strategies.

Shock

The clinical signs of shock from fluid loss include:

- Tachycardia
- Poor peripheral perfusion (cool peripheries, prolonged capillary refill time, poor pulse volume)
- Hypotension (late sign in children)
- Increased respiratory rate (respiratory compensation for developing metabolic acidosis)
- Altered mental status
- Poor urine output

The treatment of hypovolaemic shock involves an ABCDE approach and rapid intravenous administration of crystalloid. The recommended initial volume is 20 ml/kg, which may be repeated if there is an inadequate clinical response. Typically, Hartmann's or 0.9% sodium chloride is used as the initial resuscitation fluid.

Once shock is treated, attention can turn to the management of any dehydration.

Dehydration

The clinical signs of dehydration are individually unreliable and have poor interobserver reproducibility. However, taken together they provide a reasonable assessment of dehydration (see Table 19.17).

Weight loss provides the most reliable way of assessing fluid depletion but requires an accurate pre-illness weight (e.g. a child who weighs 20 kg when well, but weighs 18 kg in the ED, has lost 2 kg or 2000 ml of water, equating to 10% dehydration).

19.15.3 Management of dehydration

Firstly any hypovolaemic shock should be treated with boluses of 20 ml/kg crystalloid.

Once shock is treated the management of dehydration consists of three components:

- Daily maintenance
- Replacement fluids
- Consideration of ongoing fluid losses

Table 19.17 Clinical signs of dehydration in children

Signs/symptoms	Mild <5%	Moderate 5–10%	Severe >10%	Notes/caveats
Decreased urine output	Yes	Yes	Yes	Beware watery diarrhoea
Dry mouth	Maybe	Yes	Yes	Mouth breathers may be dry, while fluid ingestion may moisten the mouth
Decreased skin turgor	No	Maybe	Yes	Difficult to interpret in malnourished children
				Particularly unreliable in overweight children and in hypernatraemic dehydration
Sunken anterior fontanelle	No	Yes	Yes	Only useful if fontanelle patent, and in absence of disorders such as meningitis
Sunken eyes	No	Yes	Yes	Very difficult to assess, although mothers may give accurate assessment

A typical starting fluid for intravenous rehydration is 0.45% sodium chloride, which is roughly equal to the electrolyte content of stool in diarrhoea.

Daily maintenance fluids

Maintenance fluids are calculated using the formula in Table 19.10.

Replacement fluids

Replacement fluids are calculated by estimating the percentage dehydration or the known weight loss. They are replaced over a 24-hour period, unless there are electrolyte problems, in which case replacement may occur over 48 hours.

Ongoing fluid losses

Insensible fluid losses, via respiration and sweat, are approximately 10–30 ml/kg/day. The actual insensible fluid loss is related to the caloric content of feeds, the ambient temperature, humidity of inspired air, presence of pyrexia, and the quality of the skin.

Losses from stool are usually between 0 and 10 ml/kg/day, but this will be markedly increased in diarrhoea, where losses in excess of 300 ml/kg/day are possible.

Urinary losses are approximately 1–2 ml/kg/hour, but will be less initially in a child dehydrated due to gastroenteritis, but are often more in a child with diabetic ketoacidosis.

The requirement for fluid to replace ongoing losses is often judged by the response of the child to maintenance and replacement fluids (see Monitoring fluid replacement, next).

Monitoring fluid replacement

Calculations for maintenance and fluid replacement therapy are an initial estimate and careful monitoring is required.

Fluid therapy should be monitored at three to four-hour intervals using weight as an objective measure to ensure the child is gaining weight at an appropriate rate (aim to achieve a normal body weight over 24 hours). If the child is gaining weight too slowly or quickly, the administration rate should be adjusted accordingly.

Electrolytes should be monitored frequently so that the type of rehydration fluid can be adjusted accordingly.

Electrolytes

Electrolyte abnormalities may accompany dehydration. The nature of the electrolyte abnormality depends on the cause of the dehydration.

Hypernatraemia may be the result of excessive water loss (e.g. diarrhoea, diabetes insipidus), excessive sodium intake (e.g. iatrogenic poisoning, child abuse), or a combination of both (e.g. gastroenteritis and excessive sodium in rehydration fluid). If hypernatraemia is present, rehydration should occur over 48 hours rather than 24 hours, to avoid a precipitous drop in sodium levels potentially triggering cerebral oedema.

Hyponatraemia may be due to excessive water intake or retention, excess sodium losses, or a combination of both. If hyponatraemia is due to excessive water intake or retention, and the patient is not symptomatic, the restriction of fluid intake to 50% of normal estimated requirements may be adequate treatment. If the patient is very unwell (e.g. fitting) from hyponatraemia, correction with hypertonic saline may be required.

Hyperkalaemia is potentially fatal and treatment in children is the same as in adults (Chapter 12, section 12.4) with adjustments for the doses of medications (it should not be necessary to memorize the paediatric doses for the exam).

Hypokalaemia is rarely an emergency and usually results from excessive loss of potassium in acute diarrhoeal illnesses. Replacement can be oral, if tolerated, or intravenously (not at concentrations >40 mmol/L peripherally).

KEY POINTS

Dehydration is a lack of water content in the body.

Shock is an abnormality of the circulatory system resulting in inadequate tissue perfusion and oxygenation. Shock may be caused by hypovolaemia secondary to fluid losses.

Dehydration does not cause death, shock does.

Shock may result from the rapid loss of 20 ml/kg from the intravascular space.

Dehydration is only clinically evident after losses of >25 ml/kg of total body water.

Hypovolaemic shock should be treated with 20 ml/kg boluses of crystalloid with an electrolyte content that approximates plasma (e.g. Hartmann's or 0.9% sodium chloride).

Dehydration should be treated with gradual replacement of fluids, with electrolyte content that relates to the electrolyte losses, or the total body electrolyte content.

Rehydration fluid requirements are calculated based on daily fluid requirements and replacement requirements.

0.45% sodium chloride is an appropriate initial rehydration fluid.

Frequent monitoring of the child's weight and electrolytes should guide adjustments in the fluid rate and fluid type.

19.16 Ear, nose, and throat

Ear, nose, and throat (ENT) conditions are covered in Chapter 7.

19.17 Fever in children

19.17.1 Introduction

Feverish illness in children is very common, with between 20–40% of parents reporting such an illness each year. Fever is a common presenting complaint for children in the ED and a common reason for admission to hospital. Despite advances in healthcare, infections remain the leading cause of death in children under the age of five years.

Fever in young children can be a diagnostic challenge because it is often difficult to identify the cause. In most cases, the illness is due to a self-limiting viral infection. However, fever may also be the presenting feature of serious bacterial infections, such as meningitis or pneumonia. A significant number of children have no obvious cause of fever despite careful assessment. These children with fever without apparent source are of particular concern because it is especially difficult to distinguish between simple viral illnesses and life-threatening bacterial infections in this group.

NICE have produced guidance on the management of feverish illness in children and the management of urinary tract infections. Knowledge of this guidance is included in the curriculum and summarized in the following section 19.17.2.

Meningitis is covered in Chapter 15, section 15.4.

19.17.2 Feverish illness in children

Fever is a temporary elevation in the body's temperature. Fever is most commonly due to infection but it may be due to many other causes (see Chapter 15, section 15.2). This section focuses on fever due to an infective illness.

In 2007, NICE produced clinical guidelines on the management of feverish illness in children aged less than 5 years. This was the first guidance on the management of fever as a presenting illness, rather than a specific infection (e.g. pneumonia, urinary tract infection (UTI)). This makes the guidance very applicable to the ED, where patients rarely have a specific diagnosis on presentation but a constellation of symptoms. Once a diagnosis of the underlying condition is made, then the guidance specific to that condition (e.g. UTI) should be followed.

NICE guidance on managing fevers in the under fives was updated in 2013—the key areas of guidance are:

- Accurate detection of fever
- Clinical assessment to include identification of risks for serious illness (i.e. traffic light system)
- Management by non-paediatric specialist
- Management by paediatric specialist
- Use of antipyretics*

Detection of fever

Body temperature in children can be measured at a number of anatomical sites using a range of different types of thermometers. Sites used to measure temperature include the mouth, rectum, and axilla. The types of thermometers available include mercury-in-glass, electronic, chemical, and infrared.

The recommended sites and thermometers for measuring temperature in children are:

- Infants <4 weeks old: electronic thermometer in the axilla.
- Children aged four weeks to five years: electronic thermometer in the axilla; infrared tympanic thermometer; or chemical dot in the axilla.

The parental perception of fever should be taken seriously even if the child is apyrexial on assessment in the ED.

Clinical assessment of the child with fever

The initial assessment of a feverish child is very important. The majority of children presenting with fever will have either a self-limiting viral condition or an obvious cause for their fever for which specific treatment can be given. A minority will present with fever with no obvious underlying cause, and a small number of these will have a serious illness.

* Reproduced with permission from ROBERT B. SALTER, W. ROBERT HARRIS, Injuries Involving the Epiphyseal Plate, *Journal of Bone & Joint Surgery*, Volume 45, Issue 3, pp. 587–622, Copyright © 1963, Wolters Kluwer Health, Inc.

The aims of the ED assessment are to identify children with a potentially serious illness and manage them appropriately, while avoiding unnecessary medical intervention in children with minor self-limiting illness.

Initially the child should be assessed in an ABCDE manner for the presence of any life-threatening features. If life-threatening features are present, the child should be resuscitated as necessary. If no life-threatening features are present, NICE recommends the use of a 'traffic light system' to identify the absence of signs and symptoms that predict the risk of serious illness. Table 19.18 details the

Table 19.18 Traffic light system for identifying likelihood of serious illness

	Green—Low risk	Amber—Intermediate risk	Red—High risk
Colour	Normal colour of skin, lips, and tongue	Pallor reported by parent/carer	Pale/mottled/ashen/blue
Activity	Responds normally to social cues	Not responding normally to social cues	No response to social cues
	Content and smiles	Wakes only with prolonged stimulation	Appears ill to healthcare professional
	Stays awake or awakens quickly	Decreased activity	Unable to rouse or if roused does not stay awake
	Strong normal cry/not crying	No smile	Weak, high-pitched cry, or continuous cry
Respiratory		Nasal flaring	Grunting
		Tachypnoea:	Tachypnoea:
		Age 6–12 months: RR >50 breaths/minute	RR >60 breaths/minute
		Age >12 months: RR >40 breaths/minute	Moderate or severe chest recessions
		Oxygen saturations ≤95% in air	
		Crackles	
Hydration	Normal skin and eyes	Tachycardia:	Reduced skin turgor
	Moist mucous membranes	• >160 bpm <12 months • >150 bpm 12–24 months • >140 2–5 years	
		Dry mucous membranes Poor feeding in infants Capillary refill time >3s Reduced urine output	
Other	None of the amber or red symptoms or signs	Fever ≥5 days	Age 0–3 months and temperature ≥38°C
		Aged 3–6 months with temperature ≥39°C	Non-blanching rash
		Rigors	Bulging fontanelle
		Swelling of a limb/joint	Neck stiffness
		Non-weight-bearing/not using an extremity	Status epilepticus
			Focal neurological signs
			Focal seizures

Data from NICE clinical guideline 160, Fever in under 5s: initial assessment and management(May 2013) www.nice.org.uk/CG160.

traffic light system. When assessing a feverish child with a learning disability, their disability should be taken into account when interpreting the traffic light system.

As part of the assessment of a child with fever, the temperature, heart rate, respiratory rate, and capillary refill time should be recorded.

Children with fever and any of the symptoms or signs in the 'red' column are considered at high risk. Children with fever and any of the symptoms or signs in the 'amber' column and none in the 'red' column are intermediate risk. Children with symptoms and signs in the 'green' column and none in the 'amber' or 'red' columns are at low risk.

While the child is being assessed for symptoms and signs of serious illness, features that suggest a particular cause should be noted (see Table 19.19).

Management of the feverish child

The NICE guidance includes recommendations for management by non-paediatric practitioners and paediatric specialists. Therefore elements of both sections are relevant to management in the ED and could appear in the exam. The following text summarizes the main points from both these sections of the guidance.

EXAM TIP

NICE guidance uses the term 'management' to include investigations and treatments. The College glossary makes the distinction between investigations, management, and treatment.

- Investigations—specific tests undertaken to make a diagnosis or monitor the patient's condition. They may include bedside tests such as urine dipstick or blood glucose unless otherwise specified.
- Management—aspects of care including treatment, supportive care, and disposition. This does not include investigations.
- Treatment—measures undertaken to cure or stabilize the patient's condition. This includes oxygen, fluids, drugs, and may also mean surgery. It does not include investigations.

This section of the book is written to be consistent with the NICE guidance, but when answering SAQs ensure you check whether the question is referring to investigations, management, or treatment.

Green features
Children with green features and none of the 'amber' or 'red' features can be managed at home.
Oral antibiotics should not be prescribed to children without an apparent source.
If a source has not been found, urine testing should be performed.
Parents should be given verbal and written advice on how to manage the child's fever and when to seek further medical attention. Box 19.4 includes an example of discharge advice to give to the parents.

Amber features
If amber features are present and a diagnosis has been made (e.g. UTI, pneumonia), then guidance for that specific condition should be followed.

If amber features are present and no diagnosis is reached, then NICE propose two possible management plans: discharging with a safety net (e.g. written advice and/or follow-up with GP and/or direct access to out-of-hours services if further assessment is required); or admission for further investigation. The option pursued depends on the clinical assessment of the child, the social and family circumstances, and the parental concerns/anxieties.

Table 19.19 Symptoms and signs suggestive of particular causes of fever

Diagnosis to be considered	Symptoms and signs in conjunction with fever
Meningococcal disease (see Chapter 15, section 15.4)	Non-blanching rash, particularly with one or more of the following: • an ill-looking child • lesions larger than 2 mm in diameter (purpura) • a capillary refill time of ≥3 s • neck stiffness
Meningitis (see Chapter 15, section 15.4)	Neck stiffness Bulging fontanelle Decreased level of consciousness Convulsive status epilepticus
Herpes simplex encephalitis (see Chapter 15, section 15.3)	Focal neurological signs Focal seizures Decreased level of consciousness
Pneumonia (see section 19.13)	Tachypnoea (RR >60 breaths per minute age 0–5 months; RR >50 breaths per minute age 6–12 months; RR >40 breaths per minute age >12 months) Crackles Nasal flaring Chest recession Cyanosis Oxygen saturation ≤95%
Urinary tract infection (see also Table 19.20)	Vomiting Poor feeding Lethargy Irritability Abdominal pain or tenderness Urinary frequency or dysuria
Septic arthritis (see section 19.24)	Swelling of a limb or joint Not using an extremity Non-weight-bearing
Kawasaki disease (see Chapter 16, section 16.3)	Fever for more than five days and at least four of the following: • bilateral conjunctival injection • change in mucous membranes • change in the extremities • polymorphous rash • cervical lymphadenopathy

If further investigation is deemed appropriate this should include:

- Urinary testing as recommended by NICE guidance on UTIs (see section 19.17.3).
- Full blood count.
- Blood cultures.
- CRP.
- CXR if fever ≥39°C and white cell count >20 × 10^9/L.
- A lumbar puncture should be considered if the child is younger than 1-year-old.

Box 19.4 Discharge advice for parents/carers of the feverish child

Parents or carers looking after a feverish child at home should be advised:

- To offer the child regular fluids (where a baby is breastfed, the most appropriate fluid is breast milk).
- How to detect signs of dehydration by looking for the following features:
  - sunken fontanelle
  - dry mouth
  - sunken eyes
  - absence of tears
  - poor overall appearance.
- To encourage their child to drink more fluids and consider seeking further advice if they detect signs of dehydration.
- How to identify a non-blanching rash.
- To check their child during the night.
- To keep their child away from nursery or school while the child's fever persists and to notify the school or nursery of the illness.

Data from National Institute for Health and Care Excellence. *Fever in under 5s: initial assessment and management.* Clinical Guideline CG160. London: NICE; 2013, Royal College of Obstetricians and Gynaecologists.

Treatment of the child will depend upon the outcome of the investigations and ongoing clinical picture. A period of observation in hospital, for children with fever and no apparent source, may help to distinguish serious from non-serious illness.

Red features

If red features are present it is important to ensure that there are no life-threatening findings requiring immediate resuscitation (e.g. shock requiring fluid resuscitation 20 ml/kg).

Further investigation of a child with red features depends on their age:

- Age <3 months: full blood count, CRP, blood culture, urine testing, CXR (if respiratory signs), stool culture (if diarrhoea), lumbar puncture.
- Age >3 months: full blood count, CRP, urine test. Consider CXR, lumbar puncture, serum electrolytes, and blood gas.

For children with suspected bacterial infection, empirical antibiotics are recommended in the following circumstances:

- Shock
- Unrousable
- Signs of meningococcal disease
- Decreased level of consciousness
- Age <1 month
- Age 1–3 months with a white cell count <5 or >15 × 10^9/L
- Age 1–3 months who appears unwell

A third-generation cephalosporin (e.g. ceftriaxone or cefotaxime) is an appropriate initial empirical treatment. If the child is <3 months old, ampicillin or amoxicillin should be added to cover for *Listeria*.

Antipyretics

Fever is a normal physiological response to infection. Routine use of antipyretics in a child with a fever is not recommended if the sole aim is to reduce body temperature. Similarly antipyretics should not be used purely to try and prevent febrile convulsions.

Antipyretics are recommended if the child appears distressed or unwell with their fever. Either paracetamol or ibuprofen can be used to reduce the temperature in a child with fever. It is not recommended to give them at the same time but the alternative agent may be given if the child does not respond to the first drug.

Physical methods to reduce fever (e.g. tepid sponging, undressing, and fanning) take advantage of heat loss through convection and evaporation but do not treat the underlying cause of the fever; either the disease or the alteration in the hypothalamic set-point. There is little evidence to suggest these techniques are effective and therefore they are not recommended.

19.17.3 Urinary tract infections in children

Urinary tract infection is a common bacterial infection causing illness in infants and children. It may be difficult to recognize UTI in children because the presenting symptoms and signs are non-specific, particularly in infants and children under three years.

The section, 'Clinical features of urinary tract infection' is based on the NICE guidance on UTI in children.

The NICE guidance classifies UTI in children as upper, lower, atypical, and recurrent.

Clinical features of urinary tract infection

The clinical features of a child with UTI may be very non-specific and vary according to the age of the child (Table 19.20).

During the assessment of a child with a possible UTI, any risk factors for UTI and serious underlying pathology should be noted.

Risk factors for UTI/serious underlying pathology include:

- Poor urine flow
- History suggestive of previous UTI or confirmed UTI

Table **19.20** Clinical features of urinary tract infection (UTI) in infants and children

Age		Clinical features (listed in descending order of frequency)
<3 months old		Fever, vomiting, lethargy, irritability (most common)
		Poor feeding, failure to thrive
		Abdominal pain, jaundice, haematuria, offensive urine (least common)
>3 months	Pre-verbal	Fever
		Abdominal pain, loin tenderness, vomiting, poor feeding
		Lethargy, irritability, haematuria, offensive urine, failure to thrive
	Verbal	Frequency, dysuria
		Dysfunctional voiding, changes to continence, abdominal pain, loin tenderness
		Fever, malaise, vomiting, haematuria, offensive urine, cloudy urine

Adapted from NICE clinical guideline 54. Urinary tract infections in children (August 2007). www.nice.org.uk/CG54

- Recurrent pyrexia of unknown origin
- Antenatal diagnosis of renal abnormality
- Family history of vesicoureteric reflux or renal disease
- Constipation
- Dysfunctional voiding
- High blood pressure
- Enlarged bladder
- Abdominal mass
- Evidence of spinal lesion
- Poor growth

ED investigation of UTI

Urine testing should be performed in infants and children in the following circumstances:

- Those with clinical features suggestive of UTI
- Those with an unexplained fever ≥38°C
- Those with an alternative site of infection but who remain unwell

A clean catch is the recommended method for urine collection. If a clean catch is not available, then a urinary pad may be used. If non-invasive methods of urine collection are not possible, then a catheter sample or suprapubic aspiration, under ultrasound guidance, should be used.

Urine can be tested by dipstick, microscopy, and/or culture. Dipstick testing alone is unreliable in children under three years of age and therefore not recommended as the only test in such patients. In children older than three years, dipstick testing for leucocytes and nitrites is as diagnostically useful as microscopy and culture, and can safely be used. The urine testing strategies recommended by NICE for different age groups are detailed in Table 19.21.

Other investigations should be guided by the child's clinical picture as per the 'Feverish illness in children' guidance.

Emergency department management of urinary tract infection

Acute management of a child with a suspected or confirmed UTI depends on the clinical severity of the illness and the age of the child (see Table 19.22).

Infants and children older than three months with upper UTI should be treated with antibiotics for 7–10 days. Oral cephalosporin or co-amoxiclav are suitable choices. If oral antibiotics are not possible (e.g. due to vomiting) intravenous antibiotics should be used (e.g. cefotaxime or ceftriaxone).

Infants and children older than three months with a lower UTI should be treated with oral antibiotics for three days. The choice of antibiotics should be directed by local antibiotic policy. Possible options include trimethoprim, nitrofurantoin, cephalosporin, or amoxicillin.

Table 19.21 Urine testing strategies in children

Age	Urine testing strategy
<3 months	Send urine for urgent microscopy and culture
3 months to 3 years	Send urine for urgent microscopy and culture
>3 years	Dipstick testing for leucocytes and nitrites should be performed; if positive for UTI (see Table 19.24), a urine sample for microscopy and culture should be sent

Table **19.22** Management of infants and children with UTI

Age		Management
<3 months old		Refer to the paediatricians,
		Manage in accordance with the NICE 'Feverish illness in children' guidance for this age group and start parenteral antibiotics once urine for microscopy and culture has been sent.
3 months to 3 years	Clinical features suggesting UTI	Empirical antibiotic therapy should be started once urinary microscopy and culture has been sent.
	Clinical features non-specific to UTI	Children should be risk assessed using the NICE 'Feverish illness in children' guidance:
		• Red (high-risk) features—refer to the paediatricians; ensure a urine microscopy and culture sample has been sent; manage as per the NICE 'Feverish illness in children' guidance.
		• Amber (intermediate risk) features—consider referral to the paediatricians. Start antibiotics if the urinary microscopy is positive. If urgent microscopy is not available perform a dipstick, pending the microscopy results. If the dipstick is positive for nitrites start antibiotics.
		• Green (low risk)—Only start antibiotics if the microscopy or culture is positive.

Further management for UTIs

The curriculum includes knowledge of the further types of investigation that may be performed in an infant or child with UTI. The aim of imaging is to identify those children with an underlying abnormality or factor that puts them at increased risk of recurrent UTI or renal damage.

Infants and children who are asymptomatic following an episode of UTI do not routinely need their urine retesting for infection.

Further imaging in children with UTI depends on their age and type of UTI (atypical or recurrent). Children aged older than six months who respond well to antibiotic treatment within 48 hours need no further imaging.

The main options for further imaging include ultrasound, dimercaptosuccinic acid (DMSA) scintigraphy, or micturating cystourethrogram (MCUG).

- Ultrasound—evaluates the structure of the urinary tract. It can assess renal size, the presence of any obstruction of the ureter or collecting system (e.g. secondary to a calculus or congenital abnormality), and the bladder. It is a widely available technique which is non-invasive and poses no radiation risk, making it ideal for children. Ultrasound is recommended in all infants aged less than six months with UTI and children older than six months who have atypical or recurrent UTIs. Depending on the clinical picture the ultrasound may be performed during the acute illness or within six weeks.
- MCUG is considered the 'gold standard' for the detection of vesicoureteric reflux. It is only recommended in infants less than six months old with recurrent or atypical UTI.
- DMSA scintigraphy—is used to evaluate renal scarring. It is performed several months (four to six months) after UTI to allow for any parenchymal changes from acute infection to resolve. It is recommended in all infants and children with recurrent UTI, as well as those aged less than three years old with atypical UTI.

Antibiotic prophylaxis is not routinely recommended in infants and children following their first UTI. Antibiotic prophylaxis may be considered in infants and children with recurrent UTI.

KEY POINTS

NICE have produced guidance on the management of feverish illness in children. Central to this guidance is the 'traffic light system', which can be used to risk assess children and guide their further management.

The aims of the risk assessment are to identify children with a potentially serious illness and manage them appropriately, while avoiding unnecessary medical intervention in children with minor self-limiting illness.

Routine use of antipyretics in a child with a fever is not recommended if the sole aim is to reduce body temperature or try to prevent febrile convulsions.

UTI is a common bacterial infection causing illness in infants and children.

Acceptable methods of urine collection in a child include clean catch (preferred method), urinary pads, suprapubic aspiration, and catheter sample.

Urinary dipstick can be used to test urine in children older than three years.

A positive urinary dipstick result is: positive for nitrites and leucocytes; or positive for nitrites only; or positive for leucocytes with good clinical evidence of UTI.

Lower UTIs should be treated with a three-day course of oral antibiotics.

Upper UTIs require 7–10 days of antibiotics, which may need to be given intravenously initially if the child is vomiting.

Children older than six months, with their first UTI, who respond well to antibiotics within 48 hours, require no further imaging.

19.18 Floppy child

The differential diagnosis of an acutely floppy child presenting to the ED is extensive.
   The differential includes:

- Hypoxic ischaemic brain injury—due to respiratory or circulatory failure (e.g. asthma, anaphylaxis, duct-dependent heart disease)
- Epileptic seizures (see Chapter 11, section 11.6)
- Traumatic brain injury including intracranial haemorrhage and cerebral oedema (see Chapter 4, section 4.5, and section 19.5)
- Intracranial infections (e.g. meningitis, encephalitis, malaria—see Chapter 15, sections 15.3 and 15.4)
- Poisoning—either accidental or deliberate (see Chapter 17)
- Metabolic (e.g. hypoglycaemia, hypothermia, hypercapnea, renal failure, liver failure, and so on)
- Sepsis (see Chapter 15, section 15.1)

These conditions are detailed in other sections of the book as indicated here. The generic ABCDE principles apply.

19.19 Gastrointestinal bleeding

19.19.1 Introduction

Gastrointestinal bleeding in infants and children may have multiple different causes, the frequency of which varies according to the age of the child (see Table 19.23). Usually bleeding is of limited

Table 19.23 Causes of GI bleeding according to age

Age group	Upper GI bleeding	Lower GI bleeding
Neonates (age <1 month)	Haemorrhagic disease of the newborn (self-limiting bleeding disorder resulting from a deficiency in vitamin K-dependent clotting factors) Swallowed maternal blood (e.g. due to fissure on the mother's breast) Stress gastritis Coagulopathy	Anal fissure Necrotizing enterocolitis Malrotation with volvulus
1 month to 1 year	Oesophagitis Gastritis	Anal fissure Intussusception Gangrenous bowel Milk protein allergy
1–2 years	Peptic ulcer disease Gastritis	Polyps Meckel's diverticulum
Children older than 2 years	Oesophageal varices Gastric varices Mallory–Weiss tears Swallowed blood (e.g. following epistaxis)	Polyps Inflammatory bowel disease Infectious diarrhoea Vascular lesions

volume allowing time for referral to paediatrics, further investigation, and diagnosis. Very occasionally, a child presents with a large gastrointestinal (GI) bleed and they should be resuscitated in an ABCDE manner.

19.19.2 Causes of gastrointestinal bleeding

Upper GI bleeding

- Gastritis/oesophagitis—can occur in children of all ages. Gastro-oesophageal reflux is a common cause of this, as is infection with *Helicobacter pylori*. Children who are critically ill (e.g. with sepsis) commonly develop stress gastritis. Medications, both *in utero* and once born, may predispose a child to gastritis or peptic ulcers (e.g. dexamethasone to help fetal lung maturation, indometacin to maintain a patent ductus arteriosis, NSAIDs, and so on).
- Peptic ulcer disease—is the commonest cause of upper GI bleeding in children older than one year. The causes of peptic ulcer disease are similar to those for gastritis. If an ulcer is not associated with *Helicobacter pylori* infection, then a fasting plasma gastrin level should be measured to exclude Zollinger–Ellison syndrome. Zollinger–Ellison syndrome is a rare condition characterized by gastrin-producing tumours or gastrinomas, which cause excessive gastric acid secretion, leading to peptic ulcers.
- Varices—may result from portal hypertension, regardless of age. The increased resistance to portal blood flow may be due to pre-hepatic (e.g. portal vein thrombosis), intrahepatic (e.g. biliary atresia), or suprahepatic (e.g. hepatic vein thrombosis, Budd–Chiari syndrome) obstruction.
- Mallory–Weiss tear—is more commonly seen in older children following repeated, forceful vomiting.

Lower GI bleeding

- Anal fissures—are due to a tear at the mucocutaneous line and the most common cause of GI bleeding in infants. They are often associated with constipation. They cause bright red blood that streaks the stool or causes spots of blood in the nappy.
- Necrotizing enterocolitis—is rare and primarily seen in premature infants where portions of the bowel undergo necrosis. No definite cause has been found but an infectious agent is suspected, possibly *Pseudomonas aeruginosa*.
- Volvulus—is discussed in section 19.8. Intestinal malrotations lead to areas of gangrenous bowel. It should be suspected if the child suddenly develops melena, distension, and bilious vomit.
- Intussusception—is discussed in section 19.8. It is the most likely cause of lower GI bleeding in children aged 6–18 months. Colicky abdominal pain, vomiting, and 'redcurrant jelly' stools is the classic presentation.
- Milk protein allergy—causes a colitis that may be associated with occult or gross lower GI bleeding. It is the most common allergy observed in infancy and is caused by an adverse immune reaction to cow's milk. Presentation is typically soon after the introduction of cow's milk.
- Juvenile polyps—may be found throughout the colon in young children and are usually benign hamartomas requiring no treatment because they autoamputate. They cause painless lower GI bleeding.
- Meckel's diverticulum—occurs in 2% of the population. The cause of GI bleeding in Meckel's diverticulum is ileal ulceration caused by acid secretion from the ectopic gastric mucosa. Erosion into small arterioles leads to painless, brisk rectal bleeding.
- Inflammatory bowel disease—may present in childhood. Bleeding is less common in Crohn's disease than in ulcerative colitis.
- Infective diarrhoea—should be suspected when lower GI bleeding is associated with profuse diarrhoea. The two commonest pathogens in infective diarrhoea are *Shigella* and *E. coli*. If the patient has had recent broad-spectrum antibiotics, then *Clostridium difficile* should be suspected.
- Vascular lesions—include a wide variety of malformations, including haemangiomas, arteriovenous malformation, and vasculitis.

In all children with GI bleeding, the possibility of non-accidental injury should be considered.

19.19.3 Emergency department management

The management required in the ED depends on the severity of illness and the suspected underlying cause. If the child has profuse GI bleeding and is shocked, they should be resuscitated as for any shocked child in an ABCDE manner.

If the child is stable and not acutely bleeding, then referral to the paediatricians for further investigation is appropriate.

KEY POINTS

The commonest cause of upper GI bleeding in infants and children is gastritis and peptic ulcer disease. Others causes include varices, Mallory–Weiss tears, coagulopathies, and swallowed blood.

Cause of lower GI bleeding in infants and children include anal fissures, volvulus, intussusception, milk protein allergy, juvenile polyps, Meckel's diverticulum, infective diarrhoea, vascular lesions, and necrotizing enterocolitis.

19.20 Headache

19.20.1 Introduction

Headache is a common problem in children. It is estimated that up to 50% of seven-year-olds and 80% of 15-year-olds have experienced at least one headache.

Headache in adults is covered in Chapter 11, section 11.2. It is worth reading section 11.2 in conjunction with this section because there is significant overlap between headaches in children and adults.

19.20.2 Classification and clinical features of headache in children

Headache in children can be a primary disorder or secondary to a number of other conditions. Primary headache disorders include migraine and tension-type headaches.

- Migraine without aura is the most common recurrent primary headache disorder in children. Migraines are usually pulsating in quality, moderate to severe intensity, and aggravated by routine physical activity. Associated symptoms include nausea, vomiting, photophobia, and phonophobia. Compared to adults, children's migraines are of shorter duration and are more often bilateral. As a result, they can go unrecognized and therefore undertreated.
- Tension-type headaches differ from migraine in that they are characteristically pressing or tightening in nature, mild to moderate in severity, more frequently bilateral, and do not have associated nausea, vomiting, photophobia, or phonophobia. Tension-type headaches may be exacerbated or precipitated by emotional and psychological factors such as stress, anxiety, and depression.

Secondary headaches are caused by an underlying intracranial abnormality (e.g. CNS infection, intracranial haemorrhage, raised intracranial pressure, or space-occupying lesion).

Secondary headache should be considered in children presenting with new onset headache or headache that differs from their usual pattern. If the child has any of the following 'red flags', it suggests a potential secondary headache and the need for further investigation:

- Focal neurological symptoms or signs
- Reduced level of consciousness
- Acute confusion or irritability
- Seizures
- Papilloedema
- Headache that changes with posture
- Headache that wakes the child up
- Headache precipitated by physical exertion or valsalva manoeuvre (e.g. coughing, laughing, straining)
- Constitutional symptoms suggestive of underlying systemic pathology (e.g. fever, rash, tachycardia, hypotension, and so on)
- Neck stiffness
- Evidence of head trauma
- Evidence of unexplained injuries

19.20.3 Emergency department investigations for headache

A child that presents acutely with a severe headache and red flags requires neuroimaging (usually CT) and possibly a lumbar puncture.

Other investigations should be directed by the clinical picture (e.g. full septic screen, FBC, lactate, and so on). Children with a probable primary headache do not tend to require investigation in the ED and can be referred to their general practitioner or a paediatrician for further investigation and management.

19.20.4 Emergency department management of headache

The management of a child with a secondary headache depends on the underlying cause.

The management of children with intracranial infections if covered in Chapter 15, section 15.3.

KEY POINTS

Headache is a common problem in children and can be classified as primary (e.g. migraine, tension headache) or secondary (e.g. meningitis, space-occupying lesion, and so on).
Red flags for secondary headache include:

- Focal neurological symptoms or signs
- Reduced level of consciousness, acute confusion, or irritability
- Seizures
- Papilloedema
- Headache that changes with posture
- Headache that wakes the child up
- Headache precipitated by physical exertion or valsalva manoeuvre
- Constitutional symptoms suggestive of underlying systemic pathology (e.g. fever, rash, tachycardia, hypotension, and so on)
- Neck stiffness
- Evidence of head trauma
- Evidence of unexplained injuries

The management of children with intracranial haemorrhage and/or raised intracranial pressure follows the same principles as in adults (Chapter 4, section 4.5).

19.21 Neonatal presentations

The curriculum includes knowledge of the pathophysiology and resuscitation of the newborn.

Passage through the birth canal is a hypoxic experience for the foetus, since significant respiratory exchange at the placenta is prevented during contractions (typically 50–75 seconds duration). Though most babies tolerate this well, the few that do not may require help to establish normal breathing at delivery.

Newborn life-support is detailed in section 19.4, the main principles of which are:

- Dry and cover the newborn baby to conserve heat.
- Assess the need for any intervention (assess tone, breathing, and heart rate).
- Open the airway.
- Aerate the lungs.
- Perform rescue breathing if required.
- Perform chest compressions if required.
- Administer drugs (rarely required).

19.21.1 Pathophysiology of newborn cardiopulmonary instability

If a foetus is subjected to sufficient hypoxia *in utero*, it will attempt to breathe. If the hypoxic insult is not relieved, the foetus will eventually lose consciousness. Shortly after this, the neural centres controlling respiration cease to function, because of lack of oxygen, and the foetus enters a period known as primary apnoea.

Up to the point of primary apnoea, the foetus maintains a normal heart rate. Once primary apnoea develops, the heart rate drops to about half the normal rate as the myocardium reverts to anaerobic metabolism. The circulation to non-vital organs is reduced in an attempt to preserve perfusion of vital organs. Lactic acid levels increase due to anaerobic metabolism.

If the insult continues, shuddering (whole-body gasps at a rate of about 12 per minute) is initiated by primitive spinal centres. If the foetus is still *in utero*, or if these gasps fail to aerate the lungs, the shudders fade away and the foetus enters a period known as secondary, or terminal, apnoea. Up to this point, the circulation is maintained but, as terminal apnoea progresses, the increasingly acidotic environment results in impaired cardiac function. The heart eventually fails and, without effective intervention, the baby dies. The whole process takes approximately 20 minutes in the term newborn human baby.

In the face of asphyxia, a baby can maintain an effective circulation throughout the period of primary apnoea, through the gasping phase, and even for a while after the onset of terminal apnoea. Therefore the most important intervention in any asphyxiated baby at birth is effective aeration of the lungs. Provided the baby's circulation is sufficient, oxygenated blood will then be conveyed from the aerated lungs to the heart. The heart rate will increase and the brain will be perfused with oxygenated blood. Following this, the neural centres responsible for breathing will usually start functioning and the baby will start to spontaneously ventilate.

The pathophysiology of cardiopulmonary instability in newborns explains the focus on effective ventilations and the 3:1 ratio in the newborn life-support algorithm. In the vast majority of cases, aerating the lungs is sufficient to resuscitate the newborn. In a few cases, cardiac function will have deteriorated to such an extent during apnoea that the circulation is inadequate and cannot convey oxygenated blood from the aerated lungs to the heart. In this case, a brief period of chest compression may be needed. In a very few cases, lung aeration and chest compression will not be sufficient, and drugs may be required to restore the circulation. The outlook in this group of infants is poor.

KEY POINTS

The main principles of newborn life support are:
- Dry and cover the newborn baby to conserve heat.
- Assess the need for any intervention (assess tone, breathing, and heart rate).
- Open the airway.
- Aerate the lungs.
- Perform rescue breathing if required.
- Perform chest compressions if required.
- Administer drugs (rarely required).

19.22 Ophthalmology

Ophthalmologic conditions that may affect children are covered in Chapter 7.

19.23 Pain in children

Pain management in adults and children is covered in Chapter 3, section 3.6.

19.24 Painful limbs in children—atraumatic

19.24.1 The limping child

Previous MRCEM question

The limping child is a common presentation to the ED and can present a diagnostic challenge. There is an extensive differential diagnosis, some of which require urgent treatment. The differential diagnosis varies according to age and this should be considered when answering a question on the limping child (Table 19.24).

19.24.2 Clinical assessment of the limping child

A thorough history and examination should be performed to help narrow down the differential diagnosis. The possibility of septic arthritis and/or osteomyelitis should always be considered in a child with an atraumatic limp.

Important features in the history include:

- Period of onset (sudden, e.g. due to trauma, or gradual)
- Site of pain

Table 19.24 Causes of a limp in children

All ages	Toddlers (age 1–3)	Age 4–10	Adolescents (age 11–16)
Septic arthritis	Developmental dysplasia of the hip	Transient synovitis (most common age 3–5)	Slipped upper femoral epiphysis
Osteomyelitis	Toddlers fractures (non-displaced spiral fracture of lower 1/3 of tibia)	Perthes' disease	Osteochondritis
Trauma (fractures, soft tissue injuries, foreign bodies)		Leukaemia	Gonococcal septic arthritis (Chapter 5, section 5.11)
Neoplasm (the distal femoral epiphyseal plate is the fastest growing area of bone and at high risk of neoplasm)	Transient synovitis (most common age 3–5)		Physeal injuries
			Ewing's sarcoma
Sickle cell crisis			
Neuromuscular (e.g. cerebral palsy, Duchene muscular dystrophy)			
Juvenile arthritis			
Henoch–Schönlein purpura			
Referred pain (e.g. from the abdomen)			
Non-accidental injury			

- Ability to weight-bear or crawl
- Recent illnesses or other symptoms (e.g. joint pains elsewhere, rashes, fever, diarrhoea, vomiting, and so on)
- Pain at rest (e.g. waking child from sleep) or only on activity
- Past history of joint or limb problems
- Birth history (e.g. was the child born breach)
- Family history (e.g. familial tendency for developmental dysplasia of the hip)

Examination can often be difficult in a young child who is unable to localize the pain or understand what is required of them. The examination should include:

- Temperature (any history of fever should be taken seriously).
- Assessment of the child's gait while walking or assessment of the child crawling (if the child is able to crawl without discomfort, this localizes the problem to below the knee).
- Inspection of both legs for erythema, swelling, deformity, and resting position.
- Inspection for any foreign bodies in the foot which may provide a simple explanation for the limp and therefore require no further investigation.
- Inspection for any bruising or other features to suggest NAI.
- Palpation of the leg for tenderness, joint effusions, and range of movement.
- Examination of joints above and below the site of pain and the opposite leg.
- Examination of the abdomen, back, and spine.

19.24.3 Investigation of the limping child

Investigations should be directed by the history and examination. A thorough examination may detect a simple cause (e.g. foreign body in the foot), requiring no further investigation.

If the diagnosis is not apparent, then a step-wise approach to investigations is useful:

- If there is any obviously tender or swollen part, this should be X-rayed.
- If there is no obvious cause, then an X-ray of the pelvis including both hips should be performed.
- If X-rays do not reveal a diagnosis then a full blood count, ESR, and CRP should be performed. (Unfortunately normal results do not exclude septic arthritis if the clinical picture is suggestive, see Kocher's criteria in Table 19.22.)
- An ultrasound of the hip should be performed to look for an effusion, which if present can be aspirated and sent for microscopy and culture.
- A urine dipstick may be useful by revealing haematuria suggestive of Henoch–Schönlein purpura.
- A sickle cell screen should be performed if appropriate.
- Blood cultures should be performed if an infective cause is suspected.

19.24.4 Septic arthritis

Septic arthritis is also covered in Chapter 5, section 5.11.

Staphylococcus aureus is the commonest cause of septic arthritis in children. The hip and knee are the most commonly affected joints.

The child is usually systemically unwell with a fever. All movements of the joint are likely to be reduced and painful.

Differentiating transient synovitis (irritable hip) from septic arthritis can be difficult clinically especially in the early stages of septic arthritis. Kocher's criteria may be helpful to differentiate between transient synovitis and septic arthritis.

Kocher's criteria consist of four equally weighted criteria (Table 19.25) that form a clinical prediction rule.

Table 19.25 Kocher's clinical prediction rule for septic arthritis in children

Criteria	History or presence of fever >38.5°C Child not weight-bearing ESR >40 mm/h WCC >12 x 10⁹/L
Number of Kocher's criteria present	Risk of septic arthritis (%)
0	0.2
1	3
2	40
3	93
4	99

Data from Kocher M, Zurakowski D, Kasser J, et al (1999). Differentiating between septic arthritis and transient synovitis of the hip in children: An evidence-based clinical prediction algorithm. Journal of Bone and Joint Surgery. 1999 Dec;81(12):1662–70.

If the child has two or more criteria, there is a ≥40% chance of septic arthritis and the child should be admitted for intravenous antibiotics and urgently referred to orthopaedics for consideration of surgical joint washout.

If the child has one or none of the criteria, the chance of septic arthritis <3% and an alternative diagnosis should be considered.

Kocher's criteria should not replace clinical judgement but may be used to help decision-making.

19.24.5 Irritable hip ('transient synovitis')

Transient synovitis is a common cause of a painful hip and limp in a child. It can affect a child of any age but is most common between three to five years. In many cases, it appears to follow a viral illness. The child is usually systemically well and if not, septic arthritis must be excluded.

Investigations generally reveal a normal WCC, ESR, and CRP. Ultrasound may show a hip effusion; the aspirated fluid should be sent for microscopy and culture to exclude infection.

ED management is focused on excluding septic arthritis and providing symptomatic relief. If there are any concerns about the diagnosis, the patient should be referred to orthopaedics.

19.24.6 Developmental dysplasia of the hip

Developmental dysplasia of the hip is a spectrum of disorders affecting the proximal femur and acetabulum that leads to hip subluxation and dislocation. It is commoner in girls and breech presentations, and there is a familial tendency.

Neonatal screening with Ortolani and Barlow tests has increased the detection of the condition. Those at high risk (e.g. breech presentation, family history) are also screened with ultrasound.

If a child presents to the ED with a history suggestive of developmental dysplasia, joint stability should be assessed with the Ortolani and Barlow tests and the patient referred on to the orthopaedic team.

19.24.7 Perthes' disease

The aetiology of Perthes' disease is unknown, but there is a reduction in the blood supply to epiphysis of the femoral head leading to avascular necrosis. It is seen most commonly in boys aged 3–10. 15% are bilateral.

The range of movement at the hip may be reduced due to pain.

The most useful investigation is a hip X-ray, which is necessary for diagnosis and to determine the stage of disease (Figure 19.5).

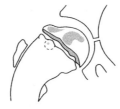

Figure 19.5 Changes in the hip in Perthes' disease.

Reproduced from Jonathan P. Wyatt, Robin N. Illingworth, Colin A. Graham, Michael J. Clancy, Colin E. Robertson, *Oxford Handbook of Emergency Medicine*, 2006, 'Changes in the hip in Perthes' disease', p. 703, with permission from Oxford University Press

X-ray changes are progressive:

1. Increased joint space on medial aspect of upper femoral epiphysis.
2. Increased bone density in affected epiphysis (appears sclerotic).
3. Fragmentation, distortion (flattening) and lateral subluxation of the upper femoral epiphysis (leaving part of the femoral head 'uncovered').
4. Rarefaction of the adjacent metaphysis in which cysts may appear.

Full blood count, ESR, CRP, and blood cultures are normal in Perthes' disease.

Patients should be referred for orthopaedic assessment and treatment.

19.24.8 Slipped upper femoral epiphysis

Slipped upper femoral epiphysis (SUFE) is a disease of adolescence and is commoner in boys. The cause is unknown but there is often a history of preceding trauma or the suggestion of hormonal imbalance. Patients with certain body types are more prone: obese adolescences with underdeveloped genitalia or tall, thin, rapidly growing adolescences with normal sexual genitalia.

Pain may be reported in the hip or the knee. Movement of the affected hip is reduced compared to the other side. The hip may be held slightly adducted, externally rotated, and shortened.

An anteroposterior (AP) pelvis and lateral hip view (or 'frog-leg' lateral) should be performed. Subtle slips are sometimes only visible on the lateral view. Trethowan's line should be drawn along the superior border of the femoral neck (Figure 19.6). Normally this line cuts through the femoral epiphysis. Caution is required when comparing findings to the 'normal' hip because the condition may be bilateral.

Patients should be referred to orthopaedics for reduction and fixation. The condition can be bilateral, so the other side may be fixed prophylactically or kept under surveillance.

19.24.9 Juvenile arthritis

Juvenile arthritis is arthritis that presents before the age of 16 years. The arthritis may be transient and self-limiting (e.g. Henoch–Schönlein purpura, rheumatic fever, or a reactive arthritis following a gastrointestinal infection) or chronic.

Juvenile idiopathic arthritis is the commonest form of chronic arthritis in children. It is an autoimmune condition but the underlying cause is unknown. Children may also develop other types of chronic arthritis such as ankylosing spondylitis, psoriatic arthritis, and rheumatoid arthritis. These conditions are covered in Chapter 5, sections 5.14 and 5.15.

The main role of the ED in the management of such conditions is the exclusion of an underlying acute problem (e.g. septic arthritis or trauma) and referral on to a rheumatologist.

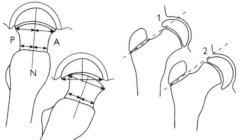

Lateral view showing normal (left) and abnormal (right)

AP view: Trethowan's sign; 1 normal, 2 abnormal hip

Figure 19.6 Slipped upper femoral epiphysis.

Reproduced from Jonathan P. Wyatt, Robin N. Illingworth, Colin A. Graham, Michael J. Clancy, Colin E. Robertson, *Oxford Handbook of Emergency Medicine*, 2006, 'Slipped upper femoral epiphysis', p. 703, with permission from Oxford University Press

19.24.10 Ewing's sarcoma

Ewing's sarcoma is a malignant bone tumour that affects children. It can occur at any age but is most common during puberty, when bones are growing rapidly.

The tumour may arise anywhere in the body but typically affects the long bones. It may metastases to the lungs and other bones, and one-third of children have metastasis at the time of diagnosis.

The most likely presentation in the ED is a pathological fracture through the tumour, following minor trauma, or as an incidental finding on X-ray.

Children should be referred on to a paediatric oncologist for further investigation and management.

KEY POINTS

Causes of a limping child include:

- All ages: septic arthritis, osteomyelitis, trauma, neoplasm, sickle cell crisis, neuromuscular, referred pain, NAI
- Age 1–3: developmental dysplasia of the hip, toddlers fracture, irritable hip
- Age 4–10: irritable hip, Perthes' disease, juvenile arthritis
- Age 11–16: SUFE, osteochondritis, physeal injuries, gonococcal septic arthritis, and Ewing's sarcoma

Septic arthritis must always be considered in any child with an atraumatic limp. Kocher's criteria (history or presence of fever >38.5°C; non-weight-bearing; ESR >40 mm/h; WCC >12 × 10⁹/L) is a recognized clinical prediction rule to help differentiate septic arthritis from transient synovitis in children.

Perthes' disease causes avascular necrosis of the femoral head. The cause is unknown. It is most common in boys aged 3–10; 15% are bilateral.

SUFE is a disease of adolescence and is commoner in boys. Trethowan's line should be drawn along the superior border of the femoral neck on the 'frog-leg' lateral to detect subtle slips.

19.25 Painful limbs in children—traumatic

19.25.1 Introduction

Musculoskeletal injuries are covered in Chapter 5 and this section should be read in conjunction with sections 5.1 to 5.7.

This section highlights injuries that are specific to children.

The possibility of non-accidental injury should always be considered in children, especially if a non-ambulatory child sustains a long bone fracture.

19.25.2 Epiphyseal injuries

There are two types of epiphyses:

- Traction epiphyses located at the insertion of muscles (e.g. base of the fifth metatarsal, tibial tuberosity, calcaneum), which are non-articular, and not involved in bone growth. Avulsion is the commonest injury.
- Pressure epiphyses located at the end of bones and involved in articulation.

19.25.3 Salter–Harris injuries

Injury to the pressure epiphyses may result in avascular necrosis or growth arrest. They are categorized into five types using the Salter–Harris classification (Figure 19.7).

- Type I—the epiphysis is separated from the metaphysis.
- Type II—a small piece of metaphysis separates with the epiphysis (commonest injury).
- Type III—a fracture occurs through the epiphysis and joins that through the epiphyseal plate.

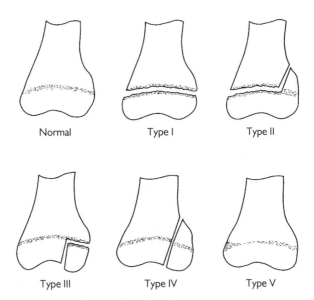

Figure 19.7 Salter–Harris classification of epiphyseal injuries.

* Reproduced with permission from ROBERT B. SALTER, W. ROBERT HARRIS, Injuries Involving the Epiphyseal Plate, *Journal of Bone & Joint Surgery*, Volume 45, Issue 3, pp. 587–622, Copyright © 1963, Wolters Kluwer Health, Inc.

Reproduced from Jonathan P. Wyatt, Robin N. Illingworth, Colin A. Graham, Michael J. Clancy, Colin E. Robertson, *Oxford Handbook of Emergency Medicine*, 2006, Salter-Harris classification of epiphyseal injuries, p. 715, with permission from Oxford University Press

- Type IV—a fracture through the epiphysis, epiphyseal plate, and metaphysis.
- Type V—a crush injury of part or all of the epiphysis.

19.25.4 Osteochondritis

Osteochondritis are a group of disorders that affect various epiphyses. Three varieties of osteochondritis are recognized: crushing osteochondritis; tractional apophysitis; and osteochondritis dissecans.

Crushing osteochondritis

Crushing osteochondritis is characterized by apparently spontaneous necrosis of ossification centres. It is mainly seen during phases of rapid growth. Patients present with pain and limited joint movement.

At the hip, it is known as Perthes' disease. Other sites include: the thoracic and lumbar vertebrae (Scheuermann's disease); the navicular bone in the foot (Kohler's disease); the lunate in the wrist (Kienbock's disease); and the second metatarsal head (Freiberg's disease).

X-rays may show sclerosis and distortion of the bone. Management is rest, NSAIDs, and orthopaedic follow-up.

Traction apophysitis

The pull of a large tendon can cause damage to the unfused apophysis to which it is attached.

Osgood–Schlatter's disease is caused by traction on the tibial tuberosity from the patellar tendon, resulting in multiple avulsion fractures. Patients report anterior knee pain typically after exercise. It is most commonly seen in boys aged 10–15. Treatment is with rest, NSAIDS, and orthopaedic follow-up. Most settle with conservative management.

A similar condition can occur on the lower pole of the patella, known as Sinding–Larsen's disease. Management is similar to Osgood–Schlatter's disease.

Sever's disease is traction apophysitis of the calcaneal attachment of the Achilles' tendon.

Osteochondritis dissecans

A small piece of articular cartilage and adjacent bone may separate (dissect) as an avascular fragment. Repeated minor trauma is believed to be the cause, which produces an osteochondral fracture. Characteristically it affects the knee (medial femoral condyle) of young adult men.

Patients present with intermittent pain and swelling of the joint. If the fragment detaches, the loose body may cause 'locking' or 'giving way' of the knee. X-ray demonstrates the fragment or defect.

Management involves rest, NSAIDs, and orthopaedic follow-up (urgently if locked).

19.25.5 Paediatric elbows

Paediatric elbow injuries often cause confusion due to the six separate ossification centres (Figure 19.8). The ossification centres appear at various intervals from age 6 months to 12 years and can be remembered by the mnemonic CRITOL.

The exact age at which each ossification centre appears is variable between children but the order of ossification is consistent.

Knowledge of the ossification centres in the elbow is particularly relevant for injuries of the internal (medial) epicondyle, where forceful contraction of the forearm flexors may lead to an avulsion. The medial epicondyle may come to lie within the joint and be mistaken as one of the other ossification centres. In order to not miss such an injury the following rule should be applied: if the trochlea is seen, there must be an ossified internal (medial) epicondyle somewhere on the

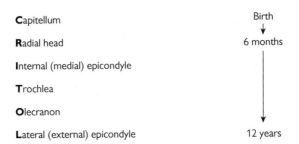

Capitellum	Birth
Radial head	↓
	6 months
Internal (medial) epicondyle	
Trochlea	
Olecranon	
Lateral (external) epicondyle	12 years

Capitellum   Birth
↓
Radial head   6 months
Internal (medial) epicondyle
Trochlea
Olecranon
Lateral (external) epicondyle   12 years

Figure 19.8 Elbow ossification centres.

X-ray. If the internal epicondyle is not located medially, then it has been displaced and will require surgical reduction (Figure 19.9).

19.25.6 'Pulled elbow' (subluxation of the radial head)

Children aged between one to five years old may sustain a subluxation of the radial head when the forearm is pulled. The radial head pulls out of the annular ligament and the child then stops using their arm. Often there is a characteristic history (e.g. a child caught by their forearm when about to fall over). If the history suggests a pulled elbow, then an X-ray is not required.

The subluxation can be reduced by flexing the elbow to 90° and then supinating the forearm fully. If this is unsuccessful, keep the elbow flexed, and pronate the arm. Occasionally a click is felt or heard as the radial head reduces. Prior to attempts at reduction the parents should have the procedure explained to them.

Following reduction, the child will usually resume using the arm within 5–10 minutes. If not, an X-ray should be performed to exclude a fracture.

19.25.7 Supracondylar injuries

Supracondylar fractures usually result from a fall on to an outstretched hand. The risk of neuro-vascular compromise (brachial artery, median and radial nerves) is particularly high in displaced fractures and requires urgent operative intervention.

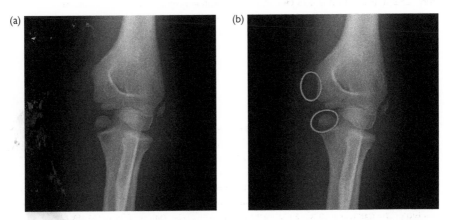

Figure 19.9 (a) Internal (medial) epicondyle avulsion; (b) internal (medial) epicondyle avulsion.
Case courtesy of Dr Ahmed Abd Rabou, Radiopaedia.org, rID: 22644

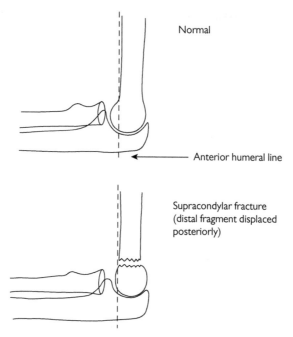

Normal

Anterior humeral line

Supracondylar fracture
(distal fragment displaced
posteriorly)

Figure 19.10 The anterior humeral line.

The detection of minimally displaced supracondylar fractures can be difficult and assessing the anterior humeral line may pick up subtle injuries. On a true lateral film of the elbow, a line traced along the anterior cortex of the humerus will normally dissect the capitellum with approximately one-third lying anterior to the line (Figure 19.10).

Most fractures are displaced, angulated, or rotated. The degree of angulation can be under-estimated and therefore measuring the angle between the capitellum and humeral shaft is useful. Normally a line drawn down the humeral shaft makes a 45° angle with the capitellum (Figure 19.11). Loss of more than 20° of this angle is an indication for surgery.

The indications for operative manipulation of a supracondylar fracture are:

- Neurovascular deficit
- >50% displacement
- >20% angulation of the distal part posteriorly
- >10% medial or lateral angulation

19.25.8 Toddler's fracture

A toddler's fracture is an oblique undisplaced fracture of the distal tibia seen in children aged one to four years old. It can result from minor trauma, sometimes with a rotational component (e.g. placing a foot awkwardly when learning to walk).

Clinical diagnosis of a toddler's fracture can be difficult. Usually the child presents with a limp or non-weight-bearing on the affected leg. The child often reverts to crawling because the injury is distal to the knee. The child is systemically well. There may be localized warmth and tenderness at the site of the fracture.

An X-ray of the lower leg may reveal the fracture, although this may not be apparent on the initial views. A repeat X-ray at 10 days should show an area of periosteal reaction of the distal tibia.

Supracondylar humeral fractures

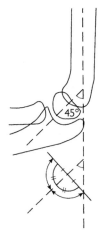

*Normal lateral view—the capitulum makes an
angle of 45° with the humeral shaft*

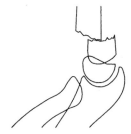

*Supracondylar fracture with >20° angulation
and ~50% displacement*

Figure 19.11 The humeral–capitellum angle.

Reproduced from Jonathan P. Wyatt, Robin N. Illingworth, Colin A. Graham, Michael J. Clancy, Colin E. Robertson, *Oxford Handbook of Emergency Medicine*, 2006, 'Supracondylar humeral fractures', p. 719, with permission from Oxford University Press

Treatment is with a long leg-plaster and orthopaedic follow-up. A plaster may be applied for symptomatic relieve if the clinical diagnosis is a toddler's fracture, even if a fracture is not seen on the initial X-ray.

KEY POINTS

The Salter–Harris classification:
- Type I—epiphysis separated from the metaphysis
- Type II—piece of metaphysis separates with the epiphysis
- Type III—fracture through the epiphysis and the epiphyseal plate
- Type IV—fracture through the epiphysis, epiphyseal plate, and metaphysis
- Type V—a crush injury of part or all of the epiphysis

The mnemonic CRITOL can be used to remember the ossification centres of the elbow. If presented with a paediatric elbow X-ray in the exam always look for the internal epicondyle, in case it has been avulsed.

There are various radiological lines that can be used to detect subtle fractures or dislocations in adults and children:

- Anterior humeral line—supracondylar fracture
- Humeral–capitellum angle—supracondylar fracture
- Radio-capitellar line—dislocation of the radial head
- Radius, lunate, and capitate line—lunate and peri-lunate dislocations
- Trethowan's line (superior border of femoral neck)—SUFE
- Bohler's angle—calcaneal fracture
- Metatarsal alignment with the cuneiforms—Lisfranc fracture

19.26 Rashes in children

Rashes in adults and children are covered in Chapter 16.

19.27 Sore throat

The causes and management of sore throats in adults and children is covered in Chapter 7.

19.28 SAQs

19.28.1 Paediatric fever and urinary tract infection

A two-year-old girl presents to the ED with a history of fever, vomiting, offensive urine, and crying when she passes urine. She is rousable but only with prolonged stimulation.

Her observations are: temperature 39°C, pulse 140, capillary refill time 4 s, respiratory rate 28, saturations 99%, blood glucose 4.5 mmol/L.

a) (i)   You are concerned she has a urinary tract infection. List four urine collection methods recommended by the NICE guidance on UTI in children. (2 marks)

a) (ii) List two of the commonest causes of UTI in children. (1 mark)

b) (i)   Microscopy of the urine sample confirms bacteriuria and pyuria. You diagnose a UTI. How long does she require antibiotics for? (1 mark) Which antibiotic would you start with and by which route? (2 marks)

b) (ii) At what age is it acceptable to use a urinary dipstick to diagnose a UTI in children? (1 mark)

c) (i)   From the information in the stem of this question, what category would you place this child on the NICE feverish illness in children traffic light system? (1 mark)

c) (ii) Which two features about this child make her this category? (2 marks)

Suggested answer

a) (i)   You are concerned she has a urinary tract infection. List four urine collection methods recommended by the NICE guidance on UTI in children. (2 marks)

Clean catch

Urine pad

Suprapubic aspiration

Catheter sample

a) (ii) List two of the commonest causes of UTI in children. (1 mark)

E. coli (must have this in answer)

Proteus

Pseudomonas

Staphylococcus

b) (i)   Microscopy of the urine sample confirms bacteriuria and pyuria. You diagnose a UTI. How long does she require antibiotics for? (1 mark) Which antibiotic would you start with and by which route? (2 marks)

This child has an upper UTI (bacteriuria and fever >38°C), therefore she requires 7–10 days of antibiotics.

She is vomiting so the antibiotics should be given intravenously.

Cefotaxime or ceftriaxone are recommended.

b) (ii) At what age is it acceptable to use urinary dipstick to diagnose a UTI in children? (1 mark)

Age >3 years old

c) (i)   From the information in the stem of this question what category would you place this child on the NICE feverish illness in children traffic light system? (1 mark)

Amber

c) (ii) Which two features about this child make her this category? (2 marks)

Capillary refill time >3 s

Wakes only with prolonged stimulation

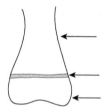

Figure 19.12 Anatomy of a long bone.

19.28.2 Paediatric musculoskeletal problems

a) On the diagram in Figure 19.12, draw a Salter–Harris II and III injury, and label two of the three arrows. (4 marks)

A seven-year-old boy presents with a limp and complaining of right hip pain. You are concerned about the possibility of Perthes' disease.

b) (i)   What is Perthes' disease? (1 mark)
b) (ii) List six other differential diagnoses for atraumatic hip pain in this patient. (3 marks)
b) (iii) List two findings on X-ray which would suggest Perthes' disease. (2 marks)

Suggested answer

a) On the diagram in Figure 19.13, draw a Salter–Harris II and III injury, and label two of the three arrows. (4 marks)
b) (i)   What is Perthes' disease? (1 mark)
        Avascular necrosis of the upper femoral epiphysis.
b) (ii) List six other differential diagnoses for atraumatic hip pain in this patient. (3 marks)
        Septic arthritis
        Transient synovitis
        Osteomyelitis
        Juvenile arthritis
        Leukaemia
        Neoplasm (e.g. neuroblastoma, Ewing's sarcoma)
        Sickle cell crisis
        Neuromuscular
        Referred pain (e.g. from abdomen)

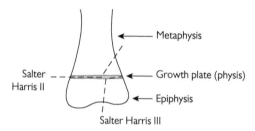

Figure 19.13 Anatomy of a long bone—answer.

b) (iii) List two findings on X-ray which would suggest Perthes' disease. (2 marks)

Increased joint space on the medial aspect of upper femoral epiphysis

Increased bone density in affected epiphysis (appears sclerotic)

Fragmentation, distortion (flattening), and lateral subluxation of the upper femoral epiphysis (leaving part of the femora head 'uncovered')

Rarefaction of the adjacent metaphysis in which cysts may appear

Further reading

British Society of Paediatric Endocrinology and Diabetes, August 2015. BSPED Recommended Guideline for the Management of Children and Young People under the age of 18 years with Diabetic Ketoacidosis.

British Thoracic Society, updated October 2011. BTS Guidelines for the Management of Community Acquired Pneumonia in Children. Available at: http://www.brit-thoracic.org.uk [Online].

Kocher MS, Zurakowski D, Kasser JR, et al., 1999. Differentiating between septic arthritis and transient synovitis of the hip in children: an evidence-based clinical prediction algorithm. *J Bone Joint Surg Am* **81**:1662–70.

National Institute for Health and Care Excellence, August 2007. NICE clinical guideline 54. Urinary tract infections in under 16s: diagnosis and management. Available at: http://www.nice.org.uk/Guidance/CG54 [Online].

National Institute for Health and Care Excellence, July 2009. NICE clinical guideline 89. Child maltreatment: when to suspect maltreatment in under 18s. Available at: http://www.nice.org.uk/Guidance/CG89 [Online].

National Institute for Health and Care Excellence, May 2013. NICE clinical guideline 160. Fever in under 5s: assessment and initial management. Available at: http://www.nice.org.uk/guidance/cg160 [Online].

National Institute for Health and Care Excellence, January 2014. NICE clinical guideline 176. Head injury: assessment and early management. Available at: http://www.nice.org.uk/Guidance/CG176 [Online].

National Institute for Health and Care Excellence, August 2015. NICE guideline 18. Diabetes (type 1 and type 2) in children and young people: diagnosis and management. Available at: http://www.nice.org.uk/guidance/ng18 [Online].

Royal College of Emergency Medicine, 2009. The College of Emergency Medicine Clinical Effectiveness Committee 2009. Best Practice for Safeguarding Children. Available at: http://www.rcem.ac.uk [Online].

Scottish Intercollegiate Guideline Network, October 2014. SIGN 141. British guideline on the management of asthma: A national clinical guideline. Available at: https://www.brit-thoracic.org.uk/document-library/clinical-information/asthma/btssign-asthma-guideline-2014/ [Online].

CHAPTER 20

Haematology and oncological emergencies

CONTENTS

20.1 Blood groups

Blood groups are genetically determined systems related to antigens on red blood cells, the most common being the ABO and rhesus groups. If an individual with a particular antigen is exposed to the corresponding antibody, agglutination occurs, resulting in haemolysis.

20.1.1 ABO group

The ABO system has four main subtypes which are defined by the presence or absence of two antigens (A and B). Individuals also have naturally occurring IgM antibodies; Anti- A or Anti-B, depending on their blood type (see Table 20.1).

20.1.2 Rhesus group

The rhesus system involves the presence of five main antigens; C, c, D, E, and e. In contrast to the ABO group, the rhesus group relates to the presence or absence of the IgG immune antibody, Anti D. Individuals who lack antigen D are termed rhesus negative. If rhesus negative individuals are sensitized to rhesus positive blood (e.g. during a mismatched transfusion or parturition), the individual will produce anti-D antibodies thus resulting in a haemolytic transfusion reaction or haemolytic disease of the newborn, respectively. In pregnancy, this is avoided by the use of Anti-D Immunoglobulin which prevents sensitization by the Foetal Red Cell D Antigen.

20.2 Transfusion

Many different blood groups types exist however the most relevant in terms of transfusions is the ABO-rhesus sub group. ABO-rhesus grouping is determined prior to a blood transfusion to prevent potentially lethal haemolysis by a process known as cross-matching.

20.2.1 Transfusion reactions

Transfusion reaction are defined as any adverse feature related to a blood transfusions. The most well-known being the immune reaction caused by blood groups incompatibility. If an individual

Table 20.1 Blood groups and associated antibodies

Blood group	Antigens on cells	Antibodies
A	A	B
B	B	A
AB	A and B	None
0	None	A and B

receives blood for which they possess antibodies against, haemolysis may occur. Although trans-fusion reactions are now rare due to the cross-matching process, they are still potentially life-threatening, being usually related to mis-administration. In the case of emergency blood transfusion, blood group O negative is used as the universal donor due to the absences of all antibodies, thus reducing the risk of transfusion-related haemolysis.

Additional adverse features related to blood transfusions include:

- Allergic reactions—to blood product of preservative
- Acquired infection—by direct transmission from donor blood of contaminated during storage
- Circulatory overload—due to sudden increase in blood viscosity (may trigger heart failure)

20.2.2 Massive transfusion

Massive transfusion is defined as:

- Transfusion of a patient's total blood volume in <24 hr period

OR

- Transfusion of half a patient's circulatory volume in one hour

The aim of treatment is to restore adequate blood volume and haemostatic components in the case of massive haemorrhage. In addition to the complications related to any blood transfusion are specific adverse features related to massive transfusions.

Blood volume replacement

Blood volume replacement should be directed towards the patient's physiological need (i.e. oxygen consumption rather that an arbitrary haemoglobin level). Over and under transfusion can exacerbate the risks associated with massive transfusion.

Coagulopathy

Massive transfusion results in a relative thrombocytopenia and coagulation factor depletion secondary to the dilutional effect of blood loss associated with blood volume replacement with packed red cells. In addition, the stress can trigger disseminated intravascular coagulation (DIC) exacerbating the coagulopathy. Thus, the use of platelet transfusion and fresh frozen plasma is also required in addition to packed red cells.

Oxygen affinity

Stored blood has a relative high oxygen affinity, thus resulting in altered oxygen delivery.

Hypocalcaemia

Stored blood contains citrate. In the case of massive blood transfusion, citrate toxicity can occur, resulting in hypocalcaemia. However, despite this, calcium replacement is not usually required.

Hyperkalaemia

During blood storage cell degradation occurs, resulting in potassium release. In the case of massive transfusion, a relative hyperkalaemia can occur.

Transfusion-related acute lung injury

The exact physiology of transfusion-related acute lung injury (TRALI) is poorly understood; however, it is defined as a syndrome of adult respiratory distress syndrome (ARDS) developing post transfusion of blood products. Symptoms usually develop within six hours of transfusion and invasive ventilation is usually required. There is associated high mortality and morbidity and is in top three causes of transfusion-related fatality. Despite this, it is usually a transient phenomenon and the majority of patients clinically improve within 96 hours.

20.3 Haemoglobinopathies

Haemoglobin consist of the oxygen carrying haem (porphyrin ring) which is bound to polypeptide globin chains. Each haemoglobin molecular consists of a tetramer of globin chains, each bound to a haem group.

Haemoglobinopthaies or abnormal haemoglobin are caused by genetic mutations coding for alpha and beta globin chains. Despite the presence of numerous haemoglobin variants, the majority of clinically significant haemoglobinoptahies involve the beta globin chain. The mutations result in the production of abnormal globin chain and thus the production of abnormal haemoglobin molecules.

20.3.1 Sickle cell disease

Sickle cell disease is one of the commonest haemoglobinopthaies worldwide, caused by a mutation in the beta globin chain resulting in the production of the abnormal haemoglobin S. *HbS* becomes crystalline at low oxygen tensions, resulting in haemolysis and microvascular occlusion. Individuals who are heterozygous are relatively asymptomatic due to the presence of the normal HbA. However, homozygous individuals form sickle cell-shaped haemoglobin molecules, leading to a chronic haemolytic anaemia and ischaemic tissue damage.

Individuals with sickle cell disease have a state chronic anaemia and experience 'crises' due to acute vascular occlusion and haemolysis. A sickle crisis or 'sickling' typically presents with acute pain in the area of ischaemia (classically long bones, abdomen, and chest). In addition, sequestration can also occur in the liver and spleen leading to pain, acute anaemia, and jaundice.

Treatment is generally conservative—avoiding triggers such as cold and low oxygen states. In a severe crises, exchange transfusions are sometimes required to reduce the proportion of circulating abnormal haemoglobin.

Patients with sickle cell can present to the emergency department in a variety of ways, depending on the cause. Common presentations include:

- Bone crisis (vaso-occlusive crisis).
- Acute chest syndrome: low-grade fever, non-productive cough, shortness of breath, haemoptysis, acute chest pain, signs and symptoms of hypoxia, signs of consolidation, new infiltrate on chest X-ray.
- Acute splenic sequestration: pallor, lethargy, hypotension, rapid splenic enlargement.
- Central nervous system (CNS) complications: stroke, presenting with hemiparesis, monoparesis, aphasia/dysphasia, cranial nerve palsies, or coma.
- Acute anaemia, presenting with pallor, tachycardia, tachypnoea, jaundice, enlarged spleen/liver, S3 gallop, congestive heart failure. Acute anaemia can be caused by bone marrow

suppression (viral or other infections); sequestration of blood in the liver or spleen; or increased intravascular haemolysis (hyper-haemolytic crisis).

Precipitants for sickle cell crises include:

- Infection
- Dehydration
- Hypoxia
- Acidosis
- Sedatives
- Alcohol
- Excessive physical exercise

Management of acute sickle cell crisis

- An acute painful sickle cell episode should be treated as a medical emergency.
- Analgesia should be offered within 30 minutes of presentation.
- Consider an alternative diagnosis if pain is reported as atypical by a patient.
- A bolus dose of a strong opioid by a suitable route of administration should be offered to all patients presenting with severe pain, or with moderate pain who have already had some analgesia before presentation.
- All patients should be offered regular paracetamol and NSAIDs in addition.
- Patient-controlled analgesia should be considered if repeated boluses of a strong opioid are needed within two hours.
- All patients on an opioid should be offered anti-emetics and anti-pruritics as needed.
- Many patient will have a personalized pain 'passport' for management of their painful crisis.

20.4 Bleeding—deranged international normalized ratio

20.4.1 Bleeding on warfarin

Warfarin is a vitamin K antagonist that is used as an anticoagulant by inhibiting the production of vitamin K-dependent clotting factors (II, VII, IX, and X) in the liver.

With an individual on warfarin who is over anticoagulated, a risk benefit analysis needs to be made. This needs to take into account the target international normalized ratio (INR) and indication for anticoagulation versus risk of bleeding.

Patients who are overanticoagulated can either have their warfarin dose reduced, stopped temporarily, or partially/completely reversed (see Table 20.2).

The decision should be made on an individual basis and through discussion with a haematologist. The discussion should involve;

- Presence of bleeding
- Indication for anticoagulation
- Risk of bleeding (patient Vs INR)
- Risk of thrombosis

20.4.2 Causes of supratherapeutic international normalized ratio

- Issues with warfarin dosage and compliance, including inadvertent over-medication
- Drug history, including prescribed drugs, over-the-counter drugs and herbal supplements (check INR 3–5 days after commencing any drug interacting with warfarin that will be administered for longer than seven days)

Table 20.2 Management of high international normalized ratio (INR)

Bleeding	INR	Management
Minor bleeding	3–6 (target 2.5)	Reduce dose or stop
	4–5 (target 3.5)	Restart when INR <5
	6–8	Stop
		Restart when INR <5
	>8	Stop
		Consider vitamin K (po/iv)
		Restart when INR <5
Major bleeding	>2.5	Stop
		IV vitamin K (5/10mg)
		Consider prothrombin complex

- Alcohol intake
- Changes to diet: reduction in vitamin K rich foods, such as leafy green vegetables; consumption of fruit juices, especially cranberry or grapefruit
- Liver disease
- Malignancy

20.4.3 Bleeding on novel anticoagulants

Novel oral anticoagulants (NOACs) directly inhibit thrombin (Dabigatran) or factor Xa (Apixibam or rivaroxaban). They are becoming popular in the management of thromboembolic risk due to the reduced associated risk of bleeding and lack of monitoring required compared with warfarin. However, there is no antidote available to reverse the anticoagulant effects and there is little evidence available on the management of bleeding patients on novel oral anticoagulant therapy. Any patient presenting with significant bleeding should be discussed with haematology regarding local management guidelines.

20.5 Oncological emergencies

20.5.1 Introduction

There are numerous different ways an individual may present with an oncological emergency, depending on the cause. See Table 20.3 for cause of oncological emergencies.

20.6 Neurological oncological emergencies

20.6.1 Metastatic spinal cord compression

Metastatic cord compression can occur from:

- Extradural tumour growth
- Peri-tumoral oedema and thecal compression
- Pathological fracture with angulation of the spinal cord
- Tumour-induced spinal arterial occlusion

Table 20.3 Oncological emergencies

Category	Causes
Metabolic	Malignant hypercalcaemia (osteolytic metastases; humoral hypercalcaemia).
	Acute tumour lysis syndrome (abrupt and massive release of cellular metabolites into the circulation after rapid lysis of malignant cells, producing the metabolic triad of hyperkalaemia, hyperphosphatemia).
	Hyperuricaemia.
	Secondary hypocalcaemia.
	Acute kidney injury.
	SIADH.
Neurological	Metastatic spinal cord compression.
	Brain metastases (raised intracranial pressure; seizures).
Cardiovascular	Malignant pericardial effusion (cardiac tamponade).
	Superior vena cava obstruction.
Haematological	Hyperviscosity syndrome (triad of bleeding, including mucosal bleeding-epistaxis, bleeding gums gastrointestinal bleeding, and purpura; visual disturbance, including central retinal vein occlusion, retinal haemorrhages and papilloedema; and focal neurological signs).
	Hyperleukocytosis (leukostasis; > 100,000/cu mm; CNS manifestations, such as headache, blurred vision, visual field defects and papilloedema; and lung manifestations, including effort dyspnoea, hypoxaemia, and respiratory distress).
	DIC.
Infections	Febrile neutropenia.
	Septic shock.
Chemotherapy side effects	Extravasation injuries: vesicants (anthracyclines; vinca alkaloids, mitomycin C); irritants (taxanes; platinum; epipodophyllotoxins; topoisomerase I inhibitors).
	Gastrointestinal: mucositis; enteritis with diarrhoea and dehydration; obstruction.

Metastatic spinal cord compression (MSCC) should be suspected and discussed with the local MSCC coordinator in any patient with an oncological history presenting with:

- Pain in the middle (thoracic) or upper (cervical) spine
- Progressive or severe unremitting lower (lumbar) spinal pain
- Spinal pain aggravated by straining
- Localized spinal tenderness
- Nocturnal spinal pain preventing sleep

Features of malignant spinal cord compression

- Back pain is the most common initial symptom. In cervical region compression, subscapular pain is noted, in the thoracic region lumbosacral or hip pain, and in the lumbosacral region thoracic pain. The back pain can be multisegmental or band-like, and is increasing in severity, with poor response to analgesic medication. The pain is increased on lying on the back.
- Radicular pain.

- Motor: progressive weakness (heaviness of legs), gait abnormalities; paraparesis (thoracic level compression).
- Conus medullaris syndrome (upper lumbar spine compression): distal lower limb weakness, saddle anaesthesia, overflow incontinence of bladder and bowel).
- Loss of bladder and bowel function is generally a late sign.

The spine should be considered to be unstable unless proven otherwise. Investigations and management should involve and be guided by the local MSCC coordinator. Imaging includes:

- MRI of whole spine, to allow definitive treatment to be planned within 24 hours, in the presence of symptoms and signs suggestive of MSCC.
- Consider targeted CT scan with three-plane reconstruction to assess spinal stability and plan spinal surgery.
- Plain radiographs of the spine should not be performed to establish or exclude a diagnosis of MSCC.

Management should involve treating symptomatic pain and preventing paralysis.

- Analgesia should be provided according to the World Health Organization (WHO) pain ladder.
- Nurse flat with neutral spine alignment, including log rolling or turning beds, with use of a slipper pan for toileting, until bony and neurological stability is ensured.
- Loading dose of dexamethasone 16 mg, followed by a short course of 8 mg bd while the treatment is being planned.
- Early discussion with local MSCC coordinator to plan ongoing management such as palliative radiotherapy or surgery.

20.6.2 Raised intracranial pressure

Raised intracranial pressure from brain metastases should be expected in any individual with an oncological history presenting with neurological signs or symptoms. Raised intracranial pressure (ICP) can occur due to the local effect of the tumour and surrounding oedema or due to the secondary complication of hydrocephalus.
   Presentation can occlude:

- Headache
- Vomiting
- Visual changes
- Motor weakness or sensory changes
- Seizures
- Altered metal state

Individuals with suspected raised ICP should be treated with high-dose dexamethasone at similar doses for spinal cord compression, in addition to simple measures such as nursing at 30°, maintaining adequate oxygenation, normocapnoea, and normoglycaemia. If impending herniation is suspected, intravenous mannitol can be given as a temporizing measure.
   Imaging of choice is contrast MRI; however, if not available CT with contrast is acceptable. Long-term management should involve discussion with their primary oncology team.

20.6.3 Seizures

Brain metastasis present with seizures in approximately 15-30% cases and should be suspected in any individual presenting with new onset seizures. Seizures can also occur due to side effects of treatment such as electrolytes imbalance or metabolic disorder such as a paraneoplastic syndrome causing hyponatraemia.

Treatment involves seizure termination with benzodiazepine. In the case of diagnosed metastasis, individuals should be loaded with an antiepileptic medication such as phenytoin.

20.7 Metabolic oncological emergencies

20.7.1 Tumour lysis syndrome

Tumour lysis syndrome (TLS) is a metabolic condition caused by the breakdown of malignant cells. It is characterized by:

- Hyperuricaemia
- Hyperphosphataemia
- Hypocalcaemia
- Hyperkalaemia

TLS can affect any individual and typically occurs in the first few days of starting chemotherapy, however it can also occur after radiotherapy, immunotherapy, and can occur spontaneously due to high tumour turnover. See Table 20.4 for risk factors for developing TLS.

Individuals thought to be at a high risk of developing TLS may be treated prophylactically with uricosuric drugs such as allopurinol.

The management of TLS is supportive and should involve hydration to prevent acute kidney injury (AKI) and electrolyte management. It is a serious and potentially life-threatening condition, which may require transfer to the intensive care unit (ITU) and haemodialysis.

20.7.2. SIADH

See Chapter 14, section 14.9.

20.7.3 Hypercalcaemia

See Chapter 14, section 14.10.

20.8 Cardiovascular oncological emergencies

20.8.1 Superior vena cava obstruction

Superior vena cava (SVC) obstruction occurs when there is an obstruction to blood flow from either external compression, thrombosis, or direct invasion. It most commonly occurs in patients with lung cancer but can also occur in lymphoma and other solid tumours. It can occur insidiously or acutely, and may be the first presentation of a malignancy.

Table 20.4 Tumour lysis syndrome risk factors

Tumour related factors	Host factors
Rapid progression	Intravascular volume depletion (dehydration)
Large tumour burden (LDH >1500 IU/ml, WCC > 50 × 10 /L)	Pre-existing hyperuricaemia
	Obstructive uropathy
Extensive bone marrow involvement	Chronic kidney disease
High tumour sensitivity to cancer chemotherapy agents	Concurrent potentially nephrotoxic medication

Symptoms relate to compression of the SVC restricting blood flow from the head, neck, and upper limbs, back to the heart and include:

- Breathlessness (acute or gradual)
- Dizziness
- Visual changes
- Swelling face/neck/head

Signs relate to venous congestion and include:

- Peri-orbital and conjunctival oedema
- Upper limb oedema
- Distended neck veins
- Distended collateral vein on chest
- Tachypnoea
- Cyanosis
- Stridor
- Papilloedema (late sign)

The diagnosis is made clinically; however, chest X-ray or CT may aid diagnosis particularly in the case of undiagnosed malignancy. Treatment is supportive and guided by the cause and severity of the obstruction. Treatments include radiotherapy, chemotherapy, and stenting. There is a possible role for the use of steroids despite the lack of evidence to support this.

20.9 SAQs

20.9.1 Blood transfusions/high INR

A 70-year-old lady presents to the emergency department with haematemesis and malaena. She has a past medical history of arial fibrillation (AF), hypertension, IHD, and she has a HR 130, BP 100/60, RR19 and sats 97% on room air.

a) She requires an urgent blood transfusion—what blood group would you give her and why? (2 marks)
b) She has received 3 units of packed red blood cells, when she complains of difficulty in breathing and her oxygen saturations begin to drop. List three complications of a blood transfusion. (3 marks)
c) Define a massive blood transfusion. (2 marks)
d) You are phoning from the laboratory with her blood results which tell you that she has an INR of 6.4. What are your three next management steps? (3 marks)

Suggested answers:

a) She requires an urgent blood transfusion, what blood group would you give her and why? (2 marks)
   - O–ve.
   - O–ve is the universal donor blood as it contains no antibodies and thus will not react to the patient's own blood.
b) List three complications of a blood transfusion. (3 marks)
   - ABO incompatibility transfusion reaction
   - Allergic reaction
   - Acquired infection
   - Circulatory overload
   - Hyperkalaemia
   - TRALI
c) Define a massive blood transfusion. (2 marks)
   - Transfusion of a patient's total blood volume in <24 hr period
   OR
   - Transfusion of half a patient's circulatory volume in one hour
d) You are phone from the laboratory with her blood results which tell you that she has an INR of 6.4. What are your three next management steps. (3 marks)
   - Give 5/10 mg IV vitamin K
   - Repeat INR
   - Order FFP
   - Call the on-call haematologist
   - Consider Prothrombin complex

20.9.2 Oncology

A 65-year-old man with a background of prostate cancer presents to the emergency department with back pain and leg weakness.

a) List three types of oncological emergency and give an example of each. (3 marks)
b) You suspect he has metastatic spinal cord compression. List three signs and symptoms suggestive of MSCC. (½ mark each)
c) List 2 causes of MSCC. (2 marks)
d) List your next three management steps. (3 marks)

Suggested answer

a) List 3 types of oncological emergency and an example of each. (3 marks)
- Neurological—MSCC, raised ICP (brain metastases)
- Metabolic—SIADH, hypercalcaemia
- Cardiovascular—SVC obstruction
- Chemotherapy related—mucositis, extravasation injury, D + V
- Infection—neutropenic sepsis
- Haematology—hyperviscosity syndrome, DIC
  (½ mark each, max 1.5 for type, and 1.5 for examples)

b) You suspect he has metastatic spinal cord compression, list three signs and symptoms suggestive of MSCC.
- Pain in middle (thoracic) or upper (cervical) spine
- Progressive or severe unremitting lower (lumbar) spinal pain
- Radicular pain
- Spinal pain aggravated by straining
- Localized spinal tenderness
- Nocturnal spinal pain preventing sleep
- Bladder/bowel disturbance
- Progressive weakness(½ mark each)

c) List two causes of MSCC. (2 marks)
- Extradural tumour growth
- Peri-tumoral oedema and thecal compression
- Pathological fracture with angulation of the spinal cord
- Tumour-induced spinal arterial occlusion (1 mark each)

d) List your next three management steps. (3 marks)
- Immobilize patient flat in a bed
- Arrange imaging—plain films/CT/MRI
- D/w oncology team
- D/w neurosurgery
- Prescribe dexamethasone 8 mg
- Prescribe analgesia for pain
  (1 mark each)

Further reading

Jones GL, Will A, Jackson GH, Webb NJ, Rule S; British Committee for Standards in Haematology. 2015. Guidelines for the management of tumour lysis syndrome in adults and children with haematological malignancies on behalf of the British Committee for Standards in Haematology. *Br J Haematol* **169**(5):661–71.

National Institute for Health and Care Excellence, Novemeber 2008. NICE clinical guideline 75. Metastatic Spinal Cord Compression in Adults: Diagnosis and Management. Available at: https://www.nice.org.uk/Guidance/CG75 [Online].

National Institute for Health and Care Excellence, June 2012. NICE clinical guideline 143. Sickle cell acute painful episode: management of an acute painful sickle cell episode in hospital. Available at: https://www.nice.org.uk/guidance/cg143 [Online].

Scottish Palliative Care Guidelines. Superior vena cava obstruction. Available at; http://www.palliativecareguidelines.scot.nhs.uk/ [Online].

CHAPTER 21

Legal aspects of emergency medicine

CONTENTS

21.1 Consent

21.1.1 Introduction

Consent is required for every examination, treatment, or intervention performed on a patient. Consent may be explicit or implied. Explicit consent is when a patient actively agrees, either verbally or in writing. Implied consent is signalled by the behaviour of an informed patient; for example, putting their arm out for a blood test. There are exceptions where consent is not required, such as emergency treatment and where the law prescribes otherwise (e.g. mental health law).

There are only a few situations where written consent is legally required (e.g. the storage and use of gametes and embryos). Verbal consent is otherwise as valid as written consent. Consent forms do not prove valid consent—they just provide some evidence that consent was obtained. Discussion with a patient regarding consent should be documented in the notes and state the purpose of the treatment, risks, benefits, and alternatives.

The key principles for valid consent are:

- The patient must be competent.
- The patient must be sufficiently informed to make a choice.
- Consent must be given voluntarily.

The GMC provides guidance on the type of information doctors should provide when gaining consent. This information includes:

- The purpose of the investigation or treatment.
- Details and uncertainties of the diagnosis.
- Options for treatment, including the option not to treat.
- Explanation of the likely benefits and probabilities of success for each option.
- The risks such as known possible side effects, complications, and adverse outcomes, including where intervention or treatment may fail to improve a condition.
- The name of the doctor with overall responsibility.
- A reminder that the patient can change their mind.

21.1.2 Who can give consent?

- The only person who can consent for a competent adult is the patient themselves.
- A young person of any age can consent to treatment provided they are considered to be competent (Gillick competent) to make the decision.
- At the age of 16 there is a presumption that the patient is able to give valid consent. However, up to the age of 18 in England, Wales, and Northern Ireland, and age 16 in Scotland, if the person is felt to lack capacity, a person with parental responsibility can give consent on behalf of the patient.
- A Lasting Power of Attorney can consent on behalf of an adult patient once capacity is lost.

21.1.3 Refusal of consent

Competent adult patients are entitled to refuse consent to treatment, even if doing so may result in permanent physical injury or death. The exception to this is where compulsory treatment is authorized by mental health legislation. Where the consequences of refusal are grave, it is important that the patient understands this. Doctors must respect a refusal of treatment if the patient is a competent adult, who is properly informed, and not being coerced.

In England, Wales, and Northern Ireland, refusal of treatment by competent under-18s is not necessarily binding upon the doctors. The courts have ruled that patients under 18 have a right to consent to treatment, but not to refuse it if this would put their health in serious jeopardy. In such circumstances, consent may be gained from an adult with parental responsibility or a court. In Scotland, it is likely that neither parents nor the courts are entitled to override a competent young patient's decision, although this has not been tested in the courts.

Cases of refused consent are best discussed with senior medical staff, the hospital legal department, and/or medical defence societies.

21.1.4 Consent for emergency treatment

Consent should be sought for emergency treatment if the patient is competent.

If consent cannot be obtained, medical treatment that is in the patient's best interest, and is immediately necessary to save life or avoid significant deterioration in the patient's health, should be provided.

If the patient has appointed a welfare attorney, or there is a court-appointed deputy or guardian, this person, where practicable, must be consulted about treatment decisions.

If the patient is under 18 years old in England, Wales, and Northern Ireland, or under 16 in Scotland, and unable to give consent due to lack of capacity or illness, anyone with parental responsibility can provide consent. If treatment is urgent and nobody with parental responsibility is available, treatment can proceed, without consent, provided it is in the patient's best interest.

KEY POINTS

The only person who can consent for a competent adult is the patient themselves.

At the age of 16 there is a presumption that a patient is able to give valid consent. However, up to the age of 18 (in England, Wales, and Northern Ireland), if the person is felt to lack capacity, a person with parental responsibility can give consent on behalf of the patient.

A competent adult can refuse consent to treatment, even if doing so may result in permanent physical injury or death.

Consent should be sought for emergency treatment if the patient is competent.

If consent cannot be obtained in an emergency, medical treatment that is in the patient's best interest and is immediately necessary to save life or avoid significant deterioration in the patient's health should be provided.

21.2 The Mental Capacity Act

21.2.1 Introduction

The Mental Capacity Act aims to protect people who lack capacity, and maximize their ability to make decisions. The Act came into full force in October 2007.

The Act is underpinned by five statutory principles:

- A person should be assumed to have capacity unless it is established that they lack capacity.
- A person should not be treated as lacking capacity unless all practical steps have been tried to enable capacity.
- A person is allowed to make an unwise decision.
- If a person lacks capacity, then decisions should be made in their best interests.
- Any decision made should be the least restrictive option.

21.2.2 Assessing capacity

Mental capacity is the ability to make a decision. The Act states that a person lacks capacity if they are unable to make a specific decision, at a specific time, because of an impairment of, or disturbance in, the functioning of mind or brain. Capacity is dynamic and a specific function of the decision to be taken. It is possible for a patient to lack capacity to make a decision about one specific issue but not about another.

Patients should always be assumed to have capacity, but if there is reason to believe a patient lacks capacity it should be assessed using the two-stage test:

1. Does the person have an impairment, or disturbance of the functioning, of their mind or brain?
2. Does the impairment or disturbance mean that the person is unable to make a specific decision when they need to?

The functional test of capacity advised in the Act is that, in order for a person to be able to make a decision, they must be able to:

- Understand the decision to be made and the information provided about the decision.
- Retain this information sufficiently long to make the decision.
- Use the information to make the decision (weigh up the pros and cons).
- Communicate their decision.

21.2.3 Advanced decisions

An advanced decision ('living will') allows an adult (over 18 years) with capacity to state how they wish to be treated if they suffer a loss of capacity. Advanced decisions usually relate to the refusal of medical treatment but can be statements authorizing or requesting certain procedures or treatments. Advanced refusals of treatment are legally binding; however, advanced request or authorizations are not, but should be taken into account when assessing best interests.

A valid and applicable advance decision to refuse treatment must be specific to the treatment in question. It has the same force as a contemporaneous decision. A Lasting Power of Attorney appointed before the advanced decision cannot overrule it, nor can the Court of Protection.

Validity of an advanced decision

In order for an advanced decision to be valid, the following criteria have to be met:

- The advanced decision must have been made by the patient when they were an adult (over 18), had capacity, and were properly informed.

- The statement should specify precisely what treatment is to be refused and the circumstances in which the refusals should apply.
- The advanced decision will only apply once the patient lacks capacity to consent to or refuse treatment.
- An advanced decision that relates to the refusal of life-sustaining treatments must be written, signed, and witnessed. The patient must acknowledge in the written decision that they intend to refuse treatment, even though this puts their life at risk.

An advanced decision may be invalid if:

- The decision was withdrawn while the person had capacity.
- After the advance decision was made, a Lasting Power of Attorney was appointed and given express authority to make the treatment decisions covered by the advanced decision.
- The person has done something that clearly goes against the advanced decision, which suggests they have changed their mind.

If the possibility of an advanced decision is raised for a patient who currently lacks capacity, reasonable efforts must be made to find out the details of the decision. This may involve contacting the patient's GP, looking at the hospital medical notes, and discussions with the patient's relatives. If emergency treatment is required, this should not be delayed to look for an advanced decision if there is no indication that one exists. If there is an indication that one exists, the validity and applicability should be assessed and the decision adhered to, if valid.

If the advanced decision is not valid or applicable, the treatment given should be in the patient's best interest.

Advanced decisions can be overruled if the patient is being treated compulsorily under mental health legislation. However, a valid and applicable advanced refusal of treatment for conditions that are not covered by the compulsory powers of the legislation must be adhered to.

21.2.4 Lasting power of attorney

The Mental Capacity Act allows people over 18 years of age, who have capacity, to appoint a Lasting Power of Attorney (LPA). The person making the LPA is referred to as the 'donor'. An LPA can be appointed to make decisions on health and personal welfare, and/or property and financial affairs on behalf of the donor should they lose capacity in the future. The LPA is bound by the principles set out in the Mental Capacity Act and must make decisions in the donor's best interest.

A valid LPA requires a signed certificate completed by an independent third party, which confirms that the donor understands the scope and purpose of the LPA and was not put under any pressure to make the LPA. The LPA must be registered with the Office of the Public Guardian.

A personal welfare LPA can make healthcare decisions for the donor once they lack capacity and can consent on their behalf to treatment and social care decisions. There are specific situations when the LPA cannot consent to or refuse treatment:

- When the donor has capacity to consent.
- When the donor has made an advanced decision to refuse treatment (unless the LPA was appointed after the advanced decision and the donor gave permission to the LPA to refuse treatment).
- When the decision relates to life-sustaining treatment and this has not been expressly authorized in the LPA.
- When the donor is detained under the Mental Health Act.

An LPA does not have the power to demand specific treatments if they are not felt to be necessary or appropriate.

All LPAs are registered with the Office of the Public Guardian, who can confirm whether a patient has a LPA or not.

If the medical team and LPA disagree on the best treatment for the patient, the case can be referred to the Court of Protection. While a decision is reached, the patient can be treated to prevent serious deterioration.

21.2.5 Court of Protection

The role of the Court of Protection is to protect individuals who lack capacity and make difficult decisions about their care and welfare.

The Court of Protection can:

- Determine whether an LPA is valid or not
- Give directions about using an LPA
- Remove an LPA
- Settle disputes over healthcare and treatment of a person lacking capacity

21.2.6 Independent medical capacity advocates

The role of an independent medical capacity advocate (IMCA) is to support and represent a person who lacks capacity in making a specific decision, who has no-one (other than paid carers) to support them.

The IMCA:

- Provides support for the person who lacks capacity.
- Represents the person without capacity in discussions about proposed treatment.
- Provides information to work out what is in a person's best interest.
- Questions or challenges decisions that they believe are not in the best interests of the person lacking capacity.
- Presents individuals' views and interests to the decision-maker.

The IMCA is not the decision-maker and cannot consent on behalf of the person but the information and views expressed by the IMCA must be taken into account.

An IMCA must be involved in decisions relating to providing, withholding, or stopping serious medical treatment. In an emergency situation, it is unlikely that there is time to instruct an IMCA so the patient should be treated according to best interest principles and any decisions clearly documented.

If the IMCA disagrees with the proposed treatment and further discussion does not resolve this, then the IMCA may use the formal complaints system to settle the case, or in more urgent cases, refer to the Court of Protection for a decision.

21.2.7 Best interests

The Mental Capacity Act states that any act done or decision made on behalf of a person who lacks capacity must be in their best interests. The Act sets out the factors that should be considered when deciding what is in a person's best interests:

- Past and present wishes and feelings.
- Beliefs and values that may have influenced the decision being made, if the person had capacity.
- Other factors the patient would be likely to consider if they had capacity.

In trying to assess the person's best interests you should:

- Encourage the person who lacks capacity to participate in the decision.
- Avoid discrimination.
- Try to identify all the issues most relevant to the person and to the decision being made.
- If possible defer the decision if the patient is likely to regain capacity.

21.2.8 Safeguarding

Safeguarding involves protecting everyone's right to be safe and stopping abuse.

At-risk adults include individuals over the age of 18 years who cannot look after or protect themselves. May include those with:

- Physical/sensory disability
- Learning disability
- Mental health problems
- Older age (elderly and frail)
- Life-limiting illness
- Alcohol/substance misuse
- Care home residents

Deprivation of Liberty safeguards relate to self-funded and privately funded residents who lack mental capacity, who are placed in care homes or hospitals for their care or treatment. They came into force in England and Wales in April 2009 under amendments to the Mental Capacity Act 2005 and were introduced following a decision in the European Court of Human Rights.

Deprivation of Liberty must encompass the definition set down in Article 5 of the European Convention on Human Rights and related case law. When someone lacks mental capacity to consent to care or treatment, it is sometimes necessary to deprive them of their liberty in their best interests to protect them from harm.

Deprivation of Liberty should not be used if a person meets the criteria for detention under the Mental Health Act 1983.

Restraint is the use of, or threat of, force to enable something to be done which the patient is resisting, or restriction of a person's movement (whether or not they resist). The Mental Capacity Act authorizes restraint if there is a reasonable belief that it is in the patient's best interests, it is believed necessary to prevent harm to the person, and is proportionate to the likelihood and seriousness of harm.

The safeguarding principles include:

- Empowerment: presumption of person-led decision and consent
- Protection: support for those in greatest need
- Prevention of harm
- Proportionality and least intrusive response appropriate to risk presented
- Partnerships: local solutions through services working with their communities
- Accountability and transparency in delivering safeguarding

KEY POINTS

Mental capacity is the ability to make a decision. Capacity is dynamic and a specific function of the decision to be taken.

The functional test of capacity, advised in the Mental Capacity Act, is that in order for a person to be able to make a decision they must be able to:

- Understand the decision to be made and the information provided about the decision.
- Retain this information sufficiently long to make the decision.
- Use the information to make the decision (weigh up the pros and cons).
- Communicate their decision.

An advanced decision which relates to the refusal of life-sustaining treatments must be written, signed, and witnessed. The patient must acknowledge in the written decision that they intend to refuse treatment, even though this puts their life at risk.

An LPA can be appointed to make decisions on health and personal welfare, and/or property and financial affairs on behalf of a person should they lose capacity in the future.

An IMCA is appointed to support and represent a person who lacks capacity in making a specific decision, who has no-one (other than paid carers) to support them.

21.3 End-of-life care—DNACPR

The GMC state that if cardiac or respiratory arrest is an expected part of the dying process and cardiopulmonary resuscitation (CPR) will not be successful, making and recording an advance decision not to attempt CPR will help to ensure that the patient dies in a dignified and peaceful manner. In the case where CPR may be successful it may also not be appropriate due to the likely clinical outcomes. When considering whether to attempt CPR, the benefits, burdens, and risks of treatment to that patient should be considered if CPR is successful. In the cases where CPR is thought to be unsuccessful or be inappropriate, discussions should be made and documented with the patient or next of kin at the earliest possible cause.

21.3.1 Patients with capacity

For patients who have capacity discussions should be made in a sensitive manner, taking into account their views and beliefs. A 'Do Not Attempt CPR' order is a medical decision and if the healthcare team believe that CPR is not in the patient's best interest, an individual's wishes can be overruled. A patient cannot demand to be resuscitated if the healthcare team feel it is not appropriate, however a second opinion will usually be required.

21.3.2 Patients lacking capacity

For patients who lack capacity, a legal proxy with authority to make decisions should be consulted. If there is no legal proxy the case should be discussed with persons close to the patient. Guidelines state that in the case of an individual lacking capacity, next of kin should be contacted for discussions regarding Do Not Attempt Resuscitation (DNAR) at the most appropriate and practical time. If the next of kin or legal proxy disagree with the healthcare professional's opinion a second opinion and legal representative may be required.

21.4 The Mental Health Act

The Mental Health Act 2007 amended the 1983 Act. It was also used to introduce 'deprivation of liberty safeguards' through amending the Mental Capacity Act 2005; and extended the rights of victims by amending the Domestic Violence, Crime and Victims Act 2004.

The 1983 Act deals with the circumstances in which a person with a mental disorder can be detained for treatment of that disorder without his or her consent. It sets out the processes that must be followed and the safeguards for patients, to ensure that they are not inappropriately detained or treated without their consent. The main purpose of the legislation is to ensure that people with serious mental disorders, which threaten their health or safety, or the safety of the public, can be treated irrespective of their consent, where it is necessary to prevent them from harming themselves or others.

The main changes to the 1983 Act made by the 2007 Act are as follows:

- Definition of mental disorder: a single definition applies throughout the Act.
- Criteria for detention: it introduces a new 'appropriate medical treatment' test which applies to all the longer-term powers of detention.
- Professional roles: it broadens the group of practitioners who can take on the functions of the approved social worker and responsible medical officer.

- Nearest relative (NR): it gives patients the right to make an application to displace their NR.
- Supervised community treatment (SCT): it introduces SCT for patients following a period of detention in hospital.
- Mental Health Review Tribunal (MHRT): it reduces the time before a case has to be referred to the MHRT.
- Age-appropriate services: requires hospital managers to ensure that patients aged less than 18 years old are accommodated in an environment that is suitable for their age.
- Advocacy: it places a duty on the appropriate national authority to make arrangements for help to be provided by independent mental health advocates.
- Electroconvulsive therapy: it introduces new safeguards for patients.

The most relevant sections of the Mental Health Act to emergency department (ED) practice are summarized in Table 21.1.

KEY POINTS

The Mental Health Act deals with the circumstances in which a person with a mental disorder can be detained for treatment of that disorder without his or her consent.

Patients in the ED who have a mental health disorder that potential requires an involuntary psychiatric admission should be assessed by an approved social worker and a Section 12 approved doctor. Section 4 of the Mental Health Act permits emergency admission for up to 72 h for further assessment.

Section 5 provides emergency holding powers for admitted patients. This section does not apply to patients in the ED.

Section 136 is a public place of safety order which can be used by the police to take a patient to a 'place of safety', against their wishes, for 72 h to enable further assessment of a mental disorder.

21.5 Confidentiality

21.5.1 Introduction

There is a legal and ethical duty to keep information about patients confidential, unless the patient consents to disclosure, disclosure is required by law, or is necessary in the public interest.

Health information should be held in accordance with the Data Protection Act 1998 and the GMC guidance on confidentiality. The information should be accurate, relevant, up to date, and held for only as long as is necessary.

When disclosure is required it should be proportional, anonymized if possible, and include only the minimum information necessary for the purpose.

21.5.2 Disclosures with consent

Before disclosing any information to a third party, the patient's consent should be sought. Consent may be implied, for example most patient understand that information about their health needs to be shared within the treating healthcare team. Implied consent is also acceptable for the purposes of clinical audit, provided patients have been made aware of this possibility by notices in the hospital and have not actively objected. Express consent is required if patient-identifiable information is to be disclosed for any other purpose, unless required by law, or in the public interest.

For the consent to disclose information to be valid, patients must be competent to give consent and provided with information about the extent of the disclosure. If a patient lacks capacity, demonstrated by the functional test of capacity advised in the Mental Capacity Act 2005, then

Table 21.1 Summary of sections of the Mental Health Act relevant to emergency department (ED) practice

Section 1	Defines 'mental disorder' as any disorder or disability of the mind.
Section 2	Compulsory admission to hospital for assessment and/or treatment.
	Duration: 28 days.
	Application: Made by the nearest relative or an approved social worker plus two medical recommendations (usually the GP and a Section 12 approved doctor).
Section 3	Compulsory admission to hospital for treatment.
	Duration: 6 months
	Application: made by the nearest relative or an approved social worker plus two medical recommendations (usually the GP and a Section 12 approved doctor).
Section 4	Emergency admission for assessment.
	Duration: 72 h.
	Application: approved social worker or nearest relative plus 1 doctor (Section 12 approved).
Section 5	Emergency holding powers for admitted patients (not ED patients).
	Section 5 (2)—doctors holding power. It does not permit treatment except in urgent situations. Duration 72 h.
	Section 5 (4)—registered mental nurse holding power. Duration 6 h.
Section 131	Informal (voluntary) admissions.
Section 136	Place of Safety order—public
	The patient can be taken to, and kept in, a 'place of safety' against their wishes for 72 h to enable further assessment.
	Grounds: a person who is in a public place and in the opinion of the police officer appears to be suffering from a mental disorder and in immediate need of care.
	Application: any police officer
	Purpose: enable the patient to be examined by a doctor and interviewed by an approved social worker.
	Places of safety: what constitutes a 'place of safety' is agreed locally and may vary. Many EDs are specifically not 'places of safety'. Once a patient has been taken to a particular 'place of safety' they cannot be transferred to another.
Section 63	Allows ancillary treatment for patients under treatment orders. For treatment of symptoms or conditions caused as a consequence of the mental disorder.
	Treatment under this Section includes medical and surgical treatment required for the physical consequences of self-poisoning or self-injury, if considered a consequence of, or a symptom of, the patient's mental disorder.
Section 12	A Section 12-approved doctor is a medically qualified doctor who has been recognized under Section 12(2) of the Act. They have specific expertise in mental disorder and have additionally received training in the application of the Act. They are usually psychiatrists, although some are GPs who have a special interest in psychiatry.

disclosure of information should be in the patient's best interest. If the patient has an LPA or IMCA, they should be consulted prior to the disclosure.

If a patient, under the age of 16 years, is able to understand the purpose and consequences of the disclosure (Gillick competent), they can give or withhold consent. If the young person refuses disclosure but this is necessary to protect the young person from serious harm (e.g. neglect or abuse) this is justifiable. The young person should be made aware of the disclosure and the reasons why.

If a young person is not competent to give consent, someone with parental responsibility may consent to the disclosure on their behalf. In a patient aged 16–17 who lacks capacity, both the Mental Capacity Act 2005 and the Children Act 1989 can apply, depending on the circumstances.

21.5.3 Disclosures required by law

There are circumstances where disclosures are a statutory requirement. In such circumstances, the information should be disclosed even without the patient's consent. The patient should be informed of the disclosure and the reason for it, unless it is not practicable to do so. No more information than is absolutely necessary should be disclosed.

Disclosures required by statute include:

- Criminal Appeal Act 1995
- Prevention of Terrorism Act 1989
- Public Health (Control of Disease) Act 1984
- Road Traffic Act 1988
- NHS Counter Fraud investigations
- Disclosures to the GMC—investigation of a doctor's fitness to practice

Other obligatory disclosures include:

- Coroner's investigations.
- Courts or litigation—a judge or presiding officer has the power to order the disclosure of information.
- DVLA—patients are legally responsible for informing the DVLA of a medical condition that may affect their ability to drive. If they refuse to do this and are likely to continue driving, then the DVLA should be contacted and the relevant information disclosed.

21.5.4 Disclosures required in the public interest

The disclosure of information about a patient without their consent maybe justifiable, if it is likely to protect individuals or society from risks of serious harm (e.g. serious communicable diseases or the prevention of them, detection or prosecution of a serious crime) or to reduce the risk of death or serious harm to the patient or a third party.

There is no agreed definition of 'serious crime'. The NHS Code of Practice on confidentiality (2003) gives some examples of serious crime (e.g. murder, manslaughter, rape, child abuse, serious harm to the security of the state or public order, and crimes involving substantial financial gain or loss). It also gives some examples of crimes where disclosure without consent is not warranted (e.g. theft, fraud, and damage to property where loss or damage is less substantial).

In all cases the balance of breaching a patient's confidentiality and the possible harm caused by this should be weighed against the benefits of disclosing the information.

The information should be anonymized if possible and the minimum, relevant information only should be disclosed.

Patient consent should be sought if possible and the patient kept informed of any disclosures, unless this undermines the purpose of the disclosure. The ultimate decision about whether or not a disclosure was made in the public interest is determined by the courts. All decisions must be justified and clearly documented.

A competent adult's wishes should generally be respected if they refuse to allow disclosure and no-one else will suffer. However, if the disclosure is to protect an incompetent patient from serious harm, there is an expectation that the relevant confidential information will be disclosed. If such information is not disclosed, this will need to be justified.

The police can request personal (not clinical) details regarding attendances to the ED if the request is made in writing on Form 826C and relates to a serious, arrestable crime (Police and Evidence Act 1984) or the Road Traffic Act 1988. The form must be signed by an Inspector or above.

21.5.5 Reporting knife and gun crime

In 2009 the GMC produced supplementary guidance on confidentiality issues relating to gunshot and knife wounds.

The GMC states that:

- You should inform the police quickly whenever a person arrives with a gunshot wound or an injury from an attack with a knife, blade, or other sharp instrument (unless the knife or blade injury is accidental or the result of self-harm). This will enable the police to make an assessment of risk to the patient and others, and to gather statistical information about gun and knife crime in the area.
- You should make a professional judgement about whether disclosure of personal information about a patient, including their identity, is justified in the public interest.

The police are responsible for assessing the risk posed by those who are harmed with, or have used, a gun or knife in a violent attack. They will assess: the risk of a further attack on the patient; the risk to staff, patients and visitors in the ED; and the risk of another attack near to, or at, the site of the original incident.

Personal information, such as the patient's name and address, should not usually be disclosed in the initial contact with the police. The police will respond even if the patient's identity is not disclosed. If the patient's treatment and condition allow them to speak to the police, then the patient's consent should be sought about whether they are willing to do so. If the patient declines consent this decision should be abided by unless, like other disclosures without consent, it is required by law or it is felt to be justified in the public interest. If there is any doubt about whether disclosure without consent is justified, the decision should be made by the consultant in charge or the hospital's Caldicott Guardian.

21.5.6 Disclosures after a patient's death

The duty of confidentiality to a patient remains after their death. There are certain circumstances where disclosure may be justified (e.g. responding to a complaint, including those made by bereaved relatives). The Access to Health Records Act 1990 allows relevant information to be disclosed to the 'personal representative' of the deceased (usually the executor of the will, or an administrator if there is no will) or anyone who may have a claim arising from the patient's death (e.g. a life insurance claim).

If the patient requested that specific information remained confidential their views should be respected, subject to those disclosures required by law or justified in the public interest.

21.5.7 Caldicott Guardian

In 1997 the Caldicott Report (named after the author Dame Fiona Caldicott) was produced, which identified weaknesses in the way parts of the NHS handled confidential patient data. The report made several recommendations, one of which was the appointment of a Caldicott Guardian, a senior member of staff with a responsibility to ensure patient data is kept secure. Each NHS organization has to appoint a Caldicott Guardian to fulfil this role.

The six key principles of the Caldicott report are:

1. Justify the purpose(s) for using the confidential information.
2. Only use it when absolutely necessary.
3. Use the minimum that is required.
4. Access should be on a strict need-to-know basis.
5. Everyone must understand his or her responsibilities.
6. Understand and comply with the law.

Since the Caldicott report, further developments in information management have occurred in the NHS, including the Data Protection Act and the Freedom of Information Act. The role of Caldicott Guardian takes into account all this legislation to ensure the NHS has the highest practical standards for handling patient information.

21.5.8 Data Protection Act 1998

The Data Protection Act defines UK law on the processing of data on identifiable, living people. It gives every living person, or their representative, the right to apply for access to their health records.

There are eight key principles that must be complied with when processing personal data:

1. Personal data should be processed fairly and lawfully.
2. Data should only be obtained for one or more specified and lawful purposes and should not be further processed in a manner incompatible with these purposes.
3. Personal data should be adequate, relevant, and not excessive in relation to the purpose or purposes for which they were collected.
4. Personal data should be accurate and, where necessary, kept up to date.
5. Personal data should not be kept longer than is needed for its intended purpose.
6. Personal data should be processed in accordance with the rights of the individual which the information concerns.
7. Appropriate measures should be taken against unauthorized or unlawful processing or destruction of personal data.
8. Personal data should not be transferred outside the European Economic Area.

Applications for access to health records by the patient, or their representative, must be made in writing or electronically to the Records Manager at the hospital, with the patient's signature. A fee may be charged for the release of the information. Requests should be dealt with promptly, within 21 days, and no later than 40 days after the request has been made. Access may be denied, or limited, where the information might cause serious harm to the physical or mental health, or condition of the patient, or any other person, or where giving access would disclose information relating to or provided by a third person who had not consented to the disclosure.

21.5.9 Freedom of Information Act 2000

The Freedom of Information Act deals with access to official information and gives individuals or organizations the right to request information from any public authority.

Under Part I of the Act, anyone can make a request for information to any public authority providing it is in writing, states the name and address of the enquirer, and describes the information requested. The authority has the duty to confirm or deny whether it holds the information, and if it does so, to supply it within 20 working days from receipt of request. Authorities are not obliged to provide information where they cannot find it without assistance.

Part II of the Act sets out exemptions where the right of access to information is not allowed or restricted. These relate to issues such as national security, law enforcement, commercial interests, and data protection.

Requests from someone about their personal information are dealt with under the Data Protection Act.

KEY POINTS

Confidential patient information can be disclosed in the following circumstances:

- With the patient's consent
- If the disclosure is required by law
- If the disclosure is required in the public interest

The police can request personal details of ED attendances if the request is on Form 826C, signed by an inspector, and relates to a serious, arrestable crime, or the Road Traffic Act.

The police should be informed whenever a patient attends the ED who has a wound sustained by a gunshot or attack by a knife.

Each hospital must have a Caldicott Guardian who is responsible for ensuring patient data is kept secure.

The Data Protection Act defines UK law on the processing of data on identifiable, living people.

The Freedom of Information Act deals with access to official information and gives individuals or organizations the right to request information from any public authority.

21.6 Driver and Vehicle Licensing Agency

21.6.1 Introduction

Patients seen in the ED may have conditions that result in restrictions on their ability to drive. It is the doctor's responsibility to inform the patient of such conditions and the duty of the patient to notify the Driver and Vehicle Licensing Agency (DVLA).

This is particularly relevant for patients discharged from the ED pending outpatient follow-up (e.g. first fits, TIAs, syncope).

21.6.2 General Medical Council guidance on reporting patients to the Driver and Vehicle Licensing Agency

The GMC has issued guidance if patients cannot or will not inform the DVLA. The GMC guidance states:

- The DVLA is legally responsible for deciding if a person is medically unfit to drive. They need to know when driving licence holders have a condition, which may, now or in the future, affect their safety as a driver.
- Therefore, where patients have such conditions, you should:
  - Make sure that the patient understands that the condition may impair their ability to drive. If a patient is incapable of understanding this advice, for example because of dementia, you should inform the DVLA immediately.
  - Explain to patients that they have a legal duty to inform the DVLA about the condition.
- If the patient refuses to accept the diagnosis or the effect of the condition on their ability to drive, you can suggest that the patients seek a second medical opinion, and make appropriate

arrangements for the patients to do so. You should advise patients not to drive until the second opinion has been obtained.

- If patients continue to drive when they are not fit to do so, you should make every reasonable effort to persuade them to stop. This may include telling their next of kin, if they agree you may do so.
- If you do not manage to persuade the patient to stop driving, or you are given or find evidence that a patient is continuing to drive contrary to advice, you should disclose relevant medical information immediately, in confidence, to the medical adviser at the DVLA.
- Before giving information to the DVLA, you should inform the patient of your decision to do so. Once the DVLA has been informed, you should also write to the patient to confirm that a disclosure has been made.

21.6.3 Common emergency department conditions and their driving restrictions

A comprehensive list of medical driving restrictions is available from the DVLA.

Table 21.2 summarizes the restrictions for common conditions that can present to the ED, where the patient may be discharged home. In such circumstances, the responsibility to inform the patient of any restriction lies with the ED doctor and should be documented in the notes.

Table 21.2 refers to the guidance for 'group 1' licence holders (e.g. drivers of cars and motorcycles). 'Group 2' licence holders (e.g. heavy goods vehicles, buses) generally have more severe restrictions, which are detailed in the DVLA guidance.

Table 21.2 Driving restrictions of common ED attendances

Medical condition	Driving restriction
First fit/single fit	Patient must inform the DVLA.
	Refrain from driving for at least six months from the date of the seizure.
	Medical review required before rstarting driving.
Alcohol-related or drug-related seizure	Patient must inform the DVLA.
	Refrain from driving for at least six months from the date of the seizure.
	Medical review required before licence is reissued to ensure an appropriate period free from alcohol misuse has passed.
Head injury (with loss of consciousness but no intracranial haematoma, skull fracture, or seizures)	No requirement to inform the DVLA.
	No driving restriction.
Simple faint (vasovagal)	No requirement to inform the DVLA.
	No driving restriction.
Loss of consciousness (syncope) and low risk of recurrence (normal ECG)	No requirement to inform the DVLA.
	No driving restriction.
Loss of consciousness and high risk of recurrence (abnormal ECG; evidence of structural heart disease; syncope causing injury; syncope while sitting or lying down, or while at the wheel; more than one episode in six months)	Patient must inform the DVLA.
	Can restart driving four weeks after event if cause identified and treated.
	If no cause identified licence revoked for six months.

Table 21.2 Continued

Medical condition	Driving restriction
Single TIA	No requirement to inform DVLA. Refrain from driving for one month.
Recurrent TIAs in a short period	Patient must inform the DVLA. Refrain from driving until three months free of TIAs.
Angina (stable)—symptoms on exertion only	No requirement to inform the DVLA. No driving restriction.
Angina (unstable)—symptoms at rest, with emotion, or at the wheel	No requirement to inform DVLA. Driving must cease until satisfactory symptom control achieved.
Arrhythmias	DVLA only need notifying if there are distracting or disabling symptoms. Must stop driving if arrhythmia has ever caused incapacity. Driving may resume when the underlying cause has been identified and controlled for four weeks.
Shock from an implantable cardioverter defibrillator	No requirement to inform the DVLA. Refrain from driving for six months.
Pre-excitation (e.g. Wolff–Parkinson–White Syndrome)	No requirement to inform the DVLA. No driving restriction.
Diabetic with awareness of hypoglycaemia	Patient must inform the DVLA. No driving restriction (unless recurrent episodes in which case driving must stop until satisfactory control is regained).
Diabetic with impaired awareness of hypoglycaemia	Patient must inform the DVLA. Driving must stop (may restart if awareness regained).

KEY POINTS

The DVLA determines whether an individual with a medical condition is safe to drive.

It is the duty of the licence holder to notify the DVLA of any medical condition, which may affect their ability to drive safely.

It is the responsibility of the doctor to inform the patient of the requirement to inform the DVLA.

The GMC has issued guidance if patients cannot or will not inform the DVLA. All efforts should be made to try and persuade the patient to notify the DVLA and to stop driving. If there is evidence that the patient is continuing to drive contrary to advice, the relevant medical information should be disclosed to the medical adviser at the DVLA. The patient should be made aware of the disclosure before giving information to the DVLA and informed in writing after the disclosure has been made.

21.7 SAQs

21.7.1 Legal

A 15-year-old girl presents to the ED requesting the 'morning-after' pill.

a) Whose criteria are used to determine if she is competent to receive contraception? (1 mark)

b) Give four of the criteria used to make this assessment. (4 marks)

A pre-alert is received about a 58-year-old lady who is septic and peri-arrest. Ambulance control informs you that the patient has multiple sclerosis and has an advanced directive refusing intra-venous fluids and antibiotics.

c) Give four criteria that you will use to determine if her advanced directive is valid. (4 marks)

d) The husband of the patient arrives and asks you to do everything to save her. Does this change the validity of the advance directive? (1 mark)

Suggested answer

a) Whose criteria are used to determine if she is competent to receive contraception? (1 mark)
   Fraser criteria

(Gillick competence is used to identify patients less than 16 years old capable of giving consent to any treatment. Fraser guidelines give the criteria to be met in order to give contraceptive advice or treatment without parental consent).

b) Give four of the criteria used to make this assessment. (4 marks)
   Fraser criteria:
   The young person understands the practitioner's advice.
   The young person cannot be persuaded to inform their parents, or will not allow the practitioner to inform the parents, that contraceptive advice has been sought.
   The young person is likely to begin or to continue having intercourse with or without contraceptive treatment.
   Unless she receives contraceptive advice or treatment, the young person's physical or mental health (or both) is likely to suffer.
   The young person's best interest requires the practitioner to give contraceptive advice or treatment (or both) without parental consent.
   (Gillick competence: the young person is able to understand the purpose and consequences of the treatment.)
   See Chapter 8, section 8.6 for further details on emergency contraception

c) Give four criteria that you will use to determine if her advanced directive is valid? (4 marks)
   Because the refusal is of life-sustaining treatment the decision must be:
   In writing.
   Witnessed.
   Signed.
   State that they intend to refuse treatment even though this puts their life at risk.
   There should be evidence that the patient had capacity when they made the advanced decision.
   The statement should specify precisely what treatment is to be refused and the circumstances in which the refusals should apply.
   The patient should now lack capacity to consent or refuse treatment.

d) The husband of the patient arrives and asks you to do everything to save her. Does this change the validity of the advance directive? (1 mark)

No. If the advanced decision is valid, it must be followed.

Further reading

Data Protection Act 1998. Available at: http://www.legislation.gov.uk/ukpga/1998/29/contents [Online].

Department of Health. The Caldicott Report 1997. Available at: https://www.gov.uk/government/organisations/department-of-health [Online].

Department of Health. The Mental Capacity Act 2005. Available at: https://www.gov.uk/government/organisations/department-of-health [Online].

Department of Health. Mental Health Act 2007. Available at: https://www.gov.uk/government/organisations/department-of-health [Online].

Department of Health. Mental Health Act 1983. Available at: https://www.gov.uk/government/organisations/department-of-health [Online].

Department of Health. Confidentiality: NHS Code of Practice. Available at: https://www.gov.uk/government/organisations/department-of-health [Online].

Department of Health. The Access to Health Records Act 1990. Available at: https://www.gov.uk/government/organisations/department-of-health [Online].

DVLA. At a glance guide to the current medical standards of fitness to drive. Available at: http://www.dft.gov.uk/dvla/medical.aspx [Online].

Freedom of Information Act 2000. Available at: http://www.legislation.gov.uk/ukpga/2000/36/contents [Online].

General Medical Council. Confidentiality: reporting concerns about patients to the DVLA. Available at: https://www.gov.uk/government/organisations/department-of-health [Online].

General Medical Council. End of life care: when to consider making a Do Not Attempt CPR (DNACPR) decision. Available at: https://www.gov.uk/government/organisations/department-of-health [Online].

General Medical Council. Consent guidance: patients and doctors making decisions together. Available at: https://www.gov.uk/government/organisations/department-of-health [Online].

General Medical Council, 2009. Confidentiality. Available at: http://www.gmc-uk.org/ [Online].

General Medical Council. Confidentiality: reporting gunshot and knife wounds. Available at: https://www.gmc-uk.org [Online].

Index

Short questions/answers are denoted by *saq/a*, and illustrations by *f*